Aspects of Face Processing

NATO ASI Series

Advanced Science Institutes Series

A Series presenting the results of activities sponsored by the NATO Science Committee, which aims at the dissemination of advanced scientific and technological knowledge, with a view to strengthening links between scientific communities.

The Series is published by an international board of publishers in conjunction with the NATO Scientific Affairs Division

A	Life Sciences	Plenum Publishing Corporation
B	Physics	London and New York
C	Mathematical and Physical Sciences	D. Reidel Publishing Company Dordrecht and Boston
D	Behavioural and Social Sciences	Martinus Nijhoff Publishers Dordrecht/Boston/Lancaster
E	Applied Sciences	
F	Computer and Systems Sciences	Springer-Verlag Berlin/Heidelberg/New York
G	Ecological Sciences	

Series D: Behavioural and Social Sciences – No. 28

Aspects of Face Processing

edited by:

Hadyn D. Ellis

Department of Psychology
University of Aberdeen
Old Aberdeen
Scotland, U.K.

Malcolm A. Jeeves FRSE

Psychological Laboratory
University of St. Andrews
St. Andrews, Fife
Scotland, U.K.

Freda Newcombe

Neuropsychology Unit
The Radcliffe Infirmary
Oxford
U.K.

Andy Young

Department of Psychology
University of Lancaster
Bailrigg, Lancaster
U.K.

1986 **Martinus Nijhoff Publishers**
Dordrecht / Boston / Lancaster
Published in cooperation with NATO Scientific Affairs Division

Proceedings of the NATO Advanced Research Workshop on ''Aspects of Face Processing'', Aberdeen, Scotland, U.K., June 29–July 4, 1985

Library of Congress Cataloging in Publication Data

Acpects of face processing.

(NATO ASI series. Series D, Behavioural and social sciences ; no. 28)
Proceedings of the NATO Advanced Research Workshop on "Aspects of Face Processing," Aberdeen, Scotland, U.K., June 29–July 4, 1985.
1. Face perception--Congresses. 2. Facial expression--Congresses. 3. Emotions--Congresses.
4. Face perception--Data processing--Congresses.
5. Facial expression--Data processing--Congresses.
6. Emotions--Data processing--Congresses. 7. Face perception--Mathematical models--Congresses. 8. Facial expression--Mathematical models--Congresses. 9. Emotions--Mathematical models--Congresses. I. Ellis, Hadyn. II. North Atlantic Treaty Organization. Scientific Affairs Division. III. NATO Advanced Research Workshop on "Aspects of Face Processing" (1985 : Aberdeen, Grampain) IV. Series.
BF241.A86 1986   153.7'5   86–12478
ISBN 90-247-3357-X

ISBN 90-247-3357-X (this volume)
ISBN 90-247-2688-3 (series)

Distributors for the United States and Canada: Kluwer Boston, Inc., 190 Old Derby Street, Hingham, MA 02043, USA

Distributors for the UK and Ireland: Kluwer Academic Publishers, MTP Press Ltd, Falcon House, Queen Square, Lancaster LA1 1RN, UK

Distributors for all other countries: Kluwer Academic Publishers Group, Distribution Center, P.O. Box 322, 3300 AH Dordrecht, The Netherlands

Printed in The Netherlands

PREFACE

In the preface to his novel "Small World" David Lodge writes:

"When April with its sweet showers has pierced the drought of March to the root, and bathed every vein of earth with that liquid by whose power the flowers are engendered; when this zephyr, too, with its dulcet breath, had breathed life into the tender new shoots .... then as the poet Geoffrey Chaucer observed many years ago, folk long to go on pilgrimages. Only these days professional people call them conferences."

At the end of June 1985 about 50 scientists drawn from a dozen different countries gathered in Aberdeen for a week to attend the first international meeting devoted entirely to studies concerning the ways humans recognise faces and read the emotional expressions written on them.

The meeting took the form of a Workshop, funded by NATO Scientific Affairs Division. So the emphasis was as much on discussing ideas and techniques as it was on presenting original experimental work. The participants were drawn from the fields of cognitive psychology, neuropsychology, neurology and computer science and all had an interest in normal or pathological aspects of face processing and a few had the additional concern of using computer technology either to mimic human face processing or to assist people to recall and recognise faces.

Faces have always been considered intrinsically interesting objects by poets and artists but did not perhaps receive the scientific attention one might have expected following Charles Darwin's "The Expression of the Emotion in Man and Animals (1872). Nevertheless, the question as to how faces are perceived was not entirely ignored: Alvin Goldstein (1983) himself one of the modern pioneers, has shown how numerous famous psychologists dabbled in the topic at some time in their careers. Systematic and sustained research, however, has only recently been undertaken which has resulted in rapid strides being made on a number of fronts. Thus, we decided that it was high time to bring together many of the prominent workers into different aspects of face processing in order for them to present their most recent work, to discuss issues of common interest, and to delineate promising areas for future study.

While the reader may gauge the success of our venture to some extent by reading the following pages, the full impact of the meeting will take some years to be felt. Ideas were exchanged both at formal and at informal meetings and plans for joint research were made by people who had previously never met. All of this was achieved in an atmosphere of great friendliness and conviviality – an ideal medium for encouraging the creative development of ideas. We don't know what Chaucer would have thought about it but we rather hope that Darwin would have approved.

HDE   MAJ   FN   AWY
Aberdeen, January 1986

ACKNOWLEDGEMENTS

The NATO Advanced Research Workshop on "Aspects of Face Processing" required the assistance and cooperation of a number of people and it is a pleasure to acknowledge their help. First and foremost, we should like to thank Mrs Jean Shepherd who did most of the administrative planning for the Workshop and collated the papers in these proceedings. Dr Rhona Flin acted as social organiser and ensured that the visit to Aberdeen was enjoyable as well as edifying. Professor George MacNicol, Principal of Aberdeen University and Professor Eric Salzen, Head of Psychology, gave us every encouragement to hold the meeting and they and their staff helped to smooth its progress at every stage. Professor Durand and Dr Di Lullo of the NATO Scientific Affairs Division were also extremely helpful and encouraging and their generous co-operation is gratefully acknowledged. Finally, we would like to thank all of the participants, many of whom came from very distant places to take part in the Workshop, everyone of whom helped to make it a scientific success and an enjoyable experience.

TABLE OF CONTENTS

X

1. INTRODUCTION

INTRODUCTION TO ASPECTS OF FACE PROCESSING: TEN QUESTIONS IN NEED OF
ANSWERS.

H.D. Ellis

1. INTRODUCTION

These proceedings of the first international conference devoted
entirely to matters concerning the identification of faces and the
interpretation of facial expressions are timely: interest in the human
face as a stimulus object in psychological research has grown quite
dramatically in recent years as figure 1 clearly illustrates.

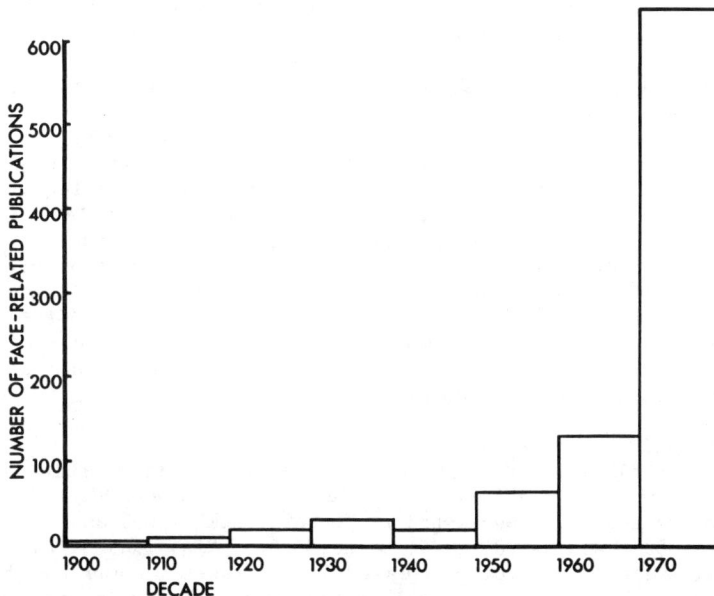

Figure 1. Growth of face-related publications, 1900 - 1980.

The 1980s has witnessed a continuation of the acceleration in published
material, including three books on face processing (Davies, Ellis and
Shepherd, 1981;   Bruyer, 1983;   Bruyer, 1986).   These books cover
psychological and neuropsychological aspects of face recognition and
emptional expressions but they do not detail the relatively novel
approach that has been aimed at devising machines capable of matching
human face recognition and this particular endeavour is bound to develop
strongly over the next decade.
Success in this latter venture is still limited, despite the optimistic

view to be found in Frederick Forsyth's latest best-seller "The Fourth Protocol" (1984). Here the difficulties of the international surveillance required to track enemy agents are explored. The denouement centres on the efforts of MI6's Miss Blodwyn, who has a legendery memory for faces, to identify the face of a soviet agent. Her success is ranked alongside the CIA's computerized face-matching system comprising memory banks with many millions of facial features. Moreover, Forsyth suggests that Miss Blodwyn's mind is organised like that of the CIA computer.

The NATO Advanced Research Workshop on "Aspects of Face Processing" was mainly concerned with the ways in which humans recognise faces. Theories as to how this very complex mechanism may operate, however, could provide computer scientists with useful ideas for designing machine systems to do the same job. By the same token, machines that work may throw light on the way the brain achieves its marvellous ability to identify faces and read emotional expressions. Fiction could become fact.

Patients with damaged brains sometimes fail to achieve efficient face processing and the detailed study of such cases has provided valuable information that has been used alongside evidence from the errors made by people with intact brains who are required rapidly to classify and identify faces. Data from both of these subject populations have been used as a basis for developing theoretical ideas on how face recognition is achieved.

While theoretical issues may dominate these proceedings the practical issues of face processing, both in the clinical and the forensic fields, are never very far away - though just how much the theory has influenced practice either in diagnosing specific disorders in brain-damaged and psychiatric patients or in establishing precepts for assisting witnesses to a crime in recalling or recognising a suspect's face is a question that is raised explicitly be some contributors who remain dubious.

In this introduction I propose now to pose a number of questions concerning face processing that may betray certain idiosyncratic qualities but that, nevertheless, should be of general interest. Many of these issues will be encountered elsewhere in the proceedings but, owing in part to limitations of time, some of them were not further developed by any discussion during the Workshop.

2.ARE FACES UNIQUE OBJECTS?

Teuber (1968) was probably the first to pose this question and his answer to it was affirmative. This view has dominated the work on face recognition subsequently published by Teubers' colleagues and students at MIT (Carey, 1981; Geschwind, 1979; Leehey, 1976; Yin, 1969, 1970;).

The idea that faces are processed by a system unique to them and qualitatively different from all other systems for perceiving and recognising non-facial objects is at the extreme end of a continuum along which shades of opinion may be discerned ranging to the position that faces are handled by the brain in no way differently from any other object pattern. An analogy supporting the belief that faces may be unique objects is not difficult to find: no one would seriously quarrel with the assertion that there exist special and unique systems for processing verbal material which have definite neuroanatomical loci, and the same may be true for faces.

Evidence for the existence of a unique face processing system arises from three principal sources, none of which by itself is very persuasive (Ellis, 1986).

Yin (1969) argued that, while faces are more easily remembered than other objects when presented in an upright orientation, when inverted they become more difficult to remember. This may point to a face system more sensitive to normally-encountered orientation than is the case for those systems processing other materials. An alternative view is that faces are simply processed to a high degree automatically and the penalty for automaticity is inflexibility (Ellis, 1975). As Rock (1974) has shown word inversion has comparably disrupting effects. Very recently Carey and Diamond (1985) have reported that the "inversion effect" can be observed in people very knowledgable about dogs: they are more disrupted by stimulus inversion than the people less practised at recognising dogs – a finding that also questions the uniqueness of faces.

A second approach is to point to the existence of patients suffering from prosopagnosia, the total inability to recognise previously familiar faces a condition which is not usually accompanied by other profound agnosia. Having said that, however, it is also true to say that in all of the published cases of prosopagnosia other cognitive defecits accompany the difficulty in recognising faces. Problems of colour recognition, topographical memory and difficulties in distinguishing exemplars drawn from within other classes of objects (e.g. foods, animals and vehicles) are all common. (But see De Renzi's paper in this volume for a case of apparently "pure" prosopagnosia.)

Prosopagnosia provides another clue to the specialness, if not the uniqueness, of faces; namely the fact that most cases involve bilateral damage to structures in the occipito-temporal region, i.e. specific brain structures which may or may not also cater for other objects.

The third approach to the uniqueness question is to argue that faces are such biologically important objects that infants come into the world prewired to be attracted by faces. A key finding is that of Goren, Sarty and Wu (1975). They claimed that neonates prefer to look at a moving stimulus with a face-like pattern in comparison with those containing no pattern or with jumbled facial features.

While it is tempting to interpret this observation as reflecting the uniqueness of faces two points need to be borne in mind. One is that, conceivably, other meaningful stimuli may also be attractive to neonates. The other is that the experiment of Goren et al. has yet to be replicated. Accordingly, Suzanne Dziurawiec and I are currently examining data collected from 30 neonates in order to see whether we obtain the same results. A positive result will be interesting but a negative one, of course, will pose the usual problem that is raised by a failure to replicate.

Hay and Young (1982) have given clearest expression to what might be termed a weak view of the uniqueness question. They suggest that face processing involves mechanisms specific to face but that other mechanisms may exist exclusive to different objects. Konorski (1967) anticipated this approach when he described 7 such mechanisms (which he termed 'gnostic units') one of which was devoted to processing facial identity and another specialized for interpreting facial expressions.

The idea, then, is that faces are handled by a special system while a number of other systems exist specialised for recognising other classes of object is not new but it remains to be unequivocally established. And it has to be admitted that some theorists prefer to assume that at least at some higher levels of analysis object classes may rely on a common system for distinguishing among exemplars within each class (e.g. Damasio, Damasio and Van Hoesen, 1982).

3.IS FACE PERCEPTION THE RESULT OF WHOLISTIC OR FEATURE ANALYSIS?

This questions is something of an old chestnut in theorising about visual perception and I will not dwell too long on the issue here. The reason for raising it is because a good deal of the research on face perception has implicitly emphasised the importance of feature information. In particular, attempts to establish which facial features attract most attention and provide useful means of discriminating faces have perhaps distracted research away from considering the face as a gestalt where inter-feature space may be just as important. Recent work by Justine Sergent (1984) has nicely illustrated the need for considering both what she terms 'component' and 'configurational' aspects of faces. By using reaction time and multidimensional scaling (MDS) techniques Sergent has illustrated the inextricable interdependence of component and configurational information so that it does not make sense to talk of either one as being more or less important in face perception: they are both important.

Such a conclusion is not necessarily inconsistent with the view that recognition involves a search of stored feature lists but seems more compatible with a wholistic mode of recognition in which the entire pattern is simultaneously processed.

Equally, the interesting suggestion, first made by Gombrich (1972) that face recognition could make use of a process akin to that employed by caricaturists to exaggerate unusual features may be reconcilable with Sergent's findings. However, attempts experimentally to support the idea (known as the 'super fidelity' theory of face recognition) have proved entirely unsupportive (Hagen and Perkins, 1983; Tversky and Baratz, 1985). That is not to deny, however, that familiar faces cannot be identified on the basis of exaggerated or even single features. Moreover, there is an interesting difference between known and novel faces with regard to the facial areas that convey most useful information. Ellis et al. (1979) found that famous individuals are better recognised on the basis of inner facial features (eyes, nose and mouth) whereas strangers seen once are equally well recognised from inner and outer features (hair and jawline). Presumably, as we interact with people we pay more attention to the expressive areas than to non-expressive ones and, as a result, become disproportionately familar with these features.

4.HOW USEFUL ARE INFORMATION-PROCESSING MODELS OF FACE RECOGNITION?

Theories or models of face processing are fairly new and most of them are couched in information-processing terms. The first detailed model, published just a few years ago by Hay and Young (1982) developed some of the ideas of Bruce (1979) and Ellis (1981). Their model shown in Figure 2, has provided an excellent framework for analysing the mechanisms underlying face recogition.

The Hay and Young model envisages face processing as comprising 3 main stages in which perceptual representation is first achieved; followed by analysis for familiarity via face recognition units which merely register that a face is known but do not contain any semantic information about the person; and then person information is accessed giving biographical and episodic information about the person. The model also accounts for the influence of other cognitive processes at different stages. It allows for analysis of facial expression etc. in parallel to identification which, of course, can also be achieved via other pathways such as voice analysis.

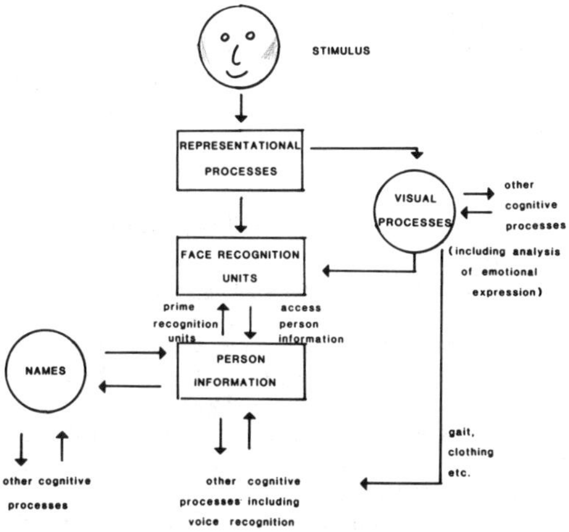

STIMULUS

REPRESENTATIONAL PROCESSES

VISUAL PROCESSES

other cognitive processes (including analysis of emotional expression)

FACE RECOGNITION UNITS

prime recognition units

access person information

NAMES

PERSON INFORMATION

gait, clothing etc.

other cognitive processes

other cognitive processes including voice recognition

Figure 2. A model of face processing (redrawn from Hay and Young, 1982)

Variation on the Hay and Young model have been published that attempt to account for hemispheric asymmetries in the processes (Ellis 1983, Rhodes 1985). The notion that the familiarity and semantic information contained within a face may be analysed at separate stages was borrowed from work on word recognition (Morton 1969) which has a more established history of model buildng (Ellis, 1981).

A number of following papers in these proceedings will amplify and refine the description I have given of the information-processing approach to face recognition and its usefulness for understanding the process will be apparent. Additional advantages may be seen when models such as Hay and Young's are used to analyse different forms of prosopagnosia (Ellis, in press).

5.ARE IDENTITY AND EXPRESSION ANALYSIS SEPARABLE?

In the Hay and Young (1982) model just discussed identity and expression analyses are shown as separate systems. Why should this be so? Ellis (1983) gives a full rationale for this suggestion. Basically the evidence comes from two sources; tachistoscopic face perception in normals; and face identification and emotional interpretation among patients suffering various forms of dementia.

Ley and Bryden (1978) found that when subjects were discriminating schematic faces exposed singly and briefly in either visual field their decisions concerning whether the face matched a subsequent one were independent of their ability to say whether the two emotional expressions matched.

Kurucz and Feldmar (1979) examined elderly dementing patients some of whom were unable to identify familiar faces but could interpret facial expressions while others had reversed problems.

Taken together these findings support, but cannot prove, the notion that identity and expression analyses are dissociable. Yet a third system may govern the extraction of information concerning words being spoken. Campbell, Landis and Regard (person communication) have studied two brain-damaged patients, one of whom can lip-read but cannot identify faces or read emotional expressions while the other cannot lip-read but can identify people and their facial expressions.

6. WHAT CAN WE LEARN FROM MACHINE FACE RECOGNITION?

In a sense this question is premature. Machines are nowhere near as good as humans at discriminating and identifying faces. No doubt this disadvantage will diminish in time and eventually computer systems such as the one Frederick Forsyth dreamed up for the CIA will become available.

Meanwhile what can be learned from the initial attempts to teach machines how to recognise faces? I do not wish to preempt John Stonham's paper so I will simply say that with Igor Aleksander and others he has developed a computer system for successfully identifying members of a set of faces independent of pose and expression. Their system (WISARD) uses fairly simply building blocks.

Other work, for example Kohonen et al. (1981), makes use of distributed "neural networks" with structured interaction to achieve face recognition. Again the emphasis is upon using fairly simple elements to achieve selective associative memory. In essence, Kohonen's approach involves a distributed network of facial information so that any face is encoded not in a localised area but, instead, is distributed throughout the entire memory.

This view is radically different from the information-processing approach adopted by most psychologists (O'Toole, 1985). The system advocated by Kohonen and others does seem to work on limited data sets and may well apply to the way the human brain operates. It is not clearly, however, whether distributed memory underlies primate face recognition. The problem remains both of explaining the apparent specificity of memory loss in prosopagnosia and accounting for the findings made by Perrett and his colleagues of single cells responsible either to facial features or whole faces located within a specific region of the temporal lobes.

7. WHAT LESSONS MAY BE LEARNED FROM DISORDERS IN FACE RECOGNITION?

I have already alluded to some of the lessons from studies of patients with particular brain lesions. In particular it is worth noting that the Hay and Young model of face processing in part derives from studies of brain-injured patients.

Other lessons to be learned from a study of impaired face recognition include the recent observations of Bauer (1984; this volume) on prosopagnosic patients who while being unable to recognise faces nonetheless, display appropriate autonomic responses to faces. These results imply that the conscious route to identification may not use the only means of registering familiarity with a face.

Bruyer et al. (1983) performed probably the most thorough analysis ever made of a prosopagnosic patient. Among their numerous findings was the observation that their patient could evince some recognition for familiar people (family and friends) while being entirely unable to identify famous faces. This may imply a functional distinction between familiar and famous faces (which are usually treated as belonging to the same class); or it may instead suggest that known faces can be arranged along a continuum of familiarity and that brain damage may obliterate memory for all but those at the extreme end of familiarity i.e. people known personally.

The role of context in face recognition is some interest to cognitive psychologists and it is interesting to note the work in France of Guy Tiberghien and his associates (personal communiciation) who have been studying a prosopagnosic patient who is extremely adept at using contextual cues to recognise people whose faces he cannot, of course, identify. This patient sometimes has trouble deciding whether any feeling of familiarity he experiences is due to face or context or both and at these times is aware of a decision process that must always play some part in normal face recognition.

8. CAN ONE IMPROVE SOMEONE'S FACE RECOGNITION ABILITY?

The face recognition skills that most of us develop are such that efforts to improve on them are doomed to failure. Roy Malpass (1981) has lucidly reviewed the literature on training programmes designed to improve both within-race and between-race recognition. His conclusion is that "While there is evidence that recognition training can bring about short-term improvement of recognition for other-race faces there is no evidence that a relatively short training programme can increase recognition performance for own-race faces; indeed the evidence points in the other direction" (p. 284). The last sentence of that quotation refers to work both by Woodhead, Baddeley and Simmonds (1979) and by Malpass himself in which training by a technique requiring subjects to attend to and classify specific features actually caused post-training recognition performance to be worse than that displayed before training!

It is possible that training techniques that focus on feature information fail to capitalise upon the rich configurational information available in a face. Indeed some studies have shown that face recognition can be improved by requiring subjects to make attributional judgements on qualities such as likeableness or honesty (Bower and Karlin 1974). However, Malpass (1981) did not find that such a global strategy when incorporated into a training programme was of any lasting value.

Given that it is very difficult, if not impossible, to improve on a lifetimes' experience of face watching what about those who have very obvious difficulties in face recognition? As far as I can tell, no-one seems to have addressed the problem, say, of prosopagnosia in the way that speech therapists approach aphasia. One reason for this is that prosopagnosia, of course, appears to be a relatively rare syndrome, with roughly one new case reported each year over the last century (Shuttleworth, Syring and Allen, 1982). A much larger number of brain-injured patients have measurable defects in face recognition, however, (Sergent, 1984); also mentally subnormal children (Harris and Fleer, 1972) and dyslexics (Langdell, 1978) have been reported as being impaired in some face recognition skills relative to normal individuals.

Taken together these different groups may sum to make a sizeable number of individuals who may benefit from some sort of training programme in discriminating and remembering faces. Andy Young and I have just begun to address this particular issue in connection with a prosopagnosic child whose social life will undoubtedly be severely handicapped if she remains unable to identify familiar people by face. Our immediate problem in her case is to get her to attend to faces in a systematic manner and to learn which features are useful discriminators. In the case of caucasian faces these are likely to be upper face features, particularly hair and eyes (Shepherd, Davies and Ellis, 1981). This approach may seem at variance with what I said earlier about feature-based training programmes but in the face of such severe problems it may prove necessary to start with such fundamental skills and to build from them. According to Carey (1981) children normally pass from what she terms a 'piecemeal' strategy when looking at faces to the 'wholistic' method used by adults and this sequence may well prove an appropriate model in case of childhood prosopagnosia (Ellis, in press).

9.HOW DOES A FACE BECOME FAMILIAR?

This is one of the most interesting theoretical questions, yet has hardly been addressed at all. It concerns the procedure by which a novel face becomes familiar and once having become familiar, how its representation in memory is updated to account for the changes that inevitably occur over time.

The face recognition units in Hay and Young's (1982) model, discussed earlier, may operate either in a threshold mode or by giving graded responses commensurate with the sensory evidence for the faces to which they belong. It may be that new faces automatically join this cerebral portrait gallery or they mave have to spend some time in a more temporary store from whence, unless encountered again, they may be easily lost. At present it is impossible unequivocally to decide between these alternatives except to note that the former possibility is the more parsimonious.

Duration of encounter is critical. Ellis, et al. (1977), for example showed a log-log linear relationship between duration of viewing and subsequent recognition accuracy for times of between 0.25 and 4 sec. Any repetition of encounter could have the effect of simply increasing duration of viewing, but whether such repetition leads to an additive increment in whatever is involved in establishing a face unit or whether the relationship is more complex needs to be established.

We do know that variety of encounter is an important factor. Dukes and Beavan (1967) showed face memory to be improved by seeing photographs of the person in a variety of poses compared with repetition of the same photograph. *extraction of invariants*

Sergent (1985) has also presented data with some incidental bearing on this question. She employed a limited set of composite faces for RT and similarity judgements and calculated MDS solutions to the data. When the faces were relatively novel she found a two-dimensional solution provided the best fit. When subjects were familiar with the faces, however, a three-dimensional (i.e. more complex) solution was best. Familiarity, perhaps, leads to a more complex representation.

Faces change over time in a lawful manner (Pittenger and Shaw, 1975). When we are in frequent contact with people we hardly notice these changes; it is on the occasionally encountered face that the wheel marks of Time's winged chariot can be seen. Even quite rapid changes may go undetected in daily encountered faces as this quotation from the son of Jan Morris, a celebrated transexual illustrates: "... the masculine appearance of my father had slowly turned into something more nebulous ... it was difficult to recall what he had looked like ... when I first saw him dressed as a woman, it seemed perfectly natural" (James Morris, "Observer" 26th Februrary 1984).

One obvious question remains and that is if the face recognition units are capable of continual adjustment how can we recognise people from photographs and film taken years ago? The answer may be that while updating the units we do not discard any of data records. Alternatively, the system may be capable of some very sophisticated transformation algorithms for backward (and forward) reconstruction.

Finally I should like to point out that almost all face memory experiments before the mid-1970s involved unknown faces. Thus subjects were only required to make familiarity judgement ("does this face seem familiar or not?"). More recent work has concentrated on memory for famous faces that have a rich semantic representation but there has been nothing published concerned with the ways in which new faces become familiar and acquire biographical and episodic associations. This gap in our knowledge must be filled before too long.

10.HOW IS FACE MEMORY ORGANISED?

This is another interesting yet, curiously, under-researched topic. If the previous question was phrased in such a way as to focus on the face recognition unit stage of the system this one will mostly address the last stage, the person information level, which may or may not be part of a more general semantic memory system.

Bruce (1983) has cleverly shown that under some circumstances semantic priming can affect familiarity decision. That is to say, the experience of one famous person may speed up RT to decide whether or not the next face is familiar or not if it is of an associate of the first person. But this provides only indirect evidence for any associate network at the semantic stage.

Equally, the work of Klatzky and her associates (Klatzky, Martin and Kane, 1982a; 1982b) indicating that face processing may be influenced by verbal labels which provide stereotypical information on fuzzy categories is also of relevance to the question - albeit at a crude level of organisation.

More direct evidence for organisation of face memory at a semantic level is provided by some recent work by Robertson and Ellis (in press). They gave subjects random photographs of 24 celebrities to rate for famousness. A day later the subjects were given a surprise recall test for the names of the individuals. The resulting lists of correct answers were then analysed mathematically for evidence of clustering (cf Bousefield's, 1953, work on clustering in verbal recall). Without going into details, the results indicate three forms of clustering: clustering by profession (i.e. tendency for actors to cluster or pop-singers to cluster); clustering by physical similarity; and clustering by an interaction of profession and appearance (i.e. actors that look alike tend to be named consecutively).

If these results have any validity they suggest that person memory may not be randomly organised but instead may involve meaningful associations based along both semantic and physical dimensions, being most powerful when the two coincide.

Even more recently I have been making tentative efforts to examine organisation by asking people to try to imagine the faces of famous people I name. By choosing personalities of modest fame it is possible sometimes to induce a 'tip of the tongue' - like state in which people can correctly recall crude physical information (usually face shape and hair colouring) but cannot form a clear image. More interestingly they sometimes report evidence of incorrect addressing whereby they get a clear image of someone who looks like the celebrity required (e.g. Robert Maxwell and Bernard Matthews - two well-known British businessmen who have similar faces) - other confusions are either nominal (e.g. Norman Tebbit for Norman Fowler, two Tory Ministers) or a mixture of name and appearance (e.g. Barbara Castle and Barbara Cartland, two elderly ladies who endeavour to keep up appearances).

11.HOW USEFUL ARE THEORIES OF FACE RECOGNITION?

One very important aspect of the preceding questions is their applicability to practical forensic and clinical problems.

The evidence is rather mixed and, in truth, it may be premature to expect much else given the novelty of theory concerning face processing and the exigencies of many practical problems that required immediate answers, or demanded pragmatic solutions at variance with what pure research had demonstrated.

An example of what I refer to may be seen in attempts over the last 10 years to examine ways of improving face recall techniques such as Photofit and Identikit. These systems require criminal witnesses to recall facial images of suspects and decompose the face feature by feature. If we initially acquire facial information in gestalt form it would be extremely difficult to perform this task - as experimental tests have shown (Ellis et al., 1975; Laughery and Fowler, 1980).

However, it is all very well to assert the inherent difficulty of facial composite systems but the Police sometimes have no other recourse than to try to use them to apprehend a suspect. The paper by John Shepherd later in this volume does point the way towards some sort of solution whereby face recognition skills allied to a computer search algorithm, based upon research into the facial features people pay attention to and can describe, provides an effective compromise. The use of identification parades has developed over the last century (Shepherd, Ellis and Davies, 1983) with little or no regard for laboratory research on face recognition. This is not entirely the fault of psychologists - although the legal profession has long been suspicious of psychologists following Muensterberg's (1908) exaggerated claims. Happily, the Devlin Committee (1976) when reporting that rules for the conduct of identity parades needed advised that overhauling and this exercise could benefit from empirical research. Many projects have since been undertaken, the results of which are at least disseminated in American courts of law by psychologists giving expert testimony concerning such things as parade composition, instructions to witnesses, and cross-racial recognition. The work of Elizabeth Loftus (1979) and Gary Wells (1978) is prominent in this endeavour (see Shepherd et al., 1983).

Applications of theory to clinical situations is equally patchy to that in the forensic sphere. Tests of face memory as a diagnostic tool have long been employed (see Benton 1980). But neurologists, perhaps, have often been unaware of psychological research that might have been useful. Some liaison on the subject of locating areas of the brain devoted to face processing has occurred with general agreement arising from lesion studies and tachistoscopic visual half field exposures (which is evident from many of the subsequent papers in these proceedings). I have also tried to use the information processing model of face processing to provide a taxonomy of the prosopagnosias which could prove useful to clinicians the successfulness of which remains to be established (Ellis, in press).

The foregoing ten questions are only some of the insistent problems besetting those interested in face processing, many more will be revealed throughout this book. Asking the right questions is difficult enough; providing answers to them is an even greater challenge - one that all of the contributers can share in years to come.

2. PERCEPTUAL PROCESSES

MICROGENESIS OF FACE PERCEPTION

Justine SERGENT

1. INTRODUCTION

One basic principle of science, which typically applies to psychology, suggests that one should never seek to explain a psychological fact by a mechanism at a higher level if it can be explained by one at a lower level (Morgan, 1894). This seems to be a reasonable principle, and it compels us to attempt to specify and understand the nature of the preliminary operations that underlie a given process. Such a principle is quite relevant to the problem of face perception, and it is with early visual processes, as well as their implications for later operations, that the present chapter will be concerned. It would be misleading, however, to begin with the idea that one can account for most of the processes underlying perception by considering only these early processes, and this is especially true of face perception. For one thing, perception is a process resulting from the interaction of the incoming information and mental states or cerebral structures, and it is therefore necessary to understand the nature and characteristics of this interaction to explain perceptual processes. For another, the human face is an extremely familiar multidimensional pattern, and our frequent exposure to such a stimulus has enabled us to develop certain processing mechanisms, which some authors (e.g, Goldstein & Chance, 1981) have referred to as "schemata," that allow access to consistent dimensions which facilitate perception and memory.

Thus, I will essentially deal with one side of this interaction, but will, toward the end, try to illustrate how the outcome of early visual operations may be relevant for understanding higher cognitive processes. The problem of early visual processing is that of understanding the nature and composition of the incoming information from which higher order operations can unfold. One first question would then be to decide on some properties of the face that can be considered as relevant during these early processes, not only in terms of its physical characteristics but also in terms of units that correspond to neural mechanisms inherent in early processes. A second question concerns the composition and description of facial information depending on the particular conditions under which a face is viewed, that is, as it can be resolved by the visual system in various situations. The answer to these questions should lead to the determination of some constraints on subsequent operations and could provide information concerning the representations on which cognitive processes take place.

In real-life situations, we are confronted with a multitude of formats of faces, and we deal with these at approximately the same level of efficiency. Whether they are three-dimensional plastic patterns or two dimensional static and schematic pictures, we consider them all as genuine facial representations. This probably indicates that a facial "schema" that assists our processing of faces must be flexible enough to accomodate a wide variety of face representations, provided they are constructed on the same invariant pattern. Yet, despite this flexibility, this schema is also characterized by a certain rigidity in that it strictly guides the way one conceives of a face. This is suggested by the considerable lack of imagination displayed in science-fiction movies in which extra-terrestrials are seldom created with a face that drastically departs from the human-face pattern, as if it could not be conceived that a face could take a shape different from the one we are used to dealing with. All this to say that what we perceive as a face can be initiated by a large variety of representations that have nonetheless an invariant configuration. The fact that most research has been conducted with 2-dimensional faces may thus not be too detrimental to our understanding of the processes underlying face perception, even if the visual system is sensitive to the particular facial representations with which it is stimulated, as we will see later.

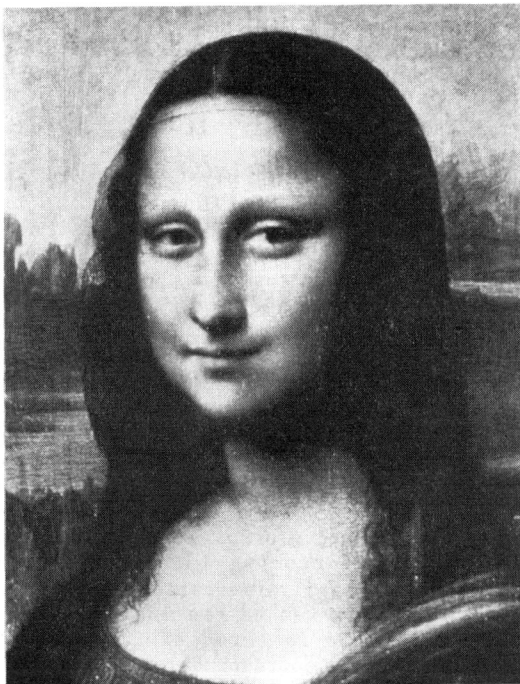

FIGURE 1. Original representation of Mona Lisa.

2. RELEVANT FACIAL FEATURES

For the moment, we may try to examine what could be the facial features that constitute the relevant dimensions of a face. Let's use the famous face shown in Figure 1 and let's try to determine what information is necessary to perceive such a pattern as a face and to carry out various operations. What seems to be most evident is that the discrete facial features, such as the eyes, the mouth, the chin, are likely relevant units on which perception is based since they are inherent components of the face and determine its individuality. In addition, we know that the visual system is particularly sensitive to variations in intensity, and these variations are typically concentrated in the facial features, which makes them important physical bases for processing. On the other hand, the availability of these facial features as such is not indispensable to recognize a face, as suggested by our capacity to identify an individual even when the facial features are blurred beyond recognition. That is, the disposition of the features within the frame of a front-view face seems to provide enough information for recognition, even though the facial features as such have no specificity with respect to the face in question. This can be illustrated in the coarsely quantized representation of Mona Lisa displayed in Figure 2.

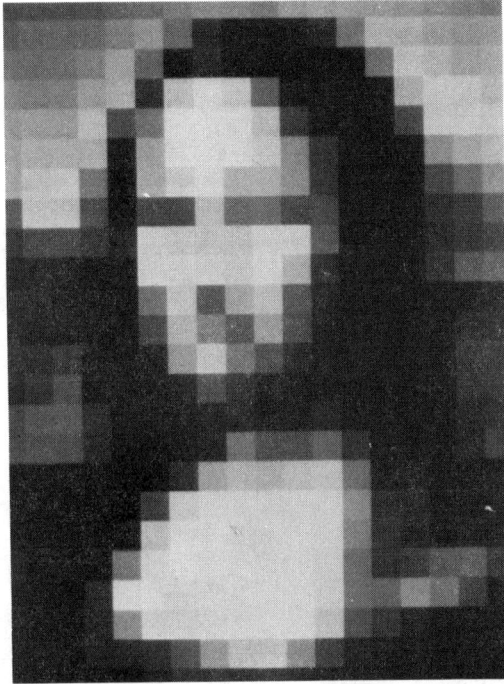

FIGURE 2. Coarsely quantized representation of the original picture of Mona Lisa (Courtesy of Ed Manning).

In this face, the intensity of each square is the average intensity of the equivalent area in the original face, so that all the fine details have been filtered out. Here, no single feature conveys enough information for recognizing the stimulus as a face, let alone Mona Lisa, and it is only the relationship among the blurred components that leads to recognition. This suggests that a face has both component and configural properties, and the configuration stems from the interaction of the components. The configuration becomes the more salient property of the face when the components are blurred, as is obvious here. This does not mean, however, that the configuration is removed when the components are not blurred, and, in a normal face, component and configural properties coexist.

2.1. Spatial composition of the face.

There is therefore some indication that different facial information is conveyed by different physical characteristics of the face, and it may be informative to examine this question in more detail to understand what the visual system is doing in early processing. Recent evidence suggests that the visual system filters information contained in a display into separate bands of spatial frequencies (De Valois & De Valois, 1981), and it has provided a new way of describing visual patterns in terms of physical characteristics consonant with the properties of early neural processing. Thus, the visual system behaves as if it comprised multiple channels and mechanisms, each selectively sensitive to a restricted band of spatial frequency and orientation. We will see later what are the temporal properties of the visual system and we may now examine its spatial properties.

We can use the coarsely quantized picture of Mona Lisa (see Figure 2) as an analogy for some of the filtering taking place in the visual system, if we consider each square here as the equivalent of a receptive field. The retina is composed of a multitude of overlapping receptive fields of different sizes, such that each point of a visual scene is encoded several times as part of different channels. Large receptive fields are activated by the low-frequency components of the picture while small receptive fields, which mainly compose the fovea, encode the high-frequency components of the display. In this particular picture, in which each average-intensity square covers a fairly large area of the face, the information about the face is carried only by the low-frequency contents, and it is clear that these low frequencies convey already a good deal of information.

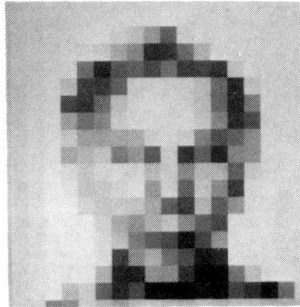

FIGURE 3. Coarsely quantized representation of an unfamiliar face.

This can be further illustrated with the face shown in Figure 3 which is probably unfamiliar to most people. Here, we can extract a fair amount of information regarding sex, age, general shape and configuration of the face, indicating, as suggested by Harmon (1973) and by Ginsburg (1978), that much of the relevant facial information is contained in the low spatial-frequency spectrum. There are, however, some high frequencies present in this picture, specifically at the edge of the square, but they can be filtered out by winking, which in fact provides a better representation of the face. (These high frequencies result from the quantization procedure and are just artificially created noise.) What is important to note at this point is that this low-frequency representation provides sufficient information concerning facial configuration but does not permit a detailed representation of the facial features. In other words, filtering out the high-spatial frequency contents makes the configuration of the face its main available property.

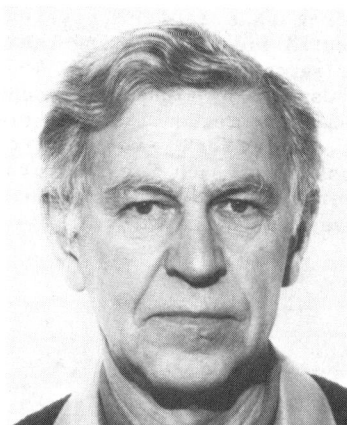

FIGURE 4. Original representation of the face shown in Figure 3.

     If we look now at the original face (see Figure 4), it is obvious that higher frequencies provide additional relevant information, particularly that about the internal features and other details of the face. What is of interest, however, is that this information is conveyed by different channels in such a way that, during early visual processing, the brain is provided with several descriptions of the face in slightly different representations corresponding to different spatial-frequency bandwidths. As we will see later, these representations do not develop simultaneously and are thus not available for processing at the same time. For the moment, however, there are three points regarding the spatial representations of a face that are worth considering further.

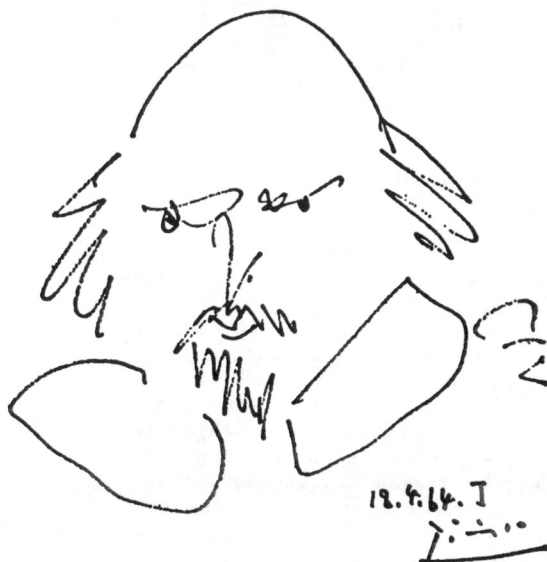

FIGURE 5. Line-drawing of Shakespeare by Picasso.

One concerns the fact that a high-filtered picture conveys quite relevant information about a face, suggesting that low frequencies may not be indispensable in the perception of faces. This can be illustrated with the line-drawing of Shakespeare by Picasso, presented in Figure 5, which is objectively composed of high-frequencies that provide sufficient information for recognition. Therefore, no particular range of spatial frequencies may be necessary as such for the perception and processing of faces. There is, however, some complications here that arise from the distribution of receptive fields across the retina, and this is the second point.

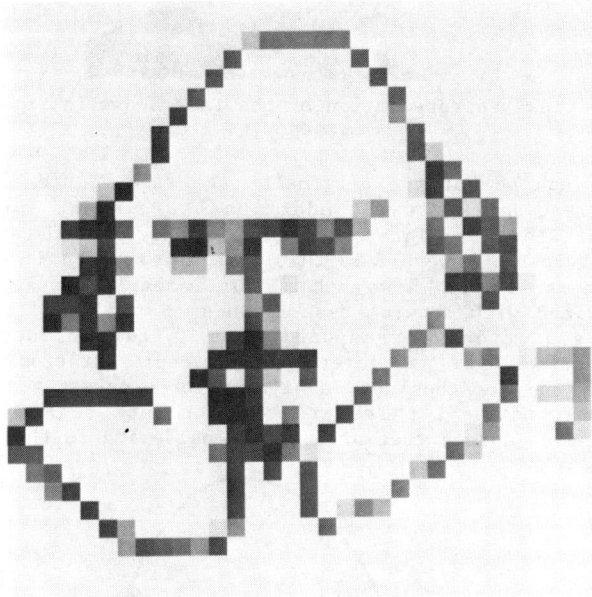

FIGURE 6. Coarsely quantized representation of the face shown in Figure 5 (Courtesy of Ed Manning).

Consider, for example, the coarsely quantized representation of the preceding line-drawing face, displayed in Figure 6. The quantization itself consists in filtering the high frequencies so that the object is described as a function of low frequencies. The face that was subjected to this quantization actually contained almost exclusively high frequency components, yet a low-pass filtering, that is a filtering that lets through only the low frequencies, results in a visible face with relevant information for perception and processing. If one applies this phenomenon to actual receptive fields, it suggests that the visual system can generate low spatial frequencies from an image that has objectively been high-pass filtered, as already suggested by Ginsburg (1978). There are, however, two conditions for this to happen. One is that the high frequencies contained in the thin lines must not be repeated over a given spatial interval, as is the case with gratings. The second condition has to do with the high contrast of the high frequencies, which is necessary for a large receptive field to be activated by a small stimulus. It may thus be suggested that whatever the objective composition of a face in terms of its physical characteristics, the visual system can always generate low frequencies which are therefore part of any description of a face in the brain.

2.2. Interaction of spatial frequencies and task demands.

A short parenthesis may be necessary at this point, concerning a recent controversy with respect to the relevance of various spatial-frequency bandwidths for face perception and processing. Several authors, among whom Harmon (1973) and Ginsburg (1978), have indicated that the low-frequency spectrum is sufficient for the processing of faces and that the high frequencies convey only redundant information. By contrast, Fiorentini, Maffei, and Sandini (1983) have suggested that the information conveyed by the high frequencies is not redundant and in fact is sufficient by itself to ensure face recognition. It seems that both views are correct, and that the controversy mainly results from a failure to take consideration of two factors that differentiate Ginsburg's and Fiorentini et al.'s studies. First, Fiorentini et al. increased the mean luminance of their high-frequency faces to achieve higher visibility of the facial features than that yielded by the usual high-pass procedure. This is a different approach from the one used by Ginsburg, and it prevents a direct comparison between the two studies since it may have increased the recognition rates for high-frequency faces in Fiorentini et al.'s study. The second point is probably more important and instructive. Ginsburg (1978) used matching tasks, that is, he presented either low-pass or high-pass unknown faces and asked the subject to retrieve the face just shown among several non-filtered faces. Fiorentini et al. (1983), on the other hand, did not use a matching task but an identification task whereby subjects were first required to learn names assigned to each experimental face and later to identify each one by name. While Ginsburg reported no difference between low-pass and high-pass faces, Fiorentini et al. obtained a higher identification rate with high-pass than with low-pass faces. They generalized their finding to all aspects of face processing while they were just testing one particular operation. In fact, Ellis, Davies, and Shepherd (1979) have shown that matching and identification may not require the processing of the same facial attributes, and that identification benefited from the processing of internal features, which, as illustrated earlier, are mainly conveyed by the high frequencies. Thus, this controversy may be resolved if one considers the particular requirements in terms of the spatial-frequency information that needs to be processed for optimal performance. While a matching task may be achieved equally well by processing the high or the low frequencies, an identification benefits from processing the high frequencies. Note that this applies to long (several seconds) viewing of the stimuli, as was the case in Ellis et al.'s and in Fiorentini et al.'s studies. The temporal properties of the visual system, as well as the resolving power of the retinal periphery, will have to be taken into account for the interpretation of results obtained with lateral tachistoscopic presentation.

2.3. Summary.

Let's now close the parenthesis, and briefly summarize what has been said so far about the spatial properties of a face. A face has both component and configurational properties that coexist, the latter emerging from the interrelationships among the former. These properties are not contained in the same spatial-frequency spectrum, and they are not equally useful depending on the type of operations that are to be implemented. By describing these properties as a function of units that characterize early visual processing, it becomes possible to specify the composition of the representations of faces that can be elaborated in the brain and from which cognitive operations unfold. The problem is now to determine the characteristics of these representations, considering that perception is a developmental process consisting of a number of conceptually distinct phases. In other words, the visual system does not instantaneously extract the entire content of a stimulus, and some physical attributes of a visual object take longer to be resolved than others. I will thus first illustrate this microgenesis of perception, and will then examine its relevance for laboratory experiments that use brief stimulus presentation and for brain-damaged patients.

3. TEMPORAL PROPERTIES

The visual system owes its great sensitivity in large part to its capacity to integrate luminous energy over time. Visual acuity develops progressively, and fine details become discernible later as energy is summed sufficiently to resolve the higher acuity requirements for these details. At a psychological level, this results in a percept of gradually increasing clarity, starting with the perception of a diffuse, undifferentiated whole which then achieves figure-ground discrimination, and finally a greater distinctiveness of contour and inner content. At a physiological level, activation of the various visual channels varies as a function of their respective integration time, and low frequencies are integrated faster than high frequencies, making the content of a percept initially a function of the low spatial-frequency spectral components of the stimulus. Although it is difficult to realize and to be aware of this developing percept given the very brief time during which integration of luminous energy takes place, I have tried to illustrate the increasing clarity of a face in such a process by filtering a single face with increasing spatial-frequency bandwidths.

3.1. Temporal development of the percept.

Figure 7 presents 9 versions of a face with increasing spatial-frequency contents by step of 0.5 octave. Face **a** has about 1.5 cycle per width and face **e** about 6 cycles per width, which is already sufficient for identifying this particular individual, as will be showed later when reporting on some results obtained with this type of filtered face. What seems to be obvious from this figure is that the increased clarity of the face in terms of information content allows for new operations to be performed. For example, while face **b**, and definitely face **c**, can be recognized as faces, they do not permit an identification and the facial features are not distinct enough even for a male/female categorization. Whereas face **e** can be accurately identified by those who know him, this cannot be acheived yet on the basis of the facial features as such. In fact, these features are not represented in face **e** in a way that would distinguish this face from other faces, and it is only the arrangement of these features within the face that serves as a basis for identification. If we now look at face **i**, it is obvious that the availability of high frequencies provides additional information that may be helpful for identification compared to face **e**. Thus, higher frequencies are not simply redundant in the processing of faces, in the sense that an increase in spatial-frequency contents of the face is accompanied by an increase in the amount of relevant information, but this is also a function of what

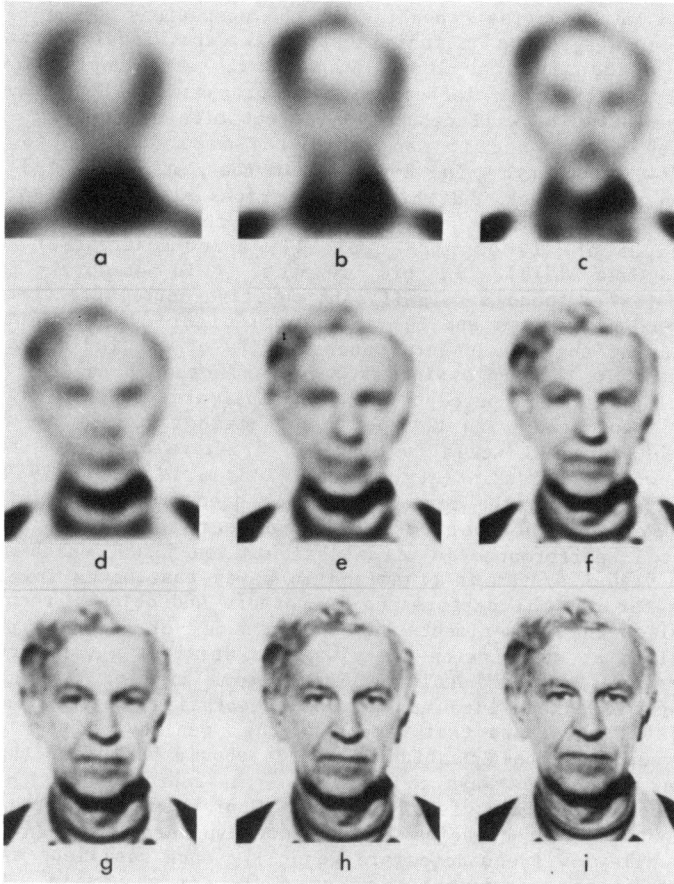

FIGURE 7. Increasing spatial-frequency contents, by 0.5 ooctave, in a face the original of which is shown in Figure 4. (As a reference, Face b contains 3.1 cycles per face width, and Face e contains 6.2 c/w.)

one has to do with the additional information. While this is true of an identification, the additional information present in face i compared to face e, for example, may be of little use if one is simply interested in deciding whether the face is that of a man or of a woman.

What figure 7 mainly illustrates is the time course of a developing percept of a face and the successive availability of additional information the use of which varies depending on the operations to be performed. This progressive integration of facial content by the visual system characterizes early processing, at least in general terms, but there are a series of factors that can influence these processes. For example, the intensity of the stimulus will determine the duration over which this integration takes place, and it can be of the order of 300 to 400 milliseconds at low intensity. The contrast of the stimulus also matters, especially when using black and white photographs since the resolution of high frequencies is made more difficult at low than at high contrast and since photographs of faces have typically a low contrast of about 0.5 (e.g., Tieger & Ganz, 1979). In this respect, it is noteworthy that Benton and Gordon (1971) found a significant positive correlation between the capacity to recognize faces and the ability to discriminate patterns of shading, indicating that the contrast sensitivity of an individual may be a critical factor in the processing of faces. Another parameter that affects the development of a percept is the retinal area that is stimulated, and projecting information in the periphery cannot result in the high level of resolution that would be obtained by stimulating the fovea. In addition, the work of Mishkin (e.g., Ungerleider & Mishkin, 1982) indicates that destruction of the foveal cortical areas in the striate cortex has detrimental effects on performance in object recognition while it leaves unaffected performance in visual orientation tasks, which may indicate that the visual system is organized in a way that makes foveal viewing necessary for optimal performance in pattern and object recognition. It may then follow that experiments based on a mode of stimulus presentation that consists of stimulating the visual system for a very brief time in a retinal area of reduced acuity implies some kind of visual sensory deficit that must be taken into account in interpreting the results.

Only some of the factors that determine the quality and the composition of the percept have been mentioned, and it should be clear that these factors interact in complex ways to determine the representation of a face that can be elaborated by the visual system. What seems to be the case is that the high spatial frequencies are the more vulnerable to any form of degradation, while low frequencies are generally more resilient and are a necessary part of the representation of a face in the brain. What is unknown, however, is the exact time course of percept development and the specific conditions that determine a particular percept. For example, stimulus integration does not stop with stimulus offset, and only the use of a backward masking may efficiently prevent the resolution of the high frequency contents. Thus, unless one uses spatially filtered faces of objectively quantified spatial-frequency composition, it is impossible to know the exact content of the incoming information that has effectively been resolved.

3.2. Limitations on temporal development of the percept in neuropsychological research.

Two further points may be worth considering with respect to the temporal integration of the incoming information. One is especially relevant to research with normal subjects and concerns the fact that processing the incoming information does not await the full development of the percept to begin (cf. Coles, Gratton, Bashore, Eriksen, & Donchin, 1985). This suggests that the information content the more rapidly extracted and integrated by the visual system will serve as a basis for early cognitive operation. In other words, these operations will initially rely on the low spatial frequencies, and they may be carried out efficiently as long as these low frequencies provide the range of information that is required for the particular processes. These early operations may serve to prepare finer visual processing of the information integrated more slowly, which would suggest some iterative rather than sequential operations in the processes mediating face perception and recognition.

The second point concerns the spatio-temporal characteristics of perception in brain-damaged patients. I will not dwell too long on this problem (see Sergent, 1984), but I would like to raise some questions regarding the nature and quality of the representation that can be constructed in a damaged brain, particularly with focal posterior lesion. There seems to be some evidence that any lesion invading cortical areas devoted to visual processing, that is occipital, parietal, or temporal, results in a disruption of the spatio-temporal capacities of the visual system. This was of course first suggested by Bay (1953), but his extreme position with respect to visual agnosia has thrown some discredit on this view. Yet, the findings hold, and they were replicated by Ettlinger (1956) who noted that bilateral visual discrimination defects may follow unilateral cerebral lesions. Specifically, what both Bay and Ettlinger found was a slower and disrupted integration of the incoming information, even in brain-damaged patients with an intact occipital cortex. That is, temporal ablation, that did not invade the optic tract and did not result in any loss in visual- field perimetry, produced sensory deficits. More recently, Bodis-Wollner (1976) observed that psychophysical measurements of the detectability of sinusoidal gratings established that in the majority of patients detection of high spatial frequencies suffers most.

It would therefore appear that early visual processes are disrupted in brain-damaged patients, and that the representations of a visual stimulus, as they are elaborated and reconstructed in the brain, may be deprived of some information that would comprise the representations in a normal brain. Independent of the processes underlying recognition, categorization or identification of the input, there seem to exist some deficiencies resulting from a defective integration during early processing. The main implication of such a disruption concerns the reduced information content of the representations on which processing is to take place, particularly with respect to the high-frequency components, and this may have to be taken into account in the interpretation of disturbances in face recognition and identification.

4. IMPLICATIONS FOR COGNITIVE PROCESSING
4.1. Relevance of sensory information for cognitive processing.

The foregoing discussion was concerned with mechanisms inherent in the early processing of visual information, and suggested a way of describing faces according to units compatible with the operations taking place during this processing. Of course, the relevance of such a description of faces for the understanding of cognitive operations rests on whether these units are still an integral part of the representations on which such cognitive operations are carried out. In other words, if spatial-frequency contents are being swallowed up, so to speak, by early visual processing, it would be of little use to study information processing in the cerebral hemispheres as a function of these units. This does not seem to be the case, however, and there is now sufficient evidence indicating that neural cells in cerebral structures underlying cognition are selectively responsive to narrow bands of spatial frequency. This has been shown by Gross for inferotemporal cells (e.g., Gross, Desimone, Albright, & Schwartz, 1984) and has been confirmed by Pollen, Nagler, Daugman, Kronauer, & Cavanagh, 1984. Pollen et al. observed that such cells were preferentially sensitive to one spatial-frequency band over the entire extent of their receptive field, and that inputs from many striate cells sensitive to a common spatial-frequency band fed into a single inferotemporal neuron. Obviously, this property does not characterize all temporal cells and there seem to be many more cells that respond to specific inputs independent of their spatial-frequency contents, but the point is that the physical attributes of the stimulus are not simply eliminated at a cognitive level. In fact, there is some evidence that physical descriptions of the input are useful and relevant to understanding perceptual performance, and Gervais, Harvey, and Roberts (1984) have recently found that confusion in letter identification were better predicted by a model of visual perception based on two-dimensional spatial-frequency contents than by models based on template overlap or geometric features.

4.2. Differential hemispheric processing of faces.

This leads us to the problem of the sensitivity of the cerebral hemispheres to spatial-frequency components and, specifically, whether a differential hemisphere sensitivity to these components could determine, or at least influence, the respective competences of the cerebral hemispheres at processing faces. It has in fact become increasingly evident during the last few years that the two cerebral hemispheres play a role in the processing of faces. While there is little doubt regarding the dominant contribution of the right hemisphere to these processes, the left hemisphere is far from being the silent partner that early research on face perception suggested it was. This is suggested by several facts: first, complete disruption of face identification, or prosapagnosia, appears to require bilateral brain injury; second, damage restricted to the left hemisphere is sometimes sufficient to impair face recognition; third, tachistoscopic experiments with normal subjects produce results suggesting that, under certain circumstances, the left hemisphere may be as efficient as, or even superior to, the right hemisphere in face perception and recognition. Such a participation of the two hemispheres in these processes poses the question of their respective role and contribution.

Among the difficulties inherent in the examination of this question, one is concerned with the diversity and heterogeneity of the tasks required from the subjects and of the particular viewing conditions under which experiments are conducted. Variations in task demands entail the implementation of different operations that may not engage to the same extent the processing competences of the two hemispheres. On the other hand, the ease with which these operations can be implemented depend on how information is represented and described in the brain.

4.3. Empirical evidence.

In order to examine this question, a series of experiments was recently conducted in which these two factors, the task demands and the spatial-frequency contents of the faces, were manipulated. The first experiment involved the presentation of 16 faces of members of the Psychology Department at McGill, with an equal number of males and females and of professors and non-professors, the latter category including secretaries, technicians, and graduate students. The subjects were graduate students of this department who had known the individuals whose face was used for at least 3 years, and they participated in each of 3 tasks on consecutive days in a counterbalanced order. The first task was a reaction-time verbal identification in which the subject had to call out the name of the face. The second task was a membership categorization, in which the subject had to press one key if the face was that of a professor and another key if the face was that of a non-professor. Since neither facial features, age or sex provide a sufficient clue as to what class a face belongs to, it can be assumed that such a membership categorization can be acheived only if the identity of the face has been accessed. This task therefore offers the possibility to examine the capacity of the hemispheres to perform face identification independent of verbal naming. The third task was a male/female categorization in which the subject had to press one key or the other depending on the sex of the face, a task that does not require accessing the identity of the face.

High-resolution faces were used and a trial involved the presentation of one face which could appear to the left, the center or the right visual field for 100 milliseconds, with a total of 288 trials preceded by 48 practice trials. Thus, the 3 tasks were conducted with the same faces, and exactly the same viewing conditions, and only the processing requirements differentiated them.

TABLE 1. Reaction times (RT, in ms), and percentage of errors (% Er.), averaged across subjects, for face identification, face-membership categorization, and male/female categorization, as a function of the three visual fields.

	LVF-RH		CVF		RVF-LH	
	RT	% Er.	RT	% Er.	RT	% Er.
Face-identif.	747	1.13	696	.33	721	1.05
Face-Members.	614	2.48	577	.92	595	2.10
Male/Female	515	1.85	490	.74	518	1.89

The results are presented in Table 1. The first important aspect is the error rate, which contrasts with previous studies in which famous faces or faces of subjects' colleagues were identified in less than 50% of the trials. This suggests that the representations of the faces that could be elaborated were of much higher quality than in earlier studies. A second aspect is the decreasing response latencies from Task 1 to Task 3, reflecting the different processing requirements of the tasks. Most important was the significant interaction between task and visual fields, suggesting that the two hemispheres were differentially influenced by variations in task demands. The simple effects of this interaction showed that latencies were significantly shorter in the right than in the left visual field in the identification and the membership categorization, while there was no significant difference between the two fields in the male/female categorization.

These results suggest that the identification of faces can be better acheived in the left than in the right hemisphere when the information to be processed is of high quality. This, however, is not simply a matter of quality since the viewing conditions and the faces were exactly the same in the three tasks, yet a significant interaction was obtained between task and visual field. At least two factors may account for the superiority of the left hemisphere in the first 2 tasks. One is the verbal naming requirement inherent in Task 1, and the access to semantic information about the faces, as well as a possible covert naming in Task 2. The second explanation, which does not necessarily exclude the verbal factor, would be that the visual analysis inherent in identifying faces, and which, as noted earlier, benefits from processing the internal features and the high spatial frequencies, is better performed in the left than in the right hemisphere because of a greater capacity of the left hemisphere to operate on high spatial frequencies. A second experiment was designed to examine which of these two factors better accounted for the present findings.

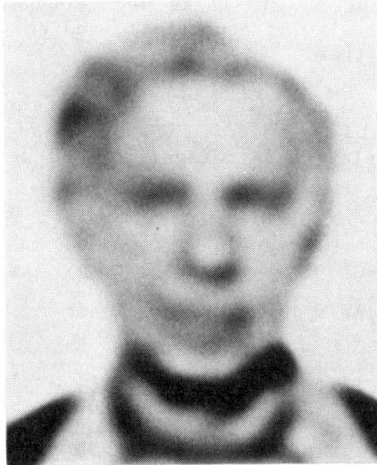

FIGURE 8. Sample of a low-pass face.

The only difference with the first experiment concerned the stimuli whose spatial-frequency composition was now controlled. Each face was first digitized and then low-pass filtered at about 6 cycles per face width so that, at the viewing distance of the experiment, they contained spatial frequencies in the range of 0 to 2 cycles per degree of visual angle (see Figure 8). To control for possible distortion resulting from the digitizing procedure, another digitized version of each face was used, containing all spatial frequencies from 0 to 32 cycles per degree of visual angle. These two versions of each face, a low-pass and a broad-pass, were mixed within an experimental session, for a total of 384 experimental trials in each of the 3 tasks. The predictions were quite straightforward. If the verbal factor was the critical one leading to a left hemisphere advantage in identifying faces, a left hemisphere superiority should still be obtained in Tasks 1 and 2 whatever the spatial-frequency composition of the faces. If, on the other hand, it was the

processing of intermediate and high frequencies that accounted for the
left hemisphere superiority in the two tasks, then filtering out these
frequency bands should eliminate the left hemisphere superiority for low-
pass faces but not for broad-pass faces.

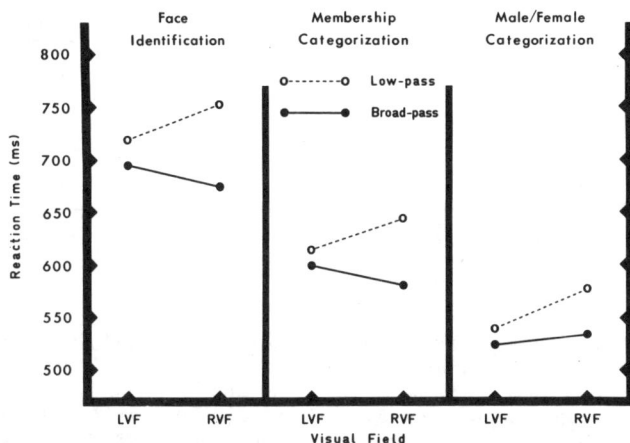

FIGURE 9. Reaction times (in ms), averaged across subjects, as a function
of visual field and face version, for each of the three tasks.

The results are presented in Figure 9 for each of the 3 tasks as a
function of face version and visual field. As can be seen in this figure,
the same pattern of results as in the first experiment obtained with
broad-pass faces, while low-pass faces yielded a left visual field/right
hemisphere superiority. This interaction of spatial-frequency by visual
field proved highly significant, suggesting that the spatial-frequency
composition of the faces may be a critical factor in the respective
processing efficiency of the cerebral hemispheres. In fact, the verbal
naming requirement of Task 1 did not seem to be determinant in this pattern of results, and the particular description of information made available for processing was the main factor in the shift of hemisphere
superiority. However, the 3-way interaction of spatial frequency, visual
field and task, indicated that the male/female categorization may not have
benefited as much as the two other tasks from the presence of high spatial
frequencies in the stimuli.

Thus, the superiority of one hemisphere over the other seems to vary
as a function of the information available and of tasks demands, and it is
worth noting that a large number of experiments used to evaluate hemisphere processing of faces have involved a matching task with unfamiliar
faces. I will just briefly mention the results of another experiment
aimed at examining further the influence of these factors and which was
conducted with the same faces in 3 different versions: broad-pass, low-pass
(see Figure 8), and coarsely quantized (see Figure 3). Two faces were
presented simultaneously in one field or in the other, and faces were made

within face-version and within sex. The task was a same-different judgement and the subjects were not from the University and had never seen the faces before. The results are shown in Table 2.

TABLE 2. Reaction times (in ms), averaged across subjects, for matching broad-pass, low-pass, and coarsely quantized faces in the left or the right visual field as a function of 'same' or 'different' judgments.

	Broad-Pass		Low-Pass		Coarsely Quantized	
	LVF	RVF	LVF	RVF	LVF	RVF
Same	523	533	530	554	616	641
Differ.	520	529	529	551	622	648
MEAN	521.5	531	529.5	552.5	619	644.5

The left visual field advantage was not significant with broad-pass faces, but it was with the two other face versions, which resulted in a significant interaction between face version and visual field. Thus, the availability of high frequencies did not result in a left hemisphere superiority in this matching task, presumably because high frequencies were not necessary for optimal performance, while low-pass filtering yielded a right hemisphere advantage, which may reflect a greater sensitivity of the right hemisphere to low frequencies.

5. CONCLUSION

What is probably the main conclusion to draw from the foregoing discussion is that the visual system provides the brain with several descriptions of facial information, that are not available at the same time and that are not equally useful depending on the type of operations to be carried out. Low frequency information is the most resilient to degradation and the visual system can generate such information even when it has objectively been filtered out in the display. In addition, low frequencies appear to convey most of the relevant information for face processing. It is interesting to note that Harvey and Sinclair (1985) have recently suggested that the memory of an unfamiliar face seems to be represented in terms of its low frequency components, which also makes our dealing with faces more likely to rely on these frequency bands. However, high frequencies are not simply redundant, at least depending on the nature of the operations or tasks to be performed, and they seem to benefit performance in tasks that require accessing the identity of a face. There is, moreover, some evidence that the two hemispheres may be differentially sensitive to the spatial-frequency contents of a face. Given the critical role of low frequencies in any processing of faces, one might expect the right hemisphere to contribute in a dominant manner to face perception and recognition. On the other hand, the contribution of the left hemisphere may become apparent in tasks that benefit from the processing of high frequencies, such as an identification, which suggests that both hemispheres are involved in the perception of faces. One should therefore expect that pros.pagnosics, who are typically defective at identifying familiar faces, should display impairment in the resolution of high frequencies.

Finally, although examining face perception, and functional asymmetry of the hemispheres as a function of spatial-frequency components available and required for processing may offer a parsimonious and coherent explanation of many findings, it addresses only one side of the problem and provides little insight into underlying cognitive operations. Nonetheless, specifying how faces are represented in early processing may be necessary to understand the nature and characteristics of subsequent operations and to determine the limitations and predispositions of the cerebral hemispheres in subserving particular processes involved in perceiving and remembering faces.

ACKNOWLEDGMENTS

The research reported in this paper is supported by the Fonds de la Recherche en Sante du Quebec, the Natural Sciences and Engineering Research Council of Canada, and the Medical Research Council of Canada. I gratefully acknowledge the contribution of Ed Manning and Gene Switkes in providing me with the coarsely quantized, and the spatially filtered pictures, respectively, and of Robert Lamarche in advising and helping me with the photographic work.

RECOGNITION MEMORY TRANSFER BETWEEN SPATIAL-FREQUENCY ANALYZED FACES

RICHARD MILLWARD & ALICE O'TOOLE

1. INTRODUCTION

The visual information that comprises a face is changing constantly. Faces age, features are altered with expression, eye-glasses are put on, and view-point and distance change almost moment to moment. Despite the variety of visual input connected with any single face, we are nearly always able to recognize faces we have seen before. In the study reported here we are interested in recognition of faces that have been spatially transformed. The specific question addressed in this paper relates to the information people use to recognize faces that are observed and tested under different spatial frequency presentations.

Marr (1982) has put together the most coherent and complete theory of visual perception to date by integrating facts from neurophysiology and psychophysics into an information-processing theory of perception. For one of our purposes - finding a mental representation of a face - his theory seems ideal. He argues for a number of levels, each of which feeds into the next higher level. His "raw-primal" sketch is a rich description of an image and consists of edges, blobs, bars, and terminators. Its importance, according to Marr, is "that it is the first representation derived from an image whose primitives have a high probability of reflecting physical reality directly" (Marr, 1982, p.,71). These primitives have attributes of orientation, contrast, length, width, and position. The raw-primal sketch is operated on by "processes of selection, grouping, and discrimination to form tokens, virtual lines, and boundaries at different scales" to yield the full-primal sketch. (Marr discusses even higher-level representations formed from the primal sketch, but for our purposes the raw-primal sketch is of central interest.)

An important idea in Marr's theory is the spatial coincidence assumption:

> If a zero-crossing segment is present in a set of independent
> VG channels over a contiguous range of sizes, and the segment
> has the same position and orientation in each channel, then
> the set of such zero-crossing segments indicates the presence
> of an intensity change in the image that is due to a single
> physical phenomenon (a change in reflectance, illumination,
> depth, or surface orientation).

In pursuing our goal of deriving a representation of an image that is consistent with some psychological processes, we wanted to look at each level of Marr's theory. We reasoned that, if the coincidence assumption were correct, then the representation derived from the lower spatial frequencies would be similar (though surely not identical) to the representation derived from the higher spatial frequencies. If similar facts, at the level of the raw-primal sketch, were extracted from each end of the spatial frequency specturm, then subjects would be able to recognize a face presented in only one-half the spectrum even though they had seen it only in the other, nonoverlapping half of the spectrum. The results of such an experiment would be a test of Marr's theory as well as give us some information about the way a face is represented mentally.

Marr argues that vision is highly modular. Although he is less precise and less extreme in his views on modularity than Fodor (1982), he still espouses the idea that vision is mostly bottom-up, is organized into a number of successively more abstract levels, and is a biologically isolated system.

> "Our approach rested heavily on the principle of modularity, which states that any large computation should be split up into a collection of small, nearly independent, specialized subprocesses. (Marr, 1982, p.325)."

Fodor would have the cognitive system (which he calls the central or horizontal system) receive only the final output of the successive stages of analysis of a module. Marr is less clear but does not seem opposed to letting the higher-level cognitive system have access to information derived at various levels. Thus, the information contained in the primal sketch is certainly available to awareness. He says, for example, "... it is interesting to think about which representations the different artists concentrate on and sometimes disrupt. The pointillists, for example, are tampering primarily with the image; the rest of the scheme is left intact, and the picture has a conventional appearance otherwise. Picasso, on the other hand, clearly disrupts most at the 3-D model level. ... An example of someone who operates primarily at the surface representation stage is a little harder - Cezanne perhaps? (Marr, 1982, p.356)."

Marr's position here is important because we must address the question of which representation, of all those computed at various levels, is necessary or, at least, sufficient, for remembering the stimulus. To address this question we must discuss what we mean by "remember". Although it is often assumed that the human memory system is separate from the perceptual system - the latter feeding into the former, this does not imply that human memory is static. The memory of a computer is a particularly bad analogy here. Human memory is not addressable in the computer sense, it is not immutable, and it is not noninteractive. Memory systems must account for interference effects, prototype abstraction, forgetting, and reconstructive processes. In a recognition memory test, we need to specify not only what the input representation is, but also how that individual representation will interact with other, already stored images. Few visual information-processing studies consider the memory component and few memory studies derive the input to memory from visual processes.

Because of the previous success of distributed-memory models in work with memory for faces (see, e.g. Kohonen, Oja & Lehtio, 1981) and because connectionist models make so much sense in other respects (see, e.g. Hinton & Anderson, 1981; Eich, 1985; Murdoch, 1979; Waltz, 1985), we assume a simple version of this class of models for our theoretical work on memory. Distributed memory models have many advantages: they give intuitive support to Gestalt ideas, allow reconstruction of the whole from the parts or from a noisy example, have a physiological rationale, and are insensitive to partial destruction of the storage medium. They have a large capacity of no fixed size and degrade gracefully when overloaded. They form prototypes, and produce inexact and fuzzy images in retrieval, just as human memory presumably does.

The distributed memory model we use follows Kohonen, Oja & Lehtio (1981) in almost all respects. The pattern vector representing the image is designated f_i. This pattern is correlated with itself by multiplying the vector by its transpose (f_i x f_i'). The result of this autocorrelation is "remembered" in a matrix, M_i. If f_i is presented again, later, then retrieval is accomplished by multiplying the input vector with the memory marix, $f_o = M_i$ x f_i, where f_o is the output vector retrieved. It can be shown that $f_o = f_i$, if f_i is presented, but f_o will represent only noise with an expectation of 0 if any other random vector is presented. When different input vectors are presented to the system to be remembered, each memory matrix is added to a common memory matrix, A, so that if n stimuli are presented, then $A = M_1 + M_2 + \ldots M_n$. If all pairs of stimuli, f_i and f_j, are orthogonal, then the value of presenting f_i to the system, computed by multiplying it by A, A x f_i, will be $f_o = f_i$ because M_j x f_i for all i and j will be zero except when i = j. Obviously the number of orthogonal vectors depends on the dimensionality of A. It is generally assumed that A is large. However, even when unrelated fs are entered into the memory matrix, they can be filtered out because they yield relatively low values and can be considered noise. Generally, unrelated stimuli will have an expectation of zero. On the other hand, note that insofar as two or more vectors correlate, they will tend to reinforce each other and can lead to a representation that "notices" the average better than the individuals, i.e. prototype learning. Faces generally correlate, which means that a new face vector will tend to produce a "face-like" vector similar to the input. Also, if the vector is incomplete or if noise is added to it, it will still tend to retrieve itself, although less well. This accounts for the ability of the system to retrieve the whole from a part.

An important question in the application of distributed memory models pertains to the encoding of the stimuli. In terms of the model, what should the elements of the vector be? One possibility considered here is that they are pixel element intensities. Another possibility is that they are some representation of lines of zero-crossings in the image. Another question concerns the degree of connectivity. The vector product discussed above represents in M the cross-product of every element with every other element. This produces a fully-connected matrix. We assume that the breadth of the association is limited to some degree and thus we enter into M only those associations (cross-products) that are within a radius of some x units in the image. (The choice here was 5 units.)

Finally, it is possible to compare the output f_o with the input vector f_i, and then multiply the matrix by corrective feedback to make f_o closer to f_i. The Widrow-Hoff (see Duda & Hart, 1973) procedure is one example of such a technique. Let $d_i = (f_i - f_o)$, where f_o is the output from applying the new input f_i to A. A is then corrected by successively iterating the correction, $A_{k+1} = cd_i f_i + A_k$. Often c is made a decreasing function of k in order to limit the number of iterations; alternatively, a maximum k can be chosen. In any case, the iteration stops when $d_i = 0$, if it does. In the simulations to be discussed here, the number of iterations was fixed at 16 and c was a constant.

2. EXPERIMENTAL RATIONALE

Our research strategy was to consider various representations based as much as possible on sensory physiology and psychophysical research and use these representations in a distributed memory model. In the research reported here, we look only at Marr's coincidence assumption. We consider a number of assumptions associated with the distributed memory model, for example, various choices for the input vector and the Widrow-Hoff rehearsal strategy. In each case, we try to find an experiment to test the efficacy of the representation and the memory assumptions.

In the experiment to test Marr's coincidence assumption, subjects were presented faces which were processed to contain only low spatial frequencies or only high spatial frequencies. Subjects were then tested by being presented these same faces for recognition in the complementary spatial frequency. A primary question is whether there is transfer from faces of only low (or high) spatial frequencies to faces of only high (or low) spatial frequencies, i.e. can subjects recognize a face presented in one spatial frequency even though they see it only in the other? Confirmation would support Marr's coincidence assumption because, according to Marr, when zero-crossings at a number of different channels all indicate the presence of a line or some other discontinuity, the visual system encodes this fact in the raw primal sketch. The "real lines" of a face are picked up by both the low and the high spatial frequencies and are represented in the raw-primal sketch. Subjects thus have common information for comparing the high and low spatial faces.

Turning to the memory model simulations, we see whether a distributed memory model can also carry the transfer results since recognition memory involves memory as well as visual information processing. By looking at raw pixel intensities we can ask whether any processing of the input is required to show transfer. That is, there might be enough in common at the pixel level between low and high frequency faces to carry the transfer from one to the other. We can also look at lines abstracted from face patches to see if a more abstract representation - one at about Marr's raw-primal sketch level - will show transfer. Without the results from the memory model we would not be able to eliminate any representation since any representation could be used for transfer. However, the memory model allows us to see if a given representation will show transfer.

2.1. Experimental Details

2.1.1. Stimuli. Photographs of 42 male and 42 female models were used as stimuli for the study. All of the models were college students and wore white drapes to hide their clothing. In the photographs, none had beards or wore glasses.

Each photograph was digitized to a resolution of 512 x 512 pixels using an Eikonix Scan 78/99 camera. Images were then multiplied by a two-dimensional Gaussian function with a period of 512 pixels. This was done to insure the quality of the filtered image by eliminating the grid-like artifacts of the photograph border present in the digitized image. Fast Fourier transforms were calculated for the images with a standard FORTRAN FFT program. High-pass and Low-pass images of each face were created by filtering the transform of the original image circularly and symmetrically from a single cutoff point and performing an inverse transform on the residual frequencies.

A cutoff of 22 cycles per image-width (512 pixels) was chosen. Frequencies above this point were eliminated in the Low-pass image and frequencies equal to or below this point were eliminated in the High-pass image. Thus, in a strict sense, no overlapping of spatial frequency information was present in the High- and Low-pass versions of a given face.

The size of the processed image was decreased to 256 x 256 pixels for display on a Conrac monitor (Model 5211C19) by sampling every other pixel. The cutoff point of 22 cycles per image-width corresponds to approximately 11 cycles per face-width since the faces spanned approximately half of the picture width (see Ginsberg, 1980 for more on c/fw). The measure of c/fw was used here because it is constant over viewing distance. Black and white slides were taken of all images from the Conrac monitor under identical conditions.

2.1.2. _Apparatus._ All experimental events were controlled by a Digital Equipment Corporation VAX 11/780 computer interfaced to two MAST System II random access slide projectors. Each subject was tested in a booth facing a projection screen on which the slides were back-projected. Prompts and instructions were presented on a video monitor, and subjects responded on a keyboard.

During the experiment, the slides subtended a visual angle of 4.77 degrees horizontally and 3.61 degrees vertically. Although contrast and luminance profiles of stimuli are often of interest in vision experiments, for a number of reasons they may not be particularly useful statistics here. First, contrast, as defined in terms of the numbers which comprise the digitized image, is not linearly related to the light intensities as displayed on the monitor. This is because the pixels of the display monitor have a nonlinear change in luminance corresponding to a linear change in those of the digitized image. Second, the faces were photographed from the monitor and there is no guarantee of linearity between luminances here either. The results, however, offer evidence that the normal, high, and low SFs are equally perceptible.

2.1.3. _Procedure and Design._ The procedure was typical of recognition memory tasks: a learning phase, in which each of a set of 42 stimuli (21 slides of male and 21 slides of female faces) was presented for inspection, was followed by a test phase in which pairs of face slides were presented sequentially in a two-alternative forced-choice paradigm. Subjects were asked to say which member of the pair of slides they had seen before. One member was always "old" and one "new". All previously seen slides were presented during the test phase so there were 42 pairs of slides in all. Presentations during the learning and test phases were for 5 seconds.

During learning, different groups of subjects were presented with face slides of different spatial frequencies. The Normal groups saw digitized photos which had not been filtered. The Low SF groups saw slides containing low SFs. The High SF groups saw slides containing only high SFs. During the test phase, all groups saw all three types of slides, one-third of each type, or 14 slides per condition. One member of the pair of stimuli was "old" in that the slide was of the same face as previously seen even though it might be of a different spatial frequency. Both test slides were always of the same spatial frequency. For each subject the order of presentation of the total set of slides was randomized, as was the order of each "old" and "new" test pair.

There were three separate experiments, which varied only in the number of presentations of each stimulus during the learning phase. In Exp. 1, each slide was presented only once; in Exp. 2, each slide was presented twice; and in Exp. 3, each slide was presented three times. All slides were presented in random order before any slide was repeated. In Exp. 1, 6 subgroups of subjects were set up to counterbalance across the three subsets of slides required when the learned slides were split into the three test conditions. Also, half the subjects saw one-half the slides as "old" and the other half of the subjects saw the remaining slides as "old". Therefore, 12 subjects were needed per learning group to balance the design. In Experiments 2 and 3, only 6 subjects were used for each group and the counterbalancing across subsets of slides was eliminated.

2.1.4. _Subjects._ The 72 subjects were Brown students and staff who were paid for their approximately one-hour participation in the experiment.

3. A SUMMARY ANALYSIS OF THE TRANSFER EXPERIMENTS

We assume that each face contains information helpful for its later recognition in both the low and high spatial frequencies (SFs). Some of that information is redundantly coded in both the low and high frequencies so that, when extracted, it represents a "common" portion of the code. This is one way to interpret Marr's spatial coincidence assumption. At the same time, there is information unique to the low and high SFs. Our experiment had subjects look at faces that were processed to contain only low, only high, or both low and high SFs - the "normal" faces. If a subject saw a high-spatially processed face and was later shown a low-spatially processed face, the only way the second face could be recognized was on the basis of common information derived from both. The following summary analysis measures the common information, the information unique to the high SFs and the information unique to the low SFs.

A number of simplifying assumptions must be made to carry out these measurements. Before listing the obvious assumptions, we wish to note that by "information" we do not mean a measure in bits derived from information theory. We are using the term somewhat loosely - its operational definition is in terms of the amount of transfer that we have observed in the recognition memory experiments. The first assumption we make is that, when looking at a face that consists only of high or low SFs, the subjects encode no more information from these high or low SFs than if they were looking at a normal face. This is not obviously true - in fact it could be wrong. Subjects could be limited in the rate at which information is extracted from the stimulus and thus, when great deal of information is present, they might encode only some fraction of it. When a low-frequency face is presented, they might encode more from the low frequencies than they would from the low frequencies when both low and high frequencies (normal) faces were presented. There might even be masking effects when both low and high spatial frequencies are present which interfere with picking up information from the high and/or low spatial frequencies.

A second assumption is that what we are calling common information is truly common and can be extracted equally well from the high or the low spatial frequency faces. There could be an asymmetry in this encoding process. Marr suggests that low spatial frequencies are used to corroborate the "edges" suggested by high SFs. This would lead to an asymmetry in encoding since the low SFs might not be as informative as the high. The whole question of which spatial frequencies carry more information is fraught with difficulty and it is not one we are focusing on here. (See Fiorentini, Maffei and Sandini (1983) for a treatment of this question.)

A third assumption is that there are not large individual differences in the encoding processes under different learning conditions. This is made purely pragmatically because we could not run subjects on the high, low, and normal SFs in the learning condition. We must therefore estimate parameters assuming homogeneity across learning conditions. We must note that the assumptions are about the system as a whole. Both visual processing and memory assumptions are mixed together in the summary analysis.

The model becomes fairly easy to derive under these assumptions. Table 1 presents the theoretical expressions for the nine cells of the experiment. Each cell represents the performance expected for a subject. The rows correspond to the learning conditions, which are tested under all three transfer conditions - normal, high and, low (i.e. the columns of Table 1). The 1st-row, 1st-column cell, for example, shows that when normal faces are presented, common information (represented by the parameter b), information from the high spatial frequencies (coded as a), and information from the low SFs (coded as c) are all present in the test with normal faces. The transfer between learning condition high (low) and low (high) depends only on the common information, b.

TABLE 1. Summary Analysis

		Testing conditions		
		Normal	Low-SF	High-SF
	Normal	a+b+c	b+c	a+b
Learning conditions	Low	b+c	b+c	b
	High	a+b	b	a+b

We use the number of faces recognized in the various experiments in each of these nine conditions to estimate the three parameters a, b, and c. The estimation technique is least squares. Although ideally we would estimate the parameters for individual subjects, the design of the experiment required a different group of subjects in each row of the table. We cannot estimate all three parameters from a single row because three values (the three columns) do not provide enough degrees of freedom to fit three parameters. Besides, the second and third row each depend on only two parameters. (Attempts to estimate parameter a from the third row and parameter c from the second row led to poorer fits overall.) These estimation problems require the third assumption above.

TABLE 2. Parameter estimations from the summary analysis

	Parameters		
	b = common	a = high	c = low
Experiment 1	.56	.11	.14
Experiment 2	.63	.11	.14
Experiment 3	.72	.10	.14
Average	.64	.11	.14

Of our three experiments, the first presented each face only once, the second twice, and the third three times. Table 2 lists the parameter estimations for all three experiments and for the average of all three experiments. (The parameters estimated from the average data are the same as the average of the parameters themselves because the theory is linear.) The parameters are proportions and indicate how many faces are recognized by the component represented by the parameter. Thus, the .11 for parameter a means that subjects recognized .11 x total number of observed faces on the basis of the high SFs. Since there were 14 faces in each condition, this amounts to 1.5 faces. The b parameter is special in that it absorbs all the chance performance – that is, it has a value of .50 due to chance. Therefore, the .56 value represents only a proportion of .06 above chance, or about .9 faces. This represents the level of common information that could be used to transfer from low to high or high to low SFs.

One interesting result is that, over the three experiments, each run with different subjects, the a and c parameters are very constant and the increased performance is taken up in the common parameter. This suggests that, however repetition improves memory, it is based on information that is common – information that can be used to recognize high SF faces from low and vice versa – and not just information associated with particular lines or shapes of the high and low SF slides.

Table 3 shows the overall goodness-of-fit of this summary analysis. We have presented the data from the average of the three experiments because they are nearly as good as Experiment 1, which showed the best overall fit. The sum of the squared deviations was 4.58, and the largest deviation (for the High-to-High transfer) 2.58. The transfer from Low-to-Low and High-to-High was better than predicted. Transfer from Low and High to Normal were lower than predicted. The discrepancies from predictions are not easy to interpret. Because of the different subjects in the three learning conditions, we cannot make a firmer judgment about how well this summary analysis describes the data.

TABLE 3. Results and summary analysis: Average of Experiments 1, 2, & 3

| | | Testing Conditions | | |
		Normal	Low	High
	Normal			
	Obs.	11.94	11.17	10.11
	Pred.	12.37	10.90	10.42
Learning Conditions	Low			
	Obs	10.36	11.61	8.67
	Pred.	10.90	10.90	8.96
	High			
	Obs.	9.56	8.81	12.03
	Pred.	10.42	8.96	10.42

Parameters: a = 1.47, b = 8.96, c = 1.95

4. MEMORY SIMULATIONS

We discussed the Kohonen distributed memory model briefly above. If we assume that information extracted by the sensory system is fed into memory and matched later with new faces, then the specification of the memory component of the system is important. Four simulations were run. The pixel simulations used only a small square (22 x 22 pixels) around the right eye, nose, and cheek. The grain of the digitized faces was also reduced to 128 x 128 pixels. For the pixel simulations, the 484 normalized pixels were fed directly into the memory model for each face stimulus. The autocorrelation matrix was not fully connected. Instead, a connectivity of five pixels was imposed on the associative matrix. The model was made to learn in three separate groups, corresponding to the experimental conditions. Twenty faces were presented for learning rather than 42 since, unlike human subjects, the model could be tested on all three test conditions without changing the memory. The test condition was simulated by presenting an "old" and a "new" face to the model and computing the cosine between the input and the output vectors from memory for each of the two input vectors. The face-vector with the larger cosine was "chosen" and the proportion correct was recorded.

The second pixel simulation introduced the Widrow-Hoff procedure in which the response to a new input vector is compared to the original vector and a correction is made. The correction is then fed back into the memory to improve what it stores for each vector. This can be considered related to "supervised learning" or rehearsal techniques. The purpose was to match the simulation to the second and third experiments in which the faces were presented more than once. In other respects the simulation was similar to the first simulation.

In the two slope simulations, the input vector was modified. Rather than using the normalized pixels, the square portion of the face, increased to 60 x 60, was divided into a 6 x 6 grid of 10 x 10 pixels each. For each of the 36 mini-squares of 100 pixels, the best fitting straight line was computed. Here we are following the ideas of Marr in generating the first step in the raw-primal sketch. (As an aside, we should note the contrast of the high, normal, and low faces were not the same; a normalization process was imposed on the digitized faces to make the line-finding algorithm comparable across the face stimuli.) The vector input to the memory matrix consisted of the slope of the single line fitted to each of the 36 regions of the face. In other respects, one simulation was similar to the first pixel simulation without the Widrow-Hoff supervised learning, while the other simulation included the Widrow-Hoff rehearsal procedure.

4.1. Results

In general, the pattern of experimental results was duplicated in a gross way by all the simulations. That is, same learning and same testing conditions were generally highest, transfer from normal faces to high or low and from high and low to normal faces were above chance with a slight edge to low spatial frequencies. Table 4 shows the correlations between the nine cells of the results matrix and the simulation matrix. All the simulations were significantly (p < .05) above chance when tested with a significance of r test with 7 dfs.

Two points should be made about the use of correlations here. One is that we cannot use a goodness-of-fit technique since the simulation does not insure that the overall level of the results corresponds to the observed level. The simulation is parameter free in its prediction and so no adjustment has been made for mean performance. On the other hand, the simulation can show a good fit because it is in line with the pattern of results even though specific predictions may be in error in fundamental

TABLE 4. Simulation results: correlations

	Simulations			
	Widrow-Hoff		No Widrow-Hoff	
	Pixel	Slopes	Pixel	Slopes
Experiment 1:	.77	.89	.79	.94
Experiment 2:	.83	.83	.81	.70
Experiment 3:	.81	.85	.74	.92
Average 1, 2, 3:	.86	.90	.83	.90

ways.   For example, pixel simulations failed in that there was slightly below-chance transfer from high to low and low to high faces. Although the subjects did not show a great deal of transfer under these conditions either, they were at least above chance.   Also, in experiments two and three, subjects were substantially above chance on these transfers. Although we did not run the simulations, there is reason to believe that just repeating the presentation of each face would not improve the pixel simulations but we are unable to say what the Widroff-Hoff procedure might do.   Hence, even though the pattern of results is good, unless the simulation can show above-chance performance in the high to low transfer conditions, it fails in a significant way.

Slope simulations are another story altogether. Here, not only is the pattern highly acceptable, even the levels are about right. The correlation of .90 is highly significant and the fit better than we could manage with fitting three parameters in the summary analysis.   That is, we ran a correlation on the predicted points from the summary analysis against the observed data and it was lower than the simulation correlation.   On the other hand, the squared difference of the error for the simulation was 12.11, but only 4.58 in the summary analysis.   The implied contradiction here is presumably due to the fact that the simulation is off in absolute level, thus increasing the squared-error while the pattern of results is more in line with the pattern of observed results.   We estimated the parameters a, b, and c from the simulation data with the resulting values of .11, .65, and .19, which are fairly close to the best-fitting parameters from the summary analysis, .11, .64 and .14.   The larger c parameter apparently reflects the higher overall performance and accounts for the squared-error differences.

What are the implications of these results? First, of course, the memory model does an excellent job of accounting for recognition memory. Second, it works better when it is given vectors that represent slightly abstracted information - slopes of lines grossly computed on grids of the face. These input vectors might be said to correspond to Marr's raw-primal sketch.   In this respect, Marr's coincidence assumption in conjunction with a distributed memory model provide a reasonable explanation of these results.

5. SUMMARY AND DISCUSSION

The goal of our research is to develop a theoretical representation for images (faces in particular) which captures what is known about subject's behavior with respect to these images. There are many phenomena to be accounted for - illusions, verbal descriptions, phenomenological awareness, prototypes, etc., and we cannot begin to suggest a representation adequate for all these phenomena. We dealt in particular with recognition memory, the representation needed to account for judgments by subjects. We began by looking at theoretical work in vision in order to base our representation scheme on results known from neuroscience and psychophysics. Marr's theory was an obvious choice of theoretical schemes. Marr argues strongly for modularity, and by that argument one would expect that fairly high-level representation schemes would result from processing a face. Comparisons between faces would then occur on the basis of these high-level representations. Another fact noticed by Marr, and one which suggested to us a way to tap some of the visual processes was the coincidence assumption. Lines in the real world provide the information needed to identify the same objects presented under different spatial frequencies. This suggested that we could study the representation problem by testing whether faces separated by spatial frequency were nonetheless represented in the same way. If they were, then subjects would have no trouble transferring between the high and the low spatial frequency faces.

Too often in psychophysics, researchers ignore the memory component of the system. Similarly, in memory work, researchers ignore the perceptual input to memory. We believe that much recent research on connectionist models has demonstrated that a distributed memory model provides a useful construct for memory. This is particularly true for recognition memory of images. So, we assumed that each face was stored in a correlation matrix which limited connectivity. We tested two different assumptions about what the visual system sent to the memory system. One was raw-pixel intensities. Although the pattern of results was not bad in this case, there was no evidence of any transfer from high to low SF faces or vice versa. Since subjects did show some transfer ability, small for Experiment 1 but increasing with repetition of faces, the lack of transfer raised questions about the adequacy of raw-pixel intensity as the correct input to memory. The second assumption was that small patches of visual space were coded as lines. These could correspond to Marr's virtual lines abstracted from zero-crossing and represented in his raw-primal sketch. When these were fed into the memory system, extremely close fitting results were obtained.

One might ask whether a higher-level representation scheme might not work just as well. We cannot argue against such a proposition. However, we can argue that we do not need to postulate a higher-level representation since we accounted adequately for the results with a distributed memory model using slopes of lines as elements of the input vectors. On the other hand, a pixel-level representation does seem to be inadequate. Thus, the visual system may compute an abstraction of at least the complexity of lines or edges and that, when used in a distributed memory model, such an abstraction is adequate to account for recognition memory of faces.

The research reported here was supported in part by two Biomedical Research Support Grants PHS-5-S07-RRO-7085-16 & -20 to Dr R. Millward who was also supported in part by the Alfred P. Sloan Foundation Grant-in-Aid 80-11-6 to the Center for Cognitive Science and the Center for Neural Science. A more detailed presentation of the data and simulations are available in O'Toole's MS thesis (1985).

REACTION TIME MEASURES OF FEATURE SALIENCY IN A PERCEPTUAL INTEGRATION
TASK.

I.H. FRASER and D.M. PARKER

1.INTRODUCTION

Research on cue saliency in facial recognition has relied heavily on
two basic paradigms which can broadly be described as (i) recognition and
(ii) recall. The recognition paradigm involves the identification of a
familiar face from one or more of its individual features or examining
the effects of alteration of particular features on identification. The
recall paradigm utilises the frequency with which fragments or features
appear in subjects descriptions of a previously presented stimulus.
Highly salient features which subjects attended to would be expected to
constitute a substantial part of their description. Recognition and
recall studies have established that particular aspects of the face are
more salient than others (c.f. Shepherd, Davies and Ellis 1981). When
caucasians view caucasian faces the hair and the eyes emerge as probably
the most important cues in both paradigms. The nose features prominently
in verbal descriptions of faces (Ellis et al. 1980, Shepherd et al.,
1977) but does not appear to be very affective as an isolated cue for
identification (Goldstein and Mackenberg 1966, Seamon et al., 1978). It
is also apparent that subjects select the hair and forehead region first,
then the eyes followed by the nose and mouth when they construct Photofit
faces and the accuracy of feature selection follows the same order (Ellis
et al., 1977). Laughery et al. (1977) and Ellis et al.(1977) report that
the amount of time devoted to the hair/forehead and eye region in
Photofit and Identikit reconstruction and when instructions are given to
sketch artists is greater than that spent on lower facial features.

It is unclear whether this preference for features of the upper face is
a consequence of subjects attending first to these regions during the
familiarization process i.e. whether it is simply a primacy effect;
whether it is attributable to the fact that hair/forehead and eye regions
are proportionally larger cues than the nose and mouth/chin or indeed
whether there is more efficient immediate processing of selected regions
of the face. Clearly these are not mutually exclusive alternatives but
there appears to be little evidence available on these rather basic
questions. Below we describe three experiments which explore feature
processing of outline drawings and whose results may illuminate these
issues. A program was written for the Apple IIe microcomputer which
allowed for rapid successive presentation of the components of a face in
which the order of component presentation was randomised. On 50% of
trials the final component in the series was omitted. This random
sequential presentation of the stimulus components was calculated to
prevent any simple processing strategy such as scanning the face from top
to bottom. Processing efficiency was measured by timing the subjects
responses (RTs) to omission of the differing components and collecting
the number and type of errors made.

2.PROCEDURE

An Apple IIe microcomputer together with a Zenith 12" monitor whose P32 phosphor was fast decaying were used as a tachistoscope to present stimuli and record subjects' responses. The stimulus (see Fig. 1) was composed of four fragments each of which was presented for 20 msc. followed by a blank interval.

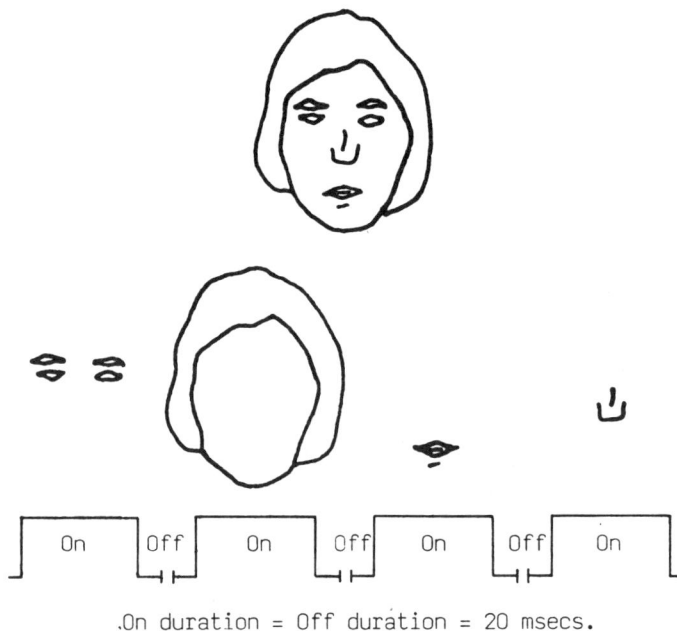

.On duration = Off duration = 20 msecs.

Figure 1. The stimulus used in experiments 1 and 3 and an example of a typical presentation sequence moving from left to right. The fragments appeared in the same position on the screen that they would have occupied if the whole stimulus had been presented simultaneously.

Subjects viewed the screen with their head supported by a chin rest from a distance of 1 metre. The stimulus subtended approximately 5°. Subjects were shown a picture of the stimulus and its subdivisions and informed that on any particular presentation one, and only one, fragment could be omitted. Their task was to indicate as rapidly as possible by pressing one of two buttons in a hand held response unit whether the stimulus was complete or incompleted. Response timing was accomplished by an internal digital clock constructed in the departments' workshop and data were printed on an Epson RX-80 printer. Before beginning the experiments proper subjects were given 10 practice trials. Subjects were required to make four sets of 100 responses with a three minute break between sets.

EXPERIMENT 1

This experiment set out to establish whether or not differences in response times were apparent when particular features, outline, eyes, nose or mouth, were omitted.

SUBJECTS
    12 subjects, 5 females and 7 males, ranging in age from 19 to 56 years
participated in this experiment.

RESULTS
    The median reaction times for all correct responses to feature omission
were calculated (for each feature per trial). A within S analysis of
variance was conducted on these medians, the independent variables were
1) 'features' - four levels relating to the four fragments of the
stimulus and 2) 'trials' - four levels corresponding to the medians of
the four sets of 100 responses. It was found that there was a main
effect for features, $F(3, 11) = 65.44$, $p < .001$. The overall means
across all trials indicated that responses were faster for the detection
of the omission of the outline (.54 sec) as opposed to the eyes (.71),
the nose (.86) and the mouth (.94). A Newman-Keuls revealed that all
features were significantly different from each other, $P < .05$. (See
figure 2).

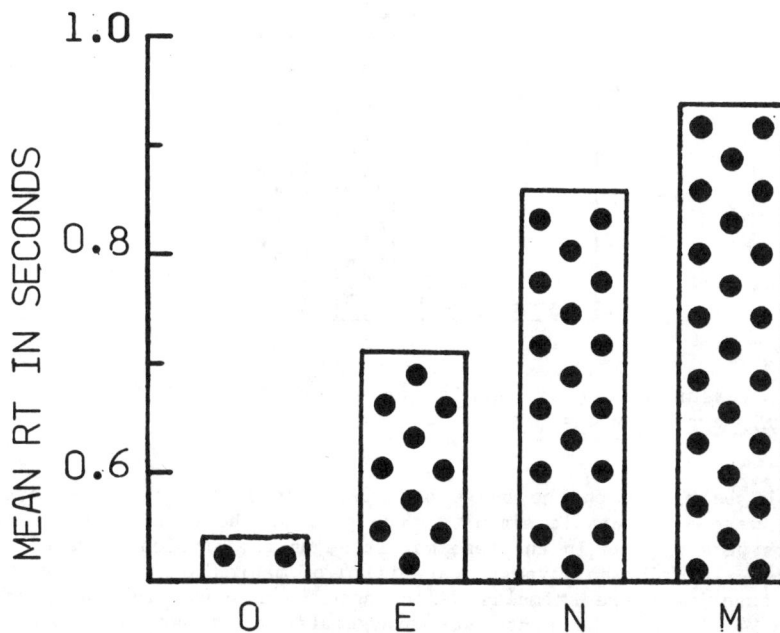

Figure 2. Mean of the median response times (RT) to feature omission. O
= outline, E = eyes, N = nose, M = mouth.

A second measure was taken of the frequency of commission errors, i.e., the errors that occur when a subject responds 'yes complete' when in fact a piece has been omitted. This measure is yet another way of assessing the difficulty involved in the detection of the absence of any one particular feature of the face. A within S analysis of variance was conducted on the frequency of commission errors for each feature per trial. There was a main effect of features with a $F(3, 11) = 16.72$ and a $P < .001$. The overall means across all trials indicated that there were fewer commission errors on average for the outline, as opposed to the eyes the nose and the mouth. A Newman-Keuls revealed that the significant difference between error frequency per feature arose when the outline and the eyes were compared to the nose and the mouth respectively. All comparisons significant at the .01 level (See figure 3). Results then indicate that there are significant differences in response times and error frequency associated with the detection of omission of particular features.

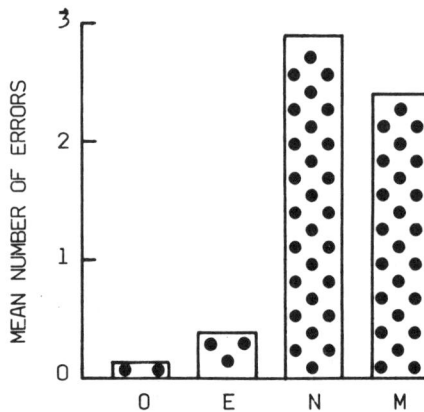

Figure 3. Mean number of commission errors for each feature   0 = outline, E = eyes, N = nose, M = mouth.

EXPERIMENT 2

It could be argued on the basis of experiment 1 that the differences observed were attributable simply to the size of the features since RTs and errors were ordered in the same magnitude on the physical size of the fragments. In order to have the capability of manipulating feature size in this experiment the stimulus was changed to a schematic happly face (see Fig. 4(a)) and the mouth was exaggerated in length to span the distance between the outer extremes of the eyes. If feature fragment size predicts RT and errors then increasing the size of the mouth should abolish or reverse the differences observed between the eyes and mouth fragments in experiment 1.

Subjects. 4 males subjects ranging in age from 22 to 56 years participated in this study.

RESULTS

The median reaction time for all correct responses to feature in omission for each feature per block of trials was obtained, and A within

S, analysis of variance conducted. The independent variables were, 1)

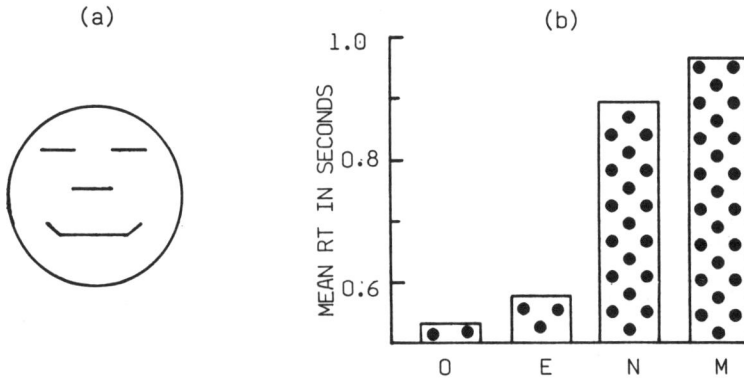

Figure 4. (a) Happy face stimulus used in Experiment 2. (b) Mean of the median response times to feature omission, 0 = outline, E = eyes, N = nose, M = mouth.

features – four levels corresponding to the stimulus fragments and 2) trials – also four levels pertaining to the medians for each set of 100 responses. There was a main effect for features, $F(3, 3) = 29.0$, P < .001. The overall means for each feature showed, that detection of omitted features, was fastest for the outline (.54 sec), followed by the eyes (.58), the nose (.87) and the mouth (.97). A Newman-Keuls revealed that the significant effects arose when the outline and the eyes were compared to the nose and the mouth respectively, with a probability less than .01 (See figure 4.)

A second analysis was conducted on the frequency of commission errors for each feature per trial. A within S analysis of variance was conducted, and a main effect of features was found, $F(3, 3) = 5.51$, with a P = .02. When the overall means for each feature was obtained, it showed that the least number of commission errors were found to involve the outline (.13), followed by the eyes (.19), the mouth (.69) and the

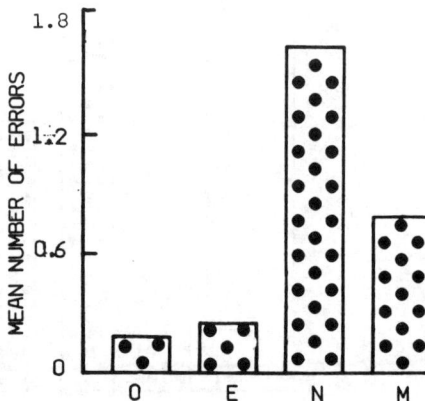

Figure 5. Mean number of errors of commision for the outline = 0, eyes = E, nose = N and mouth = M.

nose (1.63). A Newman-Keuls revealed that the significance arose, when the outline was compared to the nose and mouth, with a probability less than .05 (See figure 5.).

EXPERIMENT 3

This experiment was designed to clarify the pattern of errors made by subjects.

SUBJECTS

The study involved 4 subjects, 2 males and 2 females, ranging from 22 to 24 years of age.

APPARATUS

As noted in study 1, with the addition of a cassette recorder, which was used to store the subject's verbal responses.

PROCEDURE

The procedure was similar to study 1, with the addition of a verbal response which immediately followed the button press. One of three types of verbal responses was required, i.e., either 1) 'complete' if all the features were present, 2) the specific name of the omitted feature or 3) 'miss hit' if the wrong button was pressed, followed by an indication of the intended response. These responses were recorded and later matched to the computer printout.

RESULTS

The frequency of omission errors for each feature, per trial was calculated, and a within S analysis of variance conducted, the independent variables being features - four levels relating to the fragments of the stimulus and trials - corresponding to the frequency of errors in each set of 100 responses. There was a main effect of features, $F(3, 3) = 15.51$ with a $P = .001$. The overall means for each feature showed that most errors were caused by the omission of the nose (6.88), followed by the mouth (5.19); the eyes (1.31) and the outline (.44). Further application of a Newman-Keuls, revealed that the

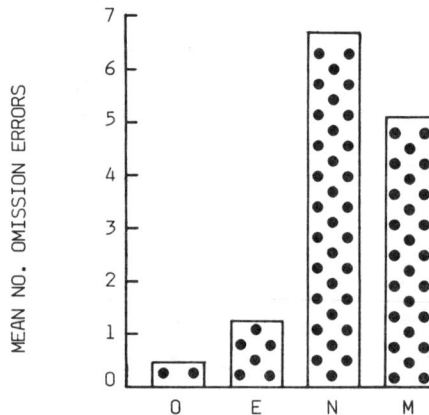

Figure 6. Mean number of omission errors for outline = 0, eyes = E, nose = N and mouth = M.

difference between features arose when the outline and the eyes were compared with the nose and the mouth respectively, the probability being far below .01 (See figure 6.0).

A further analysis was done on the commission errors, with a slight refinement over study 1 in that accidental miss hits could be eliminated from the analysis. When this was done it was evident that all errors involving the outline and the eyes, were actually miss hits and not commission errors. A within S analysis was conducted and a main effect of features was found, $F(3, 3) = 8.17$ with a $P = .006$. When the overall means for each feature was obtained it was found that all errors were distributed between the nose (2.38) and the mouth (1.69). A Newman-Keuls revealed that the significance arose when the outline and the eyes were compared to the nose and the mouth respectively, the probability being less than .05 (See figure 7.).

A third analysis was conducted on the median reaction times for all correct responses to feature omission, for each feature per trial. However unlike the previous study, two response criteria were used to yield uncontaminated results. In the first study it is clear that 'no incomplete' responses were not giving a full picture as to which piece the subject believed was missing, as opposed to what was actually omitted. However, with the aid of the verbal record responses that did not pass both criterion measures were eliminated. A within S analysis of variance was conducted and a main effect of features was found, $F(3, 3) = 4.56$ with a $P = .032$. When the overall means for each feature was tabulated it was found that the responses to the omission of a feature were faster for the outline (.61 sec), followed by the eyes (.72), the nose (.98), and the mouth (.99). When a Newman-Keuls was conducted it revealed that the significance arose when the outline was compared to the nose with a probability below .05 (See figure 8).

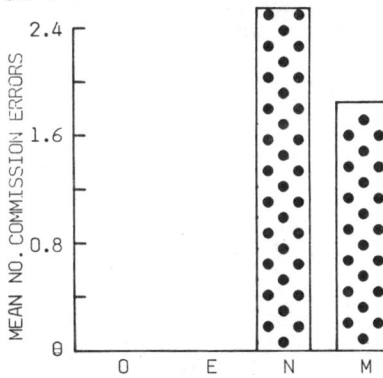

Figure 7. Mean number of commission errors for outline = 0, eyes = E, nose = N and mouth = M in experiment 3.

CONCLUSION

These three experiments indicate that clear differences in response times and patterns of errors are apparent when subjects view temporally fragmented outline sketches of faces. The randomisation of these components of the stimulus should interfere with any simple top down scanning of the face although it is possible that the fragments are stored and a more sophisticated but delayed internal scanning occurs.

The results imply that subjects are much more efficient at processing the outline and eye regions than the nose and the mouth. It appears that the

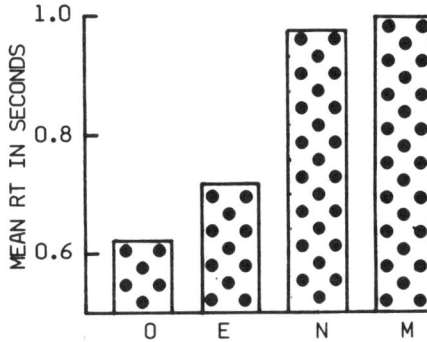

Figure 8. Means of the median response times to omission of outline = 0, eyes = E, nose = N and mouth = M in experiment 3. Data based only on correctly identified missing features.

ordering of processing efficiency is not just a product of feature size since enlarging the mouth region does not improve its property relative to the eyes (experiment 2), processing although there is a possibility that the outline is a special case since in terms of contour length and enclosed area it is so much larger than the other features. The consistency of the pattern of results and their agreement with studies of feature hierarchies studied by very different means (Shepherd et al. 1981) argues that the experiments expose some very basic aspects of the mechanisms involved in facial processing.

PERCEPTION OF UPSIDE-DOWN FACES : AN ANALYSIS FROM THE VIEWPOINT OF CUE SALIENCY

M. ENDO

1. INTRODUCTION

Pictures of human faces look different when presented upside down, and they are extremely difficult to recognise in this orientation. This phenomenon has been paid attention to by many researchers. Yin (1969) showed that recognition of human faces is disproportionately more disrupted by being presented upside down than that of other objects having properties similar to those of faces. Yin's finding has been treated as one piece of evidence for the existence of a special face processing mechanism. Hay and Young (1982) proposed that the studies concerning this specific analyser hypothesis should be divided into two aspects, namely the uniqueness to faces of the nature of the processes used; and the specificity to faces of the components of face processing systems. And they added that "there is at present little evidence to support the idea of uniqueness, but good supporting evidence for the specificity to faces of at least some components of the face processing system" (p.193).

However, the ability to perceive and remember faces is certainly excellent and represents more or less the ultimate in our capacities for discrimination and recognition within a single category of pattern (Ellis, 1981). Therefore, even if the capacities are not unique to faces, it is necessary to investigate how the perception of faces should be characterised. For this investigation, the inversion effects on perceiving faces must be an important clue.

There are two main interpretations about difficulties arising in the perception of upside-down faces. Yin (1969) and Carey and Diamond (1977) suggested that observers could not obtain the global impression of inverted faces, and that they had to recognise inverted faces using isolated features - a strategy which was used for other visual stimuli. Rock (1973, 1972) considered that the perception of human faces involves a whole set of component figures and figural relationships, whereas other complex figures are perceived only in the manner of over-all and global shapes. Accordingly, when faces are presented upside down it is not possible to visualise simultaneously how each of these would look, were they to be egocentrically upright. The distinction between the two interpretations might be shown in the ideas about the perception of orientation-free figures.

In order to clarify which aspect of the perceptual processing of faces is disrupted by inversion, it is not sufficient to study the phenomenon only by means of a recognition paradigm. It is also necessary to describe the phenomenon in detail and to investigate directly the perceptual process of inverted faces. For this purpose, we have examined perception of upside-down faces from the viewpoint of cue saliency, which indicates the relative importance of respective facial features.

2. PREVIOUS RESEARCHES

At first, cue saliency of upside-down faces was assessed and was compared with that of cue saliency of upright faces (Endo, 1982). Subjects were presented with the two faces (same or different) sequentially. When the faces presented were different, the second ones were montage photographs composed by Minolta Montage Synthesizer, which differed from the first face in one of five features, namely, hair, eyes, nose, mouth, or chin. By requiring subjects to judge "same" or "different", cue saliency was assessed by whether they could detect the change when a given feature was altered. The orientation of the faces presented were as follows: both of them were upright; rotated 180°; or only the second faces were rotated 180°.

The results showed that the detectabilities (ds) of the feature change for upside-down conditions were inferior to that for the upright condition. As to FA (false alarm) rates on each feature, for upright condition, the highest score was obtained in alterations to the nose, and the following scores those to the mouth and the chin. The lowest ones were those to the hair and the eyes. This pattern of feature saliency roughly confirms the results obtained so far (Shepherd et al., 1981). For upside-down conditions, although mean FA rates were higher in all features than those for upright ones, the increase of FA rate on lower features (nose, mouth and chin) are more remarkable than those in upper features (hair and eyes). This tendency is distinctive for the condition in which a particular feature was exchanged for dissimilar one. Although the general tendency of cue saliency is invariant in the upright and the upside-down faces, the differences in saliency between upper features and lower ones become more distinct in upside-down conditions. Inversion of faces is more influential on non-salient lower features than of salient upper ones.

Considering the implication for the perceptual process of upside-down faces from the pattern of cue saliency in upside-down faces, it can be said at least that upside-down faces could be treated as "faces", and that the first stage of the two-stage model of face recognition (Ellis, 1981) is executed for them. However, in order to make clear perceptual characteristics of upside-down faces, further studies have to be employed. For the study from the viewpoint of cue saliency, it is necessary to assess cue saliency in another experimental condition in which the state of face processing can be clarified.

In the second experiment (Endo, 1983), cue saliency in briefly presented upright faces was assessed with the same method as that in the previous study. This investigation was employed in order to examine the assumption that cue saliency in upside-down faces reveals the state of an early stage of face processing. This assumption was deduced from the fact that the inversion of faces more reduced the detectability of changes in non-salient features compared with that in salient features, and from the premise that the salient features are given processing priority to the other features.

The results showed that both the discriminability and the pattern of FA rate across features for the 250 msec presentation are very similar to those for the upside-down condition in the previous experiment. Thus, it can be said that the brief presentation of upright faces for about 250 msec has the same effect on performance as the upside-down presentation.

According to these findings, it is plausible that upside-down faces are processed to some extent by the same strategy as upright faces. But the possibility that the pattern of cue saliency can be obtained by the different strategies can not be denied so far. In the following experiment, in order to examine whether similar patterns to those obtained before still appear in such a condition that prevent an observer from adopting the global processing, cue saliency in faces is assessed on restricted visual fields.

3. CUE SALIENCY IN FACES WHEN VISUAL FIELD IS RESTRICTED

It has been shown that perceiving pictures becomes extremely difficult as the visual field is limited to a small area (Saida & Ikeda, 1979). Inui and Miyamoto (1984) showed that familiar faces could not be identified through a small window which was almost the same in size as each of the features. In this situation, observers seem not to be able to grasp the global impression, and are able only to employ a feature analytic manner. In the present experiment, cue saliency in faces was assessed in such a situation.

3.1. Method

3.1.1. Materials and apparatus.

The stimuli were all black-and-white photographs of male Japanese faces (targets), none of which had any distinctive cues (e.g. glasses), and 50 montage photographs (distractors), differed from the target in only one of five features (hair, eyes, nose, mouth, or chin). Depending on which feature was changed for a similar (or dissimilar) one, the distractors were divided into ten categories, each of which consisted of five distractors.

The apparatus for the stimulus presentation were as follows. At first, a stimulus was presented on the white screen by a projector. The picture on the screen was taken with a TV camera, which was connected to a computer display (Sharp, CZ800). Subjects observed stimulus pictures on the display. When the visible area was restricted, a white graphic pattern with rectangular window was superimposed on the stimulus face. Two sizes of the window used corresponded to about 10% or 23% of the faces (small, 5 x 4 cm; large, 7 x 6.3 cm). Through the small window, subjects could see both the eye and the eyebrow, and through the large window, three inner features at one time. Subjects could move this window area in eight directions with a control-stick.

3.1.2. Procedure.

The subjects observed the first stimulus (target) without a graphic pattern superimposed. When the subjects pressed a manual key after an interval of about 2 sec, the first face was exchanged for the second one, with or without a graphic pattern. The target stimulus was one of 11 target faces, and the test stimulus was the same face as the target stimulus or the distractor which was composed on the basis of the target. Subjects' task was to judge whether the two stimuli were the same or different and to rate the confidence of the judgement. The exposure durations of both two faces were not limited. The subjects were warned not to use the differences of lightness, size, and position of the two faces for cue to judge. Further, they were instructed to inspect all the area of the test pattern through the window.

There were two conditions concerning the orientation of the faces, namely both of the two faces presented successively were upright or rotated 180°, and there were three conditions concerning the window size, namely small, large, or without restriction. Each of the subjects was engaged in one of the six experimental conditions (2 x 3). There were 100 trials (50 "same" pairs and 50 "different" ones) for each subject.

3.1.3. Subjects.

The subjects were 48 students of Tohoku University, and eight of them were allocated to each of the 6 experimental conditions.

3.2. Results

Table 1 shows mean ds on each window condition as a function of orientation of faces. For the upright face, the scores of ds on without restriction are better than those on other window conditions. On the other hand, for the upside-down condition, all scores on each window condition show similar levels. These values are almost the same as that for the small window in upright face. A 2 (orientation) x 3 (window) ANOVA showed all

TABLE 1. Mean ds on each window as a function of orientation.

	Without restriction	Large window	Small window
Upright	2.16	1.52	1.33
Upside-down	1.26	1.13	1.34

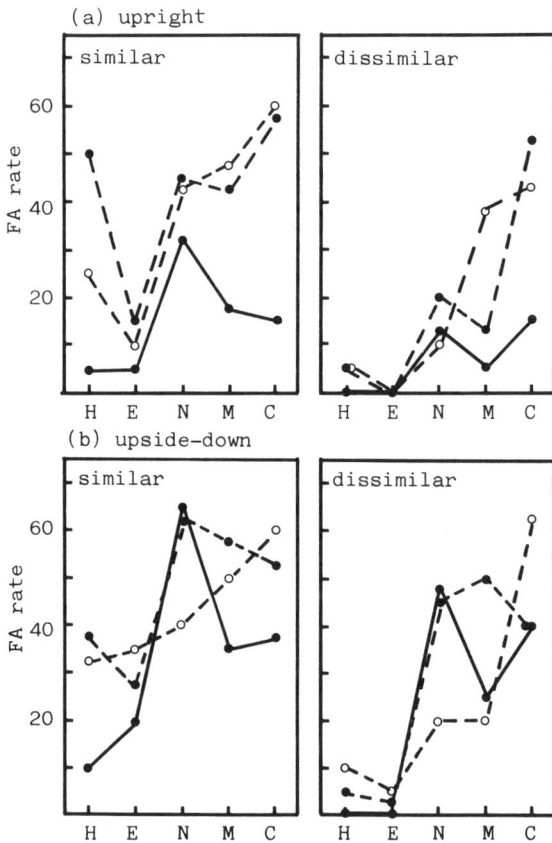

FIGURE 1. Mean FA rate on each feature as a function of orientation and similarity and window. (●———● ,without restriction; ●— — ●, large window; o— — o,small window)

significant main effects (orientation, p < .01; window, p < .05). Further, the orientation x window interaction was also significant (p < .05).

Figure 1 shows mean false alarm (FA) rates on each feature as a function of window size. For without restriction condition, the patterns of FA rate on each feature in both orientation conditions showed almost the same tendency as those in previous study. Regardless of face orientation, scores of FA rate on hair, mouth, and chin in window conditions were higher than those in the condition without restriction. But for the upside-down condition FA rate on nose with the small window was lower than that in the condition without restriction. The data of FA scores were subjected to a 2 (orientation) x 3 (window) x 2 (similarity) x 5 (feature) ANOVA with repeated measures on the last two factors. The main effects of all of the four factors were highly significant (p < .01 in all cases). And all two-way interactions except orientation x window and orientation x similarity were also significant (p < .05). Further, the three-way interaction (orientation x window x feature) achieved statistical significance (p < .01).

3.3 Discussion

The results for without restriction condition were consistent with those in the previous study mentioned above, although exposure duration of stimuli and the number of distractors were different from those in the previous study.

The detectability of feature change was reduced by restricting observers' visible area for the upright face. But window size showed no significant effect on detectability for the upside-down face. The features of hair, mouth and chin were more influenced by restriction for both face orientations. An exceptional effect can be seen in performance on nose for upside-down faces, which was enhanced by restricting visible area with small window.

Comparing the patterns of feature saliency of the three window conditions with each other, the two window conditions showed similar patterns for the up-right face. On the other hand, for upside-down face, the similarity of cue saliency patterns could be observed between the large window condition and the control one. The pattern of cue saliency on the small window and upside-down condition was the most peculiar case of all conditions. FA rate in these conditions increased monotonically with the position of altered feature being lower. These patterns seem to reveal that the faces are processed in a feature analytic manner.

The pattern of cue saliency in upside-down faces on without restriction condition is different from those on the small window condition in both orientations. This finding suggests that cue saliency in upside-down faces is different from that when faces were processed in a feature analytic manner, and that we can use global impression of faces or relationships of respective features as a cue for detection of feature alternation even if presented upside down.

These findings also show that the studies of cue saliency on faces are not necessarily treated as studies that are based on an assumption that faces may be processed in a manner of feature-by-feature analysis (Davies, 1978). We can use for face discrimination not only the changes of features itself, but also those of relationships of adjacent features and those of overall impression, which was also supported by subjects' introspections. Thus the term 'cue saliency' seems to imply the degree of contribution of features to configuration.

Restriction of visible areas has an effect on perception of upright face and upside-down ones in different ways. The effect of viewing through the larger window was more distinct on upright faces than on upside-down faces. But, the change of window size from large to small has a more serious effect on upside-down faces than on upright faces. Although upside-down faces were processed on a feature analytic manner when viewed through the small window, it cannot be said clearly that upright faces were processed in such a manner even when viewed through a small window. It is suggested that the features are finely integrated in the upright faces but somewhat loosely integrated in the upside-down faces.

4. GENERAL DISCUSSION

We have investigated the perception of upside-down faces in terms of cue saliency. The first study showed that cue saliency in upside-down faces has in some respect the same property as that in upright ones, but that the differences in saliency between upper features and lower ones become more distinct in upside-down faces because of the remarkable decrement of detectability for lower feature changes. The subsequent studies revealed that the pattern of cue saliency on upside-down faces reflects the state of an early stage of face processing, and that the pattern of cue saliency is different from that when observers cannot grasp the global impression of faces. It suggests that upside-down faces are processed to some extent by the same strategy as that used when viewed upright, and that feature integration takes place even in upside-down faces, albeit somewhat looser than for upright faces.

Considering which interpretations previously mentioned are adequate, our results seem to support Rock's one that the global processing is assumed to be the basis of form perception. However, the results obtained may be dependent on the tasks imposed upon subjects. The present study suggests that subjects can adopt a features analytic manner more easily for upside-down face processing than for upright faces. Thus when a task can be performed by processing a single distinctive feature, such as that in the usual recognition paradigm, subjects might not rely on the configuration of inverted faces. But it should be noted that even when using feature alternation technique which has been considered to force subjects to adopt feature-by-feature processing, the evidence that subjects adopted a global processing manner is revealed in the results.

3. MEMORY PROCESSES

ON THE MEMORABILITY OF THE HUMAN FACE

K.A. DEFFENBACHER

1. INTRODUCTION

Do we ever truly forget a face? Given the current state of the literature concerning memory for faces, three different answers can be framed to
this question. Consider first the work of Bahrick, Bahrick, and Wittlinger
(1975). This beautifully done piece of retrospective research examined
memory for the names and faces of a group of American high school classmates. Employing sophisticated statistical controls for variables such as
rehearsal during the retention interval, Bahrick et al. found that picture
recognition memory for the faces of former classmates held up very well
over rather extended periods of time. Recognition accuracy held at
approximately the 90% level until nearly 35 years after graduation,
whereupon it declined to about the 75% level at 48 years. Memories of this
strength have been characterized more recently by Bahrick (1984) as having
entered "permastore."

Is the underlying facial engram or trace ever truly lost? Based on the
work of Bahrick et al. (1975), the answer is, "probably not in one's
lifetime." At least this answer would be appropriate if the faces in
question were very familiar, having been encountered in a variety of
encoding contexts over a period of several years.

How resilient is the facial engram under conditions of less frequent and
less varied encounter? Bahrick (1983) has also examined recognition memory
for faces encountered over a 10-week academic term. The faces were those
of approximately 40 students per class in classes taught two weeks, one
year, four years, and eight years previously, classes taught by some 22
American university professors. The results clearly established that these
students' faces had not entered their professors' permastores. Where
chance accuracy would have been 20%, accuracy at two weeks was 69%, at one
year 48%, at four years 31%, and 26% at eight years. Under conditions such
as these, then, a facial memory trace seems bereft of useful information
after four to eight years. In the instance of casual acquaintances, then,
the question of whether the facial engram will be lost has a different
answer, "yes, over a period of several years."

Consider now the vast bulk of studies examining memory for faces as a
function of retention interval. The target faces in these studies have
been totally unfamiliar and have been viewed only once for no more than
tens of seconds. A number of individual scientists and research teams have
reviewed particular portions of this literature, a literature containing at
least 33 instances where researchers have tested for statistically significant amounts of forgetting. To these previous reviewers (Barkowitz &
Brigham, 1982; Ellis, 1984; Goldstein & Chance, 1981; McCloskey & Egeth,
1983; Shepherd, Davies, & Ellis, 1982; Wells & Murray, 1983), the literature has appeared muddled with no clear indication as to whether the engram
of the previously unfamiliar face is ever lost, much less how rapidly.

Each reviewer examined anywhere from four to eleven studies and appeared to follow the expedient of "vote counting." Studies yielding a statistically reliable effect of retention interval were counted as "yes" votes, while studies not yielding an effect of retention interval were counted as "no" votes. There appeared to be in each case roughly equal numbers of "yeses" and "noes."

What is going on here? Is the apparent muddle due to the previous reviewers examining unrepresentative subsets of the body of face memory studies? Apparently not, for pursuing the same methodology with the entire set of face memory experiments unfortunately does not clarify matters. Across all 33 experiments, there are 16 statistically significant effects of retention interval and 17 not significant effects.

2. SOME META-ANALYSES OF THE FACE MEMORY LITERATURE

The chief problem with the vote counting methodology is that it ignores too much data by concentrating on whether statistical significance is obtained and by failing to examine actual magnitudes of effect across all available studies. Consequently, I have performed several meta-analyses of the aforementioned 33 experiments to try to get a better fix on the magnitude of forgetting of the unfamiliar face seen but once.

The first effect size statistic computed was the average standard score (z score) relating to the effect of retention interval on face memory. Where exact z scores were not available for a particular experiment, one of two types of z scores was entered. If there had not been a statistically significant effect of retention interval, a z of 0.00 was entered, certainly a very conservative approach. Where there had been a significant effect, the z corresponding to the critical value for the obtained probability of a Type I error was entered, a conservative procedure, as well. The mean z obtained was 1.46. This result compares favorably with those of Shapiro and Penrod (1984) who calculated average zs for the measures of hits and false alarms separately. They found a mean z of 1.75 for hits and 1.35 for false alarms, averaged across just 16 studies in the former instance and 13 in the latter. All three effect sizes are reasonably impressive when one considers the relatively large number of null results combined in the analyses.

Though the average of 1.46 is only of marginal statistical reliability ($p < .10$), one can take advantage of the fact that this value holds across 33 independent experiments (Rosenthal, 1978). Multiplying 1.46 by $\sqrt{33}$ yields an overall or combined z of 8.38 ($p < .0001$). Hence statistically speaking, it would seem that one could safely say that the engram of faces seen but once will be weaker at longer retention intervals than at briefer ones. Will this conclusion be much affected by studies yielding null results but which have not as yet been reported or retrieved? It does not appear very likely that "file drawer" studies will soon invalidate this conclusion. Following Rosenthal's (1979) procedure, it turns out that 825 new, filed, or unretrieved studies averaging null results ($z = 0.00$) would have to exist somewhere before the overall results could reasonably be attributed to sampling bias in the experiments summarized here.

These particular meta-analyses place us on firmer ground in our quest to learn the fate of the engram for an unfamiliar face. However, such analyses still do not allow us to specify whether the engram will ever be truly lost, much less when. Can we get some idea of the forgetting function for once-seen faces?

A useful first step might be to construct a scatterplot of the data from studies that have examined face memory as a function of retention interval.

For each experiment that involved a recognition test of memory, a d' score measuring memory strength at each retention interval was obtained directly or computed after the fact. Given the vast range of retention intervals tested in the face recognition literature (one minute to 350 days), the points (n = 63) were plotted in log-log coordinates, log d' against log time in minutes. The resulting correlation coefficient is statistically reliable but not terribly impressive, r = -.31 (p < .01, one-tailed). As the sign and magnitude of the correlation coefficient indicate, there is a considerable amount of scatter in the points and the suggestion of a very modest left-to-right downward trend.

An inspection of the scatterplot suggests a plausible reason for much of the scatter. It appears that the initial memory strength (degree of learning) varies considerably across studies. This is perhaps not surprising, inasmuch as face inspection time, for instance, varies considerably across studies. At a retention interval of one minute, memory strength measured in d' units varies from 1.22 to 3.12, a dynamic range of 2.5 to 1.0. It is reasonable to suppose, therefore, that there might exist not one but a family of forgetting functions, a different function for each unique set of encoding conditions. It would be parsimonious to assume that these functions would be similar in form, differing only in vertical position on a graph. On a plot of log memory strength against log time, we might suppose that these functions would have similar negative slopes but differing y-intercepts.

Such a plot is shown in Figure 1 for two of the five studies that have employed more than two retention intervals. Presumably much of the differ-

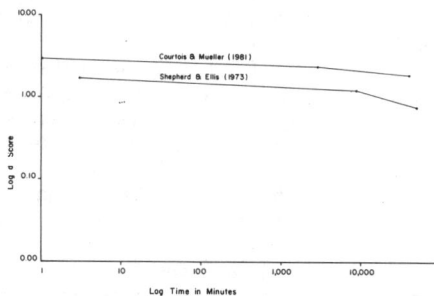

FIGURE 1. Log-log forgetting functions for two studies of memory for faces.

ence in y-intercepts for the two functions is due to there being 15 sec of encoding time for each face presented in Courtois and Mueller's (1981) study but only 3 sec in the Shepherd and Ellis (1973) experiment. One should also note the very gradual negative slopes of these two functions as well as the modest inflection at the second retention interval, the latter characteristic being a property of forgetting curves for both face recognition and associated name recognition in Bahrick's (1983) data, too.

Clearly any successful theoretical treatment of data such as these will need to account for the relatively gradual initial negative slope as well as the increase in slope at later retention intervals. A theory of forgetting having as at least one of its components a negative exponential term could account for an increased slope at later retention intervals, inasmuch as the amount of forgetting due to this component would increase with each log unit of time.

A successful theoretical account of these data should also predict that Jost's (1897) second law will be true: "If two associations are now of equal strength but of different ages, the older one will lose strength more slowly with the further passage of time." Applied to the present situation, an "older" forgetting function would be one that started out at a greater initial memory strength than a "younger" one. The forgetting curve with the higher degree of original learning would then lose strength at a slower rate than one with a lesser degree of original memory strength.

More simply expressed, Jost's venerable law proposes that the rate at which memory strength is lost continually decreases with increasing time since original learning. Hence, of two curves now at the same memory strength, the one with the greater degree of initial strength, the "older" one, will decline more slowly because it has already declined for sufficient time that the amount forgotten per unit time will have decreased to a point below that for the "younger" one. It should be noted that a theory of forgetting that includes as at least one of its components a negative power term could account for the phenomenon described by Jost's second law, a decreasing amount forgotten for each unit increase in time. It should likewise be pointed out that very recently Loftus (1985) has shown Jost's second law to be true for several studies pulled from the extant verbal learning literature.

3. WICKELGREN'S SINGLE-TRACE FRAGILITY THEORY

One might well inquire as to whether there are any extant theories of forgetting that can account both for the phenomenon of Jost's Second Law and the phenomenon of an increased rate of loss of memory strength at later retention intervals. It turns out that there is, Wickelgren's (1972, 1974, 1975, 1977, 1979) single-trace fragility theory. In its least complex form (Wickelgren, 1975, 1977), the form of the retention function is: $d' = Lt^{-D}e^{-It}$ where d' represents the strength of the memory trace at t seconds after original learning, L represents initial memory trace strength, D represents the rate parameter for a time-decay process, and I represents the rate parameter for an interference process. Of course, $e = 2.72$, the base of the system of natural or Napierian logarithms. It is also worth noting that Wickelgren's function is a gamma function, one whose properties are well known.

Instead of making a distinction between short-term and long-term memory traces, Wickelgren's theory proposes a single trace and two mechanisms that produce forgetting: (a) a storage interference process dependent on the processing of similar material prior to or subsequent to learning and (b) an interference-free time decay process. It is certainly not unusual to find a theory dealing with longer-term memories that proposes an interference process as producing forgetting. What is unusual is finding a theory that proposes that a time decay process is also involved in the loss of memories over the longer term. I shall return to this latter point a bit later.

The theory also proposes a novel hypothesis concerning consolidation. Wickelgren's notion is that memory traces have two partially coupled dynamic properties, strength and fragility. Increased strength implies increased accuracy of recognition and recall, while increased fragility implies increased susceptibility of the trace to the time-decay process but not to interference. Consolidation is assumed to be a relatively autonomous neurophysiological process that involves a continual reduction in the fragility of the memory trace over time, rather than any change in strength or availability. Hence trace fragility is greatest immediately after learning and shows a negatively accelerated decrease over time due to a corresponding negatively accelerated increase in trace consolidation. Decreasing trace fragility could therefore account for the continually decreasing amount of trace strength lost per unit time that Jost's second law demands. The negative power component of Wickelgren's forgetting function, t^{-D}, certainly seems an intuitively plausible model of the decline in trace fragility over time. None the less plausible is his neurophysiological account of this decline. Wickelgren (1979) has proposed that increases in consolidation involve a negatively accelerated repression of connections between cortical neurons and the hippocampal arousal system, consolidating memory by protecting newly connected cortical neurons from diffuse hippocampal input and thus retarding forgetting.

The interference parameter, I, is assumed to be directly proportional to the similarity of the item in question to those encountered both prior to and subsequent to original exposure. Inasmuch as the degree of such item similarity could be expected to vary greatly, one might expect that I would also vary considerably. Wickelgren (1976) reports that the interference parameter does indeed vary enormously from situation to situation, by as much as a factor of 10^6. On the other hand, one would not expect a neurophysiological process of consolidation to vary a great deal as a function of nature of the materials being learned and like variables. Indeed, Wickelgren (1976) has found the decay parameter to vary by less than a factor of 10 across studies of memory for verbal items, small variation in comparison to the variation in how long memory traces may last, more than a factor of 10^7.

Another prediction of Wickelgren's theory is of particular interest here. The contribution of the time-decay process to forgetting will decline in power function fashion with increasing trace age. Meanwhile since interference is behaving in a negative exponential fashion, it would be expected to exert an increasing influence at longer retention intervals. This might explain the apparent increase in slope at later retention intervals that was noted earlier in the instance of several long-term face memory studies. This prediction would also be in accord with a result noted by Deffenbacher, Carr, and Leu (1981). They found that for both faces and words the amount of forgetting due to retroactive interference with an item's trace in storage increased over a two-week retention interval. This increase in what they refer to as retroactive interference with item memory appears to be analogous to the unlearning phenomenon observed in interference with the recall of verbal materials.

3.1. Extant support for the theory

Though single-trace fragility theory has not as yet been applied to retention functions for faces, it is not without supporting data and arguments. Wickelgren (1972, 1974, 1975) has reported a dozen experiments he has conducted testing either the fit of empirical retention functions to theoretical ones or particular assumptions or derivations of his theory. The fit of his forgetting theory to observed retention functions is a reasonably impressive one. I have counted 35 separate r^2 statistics, averaged across three to ten subjects in each instance. The median r^2 is 0.89, the proportion of variance accounted for by Wickelgren's theoretical retention function. Though all these experiments involved "yes-no" recognition memory tasks, memory for a variety of verbal materials under a variety of conditions was tested at intervals up to two years in length. In addition, Wickelgren (1975) transformed the data of Ryback, Weinert, and

Fozard (1970) into measures of recognition memory strength for pictures of commonly encountered objects and found decent fits of his theoretical function to the forgetting functions generated by both their sober and intoxicated subjects. The r^2 statistic assessing fit to the retention function generated by sober subjects was 0.98, while for the intoxicated subjects it was 0.78.

More recently, Rubin (1982) examined memory for autobiographical details in a series of five experiments. If one assumes that his subjects encoded an equal number of events from each day of their lives, then the distribution of events recorded as a function of time can be viewed as a retention function. Wickelgren's single-trace fragility theory again fared very well indeed. The r^2 values assessing fit ranged from 0.96 to 0.97.

Despite a modest amount of supporting data for Wickelgren's theorizing, many cognitive psychologists would still appear to have difficulty in accepting any theory of long-term memory that is not a pure interference theory: All long-term forgetting is strictly due to proactive and retroactive interference. Given the well nigh universality of belief in general interference theory as a model of forgetting, a brief sketch will be presented of several powerful arguments for the inclusion of a time decay component in a theory of forgetting.

For one thing, we now have some evidence that a theory with a time decay component provides an excellent fit to forgetting functions obtained for a variety of episodic memory representations, memory for frequently encountered words (Wickelgren, 1972, 1974, 1975), frequently encountered objects (Ryback et al., 1970); and events from one's own life (Rubin, 1982). In particular, a power function time decay process nicely explains the phenomenon described by Jost's second law.

Can general interference theory provide as good an explanation of this phenomenon? It can do so only if it should turn out that greater amounts of interference were to result from shorter delays and lesser amounts were to result from longer delays between original and similar interfering material. However, studies of both recall and recognition of verbal associations as a function of delay between original and subsequent interfering learning are virtually unanimous in showing that no greater interference is obtained with shorter delays (Wickelgren, 1974, 1976). Therefore some noninterference process (time decay) that decreases in effectiveness with trace age must be involved.

Another critical task for general interference theory is to account for the considerable amount of extralaboratory forgetting that occurs in the instance of verbal lists learned alone, that is without an accompanying interfering list. Is such forgetting due exclusively to extraexperimental retroactive and proactive interference? The answer is apparently no. "We have not been able to identify the interfering associations acquired outside the laboratory which produce the loss in the singly-learned list" (Underwood, 1983, p. 238). Therefore, one might reason that a noninterference factor such as temporal trace decay is a major factor in accounting for the memory loss.

Finally, if temporal trace decay is an autonomous neurophysiological process, then increases or decreases in the general level of brain activity ought produce corresponding increases or decreases in trace decay. It turns out that forgetting occurs more slowly during the time of day when one usually sleeps than during times when the brain operates at a higher arousal level (Hockey, Davies, & Gray, 1972). If one assumes that the rate of memory consolidation depends on the rate of brain protein synthesis, then this result is nicely accounted for by the fact that plasma cortisol levels are relatively low in the early hours of the night and high at other times (Weitzman, 1977). Cortisol enhances protein degradation; hence the net rate of protein synthesis will be greater, and forgetting less, during the night, particularly the early part, than during the day. It's difficult to see how general interference theory could account for this result.

3.2. Fit of the theory to face memory data

We have only Wickelgren's (1975) replotting of Ryback et al.'s (1970) data to suggest that forgetting of nonverbal material such as faces might also proceed according to the dictates of single-trace fragility theory. My intent here is to assess the fit of fragility theory to data from the face memory literature. Table 1 contains the results of this effort for the five studies which included more than two retention intervals and which permitted appropriate d' scores to be calculated if they had not already been. In fitting the data of all five studies, the decay parameter, D, was set at 0.025. The interference parameter, I, was set at 6×10^{-8} in fitting the data of Barkowitz and Brigham (1982), Courtois and Mueller (1981), and Shepherd, Ellis, and Davies (1982); I was increased to 2×10^{-7} to fit the data of the remaining two studies, however. The predicted values of d' in the first column represent L, the initial level of memory strength. These values were estimated using the observed values given in the second column. Hence one should not be surprised at the perfect fit of theory to data in the second column.

TABLE 1. Fit of single-trace fragility theory to data from five face memory studies.

Study	Observed and (predicted) d' memory strength after various delays				
Barkowitz & Brigham (1982)	0 sec	5 min	2 days	7 days	
		1.47	1.19	1.14	
	(1.70)	(1.47)	(1.24)	(1.18)	
Courtois & Mueller (1981)	0 sec	1 min	2 days	28 days	
		2.94	2.41	1.93	
	(3.26)	(2.94)	(2.39)	(1.95)	
Shepherd & Ellis (1973)	0 sec	3 min	6 days	35 days	
		1.73	1.24	0.78	
	(1.97)	(1.73)	(1.28)	(0.74)	
Shepherd, Ellis, & Davies (1982)	0 sec	7 days	30 days	90 days	350 days
		1.92	1.62	1.47	0.00
	(2.78)	(1.92)	(1.64)	(1.17)	(0.29)
Yarmey (1979)	0 sec	1 min	7 days	30 days	
		3.12	2.44	1.47	
	(3.46)	(3.12)	(2.20)	(1.42)	

Overall the fit seems relatively good, particularly when one notes that the observed d' values are by necessity group scores, rather than being based on an average of individually computed scores such as one might obtain from continuous recognition memory experiments. The most serious lack of fit occurs for the 90- and 350-day retention intervals in Shepherd et al.'s (1982) study. From a practical point of view, however, these two discrepancies are not terribly serious in that at 90 days scores correspond to 50% correct (observed) and 40% correct (predicted); at 350 days, the observed value corresponds to 10% correct (chance), while the predicted value corresponds to 15% correct.

The face retention functions fit by Wickelgren's theory likewise conform nicely to Jost's second law. Consider just two examples from Table 1. In Barkowitz and Brigham's (1982) study, trace strength declined from an initial value of 1.70 to 1.47 in just five minutes. Starting from a much higher initial level (2.78), trace strength in Shepherd et al.'s (1982) study took a predicted 25 days to decline to a value of 1.70. Thereafter, 65 more days were required to bring memory strength down to a d' of 1.47, a striking confirmation of Jost's Second Law. Again, in Shepherd et al.'s study, initial memory strength (2.78) dropped to a d' of 1.92 in 7 days. Beginning at a value of 3.26, trace strength in Courtois and Mueller's (1981) experiment took a predicted 10 minutes to decline to a value of 2.78; the remainder of 28 days time was required to reduce strength to a d' of 1.93.

We are now in a much better position to inquire as to when the engram of the once-seen face is lost. The results of the Shepherd et al. (1982) study given in Table 1 would suggest that the engram will be bereft of any useful information whatsoever in a bit less than a year. One might well wish to question the generality of this estimate, however. Even though the decay rate may be relatively constant across a wide variety of faces, initial memory strength and the magnitude of the interference parameter certainly will vary from situation to situation. Following up on this line of reasoning, extended forgetting analyses were conducted with the data from the other four studies in Table 1. That is, fragility theory was used to predict what memory strength would have been for specific retention intervals longer than those tested in each original study. Predicted d' scores at a retention interval of 350 days were 0.18 for the Barkowitz and Brigham (1982) data, and 0.34, 0.00, and 0.00, respectively, for the data of Courtois and Mueller (1981), Shepherd and Ellis (1973), and Yarmey (1979). Based on this analysis of a body of studies where initial memory strength varied by a factor of nearly two to one and the interference parameter varied over a range of more than three to one, there indeed seems little reason to believe that a year later a once-seen face could be reliably distinguished from one never before seen.

If a once-seen face were rather typical and confusable with other faces encountered, though, generating a greater amount of interference, its engram could well be lost in much less than a year. With an interference parameter 3.33 times as great as that for the other three studies cited in Table 1, the retention functions for Shepherd and Ellis (1973) and Yarmey (1979) have predicted d' values of just 0.06 and 0.10, respectively, in only six months. To make this point more dramatically, consider two subsets of Shepherd and Ellis' data. A set of their stimulus faces was scaled as "moderately attractive," presumably rather typical. This set of faces required an interference parameter 10 times as great in value for a retention curve fit as did another set of faces scaled as "high attractive," presumably somewhat more distinctive in nature. Predicted d' values at only 35 days were just 0.27 in the former case but 1.00 in the latter.

One additional intriguing result emerges from this curve fitting exercise. The value of the time decay rate parameter (0.025) required to fit the face memory data in Table 1 is an order of magnitude smaller than the value required (0.25) to fit the data of Wickelgren (1975) in the case of frequently encountered English words and the data of Ryback et al. (1970) in the instance of pictures of frequently encountered objects. Likewise the values of the interference parameter employed here are up to an order of magnitude smaller than needed in the two studies just cited, 6 x 10^{-8} versus 6 x 10^{-7}.

So it may well be that faces are a bit special. Their forgetting functions may indeed conform to Jost's second law and also may require the same sort of theory to account for their decline and fall as for words, pictures, and life events. Nevertheless, episodic memory strength for unfamiliar faces may decline more slowly than that for autobiographic details and frequently encountered words and objects. Face memory being associated with lower values of time decay and interference parameters does not seem too surprising, however, when one considers the importance of faces as social stimuli and the relatively large amount of human cerebral cortex devoted to their processing (e.g., Geschwind, 1979).

Of course much remains to be done in assessing the validity of Wickelgren's theory as applied to the forgetting of once-seen faces. Clearly, more studies need to be done that systematically vary encoding conditions, particularly target face exposure time and target face typicality and that test memory over a greater number of retention intervals. Perhaps the most important theoretical extension of fragility theory in this context would be to determine how much additional trace strength is added back by each subsequent encounter of a particular face for n seconds. Achievement of this theoretical extension would provide rudimentary knowledge of the rate at which facial familiarity grows, knowledge of which psychology is now bereft. This theoretical extension would likewise bring us much closer to linking up the vast body of face memory studies with the work of Bahrick (1983) and Bahrick et al. (1975).

Even in the absence of such theoretical developments, continued success in validity testing of fragility theory should yield benefits in forensic application. Assuming continued stability in estimates of the time decay parameter, only two parameters would need to be estimated in any particular situation involving eyewitness identification after a period of delay. As research accumulates vis-a-vis initial memory strengths produced by various combinations of encoding conditions, it should not be difficult to produce post hoc a reasonably narrow range of initial memory strength estimates for a given forensic situation. One conservative procedure in this regard would be to assume an initial memory strength as great as the largest reported thus far in the literature, currently 3.46 (see Table 1). Estimating the interference parameter at the lowest level reported for previous studies, currently 6 x 10^{-8}, would likewise be conservative in the sense of trying not to underestimate the probability of a correct face recognition response on the part of the eyewitness.

Of course, as more face memory researchers gather typicality ratings for the target and distractor faces in their studies, more specific estimates of the interference parameter would be possible. The consulting psychologist could then simply arrange for a rating task that would include photographs of the suspect and other lineup members with a set of photographs of faces whose typicality is already known. Once an estimated d' score is obtained, one then consults a table of d' scores for M-alternative forced choice (Hacker & Ratcliff, 1979) to determine a probability estimate. For instance, employing the conservative parameter estimates previously mentioned, one arrives at d' estimates of 2.39 for a week's delay and 2.05 after a month. Given a six-alternative forced choice lineup or photospread task, for example, these values correspond to probabilities of a correct response of 0.85 and 0.77, respectively. At any event, given the current controversy concerning the proper balance that experimental psychology should maintain between general principles memory research on the one hand and ecological memory on the other (e.g., Bruce, 1985), the program of theory extension and research outlined here is another example of how both research traditions may be fruitfully combined.

FACE RECOGNITION IS NOT UNIQUE: EVIDENCE FROM INDIVIDUAL DIFFERENCES

V. CHURCH AND E. WINOGRAD

1. INTRODUCTION

An old question in cognitive psychology concerns whether separate systems for processing verbal and visual information should be postulated. In its current form, this issue takes the form of the imagery-propositionalist debate. Imagery theorists propose that visual representations or codes are constructed for certain kinds of events and that these codes are different from codes for verbal events. The propositionalists argue for a common form of representation underlying both visual and verbal events. The propositionalists differ from the behaviorists of an earlier generation in arguing for a more abstract code than inner speech. The present contribution assumes (and will provide evidence for this assumption) that, in some sense, visual and verbal information involve different processes and addresses the question of whether an additional system for processing faces should be assumed.

At least three different experimental approaches to the question of face uniqueness can be found in the literature. The first approach asks whether manipulation of the same variables has comparable effects on faces and other types of information. For example, in research on memory for faces influenced by the levels of processing approach of Craik & Lockhart (1972), it has been shown that orienting tasks have similar effects on memory for faces and words (Bower & Karlin, 1974; Warrington & Ackroyd, 1975). In this volume, V. Bruce provides another example of this approach by showing that visual search procedures as well as priming tasks yield results with faces quite similar to those obtained with other kinds of stimuli. These instances of parallel effects of procedures across stimulus classes stand in contrast to the well-known findings of Yin (1969), who reported that inversion of faces produced a greater decrement in performance than inversion of pictures of houses and aeroplanes. Yin's findings have been taken by some investigators as evidence for the uniqueness of face processing, a claim that has been criticised by others (e.g. Ellis, 1975; Goldstein & Chance, 1981). The second approach taken to the question of the uniqueness of face processing is neuropsychological and rests primarily, but not exclusively, on the existence of prosopagnosia. Prosopagnosics are brain-damaged patients who can no longer recognise people they knew well prior to brain trauma. Ellis (1975) has argued that prosopagnosia does not appear to be a purely facial deficit but, rather, is a memory deficit for difficult visual discriminations in general. Discussions of prosopagnosia are to be found elsewhere in this volume.

Another approach to the question of face uniqueness, and the one taken here, is to study individual differences. What we did was to test a large group of subjects on a variety of memory tasks, some verbal, some pictorial, and one using faces. It is important to bear in mind that the same subjects were tested on all of the tasks. By doing a correlational analysis, it should be possible to distinguish between some simple hypothetical states of affairs. Imagine that there is only a single memory system. In that case, people who are good at remembering pictures should be good at remembering words and faces as well, and people who are poor at one should be poor at the others. A factor analysis should yield only a single factor on which all the tests should load. But what if the true state of affairs is that separate systems or processes underly performance on verbal and visual tasks? Then some people should be good at remembering verbal information while others should be good at remembering pictorial information. In that case, the intercorrelations among the verbal memory tasks should be high while the correlations across the verbal and picture tasks should be low. A factor analysis should yield two factors, one on which the verbal tasks load and one on which the picture tasks load. Two memory systems would be implicated. Finally, what if memory for faces is a distinct process, uncorrelated with either verbal or picture memory? Performance on faces then should emerge in the correlational and factor analyses as a third factor. There are other logical possibilities, but these three seem to be the most reasonable to entertain at the outset.

Woodhead & Baddeley (1981) investigated this line of reasoning. They argued that if people known to be good recognisers on a face memory task performed better than bad face recognisers when these two groups were confronted with a picture memory task, then the visual nature of the tasks would be supported. Additionally, if these two groups did not differ on a word memory task, then the non-visual nature of the second task would be demonstrated. The important conclusion, of course, would be that visual memory tasks and verbal memory tasks are mediated by different cognitive processes. They did the suggested experiment using an extreme groups design and confirmed their hypotheses. Their study is ingenious and suggestive, but not entirely convincing. They had statistical problems and difficulties with ceiling effects; the lack of sensitivity in their measures makes interpretation problematic. The logic of the present study was similar to Woodhead & Baddeley's (1981) but employed a correlational approach rather than an extreme groups design.

An additional aspect of this study was the inclusion of words and pictures at two levels of concreteness-abstractness. Paivio's (1971) dual-code theory, developed to account for the greater memorability of concrete stimuli over abstract stimuli, essentially assumes that different categories of stimuli undergo qualitatively different types of encoding. According to dual-code theory, concrete words are better remembered than abstract words because they are more likely to be encoded visually as well as verbally. The logic of dual-code theory could be extended to lead one to expect that concrete words might be encoded more like pictures than abstract words. That is, it might be that the imageability of an event might be more important in determining how it is represented than whether or not it is a linguistic or a pictorial event. These considerations led to the manipulation of the imagery value of the stimuli presented.

2. PROCEDURE
2.1. Materials
2.1.1. Pictures. Ninety slides of representational paintings and ninety slides of abstract paintings were prepared. The slides were 35 mm colour reproductions of late Nineteenth and early Twentieth century works. The representational paintings were French and American impressionist and realist works. None were portraits. All depict scenes and contain easily identifiable concrete objects. The abstract paintings were European and American abstract expressionist pieces. None of these depict naturalistic scenes and few contain any concrete objects; some do contain simple

gcometric figures. Among the representational artists represented are Monet, Sisley, Corot, Whistler, and Homer. Among the abstract artists represented are Mondrian, Klee, Miro, Kandinsky, and De Kooning.

2.1.2. Faces. The face slides were black and white photographic portraits of white adult British actors of various ages. Forty-five were male and forty-five female. They were taken from a casting directory and depicted the head and shoulders.

2.1.3. Verbal materials. Three kinds of verbal stimuli were presented, high imagery (concrete) words, low imagery (abstract) words, and nominalisations. Seventy high imagery words and seventy low imagery words were chosen from the norms of Paivio, Yuille & Madigan (1968). The high imagery words all had imagery values above 6.00 while the low imagery words had imagery values below 3.61. The two sets of words were equated for length and normative frequency. Nominalisations consist of a noun and a participle, such as "carving roasts" or "howling dogs". There were forty high imagery nominalisations (mean imagery value of 5.74) and forty low imagery nominalisations (mean imagery value of 2.87) taken from Paivio (1971). Half of the nominalisations at each imagery level were object nominalisations (e.g., "studying text") and half were subject nominalisations (e.g., "bleating sheep"). It was possible to equate the high and low imagery nominalisations only on length. A complete listing of all the pictures, words, and nominalisations used in the experiment is available in Church (1984).

2.2 Method

Sixty Emory University undergraduates, of whom half were women and half were men, participated in the experiment in order to fulfil a course requirement. They were tested in small groups. The procedure followed was to present the to-be-remembered material to the subjects in a single session followed by a two-alternative forced-choice recognition memory test 24 hours later. There were seven categories of stimuli, 45 representational paintings, 45 abstract paintings, 45 faces, 35 high imagery words, 35 low imagery words, 20 high imagery nominalisations and 20 low imagery nominalisations. All of these 245 stimuli were presented at study to the subjects who were instructed to view and try to remember the slides. Each stimulus category was presented in blocked fashion but there were six different sequences used across the 60 subjects. Within each category, the items were presented in a random order. For half the subjects, the visual stimuli preceded the verbal stimuli with the order reversed for the other half. The slides were presented at a 5-second rate with a thirty second pause between successive categories.

Twenty-four hours later, the subjects were presented with 210 pairs of stimuli. For each pair, one of the slides presented an old stimulus and the other slide presented a new one of the same type. Five old slides of each type were not tested; the ones not tested had been seen at the beginning and end of each set. This left 40 pairs of representational paintings, 40 pairs of abstract paintings, 40 pairs of faces, 30 pairs of high imagery words, 30 pairs of low imagery words, 15 pairs of high imagery nominalisations, and 15 pairs of low imagery nominalisations on the test. For the paintings, each test pair consisted of an old painting (one seen earlier during study) and a distractor. The distractor was a similar work by the same artist. For the faces, the distractors were people of the same sex and approximately the same age. The verbal distractors were not paired by any similarity rule. On the test, the order of presentation of the categories for a given subject was identical to the order at study. However, the order of the stimuli within a category was a different random order from the one shown during study. During the test, each target item and its distractor were projected on the screen side by side simultaneously for ten seconds. The size of each projected image, approximately three feet by four feet since the experiment was conducted in a large lecture room, was identical during study and test. This required the use of two Kodak Carousel projectors which were stepped simultaneously by a single control. Half of the target items in each stimulus category appeared on the right hand side of the screen and half on the left. The right-left order was randomised. The subjects were given an answer booklet containing the numbers 1 through 210, the number of pairs actually tested. Beside each number was an "L" for left and an "R" for right. The subjects were required to circle the letter for each pair corresponding to the item he or she thought was the one seen during study the day before. Subjects were instructed to guess if they were not sure.

3. RESULTS

For each subject the proportion of items correctly recognised was calculated for each of the stimulus categories. The mean proportion of items correctly recognised for each category is presented by sex of subject in Table 1. It should be noted that statistical analyses of the effects of

TABLE 1. Proportions correctly recognised by item category and sex.

Sex			Items				
	PR	PA	Faces	WHI	WLI	NHI	NLI
Men	.77	.74	.77	.76	.62	.83	.82
Women	.77	.74	.80	.82	.71	.88	.80

Key: PR = representational paintings; PA = abstract paintings;
WHI = high imagery words; WLI = low imagery words;
NHI = high imagery nominalisations; NLI = low imagery
nominalisations

order of presentation of the stimuli, that is, whether paintings and faces preceded or followed verbal materials, yielded no significant effects, justifying collapsing across presentation order in subsequent analysis. It may be seen from Table 1 that, where comparison between stimuli differing in concreteness is possible, that is, for pictures, words, and nominalisations, in each case the concrete items were better recognised. The difference was significant at the .05 level for paintings, with representational paintings better remembered than abstract ones, $F(1,56) = 4.99$, and for words, with high imagery words better remembered than low imagery words, $F(1,56) = 50.19$. For nominalisations, the difference between high and low imagery items was not significant, $F(1,56) = 3.61$. There were no significant interactions involving sex and concreteness for the pictures, words, or nominalisations. The only reliable sex difference is for words; the superior performance by females is significant, $F(1,56) = 8.00$.

Tests of the main hypotheses of this study rest on the correlations among the memory tasks. It will be recalled that to the extent that within-category correlations are high while across-category correlations are low, the hypothesis of separate systems is supported. Correlations of the same magnitude would be consistent with the common processing hypothesis. Table 2 presents the correlations collapsed across sex. Included are the two categories of paintings, faces, and the three categories of verbal materials, that is, high and low imagery words and total nominalisations.

TABLE 2. Correlations among the memory tasks, collapsed across sex

	PR	PA	Faces	WHI	WLI	TN
PR	–					
PA	.478*	–				
Faces	.452*	.369*	–			
WHI	.204	.249	.262*	–		
WLI	.229	.240	.382*	.400*	–	
TN	.398*	.229	.314*	.422*	.445*	–
Sex	– .020	– .015	.124	.226	.358*	.135

Note: See Table 1 for key to abbreviations. TN stands for total nominalisations. Men (n = 30) were assigned a score of 1 and women (n = 30) a score of 2 in calculating the correlations with sex.

* p < .05

The last score is a summation of the low and high imagery nominalisations. Being based on twice as many items (thirty instead of fifteen) it was thought to be a more reliable measure; additionally, the two types of nominalisations were not significantly different in memorability. Examination of Table 2 reveals that, in regard to the paintings and the verbal materials, the four within-category correlations are larger than the six across-category correlations. Of the latter, only one is above .25, the correlation required for significance at the .05 level with these degrees of freedom. While there are, of necessity, no within-category correlations involving faces, it is notable that all five across-category face correlations are significant. Overall, the correlation matrix provides evidence for unique processing of pictures and words but not of faces.

A more powerful approach to the issue at hand is factor analysis. Factor analysis attempts to describe structure among a large number of correlations by accounting for the variability in the underlying raw data. What are identified are a limited number of factors or components, each of which is identified with a grouping of the variables (here, the stimulus categories and sex). A principal components analysis was performed and subsequently a rotated solution, achieved by an orthogonal Varimax procedure, was obtained. The rotated solution is shown in Table 3. The procedure yielded just two factors which between them accounted for 57.5% of the variability in the raw

TABLE 3. Factor loadings for six memory tests and sex: Varimax rotation.

	Factor I Visual	Factor II Verbal	h^2
Representational Paintings	.83	.94	.69
Abstract Paintings	.76	.04	.59
Faces	.65	.32	.52
High Imagery Words	.27	.64	.49
Low Imagery Words	.26	.76	.65
Total Nominalisations	.46	.54	.50
Sex	− .24	.75	.62
Eigenvalue	2.10	1.94	

Note: Men (n = 30) were assigned a score of 1 and women (n = 30) a
       score of 2.

data. Of the two factors which emerged, the first may be identified as
primarily reflecting visual memory and the second as reflecting verbal
memory. Paintings and faces load strongly on factor I while verbal
materials load on factor II. Most importantly, there is no evidence for a
separate factor associated with memory for faces. Faces load on the visual
factor with the paintings. The high loading of sex on the verbal factor
reflects the sigificantly higher recognition memory shown for words by
females (see Table 1). In the correlation matrix (Table 2), the only
correlations above .13 involving sex are those between sex and high imagery
words (r = .23) and between sex and low imagery words (r = .36).
     The factor analysis reflects the correlation matrix in showing that
whether words are imageable or pictures are labelable had no effect in the
pattern of relationships. That is, concrete and abstract words load on one
factor while representational and abstract paintings load on a second
factor. It is whether the target is verbal or visual that matters in the
factor analysis, not whether it is concrete or abstract. This is so in
spite of the finding that concreteness facilitated memory for both words and
pictures.

4. DISCUSSION
     The results reported here most strongly support the hypothesis that there
exist two sets of encoding processes, one associated with words and one
associated with pictures, each of which is mediated by different abilities.
Furthermore, the results afford no evidence for the uniqueness of face
processing. Faces seem to be processed similarly to pictures. The clearest
evidence for the face uniqueness or specificity hypothesis would have been
low intercorrelations between memory for faces and memory for pictures and
words and, in the factor analysis, a separate factor on which only faces
loaded. To repeat, such a pattern was not found. The present findings
support the conclusions of Woodhead and Baddeley (1981) that people who are
good at recognising faces tend to be good at recognising other kinds of

pictures as well, but not as good at recognising words.

A comment is in order on the sex differences found. Women showed better memory than men only for words and this was reflected in the high loading for sex on the verbal factor. In their comprehensive review of the psychology of sex differences, Maccoby and Jacklin (1974) summarise a considerable number of studies in which comparisons of memory across gender are possible. They conclude that, when a difference has been reported in verbal memory, it has favoured females in every case, with the superiority of females most evident after seven years of age. On the other hand, they found no reports of reliable sex differences in remembering nonverbal information. The present findings are consistent with this pattern and are of special interest in that all of the studies summarised by Maccoby and Jacklin assessed memory by recall. The present finding of female superiority in verbal memory is the only gender comparison we know of involving recognition memory. An encoding, rather than a retrieval, difference would seem to be implicated.

Finally, it is important to point to some specific features of the approach taken here in evaluating the conclusions drawn. Two major procedural decisions had to be made at the outset. First, the nature of the materials to be included as categories of verbal, pictorial, and facial information had to be decided. Second, a choice had to be made about the nature of the memory test. The second decision was dictated by the nature of the materials. Since a recall test for faces and abstract paintings would be difficult to administer and score, a recognition test was necessitated. In order to test recognition memory, distractor items (items not seen at study) are required. For paintings, highly similar distractors were chosen to avoid the problem of ceiling effects. Clearly, the similarity between targets and distractors was greater for the paintings than for either the words or faces. The best argument for this procedure is the comparability of the recognition memory scores shown in Table 1. A common difficulty level was the goal and was achieved within reasonable limits.

It would be interesting to know if evidence for face uniqueness would be found with an individual differences paradigm when the faces shown at study and test are not identical but, instead, show different poses of the same person. It is possible that seeing identical photographs inflated the correlation between pictures and faces. Perhaps face-specific processes would emerge when identity matching would not be possible. Obviously, the conclusions drawn here are subject to experimental test by investigators who are prepared to sample more broadly both the kinds of target information presented and tested as well as the kinds of cognitive performance demanded of the subject. The individual differences approach seems well suited to testing hypotheses about common and unique processes.

LATERAL REVERSAL AND FACIAL RECOGNITION MEMORY: ARE RIGHT-LOOKERS SPECIAL?

S. J. McKELVIE

1. ABSTRACT

Although lateral reversal of photographs of faces between presentation and test has been shown to disrupt recognition memory, the effect has disappeared when the pictures were initially turned at presentation (making left-lookers into "right lookers"). To explore the possibility that faces looking to the observer's right may be relatively impervious to the effect of reversal, two experiments were conducted. In Experiment 1, subjects viewed photographs of faces whose heads where naturally left-directed, straight or right-directed. With single-stimulus testing ($\underline{n}$ = 38), recognition accuracy was poorer for subsequently reversed left-directed and straight, but not right-directed faces; with forced-choice testing ($\underline{n}$ = 60), overall performance was superior on reversed photographs, although the effect was confined to the right-directed. In Experiment 2, half of the faces were initially presented in their natural left-looking pose, and half were initially reversed so that they became "right-lookers". For three normal ($\underline{n}$ = 66), and two reversed ($\underline{n}$ = 50) conditons, recognition performance was poorer for left-lookers than for "right-lookers" and, for both poses, it was poorer for subsequently reversed than for unchanged pictures. In both experiments, identification accuracy for the transformation on hits was above chance, but higher on normal than on reversed faces. Implications for models of face processing are presented.

2. INTRODUCTION

Despite a fairly large body of research demonstrating the importance of various subject and stimulus factors in the processing of faces (Ellis, 1975), theoretical developments have been sparse (Davies, 1978), with detailed models appearing only recently (Ellis, 1983; Hay & Young, 1982). A continuing concern, however, is whether faces are represented in memory by a feature code which contains individual aspects of the stimulus or in a more wholistic, higher-order fashion in which relationships among features are paramount (a gestalt code, Davies, 1978) or in which meaning is extracted (a semantic code, Bruce, 1982).

Perhaps the most powerful technique for comparing feature with gestalt accounts is to transform photographs of faces so as to selectively alter features or relationships. This method has shown that, although transformations which preserve pattern (inversion, change to photographic negative, lateral reversal) and which alter specific features (hairstyle, outer contour, eyes, mouth) vary in the size of their effects, they all disrupt recognition accuracy, a result which favours a feature code (McKelvie, 1983).

In one of these investigations, McKelvie (1983) reported four experiments showing that facial photographs which were laterally reversed between presentation and test were recognized more poorly than those which were kept in the normal orientation, the size of the effect (d = 0.73) being smaller than the other pattern-preserving transformations (d = 1.38, 1.15 for negative and inversion respectively). However, although the effect generalized across between-and within-subject designs, single-stimulus and forced-choice testing and prior or no prior knowledge of the change, it was not significant (d = 0.27) in a fifth experiment in which the stimuli were initially reversed at presentation, half being kept reversed (unchanged) and half being reversed back (changed) during testing. In addition, a post hoc analysis of the data demonstrated that the disruptive effect of reversal applied both to faces whose heads were turned so that the portrait looked to the left of the observer (left-lookers) and to those who looked straight ahead (full-faces), although subjects consistently recognized fewer left-lookers than full-faces. Since very few of the photographs were right-lookers, the fifth experiment created them by initially reversing the stimuli. Although the pose X transformation interaction was again not significant, inspection of the relevant scores showed that the mean proportions correct for changed and unchanged "right-lookers" (i.e. left-lookers initially turned) were both exactly at 0.67, whereas the corresponding values for "full-faces" were 0.73 and 0.78, a difference commensurate with that found with the full-faces in the other experiments. This observation suggests that faces looking to the right may be impervious to reversal between presentation and test, and that the failure to obtain an overall significant effect in this experiment may have been due to the presence of these faces.

The purpose of the present investigation was to explore this possibility by examining the effects of reversal for left-lookers, full-faces and right-lookers. This was accomplished in two experiments using two different sets of faces; in the first, all three poses were included but in the second only left-lookers and "right-lookers" (reversed left-lookers) were employed.

3. EXPERIMENT 1
3.1 Method
3.1.1.   Subjects.   A total of 98 undergraduate student (49 males, 49 females) at Bishop's University participated in this experiment, with 38 (19 males, 19 females) being assigned to the single-stimulus and 60 (30 males, 30 females) to the forced-choice testing conditions respectively. Sample sizes were increased in the second conditon since an interaction involving sex of subject and sex of face proved to be almost significant in the first.

3.1.2. Materials. The 72 stimuli were drawn from a pool of black and white photographic slides of local Quebec high school students (McKelvie, 1978, 1981). Half of them were shown at presentation and consisted of 12 with heads turned to the observer's left (left-lookers), 12 looking straight ahead (full faces) and 12 looking to the observer's right (right-lookers), sex of stimulus being equally represented in all cases; the 36 stimuli were mixed to ensure that there were no consecutive presentations of the same sex/pose combination. The remaining 36 foils were chosen without regard to pose, although they also contained equal numbers of pictures of males and of females. In the single-stimulus testing condition, the 72 pictures (with originals and foils randomly mixed) were presented one at a time and for forced-choice the 36 originals were each paired side-by-side with a foil of the same sex (originals being on the left or right on a random basis from trial to trial); however, in both cases the 36 originals were shown in the same order, which itself was different from that during presentation.

3.1.3. Procedure. Subjects in both conditions were tested in groups ranging in size from 5 to 15, and were initially instructed to view the photographed faces carefully since they would later be tested on their ability to recognize them. Each slide was then shown for 5 sec after which subjects were given recognition test instructions. They were informed that half of the original stimuli would be laterally (left-right) reversed and that during the 15 sec of each trial, they should record the following responses on the prepared answer sheet: firstly, indicate whether the stimulus was old (O) or new (N) (single-stimulus conditon) or indicate whether the old stimulus appeared on the left (L) or the right (R) (forced-choice testing); secondly, indicate confidence in the previous decision on a four-step scale from 1. certain to 2. reasonably confident to 3. somewhat confident to 4. guessing; and thirdly, if the initial response was old (single-stimulus) and for the picture judged as old (forced-choice), record whether it was in the normal (N) (i.e. original presentation) or reversed (R) orientation. The delay between presentation and test was about 10 min.

3.2. Results

Although both accuracy and confidence data were collected, only the former are presented in detail here. However, it should be noted that subjects were more confident (had lower scores) on normal ($\underline{M}$ = 1.81) than on reversed ($\underline{M}$ = 1.94) faces for single-stimulus, $\underline{t}$(37) = 2.65, $\underline{p}$ < .05, but not forced-choice testing, where there was no significant difference between normal ($\underline{M}$ = 1.99) and reversed ($\underline{M}$ = 2.01).

3.2.1. Single-stimulus testing. First of all, hits (the number of old stimuli classified as such) were analyzed with a 2 X 2 X 3 X 2 (sex of subject X sex of face X pose X transformation) analysis of variance, in which pose, $\underline{F}$(2, 72) = 3.26, $\underline{p}$ < .05, transformation, $\underline{F}$(1, 36) = 21.72, $\underline{p}$ < .01, and their interaction, $\underline{F}$(2, 36) = 8.83, $\underline{p}$ < .01, were significant. Subjects recognized more normal than reversed photographs (see Table 1), the overall effect size being d = 0.76, and post hoc tests on the six mean scores showed that subjects scored higher on normal than on reversed pictures for left-lookers, $\underline{t}$(72) = 2.58, $\underline{p}$ < .01, and for full-faces, $\underline{t}$(76) = 5.58, $\underline{p}$ < .01, but not for right-lookers. Newman-Keuls tests also showed equal accuracy on all three poses for normal photographs, but superior performance on right-lookers over left-lookers ($\underline{p}$ < .05) and full-faces ($\underline{p}$ < .01), which did not differ from each other.

Since male and female faces were equally represented among the foils, the signal detection measure d' was calculated and a 2 X 2 X 2 (sex of subject X sex of face X transformation) analysis of variance conducted. The only significant effect to appear was transformation, $\underline{F}$(1,36) = 7.52, $\underline{p}$ < .01, normal pictures being recognized better than reversed, although the sex of

TABLE 1. Mean Hit Rate in Each Condition in Experiment 1.

Method	n	Left-lookers		Full-faces		Right-lookers	
		Normal	Reversed	Normal	Reversed	Normal	Reversed
SS	38	0.76	0.66	0.83	0.61	0.76	0.79
FC	60	0.81	0.80	0.84	0.91	0.87	0.94

Note. SS = single-stimulus, FC = forced-choice.

subject X sex of stimulus interaction approached significance, $F(1, 36)$ = 2.90, $p < .10$. Inspection of the data suggested that males and females performed better on faces of their own sex, particularly for normal photographs. Individual 2 X 2 (sex of subject X sex of face) analyses supported this contention in that the interaction was significant, $F(1, 36)$ = 3.86, $p < .05$, for normal but not reversed pictures.

The mean score for accuracy (proportion of hits) of identification of orientation (normal or reversed) was .56 (SD = .17), which was significantly above .50, $t(36)$ = 3.14, $p < .01$. Performance was superior on normal (M = .61, SD = .16) than on reversed hits (M = .51, SD = .16), $t(36)$ = 2.36, $p < .05$, only the former being greater than .50, $t(36)$ = 4.24, $p < .01$.

3.2.2. Forced-choice testing. Another four-way analysis was conducted on the number of correct choices (hits, see Table 1). Significant effects were found for sex of subject, $F(1, 58)$ = 4.01, $p < .05$, females performing better than males, pose, $F(2, 116)$ = 16.45, $p < .01$, transformation, $F(1, 58)$ = 9.12, $p < .01$, and the pose X transformation interaction, $F(2, 116)$ = 3.58, $p < .05$. Subjects performed generally better on reversed than on normal pictures (d = - .43), and further post hoc tests showed that subjects correctly recognized an equal number of left-lookers and full-faces, but performed better on reversed than on normal right-lookers, $t(116)$ = 2.20, $p<.05$. In addition, Newman-Keuls tests gave no differences among the three poses for normal pictures but showed higher scores for full-faces and right-lookers (which did not differ) than for left-lookers (ps < .01) on reversed pictures.

For identification of orientation, overall accuracy was .55 (SD = .09), which was significantly above .50, $t(57)$ = 4.17, $p < .01$. Subjects performed better on normal (M = .69, SD = .13) than on reversed (M = .42, SD = .14), $t(57)$ = 9.47, $p < .01$, with the former being significantly above, $t(57)$ = 10.61, $p < .01$, and the latter significantly below chance, $t(57)$ = 4.43, $p < .01$.

3.3 Discussion

The overall significant effect or reversal in the single-stimulus condition, with subjects recognizing more normal than reversed faces, confirms the previous findings (McKelvie, 1983) using this method with a different set of pictures (Aberdeen university undergraduates); moreover, the effect size (d = 0.76) is commensurate with the value (d = 0.73) previously reported. In addition, the interaction between pose and reversal, in which subjects recognized more normal than reversed left-lookers and full-faces, but equal numbers of right-lookers, supports the contention that right-lookers may be impervious to the transformation effect.

However, in contrast to the previous finding that the negative effect of reversal was maintained with forced-choice testing, the present subjects in this condition performed equally well on normal and reversed left-lookers and full-faces, but recognized more reversed than normal right-lookers. The failure to obtain the negative effect of reversal was not entirely surprising, since the forced-choice condition permits subjects to obtain a correct response in two ways: by recognizing the old stimulus (which may be weakened by reversal) and by rejecting the foil (which is unlikely to be affected by reversal). In contrast the superior recognition of reversed over normal right-lookers was not expected. However, the pattern of results across the three facial poses was similar in both conditions, all three being recognized equally well in the normal orientation, and right-lookers being superior to the left-lookers in the reversed. This suggests that reversed right-lookers may be particularly recognizable so that, when the generally negative effect of reversal is mitigated by the forced-choice procedure, they become easier to recognize than their normal counterparts. In turn, this hypothesis is consistent with the speculation that the absence of the negative effect of reversal in the previously-published experiment in which all photographs were initially reversed, may have been due to the presence of "right-lookers".

Since these "right-lookers" were in fact reversed left-lookers, a more precise test of this explanation would entail a direct comparison of the effects of reversal between presentation and test on left-lookers and initially-reversed left-lookers, the prediction being that normal pictures would be better recognized than reversed for the former but not the latter, assuming single-stimulus testing. This was accomplished in Experiment 2. In addition, this experiment controlled for pose among the foils. Although this was not considered necessary in Experiment 1, which was designed to investigate the effect of reversal of the original pictures differing in pose, it is a requirement if the effect of pose itself is of interest.

Although only marginally significant, the interaction between sex of subject and sex of face with single-stimulus testing is generally consistent with past sex difference research (Ellis, 1975; Davies, 1978; McKelvie 1978, 1981) in which an "own sex effect" (particularly for females) has often been found. However, the forced-choice data, which was gathered with larger samples of males and females, failed to confirm the trend in the first condition, females being generally superior. Notably, the interaction was previously obtained (McKelvie, 1978, 1981) with stimuli from the present pool under forced-choice testing when the pairs were systematically matched on sex, hairstyle, pose and expression, suggesting that it occurs when testing conditions are relatively difficult. Sex differences therefore remained of interest in Experiment 2, since it employed another pool of stimuli with which the own-sex effect for females (and possibly males) had been obtained under matched forced-choice conditions (McKelvie, 1978, 1981), and since it involved single-stimulus testing, foils matched for sex and pose, and the reversal transformation, all of which might increase difficulty.

Finally, subjects were able to correctly identify the orientation of about 55% of hits, a result which is similar to that (59%) found previously (McKelvie, 1983). Moreover, they performed better on normal than on reversed hits (61% vs 51%, 69% vs 42% in the single-stimulus and forced-choice conditions respectively), which is also similar to the previous estimates (65% vs 51%). However, since the superiority of normal identification was particularly marked (42% being significantly below chance), when the overall effect of reversal was positive (forced-choice condition), it is clear that identification accuracy did not simply follow the pattern of recognition accuracy. An attempt was made to investigate this issue further in Experiment 2 by misinforming some subjects that some faces had been reversed between presentation and test, and by asking them to make subsequent identification judgements. If they continue to respond "normal" on 60 to 70% of hits, they would appear to be displaying a form of response bias rather than any discriminative capacity to identify orientation. Since faces were not reversed in these conditions, they also provided an opportunity to compare the relative difficulty of the sets of pictures to be changed or left unchanged in the transformation conditions. Although this precaution had been taken in the previously-published study of lateral reversal (McKelvie, 1983), it was not taken in Experiment 1.

4. EXPERIMENT 2
4.1 Method
    4.1.1 Subjects. A total of 116 Bishop's university undergraduate students
were tested, 66 in three normal conditions (11 males, 11 females in each) in
which no transformation occurred between presentation and test, and 50 in
two reversal conditions: 12 males and 14 females with 5 sec presentation
time and a 24 hr test delay, and 12 males and 12 females with 1 sec
presentation and a 10 min delay.
    4.1.2. Materials. The stimuli were 64 black and white slides of faces (32
males, 32 females) chosen from a pool of Quebec adults (McKelvie, 1978,
1981). All pictures were left-lookers in that the portraits were taken with
the person looking to the left of the photographer. However, for this
experiment, half of the pictures were laterally reversed to make them into
"right-lookers".   Thus, presentation and foil stimuli each consisted of 32
photographs (with eight in each of the four sex/pose combinations). The 32
presentation stimuli and 64 test stimuli were each mixed in a different
random order, with half of the originals being randomly designated for
future reversal in some conditions.
    4.1.3 Procedure. The basic procedure was similar to that in Experiment 1.
However, in the three normal (no transformation) conditions (5 sec
presentation time, 10 min test delay (labelled immediate); 5 sec, 24 hr
(labelled delayed); 1 sec, 10 min (labelled fast), all stimuli were shown in
the same lateral orientation during presentation and test, although subjects
were informed prior to the latter that half of them had been reversed, and
were required to make the same three decisions as in Experiment 1. In the
two reversal (transformed) conditions (5 sec, 24 hr (delayed); 1 sec, 10 min
(fast)), which were designed to increase difficulty, half of the original
stimuli were laterally reversed during testing, and subjects were treated in
the same fashion as in Experiment 1.

4.2. Results
    As for Experiment 1, only a summary of the confidence data will be
presented. In two (immediate, fast) of the three normal (no transformation)
conditions, confidence scores were equivalent for the set of faces to be
left unchanged and the set to be changed between presentation and test,
whereas in the third (delayed), they were lower (i.e. subjects reported
greater confidence) for the former ($\underline{M}$ = 1.69) than for the latter ($\underline{M}$ =
1.80), $\underline{t}$(21) = 2.42, $\underline{p}$ < .05. However, in both transformation conditions,
confidence scores were lower for the normal (unchanged) than for the
reversed (changed) pictures. For delayed, mean scores for normal and
reversed pictures, respectively, were $\underline{M}$ = 1.45 and 1.79, $\underline{t}$(25) = 4.85,
$\underline{p}$ < .01; for fast, the corresponding values were $\underline{M}$ = 2.13 and 2.28, $\underline{t}$(23) =
2.73, $\underline{p}$ < .01.   A separate 2 x 2 analysis of variance of the two delayed
conditions showed a strong effect of set, $\underline{F}$(1, 45) = 27.89, $\underline{p}$ < .01, but
also an interaction between condition and set, $\underline{F}$(1, 45) = 7.02, $\underline{p}$ < .01,
with the difference between sets being larger in the transformation than in
the no transformation condition. Thus, subjects were more confident on
normal than on reversed photographs, and the effect was not due to the
former simply being less difficult.
    4.2.1 Normal (no transformation) conditions. Since both sex of face and
pose were controlled on the foils, the hits (number of old stimuli
classified as old) and false-alarms (number of new stimuli (foils)
classified as old) were converted to d' scores (see Table 2). A 3 X 2 X 2 X
2 X 2 (conditon X sex of subject X pose X set X sex of face) analysis of
variance gave significant effects of condition, $\underline{F}$(2, 60) = 38.50, $\underline{p}$ < .01,
pose $\underline{F}$(1,60) = 16.92, $\underline{p}$ < .01, and the condition X set interaction, $\underline{F}$(2, 60)

TABLE 2. Mean d' Score in Each Condition in Experiment 2 (Hit Rates in Brackets)

Condition	n	Left-lookers		"Right-lookers"	
		Set 1	Set 2	Set 1	Set 2
No Transformation					
Immediate	22	2.75 (0.84)	2.26 (0.84)	3.02 (0.82)	3.02 (0.82)
Delayed	22	2.43 (0.80)	2.13 (0.74)	2.72 (0.81)	2.50 (0.79)
Fast	22	0.90 (0.57)	1.06 (0.64)	1.33 (0.61)	1.60 (0.67)
Transformation					
Delayed	26	2.66 (0.70)	2.09 (0.58)	3.07 (0.68)	2.47 (0.52)
Fast	24	1.09 (0.84)	0.66 (0.71)	1.29 (0.89)	0.71 (0.75)

Note. Set 1 was presented normally (unchanged) and Set 2 reversed (changed) in the two transformation conditions.

= 3.74, p < .05. Post hoc tests showed that the scores in the fast condition were lower than in the other two (ps < .01), which did not differ; and scores on left-lookers were lower than those on "right-lookers". The interaction effect was the result of equivalent scores on the two sets of photographs in the immediate and delayed conditions, but lower scores in Set 1 (later to be kept unchanged) than in Set 2 (later to be changed) in the fast condition, $t(60)$ = 2.19, p <.05; effect size was - 0.51.

Two effects involving sex variables were also significant. Male faces (mean d' = 2.33) were generally easier to classify as old or new than female faces (mean d' = 2.04), $F(1, 60)$ = 6.91, p < .01; however the interaction between sex of subject and sex of face, $F(1, 60)$ = 6.77, p < .05, showed that this effect was confined to males, the four mean scores being as follows: male subjects on male faces (2.60) and on female faces (2.01); females on male faces (2.07) and on female faces (2.07). Notably, separate d' analyses in each of the three conditons showed that, although the data followed this trend in all of them, the pattern was only significant under the fast treatment.

The main effect of pose, in which subjects obtained higher scores on "right-lookers" than on left-lookers was further investigated by conducting a 3 X 2 X 2 (condition X pose X set) and a 3 X 2 (condition X pose) analysis on hits and false-alarms respectively. For hits, the only significant effect was condition, $F(2, 63)$ = 5.58, p < .01, and for false-alarms, condition, $F(2, 63)$ = 7.47, p < .01, and pose, $F(1, 63)$ = 8.67, p < .01. Subjects performed more poorly in the fast condition than in the other two on both criteria, and had more false-alarms on left-lookers than on "right-lookers".

When asked to identify whether each face classified as old was normal or reversed, the mean proportions of "normal" responses in the three conditions were as follows: M = .68, SD =.12 (immediate); M = .65, SD = .13 (delayed); and M = .62, SD = .13 (fast). All three mean values were significantly greater than .50, $t(21)$ = 6.64, 5.21, and 4.26 respectively (ps < .01).

4.2.2 Reversed (transformation) conditions. Another five-way analysis of the d' data (see Table 2) for the transformation conditions gave significant effects for condition, $F(1, 46)$ = 75.78, p < .01, and transformation, $F(1,$

46) = 24.93, p < .01. Inspection of Table 2 shows that subjects performed better in the delayed than in the fast condition, and on the normal than reversed pictures. On the basis of normal and reversed hits, the effect sizes for the two conditions respectively were d = 0.69 and 0.92. Although the overall effect of pose was only marginally significant, F(1, 46) = 3.80, p < .06, performance on left-lookers being slightly poorer than on "right-lookers", separate analyses of hits and false-alarms showed that, on hits, subjects performed better on "right-lookers" than on left-lookers only in the delayed condition, t(48) = 2.19, p < .05, but that, in both conditions, they made more false—alarms on the left-lookers than on the "right-lookers", F(1, 48) = 4.90, p < .05. Neither the main effect of sex of face, or its interaction with sex of subject, were significant.

For identification of orientation, overall accuracy was .66 (SD = .13) and .61 (SD = .11) for the delayed and fast conditions respectively, both of which were above .50, t(25) = 6.02, t(22) = 4.80, ps < .01. In both cases, subjects performed better on normal than on reversed pictures, the values being as follows: M = .70, SD = .18, normal delayed; M = .61, SD = .17, reversed delayed, t(25) = 2.19, p < .01; M = .72, SD = .12, normal fast; M = .45, SD = .26, reversed fast, t(22) = 3.96, p < .01. Both normal mean proportions were significantly higher than .50, t(25, 22) = 5.75, 8.79, respectively, ps < .01, as was the reversed mean in the delayed condition, t(25) = 3.30, p < .01.

5. GENERAL DISCUSSION

In both transformation conditions in Experiment 2, subjects obtained higher accuracy (d') scores on normal than on reversed faces, effect sizes being 0.69 and 0.92 (or 0.92 + 0.51 = 1.43 if allowance is made for increased difficulty on Set 2 in the fast no transformation condition). These findings replicate the negative effect of reversal reported previously (McKelvie, 1983; Experiment 1 here) with a third set of pictures, and permit a revised estimate for the general size of effect of this manipulation. In view of the current practice in meta-analysis research (e.g. Feltz & Landers, 1983) to include all d values, whether positive, zero or negative, the five d values from McKelvie's (1983) investigation were combined with the four here to obtain an overall mean effect size estimate of 0.57 (or 0.63 if the larger of the two above alternatives is chosen). This number is similar to the estimates of 0.46 for expression change and of 0.75 for mouth removal, but is lower than those (1.38, 1.15) for photographic negative and inversion transformations (McKelvie, 1983). Taken together with the latter two, however, the present result provides further evidence against a simple gestalt code for face representation, since all three transformations leave patterned relationships in the photographed face intact. Notably, the finding contrasts with a lack of effect of reversal on heterogeneous (Standing, Conezio, & Haber, 1970) or homogeneous (Kiphart, Sjogren, & Cross, 1984) pictures of varied scenes or football incidents respectively, suggesting that the latter sets of stimuli may involve a gestalt code.

In Experiment 2, the negative effect of reversal applied to both left-lookers and "right-lookers". The former result confirms the previous post hoc analysis with faces in this pose (McKelvie, 1983) and the present deficit on them in Experiment 1 (single-stimulus condition). However, the latter finding suggests that, although genuine right-lookers (Experiment 1) may be impervious to reversal, reversed left-lookers are not. Furthermore, it implies that the failure to obtain a significant effect of reversal between presentation and test when all pictures were initially turned (McKelvie, 1983, Experiment 5), was not simply due to the presence of resistant "right-lookers".

At the same time, Experiment 2 demonstrated greater recognition accuracy on "right-lookers" than on left-lookers, due mainly to a lower false-alarm rate on the former. Thus, faces which look to the observer's right seem to be relatively easy to detect as novel, and also seem to be relatively easy to recognize when reversed (Experiment 1). Indeed, the overall pose effect in Experiment 1, in which performance on right-lookers was generally higher than that on left-lookers and full-faces (because of the reversed performance) might have been increased if pose had been controlled on the new pictures (foils). Some caution should be exercised before concluding that these data constitute evidence that faces directed to the observer's right are "special", since pictures in all three poses were equally well recognized in the unchanged conditions in Experiment 1, and since both sideways poses were affected by the transformation in Experiment 2, but the notion is consistent with some evidence that this pose is less common in portraits (Fisher & Cox, 1975; Humphrey & McManus, 1973). Although word frequency and face typicality may not represent the same underlying dimension (Light, Kayra-Stuart, & Hollander, 1979), both variables are related negatively to recognizability (words: Morris, 1978, Wolters, 1980; faces: Courtois & Mueller, 1981; Light et al., 1979), which may reflect variations in inter-item similarity (Light et al., 1979). Right-lookers may be special in that they are less similar to each other than left-lookers or full-faces.

In the three normal conditions of Experiment 2 taken together, and in the more difficult fast condition considered alone, there was an "own sex effect" for males, the best performance on the four sex of subject/ sex of stimulus combinations occurring for males on male faces. Although this result is consistent with some of the patterns previously found with pictures from this pool (McKelvie, 1978, 1981), where originals and foils were also matched on sex and pose, it may not simply be a function of task difficulty, as hypothesized. In the two transformation conditions, which included an extra element of difficulty in the form of reversal between stimulus and test, the sex interaction disappeared. Examination of Table 2 shows that, although reversed pictures were less well-recognized than normal ones in the delayed condition, overall d' ($\underline{M}$ = 2.56) was not lower than the corresponding value ($\underline{M}$ = 2.44) for the no transformation condition; however, the two fast conditions differed ($\underline{M}$ = 0.94 and 1.24), with performance in the presence of the transformation being the poorest of all. But a separate analysis of these data gave no sign of the sex interaction. The circumstances under which it appears therefore remain unclear.

Identification performance in the transformation conditions in Experiment 2 was slightly higher (66%, 61%) than in Experiment 1 (about 55%), but was closer to the levels (about 59%) reported originally (McKelvie, 1983). Moreover, proportion correct was again higher on normal (70, 72%) than on reversed (61, 45%) pictures. Of most interest, however, was the finding that subjects in the three no transformation conditions, who were led to believe that reversal was occurring, reported "normal" responses at about the same rate (62, 65, 68%) as with normal stimuli in the other conditions. Considering all of the identification estimates together, only one of the reversed values (61% in Experiment 2 here) was greater than chance, and all the normal ones fell in the 60 to 72% range, despite positive, zero and negative effects of reversal on recognition accuracy and, in Experiment 2, the complete absence of the transformation between stimulus and test. Similarly, although Klatzky and Forrest (1984) failed to show a significant effect of lateral reversal on hit rates for famous or nonfamous faces, they found that identification accuracy was above chance, and generally higher on normal (about 82%) than on reversed (about 46%) pictures. These results suggest that subjects could not identify orientation accurately but, rather than guessing whether or not the picture has been turned, they adopted a response strategy in which they tended to report a familiar-looking face as unchanged. Since subjects were generally more confident ⟍on normal than reversed faces, they may have been more likely to identify the former than the latter as normal.

In conclusion, the present experiments replicated the generally negative effect (McKelvie, 1983) of lateral reversal on recognition accuracy, but showed that it could be removed with forced-choice testing and with faces initially looking to the right of the observer. Since left-right reversal leaves patterned relationships intact, the latter result, if replicable, suggests that right-lookers may be processed in a gestalt fashion, whereas left-lookers and full faces may be coded more in terms of features. Finally, although subjects were able to identify orientation at an above-chance level, their performance seems to reflect a response strategy rather than a discriminative capacity.

CONTEXT EFFECTS IN RECOGNITION MEMORY OF FACES:
SOME THEORETICAL PROBLEMS

G. TIBERGHIEN

1. INTRODUCTION

By context effects we mean, in a very general way, modifications of the characteristics of specific and oriented behavior under the influence of secondary changes in the conditions under which it arises. Such effects often have an inhibiting influence on observed performance. Context effects are very common since they have been shown to exist in motor activity (Greer & Green, 1983; Reeve & Mainor, 1983), in sensory processes and perceptual activity (N.H. Anderson, 1975, 1979; Antes & Metzger, 1980; Birnbaum, 1974), in memory and learning (Horton & Mills, 1984; Perlmuter & Monty, 1982), in problem solving (Medin & Schaffer, 1978), and in speech production and understanding (Bowey, 1984; H.H. Clark & Carlson, 1981; Underwood, 1977). It is obvious that these various manifestations of context effects cannot all be simply reduced to the same psychological processes or referred back to the same explanatory models. All the same the wide application of the concept of context incontestably denotes an explanatory and descriptive significance (Tiberghien, 1985). Moreover, in the field of memory, the behavioral reality of context effects is no longer seriously questioned. It is indeed well known that the modification of conditions of retrieval of a memory trace with respect to the conditions of memorization has a definite influence on the probability of recall or recognition (for review; Lecocq & Tiberghien, 1981; Tiberghien & Lecocq, 1983). This fact had been suggested quite early on by the Gestalt theory but it was several decades before all the consequences were drawn and admitted that a theory of forgetting cannot do without a context law (Hoffman, 1985; Jenkins, 1974; Norman, 1969). And again it was several years before this law was clearly formulated by Tulving (1973, 1974, 1983) under the name of encoding specificity principle. According to this law the efficiency of memory retrieval cues depends on their similarity to events having taken place at time of encoding. The encoding specificity principle thus predicts interaction between encoding and retrieval conditions and it is the presence of such interaction which constitutes the operational indicator of the presence of a context effect. The encoding specificity principle is thus a context law, the validity of which has been amply confirmed in recent years.

However, this principle is basically descriptive and gives no indication of the way contextual information functions. It is clear, to begin with, that sources of contextual information can vary. The general characteristics of the environment in which memorization takes place constitute what could be called a situational context (Dolinsky & Zabrucky, 1983; Smith, 1973; Smith, Glenberg & Bjork, 1978). The more specific characteristics of the task and of the activity of the subject (expectations and attention) constitute what can be called mental context and, finally the motivation and emotional state of the individual doubtless provide a motivational context (M.S. Clark, Milberg & Ross, 1983; Leight & H.C. Ellis, 1981). The global context effect so often described results, therefore, from the interaction of these sources of contextual influences and it is by no means certain, if we take this stand-point, that their modes of functioning are strictly equivalent. In this chapter however, we will in the main deal only with the two former classes of context effects and for these we will attempt to designate the most significant functional properties.

The study of the dynamics of context effects in human memory can be done on extremely varied material. Two classes in particular have provided the basis for a large number of investigations: linguistic material (words, sentences, texts) and non linguistic material (objects, scenes, faces, motor sequences). Though context effects have been demonstrated and studied mostly on linguistic material, it must be recalled that this raises extremely delicate theoretical problems. Indeed, it is virtually impossible to dissociate unambiguously the episodic and semantic components of linguistic material. But context effects derive from the spatio-temporal organisation of unique events, even though they may, as we shall see, be modulated by certain semantic characteristics of the situation. Further, if we restrict ourselves to isolated lexical items, it can be maintained that to each of these corresponds a semantic representation which has been built up on the basis of many utilisations in extremely varied linguistic and non-linguistic contexts. In other words, the contextual specificity of a word is relatively low, lower certainly than that of a scene or an object which is associated with much more definite spatio-temporal conditions. From this point of view faces are of considerable methodological interest because they have a much higher degree of contextual specificity than mere lexical units. This means it is possible with this type of material to delimit clearly the episodic and semantic elements which determine memory representation. As Watkins, Ho & Tulving, 1976, says there is always confusion between the episodic occurrence of a word and the permanent semantic representation it refers to. A non-familiar face, on the contrary, does not have any memory representation but can constitute a perceptual event in specific spatio-temporal context. This possibility of dissociating the episodic and semantic elements of face memory probably accounts for the interest shown in systematic psychological study of context effects in the memory of faces (other reasons for this "fascination" of faces for psychologists have been evoked by Goldstein, 1983). Here I shall present experimental results which may provide the beginnings of an answer to the question of the nature of the psychological processes which give their scope and significance to the context effects generally observed in memory recognition of face (Baddeley, 1979; Bruce, 1982; Brutsche, Cisse, Deleglise, Finet, Sonnet & Tiberghien, 1981; Keer & Winograd, 1982; Memon, 1985; Memon and Bruce, 1985; Patterson & Baddeley, 1977; Tiberghien, 1983; Watkins et al., 1976). The approach adopted here is resolutely functional-ist, the aim being to construct a genuine dynamics of context effects which may eventually improve our understanding of face representations in human memory.

2. CONTEXT, DECISION AND SEARCH IN MEMORY RECOGNITION OF FACES

Theories of human memory capable of integrating context effects can be very roughly divided into two main categories: models which we can refer to as "resonance" models and those we can refer to as "reconstruction" models, the former explain recognition and recall by "non-conscious" interaction, the exact mechanism of which is unknown, between the content of a memory trace and the representation of contextual characteristics of the recognition situation. In this view the probability of successful retrieval is supposed to depend on the compatibility between trace content (including, naturally, the cues of the memorization context) and the content of the objective recognition or recall situation. The theory of synergistic ecphory (Tulving, 1976, 1982, 1983) is a choice example of this type of theory (see also Ratcliff, 1978), the "holographic" models of memory and the models of distributive memory also belong, if we take only most important features into consideration, to this class of theory (Cavanaugh, 1976; Eich, 1982; Murdock, 1982, 1983; Pike, 1984; for review, Roediger III, 1980). One of the important features of these theories is that they postulate more or less automatic access to memory information and claim that context is an integral part of memories. The second type of theory on the other hand postulates a memory search which is oriented by context and could be likened to activation of a semantic network or to an intentional search for markers in an association network (Anderson, 1976; Anderson, 1983) or, finally to a "backward" or "forward" search for mnesic and contextual representations (Mandler, 1976, 1980).

It is, however, probable that both types of mechanism can co-exist in human memory. In a model worked out a few years ago Tiberghien, Cauzinille & Mathieu (1979) put forward the hypothesis that memory recognition can result to begin with from a rapid automatic process giving rise to a strong feeling of subjective certainty. The efficiency of this process would then depend on the overall familiarity of the recognition situation i.e. an interaction between the familiarity of the target and that of the accompanying context. When this "resonance" process fails, the subject might engage in an intentional search process in order to recall another mental state which might enter into resonance with the recognition situation (this "conditional" search would be analogous to the "recollection" of Baddeley, 1982). This hypothesis could, of course, be formulated in other terms but what counts here is the duality proposed between a rapid decision process based on the familiarity of the recognition situation and a longer deliberate process guided by semantic and episodic associations between memorization and retrieval contexts. The distinction brought in by Jones (1978) between intrinsic retrieval (where target and context "contain" each other) and extrinsic retrieval (where the relation between target and control has to be retrived) is probably another way of formulating the same hypothesis within the conceptual frame work of "redintegration". In the same way Donaldson's model (1981, p.312) puts forward a similar idea since he supposes that, first, familiarity of a situation is estimated and then begins a search for the representation of face memory, the orientation of which is determined by the degree of familiarity of the context.

If the foregoing analysis is valid it should be possible to show that slow recognition is affected by a modification of context between study and retention testing whereas rapid recognition is not particularly affected. Experimental results consistent with this hypothesis were obtained recently by Peris (1982) and Peris & Tiberghien (1984). In this investigation subjects study and memorize incidentally several female faces. Each face is associated with a Christian name pronounced by a different feminine voice. Thus there are two contextual cues: a semantic one (name) an episodic one (voice). Ten minutes after the end of the study period there is a recognition test. Faces are to be recognized with the same name and same voice or the same name and a different voice or a different name and the same voice or, finally, with different name and voice. There are of course new faces associated with these different context conditions. This experiment gives a particularly interesting result if we dissociate rapid and slow recognitions (Fig. 1). Indeed here it can be observed that the change of context affects the probability of slow hits only. There is no context effect on the probability of correct rapid recognition. The data

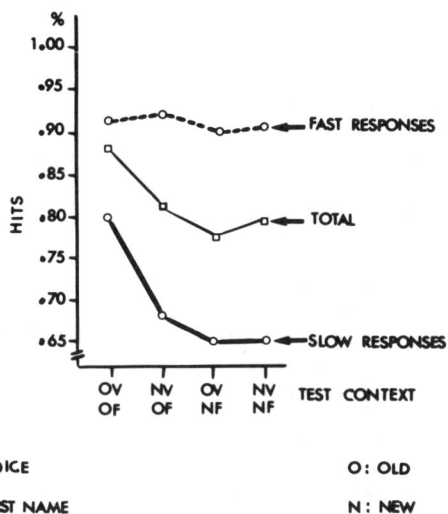

FIGURE 1. - Percent correct recognitions of faces, by context change, and speed of response (Peris & Tiberghien, 1984)

from this experiment is consistent with the principle of encoding specificity, but for correct slow recognition only. It is probable that most slow answers are the result of a search process, whereas most rapid answers result from a simple decision based on familiarity.

Though there are other possible interpretations, based on a mere time-lag in the processing of contextual data (H.D. Ellis, 1985) or on differential sensitivity of the context to holistic and analytic processing (Thomson, 1984), the data is consistent with the hypothesis of a double recognition mechanism, one rapid and little affected by context changes, another slower but affected by such changes. However, it should be noted that the foregoing dissociation was not obtained for false recognition, which suggests that the association of an "old" context with a "new" face has different and probably more complex effects than those of the association old context/old face.

3. CONTEXT AND FAMILIARITY IN FACE RECOGNITION

The above experiment suggests that context variations affect above all the process of memory search. However, the fact that this dissociation only comes to light on hits, and not on false recognition, is really puzzling. This pattern of results is however quite frequent and though context effects do have an influence on the proportion of hits, results are much more contradictory with regard to false recognitions. Indeed, some researchers have observed a context effect which concerns both correct and false recognitions (Davies & Milnes, 1982; Donaldson, 1981; Winograd & Rivers-

Bulkeley, 1977) but others have found them only for correct recognitions (Brutsche et al., 1981; Bruce, 1982). In view of this, how can the divergencies be accounted for? It may be - contrary to our original hypothesis - that recognition context has a double effect: the familiarity of an "old" context combined with familiarity of the face to be recognized might add to the overall familiarity of the situation, this effect being quite analogous to a "response bias" (Bruce & Young, 1985); but an "old" context can also serve as a cue for retrieval of the original encoding conditions, this effect being then a memory effect in the strict sense. Thus the association of a context with a face might act on the predecision and consequently on the proportion of rapid recognitions but it might also affect the process of memory search as such and modify the proportion of slow responses. It might be that this double context effect does not work in the same way in the recognition of "old" and of "new" faces. Indeed the increase in familiarity, brought about by the presence of an old context is different for an old (already familiar) face than for a new (non-familiar) face. The outcome is that the "response bias" effect of context is probably greater for new than for old faces. A mechanism of this sort could, moreover, explain as well the facilitation effect of an old context in irrelevant association with an old face (Baddeley, 1982; H.D. Ellis, 1985). In the same line of thinking, the "cuing" effect of the context is perhaps different for old and new faces. In the former case, if recognition conditions permit recall of those of the memorization of the target this can only enhance the probability of correct recognition. Things are rather different for a new face, where the context cues make it possible to retrieve encoding conditions and notice that the face associated with these context cues is not the same as the old face retrieved from memory. In other terms, an old context associated with a new face might very well increase the probability of a correct rejection. Thus this double function of an old contextual cue could lead only to an increase in correct recognition (hits) but could increase either the proportion of false recognitions (bias effect) or that of correct rejections (memory effect).

If the above analysis corresponds to psychological reality it should be possible to manipulate certain situational factors in order to enhance the retrieval of study conditions on the basis of a context cue associated with a new face. An experiment done by one of my students (Peris, 1985, personal communication) has contributed extremely suggestive data on this point. He presented his subjects with 12 faces associated with 12 different feminine Christian names. The photographs used were all in colour and showed a front view of the faces. During subsequent recognition testing 24 photos (12 old, 12 new faces) in black and white are presented to the subjects. This time the faces are shown in profile and subjects are required to recognize the "person" studied earlier. They are moreover informed that some lures have same names as the old faces. The particularity of this experiment lies in the fact that 12 lures are presented as a block before the 12 old faces. Half the lures are presented without name, half with an "old" name. They are presented in alternation. The "old" faces are also presented in alternation accompanied by the corresponding old names or without names. The aim here was to increase the contrast between faces to be recognized (black and white profiles) and memorized faces (coloured front views), a manipulation which was aimed at reducing considerably the familiarity of all the faces. The order of presentation of the faces (new faces presented before old faces) was meant to enable us to study in priority the responses to new faces without contamination from responses to old faces such as usually occurs in habitual recognition procedures. Under such conditions, if a subject is confronted with a new face associated with an old name, he has only to remember the name was associated with a face in coloured front-view in order to identify a mis-match immediately and produce a correct rejection. In other words, in a paradigm of this sort it is to be expected that the rate of false recognitions would be lower when the face is accompanied by an old context than in the opposite case. This was in fact found to be so. The rate of false recognitions is only 11% when an old context is associated with a new face and 28% when a new face is not associated with any context (Table 1). The phenomenon is moreover strongly

TABLE 1. Percent correct and false recognitions of faces, by associative verbal context, and similarity between old and new faces (Peris, 1985 unpublished).

Similarity Between Old and New Faces		Associative	Context
		Present	Absent
Low	% hits	.94	.71
	% FR	.00	.33
High	% hits	.86	.86
	% FR	.21	.23

influenced by list context : the order of presentation of persons (names) associated with new faces could be the same as or different from that of study.

4. INDEPENDENT AND INTERACTIVE CONTEXTS IN FACE RECOGNITION

Both the above experiments therefore are consistent with the hypothesis that face recognition may be the product of a double mechanism of decision and of memory search. The first experiment (Peris & Tiberghien, 1984) showed that the associated context affected the probability of a correct slow recognition and had no effect on the probability of correct rapid recognition. This data provides an argument in favour of the hypothesis of a specific action of context on memory search, the decision process being deteriorated only by variations in overall familiarity of the situation. However, the effect was not noted for false recognition and we felt compelled to ask why these context effects were much less consistent with new faces than with old. The second experiment (Peris, 1985) contributes evidence in favour of the interpretation that an old context might favour false recognition by enhancing the overall familiarity of the situation but might also favour correct rejection by providing access to original study conditions and to the representation of the old face earlier associated with the perceptually available context. The heterogeneity in results generally observed could thus arise from the varying degrees of mixture of the two processes under varying experimental conditions. When recognition testing only applies to new faces, where familiarity has been drastically reduced by manipulating angle of view and colour and when contextual conditions of access to original information are optimal it is found that an old context can largely reduce the proportion of false recognitions.

However in these two experiments the contexts used were relatively independent from the target. But we know that Baddeley (1982) upheld a distinction he considered essential between independent and interactive contexts (see also: Begg & Sikich, 1984; Godden & Baddeley, 1980). In his view, a context which is independent of the target may affect recall but not recognition, whereas an interactive context may act just as well on both these indicators of memory trace. Nonetheless, it must be admitted that it is particularly difficult to reach agreement on a set of criteria to decide whether or not a context is independent or not from the face to be recognized, all the more so in view of the fact that the interactive nature of the context does not depend solely on the objective properties of the memorization or retrieval situation but also on the aims and expectations of the subject, the orientation of his attention and the depth of the encoding process he applies (Baddeley & Woodhead, 1982; Bower & Karlin, 1984; Memon & Bruce, 1983; Parkin & Goodwin, 1983). In fact the distinction has only relative value and when a context effect is observed in recognition it can always be explained a posteriori by the assertion that in reality context interacted with the face. In an experiment done by Peris (1983) he set out to control simultaneously an independent and an interactive context. In this study subjects were required to memorize faces of people (without clothing cues) photographed in three quarter view holding a specific object (telephone, pick, etc.). On the white wall behind, there was always a poster of which only the bottom quarter was visible. In recognition testing the "old" persons were to be recognized mixed with other new ones. The object associated with the "old" persons could be the same as what they were holding in study presentation, or different. New persons could hold objects used or not at the study stage. The posters could also be the same as or different from those used in study series. Results obtained show a very significant inhibition effect of change of object associated with the person and an absence of effect of modifications of the poster; and no interaction between these two types of contextual change (Table 2). It seems therefore that only the change of interactive contexts is likely to affect face recognition. As in the earlier experiments we do not obtain context effects on false recognitions. This result seems therefore at first sight perfectly consistent with Baddeley's analysis and with the results he obtained in a situation of memory recognition of faces. However during his investigation Peris also recorded the points of eye-fixation at the moment of recognition by means of a NAC eye-recorder. It is therefore possible to distinguish the frequency of hits according to whether they are preceded or not by foveal eye-fixation on the context. It was found, on one hand, that the interactive context is much more often fixated than the independent, and, on the other, that the frequency of hits is lower when preceded by an eye-fixation than in the opposite case, which would seem to indicate that the response obtained in such conditions results from a state of greater uncertainty requiring a more thorough perceptual analysis of the scene. Finally, it was found that a context effect is manifested only after an eye-fixation and its amplitude is about the same whether the context is independent or interactive. Here also, the

TABLE 2 – Percent correct recognitions of faces, by context change, type of context, and eye-fixation of retireval context (Peris, 1983, unpublished).

| | Context | | Difference |
	Old	New	
Interactive context			
Eye fixation	.81	.64	.17
No eye fixation	.84	.76	.08
Mixed	.83	.70	.13
Independent context			
Eye fixation	.62	.48	.12
No eye fixation	.79	.75	.04
Mixed	.76	.73	.08

data reinforces the hypothesis of a double recognition mechanism based on a rapid predecision not requiring extra eye-fixation and for this reason unaffected by context changes, or based on a slower search process, requiring additional seizure of information from context and for this reason affected by context change. Finally, in contradiction with Baddeley's analysis an effect of independent context can be observed in a recognition situation on certain types of response.

5. SEMANTIC DETERMINANTS OF CONTEXT EFFECTS IN FACE RECOGNITION

It is known that context effects have provided empirical basis for the classical dichotomy between episodic and semantic memory (Tulving, 1984). Context effects are obviously one of the most spectacular manifestations of this principle of encoding specificity, i.e. of the spatio-temporal specificity of operations of encoding and retrieval. It has been found useful from a heuristic standpoint to posit quite firmly these two classes of memory representation. However it must be admitted today that it has not been possible to demonstrate any qualitative difference between episodic and semantic representations. The former probably encode semantically specific referential and temporal properties which should more properly be considered as sub-sets of semantic representations (Lieury, 1979; Tiberghien, 1984; Tulving, 1984, 1985). Further, the study of face recognition makes it possible to show the interaction between episodic and semantic determinants of context effects. Thus in an investigation done by Klee, Leseaux, Malai & Tiberghien (1982) subjects were required to memorize female faces. These were associated with different landscapes (mountains, town, etc.). A week later they were asked to recognize the old faces among new ones. The study was incidental and in the recognition each face was associated with an old or new landscape. In the latter case the new context might be strongly or weakly semantically associated with an earlier study context (for example, if a face had been studied in a mountain landscape, it was presented in another mountain landscape or in a green countryside landscape). We had one-within subject design and the experimental factor was defined by the relation between study and recognition context : unchanged, changed with strong semantic association between study and recognition context and changed with weak association between study and recognition context. The results show that a changed context which maintains semantic association between study and testing context has no inhibiting effect on the proportion of hits. Furthermore, there is an inverse proportion between the probability of correct rejections and the consistency between test and study contexts (see Fig. 2). A result of this sort is not negligible because it

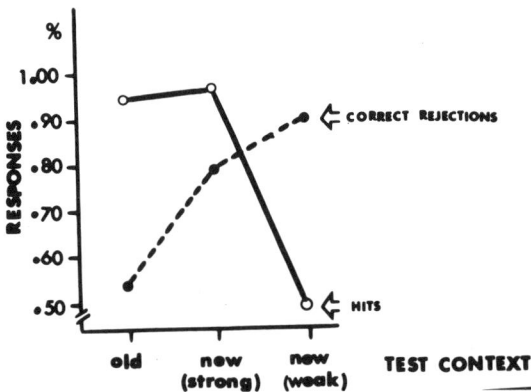

FIGURE 2 - Percent hits and correct rejections, by strength of semantic association between test and study contexts (Klee et al., 1982).

tends to show that it is not so much the context change as such which affects recognition but the absence or weakness of semantic relation between recognition context cues and those of the initial memorisation. This fact is moreover confirmed by an examination of latency of correct recognition and of correct rejection in relation to semantic association between contexts (see Fig. 3). It can be noted that a changed context always increases the latency of correct recognitions and always decreases that of correct rejections. The rise in latency of correct recognitions when there is strong semantic association between a new (test) context and the old (study) context is however not correlated with the stability of the frequency of correct recognitions. However if there is a weak semantic association between new test context and old study, the rise in latency is

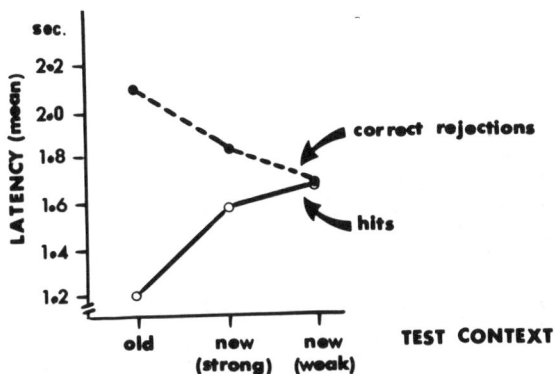

FIGURE 3 - Latencies of hits and correct rejections, by strength of semantic association between test and study contexts (Klee et al., 1982).

negatively correlated with the decrease in frequency of correct recognitions. The explanation for this pattern of correlations might be the following: in the first case the increase in latency of correct recognitions could be considered as an indication of a process of successful search whereas in the second case it could be taken as an indication of an unsuccessful search process.

The experiment carried out by Peris & Tiberghien (1984) already presented earlier also illustrates the interaction between the semantic component of context (Christian name) and the prosodic component (voice). Indeed it is clear that it is the change of name between study and retention test which contributes most to the deterioration of recognition. The voice change has an inhibiting effect only if the Christian name is not changed between study and retention test. Thus a change of semantic context has much more marked effects than a change of prosodic context. The action of the latter is only manifested if the semantic context is not modified. Things work out as if there were a - probably ecologically determined - hierarchy of contextual cues; the individual detecting change in the cue that ranks highest in the hierarchy.

In another investigation (Chave, 1982) subjects incidentally memorized faces of women associated with a name of a profession. The names could be general (for example, "doctor") or specific (for example, "pediatrician"). Ten minutes after the end of study there was a recognition test. The faces to be recognized were associated with the same contextual cue or with a diferent one. In the latter case the test context could be more specific than that of study (for example, "captain" instead of "soldier") or more general (for example, "shopkeeper" instead of "grocer") or, of course, be without semantic relation with study context (for example, "writer" instead of "sailor"). The results of this experiment show that recognition is better after a general encoding than after a specific encoding (see Fig. 4).

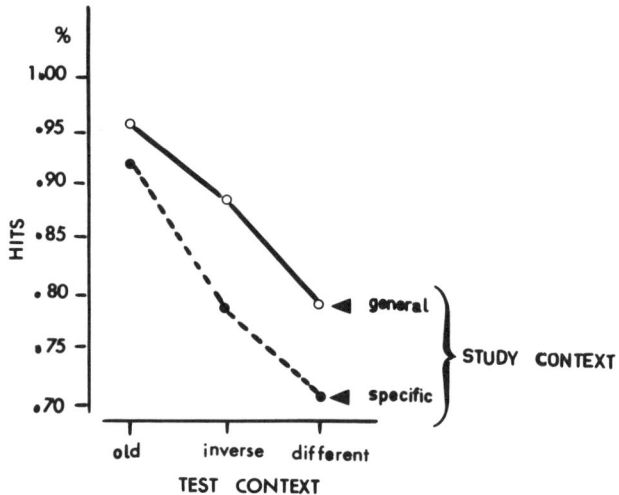

FIGURE 4 – Percent correct recognitions of faces, by semantic specificity of study context, and semantic relation between test and study contexts (Chave, 1982, unpublished).

A more detailed analysis shows that this effect is statistically significant only when the test context is more specific or more general than the study context. Our tentative explanation for this fact is the following: the features of the mental representation of a general job are always included in the mental representation of a more specific job but the reverse is not true. In these conditions it is probably easier to search for and to retrieve the general features from the specific features than the opposite. In the first case, the probability of a successful search for the study context is very high; in the second case a successful search is uncertain. The contextual effect in this experiment is thus affected by the semantic relation between test and study context. This ineraction between change of context and semantic relations between contexts is, in our opinion, the result of a facilitation of the conditional search process when the subject has to recognize a face with a contextual cue which is more specific than the encoding cue associated with this face during the study. In other terms, too specific an encoding is not necessarily the best state of affairs for future recognitions.

6. NEUROPSYCHOLOGY OF CONTEXT EFFECTS IN FACE RECOGNITION

The investigations described above were all done with normal subjects. It is generally considered, though the integration of experimental data is particularly difficult (Moscovitch, 1979; Sergent & Bindra, 1981; Sergent, 1983, 1984), that the processing of facial data seems to involve the right brain-hemisphere more than the left (Bradshaw & Nettleton, 1981; Bruyer & Velge, 1980; H.D. Ellis, 1983; Gazzaniga & Smylie, 1983; Hay, 1981; Landis, Cummings, Christen, Bogen & Imhof, 1985; Young, Hay, McWeemy, A.W. Ellis & Barry, 1985). However contextual information associated with the face can be preferentially processed by right or left hemisphere depending on their nature, linguistic or non linguistic. If this be the case we may ask how contextual dynamics are likely to be affected by localized damage to different centers of the Central Nervous System. In an explanatory investigation, Carrillo (1985) studied 36 patients suffering from brain damage of sometimes greatly varied extent and etiology (Korsakoff, confusional syndrome, extra-pyramidal syndrome, Alzheimer's disease). The only point all these patients have in common was that they had all showed similar difficulties with classical memory tests (anterograde amnesia, recall difficulties, recognition difficulties). The experiment consisted in presenting to the subjects and to a control group of normal subjects a series of photographed faces superimposed on various landscapes. At later testing faces were presented in the same context or in a different but semantically associated context (if the face had been studied in a mountain landscape, it was presented in another mountain landscape, for example) or, finally, in a different context without relation to the study context (face studied in a mountain landscape, presented in an urban landscape). Under these experimental conditions it was found that brain-damaged subjects consistently obtained fewer correct recognitions (particularly of high certainty) than normal subjects; both groups were equally perturbed by change of context between study and recognition and the interaction between group and context was significant (Table 3). This interaction is

TABLE 3 - Percent correct recognitions of faces, by context change, and groups of subjects (Carrillo, 1985, unpublished).

		Context Recognition		
		Unmodified	Modified but Related	Modified but Unrelated
Control	% Hits	.94	.75	.45
(n = 37)	% FR	.19	.16	.15
Brain-Damaged	% Hits	.66	.60	.38
Patients	% FR	.35	.38	.28
(n = 36)				

particularly interesting because it suggests that the performance of brain-damaged patients is significantly poorer than that of normal subjects only if context is <u>not</u> modified between study and recognition test. It would seem that the presence of the "old" context perturbed the recognition capacities of brain-damaged patients.

Over the last two years, Tiberghien & Clerc (1985) have also studied a particularly "pure" case of prosopagnosia (Mr A.H.). The series of experiments he underwent consisted in getting him to memorize series of faces associated with varied contexts and then asking him to recognize them either in the same or in modified contexts. Depending on experiment design the faces to be recognized and the lures could be non-familiar (unknown) or familiar. Here familiarity was induced by a phase of familiarisation which preceded the actual experimental procedure. A.H.'s performances were compared with those of a group of normal subjects to whom we applied the same experimental procedures. The normal subjects' performances were quite classical (see Fig. 5). Recognition of familiar faces was better than that

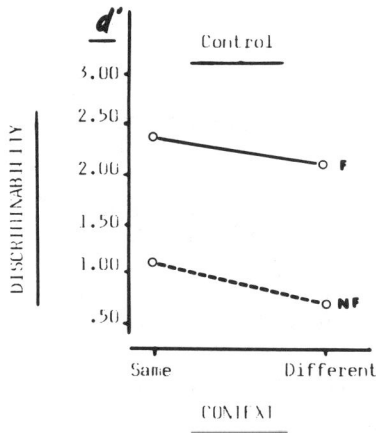

FIGURE 5 - Discriminability Parameter (d'), by strength of semantic association between test and study contexts, and face familiarity for control subjects (Tiberghien & Clerk, 1985).

of non-familiar faces; change of context perturbed recognition and there was no interaction between these two factors. A.H.'s results, on the contrary, were quite a-typical and characterized by an inversion of the usual context effects since his capacity for face recognition was better in conditions where context was modified between study and test than when it remained unchanged (see Fig. 6). Furthermore there appeared to be a strong

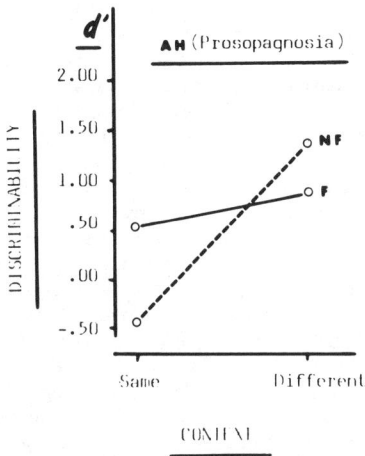

FIGURE 6 - Discriminability parameter (d'), by strength of semantic associa-tion between test and study contexts, and face familiarity for the prosopag-nosic patient A.H. (Tiberghien & Clerc, 1985).

interaction between familiarity and context in his case. Results like this pose a difficult problem of interpretation for any theory that aims at explaining prosopagnosia by the malfunctioning of processes of represent-ation, encoding or retrieval of contextual information (Damasio, 1985; A. Damasio, H. Damsio & Van Hoesen, 1982; Huppert & Piercy, 1982; O'Keefe & Nadel, 1978; for an overview; Mayes, Meudell & Pickering, 1985; Stern, 1981; Wickelgren, 1979; Winocur & Kinsbourne, 1978). They also raise difficulties for any theory that tries to explain the syndrome by the disturbance of a mechanism of estimation of familiarity of the face to be recognized (Blanc-Garin, 1984; Gaffan, 1976). Further, such data throws serious doubt on the hypothesis of complete independence of context and familiarity variables (Bartlett, Hurry & Thorley, 1984). In fact it seems impossible to explain these results without assuming that familiarity of context and that of the face interact to give rise to an overall feeling of familiarity. We have already mentioned this "bias" effect of context in an attempt to interpret the contradictory context effects for false recognition. The origin of A.H.'s functional difficulties could lie in his incapacity to dissociate in the overall feeling of familiarity what is due to context familiarity and what is due to that of the face (see Luaute, Bidault & Thionville, 1978, p.808). This relative estimation of familiarity would be made easier if the recognition contexts were different from that of study since the familiarity of the "old" face would then be easily discernible. Association with an unchanged (therefore familiar) context obviously reinforces the overall feeling of familiarity and thus facilitates recognition; on the contrary association of an unchanged (familiar) context with a non-familiar face creates a discrimination conflict in the estimation of the origin of the feeling of familiarity. We have a quite symetrical situation when it is the context that changes.

These neuropsychological investigations point up the theoretical importance of research into the possibly differential nature of processing of focal and contextual information by the two brain hemispheres, Semnes (1968) argued in favour of a hypothesis of differential neuronal organisation for each hemisphere : the left hemisphere being characterized by highly focalized representation of elementary, sensory and motor functions, the right by more general, overall, diffuse, vague representation. If this hypothesis is correct there should be clear repercussions on the processing of focal and contextual information. As far as we know not much systematic investigation has been done in this direction. However Versace (1983) did obtain suggestive results on normal subjects by using a tachistoscopic paradigm which made it possible to present focal information (Christian name) in the right or left visual field accompanied or not by a context (face) in the right or left visual field, this context could be retained or not at testing and presented in the same or different visual half-field. The author shows that memory recognition is optimal when focal information is studied in the right visual field, recognition not being affected by the half-field used for testing. He shows moreover that when recognition takes place in the presence of a context it is always better when focal information appears in the same visual half-field in study and recognition testing. It is therefore not impossible that there may be a complex interaction between the process of contextualisation and the relative specialisation of brain hemispheres. If such turned out to be the case it is obvious that this would have to be taken into account in the interpretation of respective roles of hemispheres in memory recognition. All the more so in view of the fact that the status of focal information and contextual information has obvious repercussions on their perceptual processing and in particular on the extraction of utilisable spatial frequencies (Sergent, 1984, 1985a, 1985b; Versace & Tiberghien, 1985).

7. CONCLUSIONS

The existence of context effects in memory recognition in general and in face recognition in particular has today been well established experimentally. The aim of research is now to give an account of the dynamics of these context effects and of their role in the general functioning of human memory. Face recognition can probably be achieved in two distinct ways: either by a highly rapid and automatic predecision process giving rise to an overall feeling of familiarity or non-familiarity accompanied by a high degree of subjective certainty. The efficiency of this process depends essentially on the familiarity of the face and is only secondarily affected by context, the familiarity of which may however interact with face familiarity and thus contribute to the resulting overall feeling of familiarity. This "bias" introduced by context familiarity is probably relatively slight when the familiarity of the face is higher (known, famous faces) but can become more marked when the face is unknown or unfamiliar but must be recognized in a familiar context. This probably explains the often contradictory effect of context on false recognition, an effect well known to psychologists working on problems of eye-witness testimony in legal proceedings, and known as "unconscious transference" (H.D. Ellis, Davies & Shepherd, 1977; Loftus, 1975). Rejection of this principle would mean throwing doubt on the principle of encoding specificity, as indeed a new face, not having been previously encoded, should therefore never benefit from facilitation effect of an old context with which precisely it has never been associated.

The second mode of face recognition much more closely resembles an activity of mental reconstruction guided by context. It occurs when the predecision process has failed and consists in an attempt to retrieve the original encoding context on the basis of the present recognition context. This conditional memory search is mainly affected by the context and its episodic and semantic properties. The existence of a general or specific semantic relation between recognition and study contexts is a decisive factor of the success of this type of search. The degree of interaction of face and context is also an important factor in the emergence of these context effects since, according to the degree of attention the subjects accords it, it determines the success or failure of retrieval of the original encoding situation. The strength of action - inhibiting or facilitating - of an independent context depends much more on the orientation of attention and the depth of processing to which perceptual data is subjected. In any case, in a given recognition situation, there is probably and ecological hierarchy of perceptual and semantic cues and the activity of the subject is greatly modulated by changes in cues which rank highly in this hierarchy. However if the existence of a semantic link between recognition and study context is a critical condition of the probability of success of the memory search process guided by context, this analysis applies in the strict sense to old faces alone. Indeed when a new face is associated with an old context search activity can very well lead to retrieval of the representation of the whole set of original study conditions and to the recognition of the fact that the context was accompanied by a different face from the one perceptually available - the lure. In other words, for old faces a change of context, by preventing retrieval of the old context and thus lowering the overall sense of familiarity of the recognition situation has a cumulative strongly inhibiting effect on performance. On the contrary, for new faces, an old context may prevent a false recognition by making it possible for the subject to retrieve the face formerly associated with the context; but it can also increase the probability of a false recognition by raising the overall familiarity of the recognition situation. Probabilistic mixture of these two factors makes it possible to understand the remarkable stability of context effects for correct responses (hits) and the considerable instability of context effects in false recognition.

This analysis throws doubt on the postulate according to which familiarity depends solely on the frequency of earlier experiences and is independent of the context of these experiences (Bartlett et al., 1984; Mandler, 1980). The interaction between context and familiarity observed in the prosopagnosia of A.H. could justify such a doubt. It seems that there are three fundamental problems which have been relatively neglected of recent years the solution of which would be theoretically decisive:

a) Classical research has so far opposed familiar and non-familiar faces and it is clear that context effects only massively influence the latter (Davies & Milnes, 1982; Klatzsy & Forrest, 1984), but to my knowledge context familiarity has never been systematically controlled, which could be justified only if we consider there is no interaction between context and familiarity. However, in a verbal learning situation, Malmi (1977) has shown that the increase of context frequency improves the hits percent and interacts with the target frequency (see also; Hintzman & Stern, 1978). The existence of interaction between familiarity and context was suggested by Mandler (1972, pp.141-142) since he considers that "we recognize a person we met the day before on the sole basis of currency information but we recognize the face of someone not seen for several years only on the basis of a search involving contexts and categories". We have presented some experimental data which gives evidence in support of the hypothesis of an interaction between these two factors;

b) Furthermore, in classical memory face recognition situations, context and face familiarity must be combined in a complex manner to produce the overall feeling of familiarity (Rheingold, 1985, p.15). Is absolute estimation of this overall familiarity sufficient to induce relevant recognition or does the individual need to be capable of estimating relative familiarity i.e. the respective contributions of the different elements of the situation to the overall feeling? The prosopagnosia case we presented shows that a distinction of this sort can have considerable theoretical relevance;

c) Finally, the concept of familiarity is today still rather poorly defined since it can be just as easily taken to refer to ecphory similarity (Tulving, 1981), or situational frequency of an experience, or production of associations or situational recency (Morton, 1981, p.231). We can moreover ask if there are not several types of familiarity: it is not certain that repeated presentation of a face in an unchanging context gives rise to the same feeling of familiarity as that produced by repeated presentation of the same face in varying contexts. In the first case the resulting facial representation is highly dependent on contexts and we can be tempted in this case to speak of "episodic" familiarity; in the second case the resulting facial representation becomes relatively independent from context by very reason of its equivocality and here one can be led to refer to "semantic" familiarity. This reasoning concurs with the proposition of Jacoby & Witherspoon (1982) who consider the distinction between episodic and semantic memory should be referred back to a continuum of greater or less sensitivity to contextual influences. This way of interpreting the role of familiarity also concurs with the viewpoint of Thomson, Robertson & Vogt (1982, experience 5, p.148) who demonstrate experimentally that for non-familiar faces it is the context which defines the person. Besides which, the concept of contextualisation could account rather neatly for the transformation of episodic face representation into semantic. Viewed from this angle the structure of face representations is perhaps much closer to that of verbal representations than to that of objects and scenes since the contextual specificity of possible occurrences of these events (words, faces, objects, scenes) rises along a continuum of which the limits would be the extreme degrees of contextual autonomy and dependence. The greater or lesser degree to which experimental data is affected by contextual influences probably largely accounts for observed differences in recognition of words, faces, objects and scenes (Deffenbacher, Carr & Leu, 1981). For the moment therefore nothing justifies the postulation of a specific system for the representation and retrieval of faces (see; H.D. Ellis, 1975; Hay & Young, 1982).

4. COGNITIVE PROCESSES

RECOGNISING FAMILIAR FACES

V. BRUCE

1. INTRODUCTION

Much of the research in the area of face recognition has explored the processing of and memory for previously unfamiliar faces. Such research has provided us with important information about hemispheric specialisation in face processing (Ellis, 1983, and Rhodes, 1985 give reviews), the kinds of visual information which might be extracted from faces (e.g. see Sergent, 1984, and this volume), and, of most applied relevance, the factors which may influence an eyewitness's ability to identify a suspect from a line-up or photograph file (see review by Deffenbacher & Horney, 1981). However, such research in isolation cannot tell us about the cognitive processes involved when we recognise a _familiar_ face. Experiments on letter recognition or memory for nonsense syllables do not reveal semantic levels of processing which are involved in word recognition, nor do they inform us of the relationship between perceptual and semantic classification. In the same way, by studying only the processing of unfamiliar faces we will not learn about the totality of perceptual and cognitive processes which operate when we recognise the faces of our friends.

I have argued this often and have been accused by our host (e.g. Ellis, 1981) of likening unfamiliar faces to nonsense syllables, and faces to words. The first comparison is not a valid one, though I do think that studying the processing of unfamiliar faces may be analogous to studying the processing of complex neologisms, which a reader must attempt to interpret in terms of knowledge of known words. The second analogy, between familiar face recognition and word recognition, I am to clarify in this paper.

There are two distinct senses in which one can claim that comparisons can be made between face and word recognition. Firstly, I will argue that to get to grips (theoretically) with face recognition requires the same methods and conceptual tools which have proved successful in tackling the word recognition problem. Thus, while much in the literature on remembering unfamiliar faces is concerned with effects of such variables as exposure duration, list-length and delay. In my own work on the recognition of familiar faces I have been interested in the effects of recent exposure to the face, or to the face of a closely associated person. Rather than record percent correctly recognised, in my work the dependent variable of interest is generally the latency with which a judgement of familiarity can be made, in tasks resembling the lexical decision task much-loved in research into word recognition. Secondly, and perhaps more contentiously, I will argue that the similarities which are observed between the results obtained with words and with faces in similar studies, point to important similarities in the kinds of cognitive processes which deal with these very different types of material. There are differences too, and models of the face recognition process must accommodate both these similarities and these differences.

Over the past ten years I have conducted experiments on familiar face recognition in which I have examined:

a) The processes involved in searching for specified targets;
b) Repetition effects in face recognition (Identity priming); and
c) Semantic priming.

In this paper I will first briefly review the results I have obtained in each of these three areas, and then describe in more detail a recent experiment in which the time course of identity priming is compared with that of semantic priming.

2. REVIEW OF RESEARCH RESULTS

2.1. Semantic influences in search for specified targets

It has often been observed in studies of verbal processing that when a subject is required to make a decision which logically requires scrutiny only of a word's physical characteristics, semantic information can influence performance. The classic demonstration of this is the Stroop effect.

In a slightly different situation, where subjects are required to find a specified target word amongst an array of other words (Henderson & Chard, 1978) or decide to each of a series of words whether it is one of a specified target set (Bruce, 1981), the semantic characteristics of distractor items can also influence decision time, even though at an intuitive level, such influences should be redundant. For example, if one is searching for the words OAK and ELM, on encountering the distractor item MAPLE, sufficient evidence of its physical features should have been accrued to reject it as a target before a full semantic representation has been accessed.

An experiment of my own (Bruce, 1981) serves as an example here, and investigates the relative importance of visual and semantic similarity between distractor items and the target set in a serial classification task. Subjects were presented with a series of words and non-words and required to respond positively if each was one of the set RAT, DOG, MOLE or BOAR. The typeface and case of targets and distractors were varied, so that subjects could not look simply for a constant pattern of letters. Some of the distractor items were visually similar to the target words, while others were dissimilar. Some were other animal names, while others were unrelated, or non-words.

I found that rejection latency was influenced both by visual similarity (words like RAG and BOG took longer to reject than COAT or SIREN), and by semantic similarity (CAT and HOG took longer to reject than RAG and BOG), but that there was no interaction between these factors. The semantic similarity effect was as great for visually dissimilar as for similar words. There was, however, no effect of familiarity per se. Non-animal words and non-words were rejected equally quickly.

Such a result is not consistent with a model of the rejection process which involves first checking the visual features of each encountered item and then checking its meaning only if the first tests fail to confirm or disconfirm the presence of a target item. However, if we suppose that the visual feature checking process induced by the subject's task continues alongside automatic recognition of target words via the mental lexicon, and that both send outputs to a central decision process, then such effects can be adequately accounted for. One must only assume in addition that activation spreads from the lexical representations of target items to those of closely associated items to explain the semantic similarity effects here. There will therefore be a tendency to respond 'yes' wrongly) to related distractor items, due to the lowered thresholds for recognition of such items, so that more extensive visual feature analysis must be applied in order to compensate and successfully reject such items. The proposal that lexical representations might be 'primed' for recognition through processes of 'spreading activation' is quite common in the literature on word recognition (cf. Collins & Loftus, 1975; Meyer, Schvaneveldt & Ruddy, 1975).

The experiment I have described with words followed up a similar one that I had conducted earlier with faces (Bruce, 1979, experiment 2). In the faces task, subjects viewed a series of faces, some familiar and others not, and had to respond positively when there appeared any one of four specified target politicians (whose poses varied from one occurrence to another). Rejection latencies were slowed if distractors were visually similar to targets, and if they were other politicians, but the two effects were independent. There was no effect of familiarity per se. Non-politicians took the same time to reject as unfamiliar faces. The interpretation of such results is similar to that offered for the effects in word recognition. Scrutiny of individual features of each face for remembered characteristics of the target faces proceeds in parallel with automatic recognition of target faces via the 'lexicon' of face representations.

In 1982 Hay and Young published a model of face recognition in which they explicitly suggested that faces might be recognised via a set of face recognition units somewhat analogous to logogens, (Morton, 1969, 1979) which mediate access of semantic information about personal identity held in a separate store. Such a suggestion provides an explicit mechanism to mediate the semantic effects in visual search tasks. The subject's concentration on detecting the faces of the familiar politician targets leads to lowered thresholds in the face recognition units corresponding to these items. This attention to the targets, and the frequent recognition of the politicians, will lead to activation spreading to related nodes in semantic memory and thereby lowering the thresholds to faces of related people.

Over the last two years I have tried to test further the analogy between face recognition units and logogens by exploring whether the results in different experimental situations are consistent with the predictions of a model of the logogen type.

2.2. Repetition effects (Identity priming)

Morton (1969, 1979) has tested and extended his theory of word recognition by exploring the way in which prior exposure to an item facilitates later recognition of that same item. In the logogen model, each lexical representation of a word (more strictly, morpheme) has a threshold which must be exceeded for recognition to occur. Once fired, the threshold is lowered, and only slowly returns to a value just below its original one (thus accounting for word frequency effects in the long term). It should therefore be easier to recognise the same word again soon after an initial encounter compared with a condition where no such earlier encounter has taken place.

Such results are indeed obtained (e.g. Neisser, 1954; Winnick & Daniel, 1970). Earlier exposure to a written word facilitates its later recognition, even in a quite different typeface (Clarke & Morton, 1983). However, naming a picture does not facilitate later recognition of the word (Winnick & Daniel, 1970; Morton, 1979), and hearing a word has less of an effect than reading it (Clarke & Morton, 1983) which led Morton (1979) to suggest that there were separate input recognition systems for heard words, seen words and pictures. Following from this, Warren & Morton (1982) examined identity priming in picture recognition, and found that there was no facilitation of picture recognition through prior naming of the word which labelled the pictured object. However, earlier presentation of the same or a different picture of an object led to reduced thresholds in later tachistoscopic recognition of these pictures, compared to a control condition in which there was no prior exposure of any kind.

The observation that the degree of facilitation obtained in the 'different' picture condition was uncorrelated with the degree of difference between the two pictures used (as rated by other subjects), led Warren and Morton to attribute the effect to priming at the level of 'pictogens' – threshold devices which respond when any pictorial instance of their represented category is presented. Warren and Morton attributed the additional advantage of retesting with same pictures (compared with different) to an additional, pictorial memory component.

Bruce & Valentine (1985) conducted an analogous experiment using famous faces. When recognition in the test phase was measured in terms of tachistoscopic recognition thresholds, the results departed from those of Warren and Morton, showing facilitation following earlier presentation of a celebrity's name as well as from his or her face. However, since the criterion for correct recognition in the tachistoscope was correct naming of the famous person, it is perhaps not surprising to discover that earlier reading of this name is facilitatory. Face names, unlike object names, pose significant retrieval demands. We therefore moved to a different kind of test phase in which familiarity decisions were required to each of a series of faces. Here there was no requirement for subjects to name faces at test. Half of the test series were familiar faces, and of these, some were novel (control), some were the faces of people whose names had been read 20 minutes earlier, some were different pictures of people whose faces had been named earlier, and some were the same pictures of the rest of those faces.

Results of the second of two experiments making use of this methodology showed a non-significant difference between the name and control conditions, and significant facilitation of 80 msecs in the different condition and 139 msecs in the same condition. Like Warren and Morton, we found no correlation between facilitation in the different condition and the rated similarity between the pairs of pictures used.

This result is therefore consistent with facilitation at the level of face recognition units, which are not accessed by names, and which selectively respond to individual faces in any view. Like Warren and Morton, we attribute the additional advantage of same compared with different conditions to a pictorial memory component. Here there is one contrast with the word recognition literature, where there is little difference in the facilitation obtained from words in the same or a different typeface (Clarke & Morton, 1983; see also Scarborough, Cortese & Scarborough, 1977).

It seems reasonable that one should pay attention to, and hence retain details of the particular instance of an object seen. Warren and Morton's task involved recognition at a basic level (Rosch et al., 1976), but one needs to know, not just that a 'dog' was seen, but what kind of dog, and whether it looked friendly or hostile. Likewise, for face recognition, while recognising a person's face irrespective of view is an important task, we need also to pay attention to the particular view of a face to assess its expression, attentiveness, and so forth. In comparison, details of a particular typescript are relatively unimportant to most readers, except perhaps when proof-reading or identifying a particular, known handwriting.

2.3. Semantic priming in face recognition

In the logogen model, an appropriate context should facilitate word recognition by lowering the thresholds of the logogens corresponding to contextually appropriate words following processes of spreading activation within the cognitive system (where semantic representations are held). Many demonstrations of facilitation by appropriate prior context can be found in the literature on word recognition. Specifically, in lexical decison tasks, it has frequently been shown that subjects are faster to decide that a given letter string is a word if it is immediately preceded by a semantically related word (e.g. NURSE preceded by DOCTOR) than if preceded by an unrelated word (NURSE preceded by BUTTER) (e.g. Meyer et al., 1975; Neely, 1976; De Groot, 1984).

In an earlier paper (Bruce, 1983) I presented the first demonstration of a similar effect in face recognition. As in lexical decision, subjects were required to make a series of familiarity judgements (respond yes if familiar, no if unfamiliar) to each of a sequence of faces which appeared one every 5 secs. Embedded within this series, unknown to the subjects, were ten 'critical' faces (target items). Five of these were familiar targets preceded by appropriate 'partners' (e.g. the face of Ernie Wise preceded by that of Eric Morecambe: the two form a well-known British comedy duo). The other five were control items which were familiar targets preceded by unrelated familiar faces. The faces which appeared in the 'related' and 'unrelated' conditions were rotated between subgroups of subjects. Familiarity decisions to faces preceded by related items were made on average 126 msecs faster than judgements to those same items when preceded by unrelated faces.

Bruce and Valentine (in press) have proceeded to explore this in more detail. In these experiments we moved to a situation in which prime faces (e.g. Prince Charles) and target faces (e.g. Princess Diana) were explicitly presented in pairs, with a response required to the second member of each pair only. This allowed us to include a neutral prime condition against which to assess the effects of both related and unrelated primes, and also to reduce substantially the prime-target stimulus-onset asynchrony (SOA) in order to explore the time course of any facilitatory effects (cf. Neely, 1976; De Groot, 1984). In our first experiment we showed that significant facilitation (related condition faster than neutral) and no inhibition (unrelated condition equal to neutral) was present for SOA's of 250, 500 and 1000 msec. There was a (non-significant) trend towards greater facilitation with increasing SOA.

The facilitation observed at 250 msec is consistent with a priming effect mediated by 'automatic' processes of spreading activation. In terms of Hay & Young's (1982) model, this could operate as follows. Recognition of the prime face leads to activation spreading to related nodes within semantic memory, which may in turn lead to the lowering of the thresholds of face recognition units corresponding to contextually appropriate faces. Further evidence for the priming effect operating at a relatively early stage in face processing was given by an experiment in which a priming effect of greater magnitude was obtained when target items were blurred. An interaction between stimulus quality and semantic priming has also been found in the literature on word recognition (e.g. Meyer et al., 1975).

The results of such experiments on identity and semantic priming strengthen the analogy between word recognition and face recognition in two ways. Firstly, we have shown that the two kinds of material give similar results in tasks making similar cognitive demands. Secondly, the result obtained with both kinds of material are compatible with models of recognition in which recognition units mediate between the visual analysis of an encountered item and the access of its semantic representation.

In the next section of this paper I turn to describe in more detail a recent experiment which further strengthens the analogy between face and word recognition in terms of the similarity of the results obtained, while at the same time posing problems for the simple explanation of both the identity and semantic priming effects in terms of threshold lowering in face recognition units.

3. THE TIME COURSE OF IDENTITY AND SEMANTIC PRIMING

3.1. Introduction

The experiments by Bruce & Valentine (1985) have shown that significant identity primig is found with delays of 20 minutes or more between the first and second presentation of a familiar face. The experiments by Bruce (1983) and Bruce & Valentine (in press) have shown semantic priming between related faces operating at intervals of 5 seconds or less. If both effects are explicable through reduced thresholds in recognition units, then we might expect the effects to decay in similar ways over time.

Dannenbring & Briand (1982) made use of this logic to compare the time course of semantic priming and the repetition effect in word recognition, by using a lexical decision task. Decision times to individual items in their experiment were examined as a function of the type of earlier exposure that had been given, and the lag between first and second exposure. Words were either novel (no prior exposure) or had earlier been preceded by the same word (repetition) or a related item (semantic priming). Non-words were also either novel or were repeated. The lag between first and second presentation of repeated items, or associatively related pairs, was varied from 0 intervening slides (about 4 secs, depending on subjects' decision latency), through 1, 5 and 16 intervening slides (about 8, 20 and 64 secs). Dannenbring and Briand found that there was a significant repetition effect at all lags tested, with no evidence of this diminishing as lag was increased. In contrast, semantic priming was smaller in size, and only significant at lag 0. Dannenbring and Briand use their results to question contemporary accounts of semantic priming (Posner and Snyder, 1975) and word recognition (Morton, 1979). If repetition of an item leads directly to threshold reduction, and presentation of a related item leads indirectly (via the semantic system) to threshold reduction, then the effects of this threshold reduction should be the same whatever the delay between members of a 'pair'. Semantic priming effects might be smaller than repetition effects (due to activation spreading diffusely within the semantic system and thus leading to small effects on the thresholds of several items), but it should not decay differentially. In addition, Dannenbring and Briand's replication of an often-observed repetition effect for non-words poses further problems for a model of this kind.

We conducted an analogous experiment to compare the time course of semantic and identity priming in the recognition of familiar faces. There were some differences in our procedure which were necessary due to the small pool of stimulus items we used. Lag was varied between groups of subjects, and we did not investigate repetition effects for unfamiliar faces.

3.2. Method

3.2.1. Subjects: Our final sample of subject comprised 64 members of the general public recruited by local advertisement to take part in other, human factors, experiments. Subjects were discarded and replaced where they were insufficiently familiar with the target faces used or if they had unduly long decision times (see results for the criteria of accuracy and latency used).

3.2.2. Materials: Pictures of familiar faces were obtained from a wide variety of sources: magazines, photographic libraries etc. We selected 20 target items for the experiment, each available in two different views, and for each of which an associated face was available (e.g. target Prince Charles, associate Princess Diana). Each pair of related items was then put together with a third, unrelated item to serve as 'prime' in the control condition (e.g. target Prince Charles, associate Princess Diana, unrelated Magnus Pike, a popular television scientist). The familiar faces used are listed in the Appendix.

Of the 20 related pairs used, associative strengths were available for 19 of them. These were obtained independently by asking 16 student subjects to write down, to each of a series of names, any other names that each reminded them of. The target items used here were mentioned as primary associates to the primes used on an average of 66% of occasions.

A further five familiar filler items were also obtained, and 60 unfamiliar faces were obtained from the same sources as the familiar faces. A further 20 familiar and unfamiliar faces were obtained for use in practice trials.

All faces were copied through a circular mask which excluded most of the background and clothing, to form 35 mm monochrome slides.

3.2.3. Design: The test series comprised 120 slides, presented in two blocks of 60 slides each (each preceded by 10 practice items). Within the 120 experimental trials, each subject saw five of the target faces in each of four conditions:

a) Control: The target was immediately preceded by an unrelated familiar face.

b) Related: The target was preceded by a related familiar face.

c) Identity (diff): The target was preceded by a different picture of the same person.

d) Identity (same): The target was preceded by the same picture of the same person.

Faces were rotated around conditions a–d so that all faces appeared in all conditions between subgroups of four subjects.

For each of the non-control conditions b–d, the lag between presentation of first and second members of a pair was varied between groups of 16 subjects. At lag 0 (5 secs), targets immediately followed the appropriate partners. At lag 1 (10 secs) there was one intervening slide which was always an unrelated familiar face (to allow comparison with the control condition). At lags 3 and 11 (20 secs and 60 secs respectively) there were 3 and 11 intervening slides, but again the one which immediately preceded the target was always an unrelated familiar face. Thus targets were always preceded by a familiar face, so that there was response repetition in all conditions. What varied was whether there had been an earlier presentation of the same or a related person, and how far back this had occurred. (Repetitions always occurred within a block of 60 experimental trials).

A single slide order was generated for all subjects at one lag, such that pairs were placed unsystematically within the sequence of unfamiliar and filler familiar items, and that long runs of familiar and unfamiliar faces were avoided. At lag 0, all other unrelated familiar faces (from targets in conditions b to d) plus the five filler items were used along with unfamiliar items to fill up the sequence. At the other three lags, only the familiar fillers and the unfamiliar items were free to vary in position once the pairs had been placed. Variation in slide order between subjects was created first by the rotation of target items around conditions, and second by reversing the order of blocks of slides between pairs of subjects.

The dependent variable of interest was the time to respond positively to the 20 target items as a function of condition and lag.

3.2.4. Apparatus: Slides were projected onto a white wall in front of the subjects from a Kodak SAV 2020 projector controlled by a Rockwell AIM-65 microcomputer. This was interfaced to a purpose-built group-testing apparatus with its own hardware clock, which allowed both decisions and latencies (1 msec accuracy) to be recorded from more than one subject simultaneously. Subjects signalled their responses via silent touch-sensitive push-buttons, to minimise competition between subjects tested together. The microcomputer was programmed to present each slide for 2 secs, followed by a 3 sec interval (total slide-onset asynchrony was 5 secs) and to record as void any responses whose latencies exceeded 2000 msec from the onset of a slide. Faces subtended about 5 degs. visual angle at the subject's seat.

3.2.5. <u>Procedure</u>: Subjects were tested singly or in pairs. They were each given two push-buttons to signal 'yes' and 'no', and instructed to press these firmly to obtain tactile feedback. They were instructed that they would see a series of faces, one every five seconds, and that they were to press 'yes' if they recognised the face and 'no' if they did not. They were asked to press one or other button as quickly as possible without sacrificing accuracy, and were also warned that faces might sometimes be repeated. A short break was given between the two blocks of trials, while slide magazines were exchanged and the computer reset. Each block was preceded with 10 practice trials to allow for warm-up effects.

3.3 <u>Results</u>

Our pool of subjects showed great variation in age and produced decisions of variable speed and accuracy. Without inspecting latencies, we discarded and replaced any subject who made more than two errors (out of max. five) to targets in any of the four conditions of interest. This ensured that three correct response latencies were available to calculate a subject mean latency in each condition. We also discarded and replaced a further nine subjects whose average latency in any cell exceeded 1500 msecs.

The mean response latency to recognise familiar targets correctly in each condition of the experiment was calculated and the group means are shown in Table 1.

TABLE 1. Group mean response latencies (msec) and total errors (in brackets) in each condition.

| Condition: | Control | Related | Identity | |
			Diff picture	Same picture
LAG				
0	1039 (10)	952 (2)	945 (6)	856 (6)
1	1027 (7)	992 (4)	957 (4)	873 (4)
3	1036 (10)	1023 (9)	901 (8)	935 (7)
11	975 (9)	959 (6)	802 (4)	765 (4)

A 4 (lag) x 4 (subject group) x 4 (target condition) mixed design analysis of variance was conducted on the subject mean response times in each condition. This showed a highly significant effect of prime type ($F(3,44) = 32.22$, $p < 0.0001$) and a significant interaction between lag and prime type ($F(9,144) = 1.96$, $p < 0.05$). Two further interactions involving subject group were also significant. There was a significant interaction with prime type ($F(3,144) = 3.23$, $p < 0.01$), suggesting some variability in the recognisability of targets in the four different groups of slides (cf. Bruce, 1983). The three way interaction was also significant ($F(27,144) = 1.64$, $p < 0.05$). There is clearly then some variability in the effects from subgroup to subgroup. Given that each subgroup comprised only four subjects, and that each slide group consisted of only five slides, this is perhaps not too surprising. The effect of lag was not significant (p = 0.14) despite the trend in Table 1, where subjects in the lag 11 condition appear to be responding more quickly than those in the other three conditions.

Our main interest is in the interaction between lag and prime type. Given the significant interaction between these factors, we went on to compare each condition (b-d) with control, separately at each level of lag, using the within-subjects error term from the overall analysis of variance. For each of these planned comparisons, we calculated the one-tailed probability and compared this with a criterion of p = 0.05/3 = 0.017, in order to adjust the criterion of significance for the three comparisons made at each level of lag. Following such analysis, the pattern of significant effects is as shown in Table 2.

Examining this table, we find that there are significant effects of identity priming in all but one case (different picture at lag 1), where the effect is marginal. There is certainly no evidence of any reduction in the identity priming over the range of lags tested.

TABLE 2. Mean difference (msec) between each condition and control. (* = p ~ 0.017; ** = p ~ 0.002; *** = p ~ 0.0002)

| Condition | Related | Identity | |
		Diff picture	Same picture
LAG			
0	87 *	94 *	183 ***
1	35 n.s.	70(p = 0.02)	154 ***
3	13 n.s.	135 ***	101 **
11	16 n.s.	173 ***	210 ***

Like Bruce & Valentine (in press) we find that there is generally greater identity priming from same pictures compared with different pictures. In contrast to the persistent effects of repetition, there is a significant effect of semantic priming only at lag 0.

3.4. Discussion

This experiment has shown that semantic priming of familiar faces does not persist beyond 5 secs SOA, in a situation where longer intervals are filled with intervening slides. Repetition effects, in contrast, are robust and persistent over the 60 second interval tested here. These results therefore mirror those obtained by Dannenbring and Briand in lexical decision.

The semantic priming found at lag 0 is rather smaller in size than that reported by Bruce (1983) using 5 secs SOA (average 126 msec). However, Bruce & Valentine (in press, Experiment 3) used the same face pairs as those tested above (though not all tested in the same order of associate and target), and found a difference of 97 msec between related and unrelated conditions at 1000 msec SOA, which is very comparable with the 87 msecs found here. The small size of the semantic priming effect obtained here might be due to the relative rarity of related pairs among the sequence of slides presented to subjects. In only five out of 60 familiar faces had an associate been recently seen. This would probably serve to minimise, or eliminate completely, any effects of conscious anticipatory strategies on the part of the subjects, which might contribute to semantic priming effects at longer SOAs and in situations where there is high cue-validity (cf. Posner & Snyder, 1975; de Groot, 1984).

While it could be argued that a 'weak' semantic effect is more likely to dissipate quickly than a 'strong' repetition effect, we must note that the size of the effect in the Identity (different) condition was comparable with the semantic priming effect at lag 0, and was only marginally significant at lag 1.   Nevertheless, we were able to show clear evidence of identity priming at the longer lags tested.

One way in which to accommodate the apparently different effects of semantic and identity priming is to propose that they stem from different components of the face recognition system, with identity priming seen as a face recognition unit effect, and semantic priming requiring a post-access explanation.   Such a position would entail that we abandon Hay & Young's (1982) position that face familiarity decisions can be made purely on the basis of activity within the face recognition units.

Recently, Andy Young and his colleagues (Young, Hay & Ellis, in press; Bruce & Young, in prep) have suggested that face recognition units be seen, not as threshold devices, but as devices which signal the degree of resemblance between their input and the face whose representation they hold. These 'resemblance activators' would send outputs to a central decision process.   Such a modified mechanism could still accommodate repetition effects through modification of the overall firing level of a face recognition unit.   Contextual effects, however, might be seen as operating via the decision process, rather than directly influencing the activity within face recognition units.   Such a conception of recognition units clearly departs from the original logogen type, but may be worth developing further in order to explain satisfactorily the pattern of results obtained in priming studies using faces and also those using words.

4. GENERAL DISCUSSION

This paper has covered a range of experimental results in which results are found in the processing of familiar faces which strongly mirror those found in the literature on word recognition.   Perhaps our results simply reflect explicit naming of the faces?

We think not.   Note that in identity priming (Bruce & Valentine, 1985), exposure to the name of a celebrity does not influence subsequent familiarity decisions to a face.   This suggests that subjects do not need to name faces in order to respond in such speeded familiarity decision tasks. Decisions which require faces to be named are made much more slowly than those which require familiarity judgements (Young et al., in prep. and Young, this volume), and naming faces is a notoriously error-prone process (Young et al., in press).   We think the similarities in recognition of faces and words reflect something more interesting than verbal mediation of face recognition processes.

Our position is that the similarities observed reflect fundamental similarities in the way in which processes of perceptual classification and semantic classification are organised with respect to each other.   The 'recognition unit' metaphor has proved useful in understanding such processes, although as we have seen, it encounters difficulties in accommodating the full pattern of priming effects.

5. ACKNOWLEDGEMENTS

The research described in this paper has been supported by a grant from the Economic and Social Research Council (ref. HR8757). Tim Valentine and Deborah Hellawell collected the data in the main experiment reported here.

6. APPENDIX: Familiar faces, associates and unrelated items. (Some of the names given are those of fictitious characters, where these are more familiar than the actors or actresses who play them.)

TARGET	ASSOCIATE	UNRELATED
Sue Ellen	J.R.	Margaret Thatcher
Sid Little	Eddie Large	Liza Minelli
Bobby Ball	Tommy Cannon	David Bellamy
Felicity Kendall	Richard Briers	Marilyn Monroe
Terry Scott	June Whitfield	Sue Lawley
Jayne Torvill	Chris Dean	Meryl Streep
Stan Laurel	Oliver Hardy	Noel Edmonds
Ernie Wise	Eric Morecambe	Dennis Healey
Captain Kirk	Mr Spock	Woody Allen
Prince Philip	The Queen	Jan Leeming
Bodie	Doyle	Cliff Richard
Prince Charles	Princess Diana	Magnus Pike
Ronnie Corbett	Ronnie Barker	Michael Foot
George Cole	Dennis Waterman	Ronald Reagan
David Steel	David Owen	Jimmy Saville
Sebastian Coe	Steve Ovett	John Wayne
Larry Grayson	Isla StClare	Elvis Presley
Roger Moore	Sean Connery	John Cleese
Jimmy Connors	Bjorn Borg	Terry Wogan
Paul Newman	Robert Redford	Michael Parkinson

FACE RECOGNITION : MORE THAN A FEELING OF FAMILIARITY?

D.M. THOMSON

1. INTRODUCTION
The object of this paper is the resolution of apparent contradictory claims emanating from infant and child studies of face recognition. Findings of infant studies suggest that by seven months of age the infant possesses sophisticated skills in face recognition (Cohen, Deloache & Pearl, 1977; Fagan, 1972, 1973, 1976, 1977). Fagan (1976) claimed that seven month-old infants are able to recognise a photograph of a face after having previously observed a photograph which depicted that face from a different angle. In contrast, findings from child studies suggest that initially the recognition system is not very proficient and it is only during adolescence that it reaches adult proficiency (Carey, 1981; Carey, Diamond & Woods, 1980; Diamond & Carey, 1977; Flin, 1980; Thomson, 1984). Diamond & Carey (1977) have shown that children under the age of 10 years experienced great difficulty in recognizing a photograph of a person when that person was wearing different headgear. Thomson (1984) found age and context effects on person recognition interacted.
It is argued that the apparent contradictions can be attributed to the failure to distinguish between different meanings of face recognition and the use of different experimental paradigms. It is proposed that the findings of infant and child studies can be incorporated within a three-process model of face recognition

1.1. Meanings of face recognition
Four different meanings of face recognition can be distinguished. The first meaning of face recognition concerns whether the observer knows that a particular shape or form is that of a face. The second meaning of recognition has to do with whether the observer knows that a particular face has been seen before. The third meaning is similar to the second but it is not just whether the observer knows that a particular face was seen before but whether it was seen before at a particular time or place. The fourth meaning of face recognition refers to the observer's knowledge of the name or identity of the face. It is with the second and third meanings, knowing a face has been seen before, that is the concern of this paper.
Two other uses of the word recognition can be distinguished. Recognition may be used in the sense that the perceiver decides, whatever the basis, that he or she has perceived that face or object before. The second use of the word recognition is when the term is used as a synonym for a feeling of familiarity. It is argued that the latter meaning should be avoided, the observer may know that he or she has seen the face or object before in the absence of feeling of familiarity and, conversely, the observer may know that he or she has not seen the face or object before even when that face or object evokes feelings of familiarity in the observer.

2. FACE RECOGNITION AND IDENTITY CONSTANCY

Attainment of identity constancy would appear to be a necessary precondition for face recognition. Identity constancy refers to the knowledge that a face is still the same face despite the fact that that face may look quite different. Piaget (1954) and Bruner (1966) have noted that very young children respond to transformed objects as if those transformed objects were different objects even when the children have the opportunity of observing the transformations. The concept of identity constancy of faces is probably attained much sooner than identity constancy or other objects because the observed person will quickly confirm or disconfirm the child's judgment. Essentially there are two fundamental rules the child must learn: if a face (person) is observed continuously it will be the same face (person) regardless of the transformations. The second rule is that no matter how similar two faces (persons) are they cannot be the same face if the two faces (persons) co-exist.

In face recognition tasks, the observer has not had the faces under continuous surveillance. The observer whose recognition is being tested does not know whether the face now before him or her has or has not been transformed. Thus the two basic questions confronting the observer are: how different can two representations be and still be representations of the same face, and how similar can two representations be and yet be representations of different faces?

3. THREE-PROCESS MODEL OF FACE RECOGNITION

It is proposed that the face-recognition system comprises three processes: a familiarity process, a cognitive process and a decision process. When an individual observes a face, information generated by the familiarity and cognitive processes passes to the decision system. The decision process combines the information generated by the familiarity and cognitive processes in some fashion and on the basis of this combined information the face is judged as one which has been seen before at the specified time and place or the face is adjudged as being new. This three-process model of face recognition is very similar to episodic word-recognition models, see for example, Atkinson & Juola, 1974; Gillund & Shiffrin, 1984; Jacoby & Dallas, 1981; Mandler, 1980; and Tiberghien, 1976.

3.1. The familiarity process

The familiarity process is a fast automatic system. The familiarity process receives its name from the feeling it generates. It is postulated that this process is "hard-wired", that is, it is a process with which everyone is endowed. It attempts to match the representation of a face presently being perceived with a mnemonic representation. The more similar the present perceptual representation is to one or more mnemonic representations, the greater the feeling of familiarity. All perceptual representations of faces and hence all mnemonic representations of faces are assumed to be a product both of sensory information, for example, visual stimulation, and memory information, for example, previous experiences such as instructions, together with immediately preceding objects and the process involved in the generation of the representation from the sensory and memory information (compare Kohlers, 1973).

Assuming that the perceptual representation of a face depends on the context in which a face appears, then if the context of a face changes then feelings of familiarity should be reduced and faces will be less likely to be judged as old. In a series of experiments my colleagues and I (Thomson, Robertson & Vogt, 1982) found that faces were more accurately and confidently recognized when the original context of the faces was restored.

A student of mine, Joanne O'Hara, has made a more direct test of the effect of context change on feelings of familiarity. Her subjects were asked to rate their feelings of familiarity of faces in the test phase. Joanne found that faces whose context had been re-instated were rated as more familiar than those faces whose context was changed. Recognition responses to faces which evoked strong feelings of familiarity were faster than responses to faces which did not evoke strong feelings of familiarity.

One implication of this analysis of face recognition is that the familiarity process is likely to be the process which underlies Tulving and Thomson's (1973) encoding specificity principle.

3.2. The cognitive process

The cognitive process can be characterized as a problem solving one. It involves active conscious searches of the memory store. One such search is to locate representations which contain any or all of the features of the face presently being observed. Once a representation has been located, other features of that representation are retrieved. Information about the number of matching and mismatching features is made available to the decision process. Another search may be made by tne cognitive process to retrieve temporal and contextual information. The cognitive process also attempts to provide circumstantial evidence, such as the likelihood of the presently observed person being the same person as one previously observed, and whether the observed person appears to recognize the observer. Any or all of this information may be retrieved and transmitted to the decision process.

3.3. The decision process

The decision process makes its "knowing" or recognition judgments on the basis of the information transmitted by the familiarity and cognitive processes. Note that the familiarity and cognitive processes are assumed to operate in parallel (compare Atkinson & Juola, 1974; Gillund & Shiffrin, 1984; Johnston, Dark & Jacoby, 1985; Mandler, 1980). Further, there is a flow of information between the familiarity process and the decision process. Thus, evocation of a strong feeling of familiarity by a face may prolong or renew a search by the cognitive process to determine when and where that face was previously observed. Conversely, retrieval of contextual information by the cognitive system may result in a face which did not evoke feelings of familiarity, now doing so.

There are also non-memory factors which influence the decision process. These non-memory factors can be subsumed under the head of criterion factors. For example, I have shown that the number of faces "recognized" was increased or decreased by varying instructions given to observers just prior to the recognition test (Thomson, 1981).

The interaction of the familiarity process and the cognitive process is illustrated nicely by an observation of Piaget (1951). Piaget relates that he and his daughter were taking a walk one day when they stopped to examine a slug which was crossing the path. They resumed their walk when the child excitedly pointed to another slug also on the path and exclaimed, "There is that slug again, daddy". Piaget explained the child's false recognition of the second slug as evidence of the child being unable to distinguish between an individual slug and the general class of slugs. While Piaget's assessment of the child's lack of understanding of class of objects and instances of class may be correct, it is likely that Piaget's conclusion that the second slug was a different one was based on his knowledge that the first slug could not have travelled quickly enough to be in the location of the second slug.

The relative weight given to information provided by the familiarity and cognitive process is demonstrated in a field study of mine. The parents of one of my students had flown from Australia to London. Soon after, and unbeknown to the parents, their daughter and a companion also travelled to London. The daughter and I arranged that she stand at a bus stop near her parent's lodgings; the companion was to stand some distance away and observe. The daughter and the companion later reported that when the parents emerged from their lodgings and saw their daughter they stopped abruptly. The father then approached the daughter and said hello to her. She turned to face him, and as instructed, looked straight through him. His greeting choked in his throat and he lamely concluded, "I am terribly sorry, I thought you were someone else".

Before I leave this example, the importance of the observed person's behaviour for face recognition in everyday life cannot be overestimated. If the person being observed gives some indication that he or she recognizes the observer then recognition is facilitated. The response of the observed has already been alluded to in connection with the child's attainment of identity constancy. It is the observed person's (or animal's) response which makes recognition of humans in real life so unique.

4. RESOLUTION OF FINDINGS OF INFANT AND CHILD STUDIES

A comparison of infant and child studies reveals an important fundamental difference which may account for the conflicting claims about face recognition. This difference has to do with the meaning given to recognition. Infant studies, which typically use preference or habituation paradigms, would appear to equate recognition with familiarity and take no account of the source of the familiarity. Child and adult studies, which typically require a decision as to whether a face occurred at a particular time or in a particular context, would appear to equate recognition to a response based not just on familiarity but also other information. In terms of the theoretical analysis outlined earlier, face recognition tasks used with children and adults tap both the familiarity and cognitive processes.

I attribute the improvement of children's face recognition as a function of age (Diamond & Carey, 1977; Flin, 1980, Thomson, 1984), to the increasing efficiency of the cognitive process. I have investigated recognition of faces as a function of age and context in a series of experiments (Thomson, 1984). Recognition of faces was tested when the context of the faces remained the same as when the face was previously presented, or the context was changed. Faces which appeared as lures were depicted in contexts seen in the study phase or in new contexts (see Thomson, Robertson & Vogt, 1982, for description of the context manipulation). The pattern of results which I obtained is most instructive. When the context of a previously seen face remained the same the performance of 5 year olds was the same as that of adults. When the context of previously seen faces changed, 5 year olds responded as if the face was a new one, the recognition of these faces by 6 and 7 year olds was somewhat better and that of 11 year olds was indistinguishable from that of adults. For the lures, false recognition of new faces in new contexts was much the same for all age groups but false recognition of lures depicted in a previously seen context was uniformly very high until 11 years of age. The pattern of false recognition responses is consistent with the observations of Piaget (1954) and Mosher & Hornsby (1966) of the inability of young children to systematically examine and evaluate relevant features. It is only at about 12 years of age when Piaget's formal level of operation is reached that a list of features will be systematically abstracted and retrieved during the recognition test. This abstraction of features and testing is part of the cognitive process.

For adults the information from the cognitive process predominates whereas for young children and infants responses are likely to be made on the basis of feelings of familiarity.

Finally, it should be noted that the explanation I am proposing is the reverse of the one offered by Carey and her colleagues (Carey, 1981; Carey, Diamond & Woods, 1980; Diamond & Carey, 1977). Carey and her colleagues claim that until adolescence global or complete processes of face recognition are unavailable; before that, the child must use a "piecemeal" approach. I maintain that it is the total information pattern which generates familiarity, and the abstraction and testing of features, the piecemeal approach, emanates from the cognitive process.

GETTING SEMANTIC INFORMATION FROM FAMILIAR FACES

A.W. YOUNG, D.C. HAY & A.W. ELLIS

1. INTRODUCTION

When we see the face of someone we know, we are able to access all sorts of stored information; 'She goes to the same pub as me', 'Her name's Susan Smith', 'She wasn't there last night', and so on. How is this achieved?

The question is deceptively simple. So much so that until recently psychologists did not often ask it. In this paper we will summarise the findings of some of our own studies, and outline the theoretical position that we are developing in an attempt to explain how people access semantic information and names from familiar faces.

We begin by outlining some of the different kinds of information we can get from faces, and consider these as being represented in different types of information code (see Bruce, 1983). We will distinguish structural codes, expression codes, visually-derived semantic codes, identity-specific semantic codes, and name codes.

Look at the face shown in Figure 1A. It is easy to see the shape of the face, the nose, the chin, the hairstyle, and so on. Thus we must have access to structural codes that can describe the face's surface form. It is also easy to see that the person is smiling a little, though the smile does not perhaps look entirely spontaneous. Hence we must also have access to derived expression codes.

The face in Figure 1A should be unfamiliar to most people. Even so, there is some 'semantic' information that can be obtained from it. We can see that it is probably a man's face, and that he does not look to be very old (some of the ways in which age and sex judgements can be made to faces are described by Enlow, 1982). We can also make attributions. We might, for instance, think that he looks a friendly sort of person, or that he looks intelligent. In addition, we can relate the face to our own occupational stereotypes, thinking perhaps that he looks like the sort of person who might be a journalist or teacher (Klatzky, Martin & Kane, 1982a, 1982b).

All of these types of semantic information have been arrived at on the basis of the person's appearance, thus we will refer to them as involving visually-derived semantic codes.

There are, however, some kinds of information that we cannot get from unfamiliar faces. We do not actually know that the person whose face is shown in Figure 1A really does have the characteristics we attributed to him, we do not know what he does for a living (since occupational stereotypes are not reliable indicators of this), we do not know where he lives, and we don't know his name. In contrast, although Figure 1B shows a person of the same sex and age as Figure 1A, if we recognise the face in Figure 1B we will know that he is an athlete and that his name is Sebastian Coe. Thus we have been able to access identity-specific semantic codes (athlete, runner, Olympic medallist, etc.) and a name code (Sebastian Coe).

It is clear, then, that structural codes, expression codes and visually-derived semantic codes are available to both familiar and unfamiliar faces,

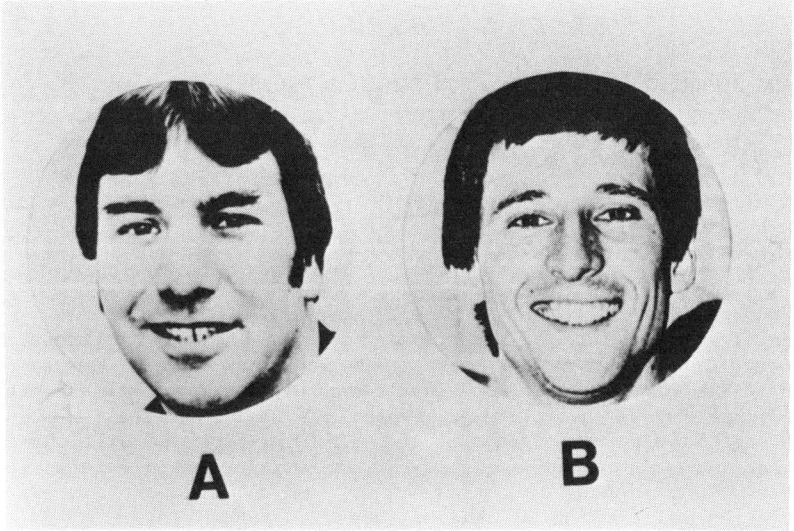

FIGURE 1. - (see text for explanation)

but that identity-specific semantic codes and name codes can only be accessed from the faces of people we know. The main question that we will address in this paper concerns the sequence in which these codes are accessed. Our proposal is shown in schematic form in Figure 2, which is derived from the model put forward by Bruce and Young (1985).

We maintain that a face recognition unit exists for each of the faces known to an individual. Each of these face recognition units contains a stored description of the appearance of the face of a known person. When we look at a face, each face recognition unit signals the degree of resemblance between structural codes describing the seen face and the description stored in the recognition unit (A.Ellis, Young & Hay, in press). When a certain degree of resemblance to one of these stored descriptions is signalled, we will think that the face seems familiar. Identity-specific semantic codes describing the known person are then accessed, and finally the appropriate name code is retrieved.

For present purposes, the key features of this model of how a familiar face is identified are that a recognition unit responds to the face's surface form and signals that it looks familiar, and that identity-specific semantic codes and name codes are subsequently accessed in sequence. We maintain, however, that expression codes and visually-derived semantic codes are formed independently from the part of the system that determines the face's identity. Both neuropsychological studies and studies of normal subjects are consistent with this type of model (Hay & Young, 1982; Bruce, 1983; H.Ellis, 1983, in press a, in press b; Bruce & Valentine, 1985, in press; Rhodes, 1985; A.Ellis, Young & Hay, in press). In this paper, however, we will concentrate on studies of normal subjects, and in particular on the structural codes   face recognition units   identity-specific semantic codes   name codes sequence for familiar face recognition shown in Figure 2. We will begin by examining everyday errors and

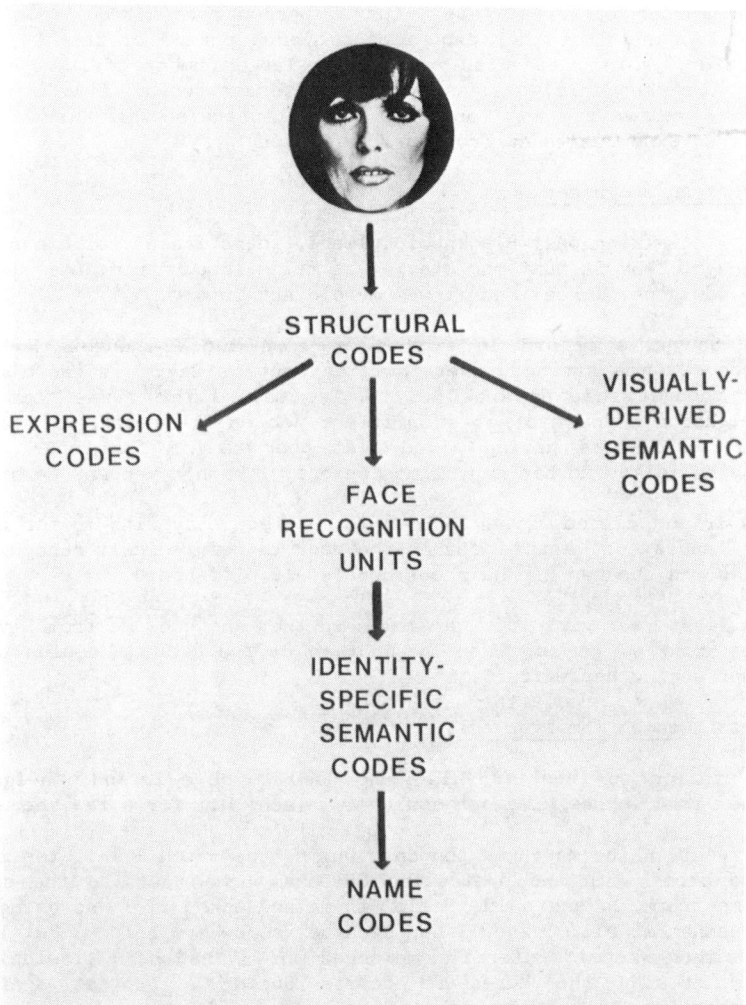

FIGURE 2. - Sequence in which different types of information are obtained from familiar faces

difficulties, and then turn to consider the results of formal experiments. The experimental studies will be described in three sections, concerned with familiarity and semantic decision latencies, categorisation and naming latencies, and interference between faces and printed names.

2. EVERYDAY ERRORS AND DIFFICULTIES

Everyday errors and difficulties in recognising people, which we will call 'slips', have received little attention from researchers, yet they form a potentially rich source of insight into the processes underlying recognition. In order to investigate slips in person recognition we asked people to note down any that they experienced over a period of time (Young, Hay & Ellis, 1985). This exercise produced a large number of records of slips that we were then able to classify into different types. Only some of these types are relevant here, and we will illustrate them with previously unpublished examples taken from our diary study:

2.1 Person unrecognised

"I was walking past Blackpool College, where I used to be a student. I thought 'Why is that man staring at me?' About ten minutes later, when he was gone, I realised it was my old Art tutor".

"I bought a record in a shop in town and I thought the assistant behaved in a strange, over-familiar sort of way. It was almost as if he thought that he knew me. A few days later I was told that our neighbour's son had got a Christmas job on the record counter in that shop. Despite having lived next door to him for three years, and having talked to him many times before, I hadn't recognised him!".

"A friend called Jayne decided to come and stay with me for a few days in Lancaster. When I opened the door to her I didn't recognise her at first as she had her hair cut completely different".

"A first year girl from Cartmel said that she knew me from Liverpool as she used to go out with my brother Jeffrey, but I couldn't remember ever seeing her before".

2.2 Person seemed familiar only

"I failed to identify R.H., who used to be a friend's neighbour. I knew that I knew him, but couldn't 'place' him for a few seconds".

"I went on the march in London. During the march I left the main march and stood with the protesting Greenham women outside the courts. A woman came up and said 'Hello' to me and asked if I was going to go to Greenham at all. I knew I had seen her somewhere before, but I couldn't remember where. Later I remembered that I had been linking arms with her outside the Morecambe courts during a protest against some Lancaster women being tried for lying in front of the town hall in Lancaster, in support of other Greenham women".

"I saw the barman from the Trades Hall when I was in town shopping. I could remember knowing that I knew him, but I couldn't remember where from".

"I took an exhibition down to the Sugar House in the morning. I recognised one of the cleaners but I couldn't remember where I had seen her before. Later I remembered that she used to clean our kitchen in Grizedale".

2.3. Difficulty in retrieving full details of person

"In a store I spoke to a woman at the checkout. I knew her face, knew her child came to playgroup, but couldn't remember her name. She used my name a few times – I still couldn't remember her name. I only remembered her name when retelling the story to a workmate".

"I was reading the Radio Times. I saw a photograph of an actor I knew, but couldn't remember the name. I thought it was Paul something. I knew the name well (Paul Scofield), and just had to wait till it popped into my mind; I expected it to come in a few seconds".

"I went to the Union meeting. When somebody got up and spoke I recognised that I knew him from the first year, but I couldn't remember his name".

"I recognised a woman on Jackanory as one of the actresses from Rock Follies; but I couldn't remember her name. I had to be told it was Julie Covington".

These types of slips are fairly common, and we are sure that most people will be able to recognise them in their own experiences. They fit easily against a sequential model such as that shown in Figure 2. In terms of this model, the first (person unrecognised) type of slip arises when structural codes fail to activate a recognition unit, the second (person seemed familiar only) type arises when a recognition unit has been activated but identity-specific semantic codes cannot be accessed, and in the third (difficulty in retrieving full details of person) type identity-specific semantic codes have been accessed but the name code remains unavailable.

The examples of the 'difficulty in retrieving full details of person' slips that we have given here all involve difficulty in retrieving a person's name. These form the large majority of errors of this type (Young et al., 1985). Occasionally, however, it is not the name but some other detail that is sought. We might, for instance, find ourselves watching Clint Eastwood in a film and then having difficulty remembering some of the other films he has been in. When experiencing this problem, we are perfectly well aware who Clint Eastwood is (actor, cowboy films, detective films, etc.), it is only information that is not essential to determining his identity that is sought. For this reason we have sometimes used a conception of 'person identity nodes' to draw attention to the idea that certain identity-specific semantic codes are more important to name retrieval than others (e.g. Young et al., 1985) but this has been omitted from the present discussion for the sake of simplicity.

It is clear, then, that the sequential model shown in Figure 2 can account for some of the slips that commonly occur in face recognition. In addition to its ability to account for such slips, a sequential model is also supported by the fact that it is possible to invent descriptions of types of slips that do not actually happen. We do not, for instance, find ourselves thinking 'I can remember that his name's John McEnroe, but who is he?' Such slips could arise if identity-specific semantic codes and name codes were accessed in parallel, or if name codes were accessed before identity-specific semantic codes. The fact that they do not occur lends support to the idea that name codes are accessed from faces via intervening identity-specfic semantic codes. Similarly, we do not find ourselves thinking 'That's the person who owns the newsagent's shop, but her face doesn't look familiar'. The absence of such experiences supports the view that the face's familiarity must be determined before identity-specific semantic codes can be accessed.

Everyday slips in recognition are thus consistent with a model of the type shown in Figure 2. We turn now to examining the results of our experiments.

3. FAMILIARITY AND SEMANTIC DECISION LATENCIES

We have suggested that when we look at a face its familiarity can be determined from the outputs of recognition units that respond to the face's surface form, and that identity-specific semantic codes are accessed via these face recognition units.

A simple way of testing these views is to compare latencies for familiarity decision and semantic decision tasks. If decisions as to whether or not faces are familiar can be based on recognition units that respond to the surface forms of seen faces, then they should be taken more quickly than decisions that demand access to identity-specific semantic codes. To test this prediction we compared response latencies for deciding whether or not a face is familiar to latencies for deciding whether or not a face belongs to a politician. Slides made from photographs of three types of face were used as stimuli in our experiment; these were the faces of politicians, television personalities, and unfamiliar people. These faces were carefully matched so that the politicians, television personalities, and unfamiliar people did not show general differences in appearance. This was done to prevent subjects' being able to rely on visually-derived semantic codes.

The experiment is described in more detail by Young, McWeeny, Hay and Ellis (in press, Experiment 1). Faces were presented one at a time. Half the experimental subjects were asked to decide whether or not each face was familiar (familiarity decision), the rest of the subjects were asked to decide whether or not each face belonged to a politician (semantic decision). The familiarity decision condition involved a set of sixteen politicians' faces, a set of sixteen television personalities' faces, and two sets of sixteen unfamiliar faces, whereas the semantic decision condition involved two sets of sixteen politicians, a set of sixteen television personalities, and a set of sixteen unfamiliar faces. For any particular subject, the faces occurred in an unpredictable order and were not repeated during the course of the experiment (i.e. each face was used in one trial only).

Manual reaction times from this experiment are shown in Table 1. The reason why one set of politicians' faces was not used in the familiarity decision task and one set of unfamiliar faces was not used in the semantic decision task was to maintain the same proportion of correct 'Yes' responses (50%) in both conditions. The results show that semantic decisions do indeed take longer than familiarity decisions. This is the case even for those faces (set 1 politicians and set 1 unfamiliars) to which subjects made the same (in terms of 'Yes' or 'No') responses in each condition (type of decision, $F(1,22) = 8.53$, $p < 0.01$).

The fact that familiarity decisions can be taken more quickly than semantic decisions is consistent with the view that familiarity can be determined from the outputs of face recognition units that respond to the surface forms of seen faces, whereas the semantic decision task used in the experiment required additional access to identity-specific semantic codes. A further experiment, which we will not describe here (Young et al., in press b, Experiment 3) showed that familiarity decisions are taken more quickly to politician's faces than semantic decisions even when subjects are well practised at responding to a small set of photographs. The effect is thus a robust one, since it arises even under conditions likely to maximise subjects' efficiency in performing the task.

TABLE 1. Reaction times (in milliseconds) to faces for familiarity decision and semantic decision tasks.

	Politicians		TV Personalities	Unfamiliar	
	Set 2	Set 1		Set 1	Set 2
Familiarity decision	–	775	772	826	855
Semantic decision	930	915	941	1051	–

The view that familiarity decisions can be based on face recognition units whereas semantic decisions require an additional sequential access of identity-specific semantic codes also predicts that it should be possible to identify factors that can affect semantic decisions without affecting familiarity decisions (i.e. affect the later part of the sequence only). This prediction can be tested by comparing reaction times for familiarity decisions and semantic decisions when familiar faces used in the experiment come from consistent (all politicians) or from mixed (politicians and television personalities) semantic categories. We would expect semantic decisions to be faster when the familiar faces are drawn from a consistent semantic category, but we would not expect this factor to influence reaction times for familiarity decisions because it does not change the range of surface forms of the stimulus faces.

TABLE 2. Reaction times (in milliseconds) to faces for familiarity decision and semantic decision tasks performed under conditions involving consistent or mixed categories of familiar faces.

		Politicians	TV Personalities	Unfamiliar
Consistent category familiar faces	Familiarity decision	784	–	950
	Semantic decision	801	–	910
Mixed category familiar faces	Familiarity decision	798	789	916
	Semantic decision	918	971	999

To investigate this prediction subjects were asked to carry out familiarity or semantic decision tasks to a series of faces of politicians and unfamiliar people (consistent category conditions) or to a series of faces of politicians, television personalities and unfamiliar people (mixed category conditions). Thirty-two politicians' faces, sixteen television personalities' faces, and thirty-two unfamiliar faces were used. The experiment is described in more detail by Young et al. (in press b, Experiment 2). As can be seen from Table 2, the predicted interaction was found ($F(1,60)$ = 4.54, p < 0.05). Reaction times for semantic decisions with mixed category familiar faces were longer than reaction times in the other conditions, which did not differ from each other. Thus the use of consistent cateogory familiar faces made semantic decisions faster whilst having no effect on the speed of familiarity decisions, as our model predicts.

4. CATEGORISATION AND NAMING LATENCIES

Everyone has their own name, and we often need to make use of people's names. Thus the ability to put names to faces might be expected to be well practised and virtually error free. Sadly, however, this is far from being the case. Everybody knows that there are occasions on which they can remember virtually anything about someone except her or his name, and when this happens people will often find that retrieving the name they want is apparently blocked by the continual intrusion of a name that they know to be wrong (Yarmey, 1973; Reason & Lucas, 1984).

As we have already explained, the existence of such slips suggests that name codes can only be accessed from faces via intervening identity-specific semantic codes. This idea implies that naming latencies for faces should be longer than semantic decision latencies. We have investigated this prediction in a series of experiments that also compared the properties of faces and written names (Young, McWeeny, Ellis & Hay, in press). In one of these experiments (Young et al., in press a, Experiment 2) subjects categorised faces or handwritten names as being those of politicians or nonpoliticians (saying 'Yes' to politicians and 'No' to nonpoliticians), or named them aloud. Trials with faces or with written names were arranged into separate blocks, and none of the people whose names or faces were used as stimuli was repeated during the course of the experiment. Results are shown in Table 3.

The interaction of stimulus type (faces or names) and subject's task (semantic decision or naming) is highly significant ($F(1,30)$ = 274.16, p < 0.001). As predicted, semantic decision latencies for faces were faster than naming latencies. For written names, however, naming latencies were faster than semantic decision latencies. This implies that the way in which name codes (i.e. the output codes that can allow a name to be pronounced) are accessed from written names is quite different from the way in which they are accessed from faces.

Further experiments involving small sets of stimuli with which subjects became well practised (Young et al., in press a, Experiments 3 and 4) showed that the same form of interaction is obtained. The findings can be related to those of studies using comparable tasks with visually presented objects and words (e.g. Potter & Faulconer, 1975). Pictures of objects, like photographs of faces, can be categorised more quickly than they can be named whereas printed words, like written names, can be named more quickly than they can be categorised.

TABLE 3. Vocal response latencies (in milliseconds) for semantic decision and naming tasks involving faces or written names.

	Faces		Names	
	Politicians	Nonpoliticians	Politicians	Nonpoliticians
Semantic decision	945	923	986	965
Naming	1293	1286	710	707

5. INTERFERENCE BETWEEN FACES AND PRINTED NAMES

Interference paradigms provide a way of examining the extent to which different kinds of information are automatically extracted from a stimulus. The technique derives from Stroop's (1935) work on colour-word interference, which can be adapted to look at other types of interference effect. In essence, a subject is asked to respond to a target stimulus of a particular type and to ignore a simultaneously presented distractor stimulus of a different type. The extent to which the distractor stimulus interferes with the response to the target gives some indication of the extent to which the distractor is automatically processed. The usual way of assessing the size of the interference effect is to compare response latencies for target processing in target + distractor conditions to response latencies for processing targets presented without an accompanying distractor.

We have examined interference betwen faces and names in naming and categorisation tasks. Photographs of faces were combined with printed names to produce different types of stimuli:

i.   Same person: a face and the same person's name.

ii.   Face only or Name only: a condition in which a face was presented without an accompanying name, or a name was presented without an accompanying face.

iii.   Unrelated: a face and an unrelated name, belonging to a person drawn from a different semantic category.

iv.   Related: a face and a related name, belonging to a person drawn from the same semantic category.

Examples showing the way in which faces and names were arranged on our stimuli are shown in Figure 3.

The experiments we will describe here are taken from a series conducted by Young, Ellis, Flude, McWeeny and Hay (1985). Names and faces of six politicians and six pop stars were used. Only one photograph of each person's face was employed, so that subjects were well practised at recognising it. The names and faces of the six politicians and six pop stars were made into stimuli of each of the types described; thus the same names and faces were used in each condition of the experiment, and only the way in which the faces and names were combined with each other differed across conditions.

132

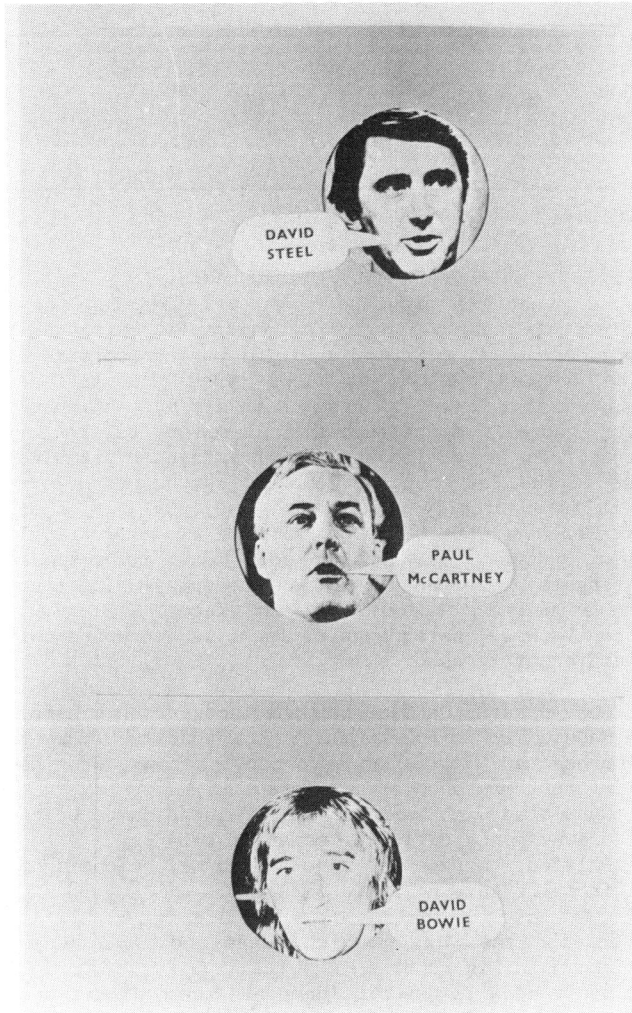

FIGURE 3. Examples of arrangement of face + name stimuli for same person (top; David Steel's face + David Steel's name), unrelated (middle; Tony Benn's face + Paul McCartney's name) and related (bottom; Rod Stewart's face + David Bowie's name) conditions.

We will consider the naming task first. Subjects were asked to name the faces and disregard the printed names in one block of trials, and to name the printed names and disregard the faces in the other block of trials. Vocal response latencies are shown in Table 4. There is a clear interaction between the type of stimulus to be named and the nature of the distractors ($F(3,33) = 36.36$, $p < 0.001$). Put simply, the presence of irrelevant names interferes with face naming, but the presence of irrelevant faces has no effect on naming. Latencies for face naming are slowed by the presence of either unrelated or related printed names, but the interference effect is greater in the case of the related names. Similar findings are reported by Young, Flude, Ellis and Hay (in press).

TABLE 4. Vocal response latencies (in milliseconds) for naming faces or printed names accompanied by different types of distractor.

	Same Person	Face only or Name only	Unrelated	Related
Face naming	859	895	993	1045
Name naming	615	625	622	624

In our categorisation task, subjects were asked to categorise the faces as politicians or nonpoliticians, saying 'Yes' to politicians and 'No' to pop stars. The task was again performed with instructions to categorise the faces and disregard the printed names in one block of trials, and to categorise the names and disregard the faces in the other block of trials. Vocal response latencies are shown in Table 5.

TABLE 5. Vocal response latencies (in milliseconds) for categorising faces or printed names accompanied by different types of distractor.

	Same Person	Face only or Name only	Unrelated	Related
Face categorisation	712	707	742	708
Name categorisation	789	821	875	815

There is a significant interaction between the type of stimulus to be categorised and the nature of the distractors ($F(3,33) = 3.32$, $p < 0.05$). In this case, however, the presence of irrelevant names does not interfere significantly with face categorisation. In some of our other experiments, names have interfered significantly with face categorisation, but the interference with name categorisation created by the presence of irrelevant faces is always greater. The interference effect on name categorisation derived from the presence of unrelated faces, which can be considered as being linked with the incorrect response.

The politician or nonpolitician categorisation task used is comparable to the semantic decision task used in our investigation of categorisation and naming latencies, but politicians and pop stars form occupational categories whose faces might be expected to differ in general appearance (age, hairstyle, etc.). Thus it would be possible for subjects to make use of visually-derived semantic codes in categorising the faces. However, further experiments that we will not describe here show that the same pattern of interference effects is found even when the possibility of using visually-derived semantic codes has been eliminated.

In interference tasks, then, irrelevant names interfere with face naming, and irrelevant faces interfere with name categorisation. As with our experiments on categorisation and naming latencies this pattern is comparable to that found for objects and words; photographs of faces show similar properties to depicted objects and printed names show similar properties to other printed words (Rosinski, 1977; Smith & Magee, 1980).

In our experiments, as in many others, it is noticeable that the pattern of interference effects tends to run in the direction of the stimulus that can be processed more quickly interfering with the stimulus that is processed less quickly. However, it is now thought that relative processing speeds are not in themselves a sufficient explanation of interference effects, since similar patterns of interference can be found even when differences in processing speeds have been eliminated (Dunbar & MacLeod, 1984; Glaser & Dungelhoff, 1984). A more promising approach would seem to be to argue that interference effects depend on the ease with which the stimuli can be recoded into a form suited to the task being carried out. In terms of this hypothesis, our findings demonstrate that faces are recoded into a form that is well suited to the categorisation task, and names into a form well suited to the naming task.

6. SUMMARY

In this paper we have tried to demonstrate that a functional model such as that shown in Figure 2 can help in understanding how people get semantic information from familiar faces. We have concentrated on the idea that stored information is accessed in a structural codes —— face recognition units   identity-specific semantic codes —— name codes sequence, and shown that this sequence can both predict and account for a number of findings:

a. Everyday slips often take the form of an apparent 'block' in proceeding from one part of the sequence to the next. Slips that would be inconsistent with this sequence do not occur.

b. People are able to classify faces as familiar more quickly than they can classify them by occupation. This finding is consistent with the idea that familiarity decisions can be based on face recognition units, whereas classification by occupation (e.g., as politicians or nonpoliticians) demands additional access to identity-specific semantic codes. It is possible to identify factors that can affect semantic (politician or nonpolitician) decisions without affecting familiarity decisions.

c. People are able to classify faces by occupation more quickly than they can name them. This finding is consistent with the idea that identity-specific semantic codes are accessed more quickly than name codes from familiar faces.

d. The face-name interference paradigm shows that seen faces are recoded into a form that interferes with printed names in categorisation tasks, but that does not interfere with printed names in naming tasks. In naming tasks faces are themselves vulnerable to interference from printed names, yet they are resistant to such interference in categorisation tasks. The findings are consistent with the view that the semantic information needed for categorisation tasks is more readily derived from familiar faces than the name codes needed for face naming.

Thus the model shown in Figure 2 provides at least an approximation to what happens when we recognise a familiar face. Whether or not this model proves to be correct in all details, it has led to studies that have provided data that any adequate account of face recognition will need to explain.

ACKNOWLEDGEMENTS
The studies described here have been supported by the ESRC (grant C 0023 2075) and by Lancaster University's Research Grant Fund. We are grateful to the Press Association and to the Lancashire Evening Post for assistance in obtaining suitable photographs for use as stimuli in our experiments, and for permission to reproduce photographs used in the Figures. We are also indebted to Brenda Flude and Kate McWeeny for their contributions to the studies and ideas presented.

WHAT HAPPENS WHEN A FACE RINGS A BELL ? : THE AUTOMATIC PROCESSING OF
FAMOUS FACES

D.C. HAY, A.W. YOUNG and A.W. ELLIS

1.INTRODUCTION

One of the earliest and most fundamental decisions that can be made when
viewing a face is whether or not this has previously been encountered. It
is only recently, however, that psychologists have concentrated their
attention on the problem of how familiarity influences the types of
processing and storage involved in face recognition. What will be attempted
here is; to explore what is meant by familiarity, to highlight how and
where familiarity might produce processing changes, and to report the
findings of an experiment which attempted to investigate two of these
proposed loci.

Evidence is now converging from a number of sources suggesting that
familiar and unfamiliar faces are processed differently. Clinical evidence,
from patients who exhibit face processing deficits, had for some time
suggested that dissociatable deficits might exist (see Benton, 1980 for a
review of this evidence). This view gained more credence when Malone,
Morris, Kay and Levin (1982) published details of two case studies
indicating the existence of a double dissociation between disorders of
familiar and unfamiliar face processing.

It is against this background that recent models of the face processing
system have sought to separate the processing of familiar and unfamiliar
faces (Bruce and Young, 1985; Ellis, 1983; Hay and Young, 1982). These
share many similarities and all postulate a collection of stored visual
representations of known faces. These will be referred to here as face
recognition units (FRU's) and are seen as operating in parallel with an
additional set of visual processes. These are used in the handling of both
familiar and unfamiliar faces. FRU's, therefore, exist only for familiar
faces and are seen as both storing the internal visual representation and
conducting the necessary comparisons between the incoming stimulus
information and this stored representation. In addition, they are seen as
being only one of a number of different types of input code (others being,
for example, the name input and the voice input codes) which may activate a
node containing the semantic information relevant to that face. In the
following discussion these are termed person information nodes (PIN's) and
may, in turn, activate a name output unit (NOU) which is capable of
generating the appropriate name output code (see Hay and Young, 1982 and
Bruce and Young, 1985 for a fuller account of these models). Such a serial
accessing system is found to correctly predict the types of errors, slips
and failures in recognizing faces, observed both in everday life (Young,
Hay and Ellis, 1984) and in laboratory studies (Hay, Young and Ellis, in
preparation). In addition, the time to make familiarity, semantic and name
judgements also exhibit a systematic increase in accordance with the
model's predictions (Young, McWeeny, Hay and Ellis, 1985; Young, McWeeny,

Ellis and Hay, 1985). However, there is little direct evidence avaliable which relates familiarity specifically to faces, although this precise problem has been of interest to experimenters in other branches of psychology; in particular, to those investigating word recognition (e.g. Atkinson and Juola, 1974; Mandler, 1980). In fact, many of the concepts and approaches currently used to investigate the face recognition system have been borrowed unashamedly from the field of word recognition. While this has proved both useful and rewarding as a means of quickly tackling the problem, it quickly becomes apparent that some concepts may be more useful than others. When examining the effects of familiarity what seems to emerge is that familiarity, when applied to faces, is a much broader concept than when it is applied to words.

1.1.What is familiarity ?

Before considering the possible mechanisms by which familiarity influences recognition, it is worth considering what is meant by the term familiarity. Mandler(1980), for example, prefers to define this as occurrence information treating familiarity as synonomous with frequency. Thus, the more frequently a word (or a face) has been encountered the higher the associated familiarity value. Consistent with other researchers Mandler(1980) also assumes that familiarity may be viewed as a continuous dimension ranging from "never seen before", to, "very familiar" (Atkinson and Juola, 1974). These simplifying assumptions have proved useful in the field of word recognition and make intuitive sense but may, however, not be so useful when adopted for face processing models.

The first distinction to be made is that, unlike words, there can be different types of face familiarity. For example, familiarity as it relates to real people such as friends and relatives who are encountered in our daily lives. However, it is also possible to use this term to refer to media personalities who are normally only encountered via television, films, newspapers, magazines etc. (e.g. Yarmey, 1973). What little evidence exists, suggests that such media personalities are treated similarly to known individuals, since these two populations produced similar patterns of errors, slips, and failures in a diary study of everyday face recognition (Young, Hay and Ellis, 1985). The term 'familiar face', however, has been applied in other ways with little thought to how this relates to the above types of familiarity. Umilta, Brizzolara, Tabossi and Fairweather (1978), for example, explored the effects of 'familiarity' in a visual-half field study by allowing subjects to view the same photographs of the same four faces over a period of days. It is debatable whether it was familiarity of the photographs (which Hay and Young, 1982 termed stimulus effects) which increased, or the familiarity of the individual faces, or both. Such a process of repitition is likely to be important in faces becoming familiar, but the effects differ from the natural process in two ways. First, by artificially restricting the level of detail of the internal representation, and second, by preventing this being associated with realistic semantic information.

Leaving aside problems associated with the type of stimulus materials involved, there also exist problems in viewing familiarity as being equivalent to frequency. Hay, Young and Ellis (in prep.) presented photographs of famous and unfamiliar faces and asked subjects to state whether each; was familiar, what the occupation was, and to produce a name. These responses were examined and on a second visit each subject was presented with each of the faces again. Subjects were asked to volunteer the same information. When presented with a face which had originally produced an error subjects were informed of the fact and given cues to elicit how much information, of all types, was available to the subject but not recalled. This was also done when subjects failed to recognize a famous face. For each error and failure subjects were also asked to explain why they thought that difficulty had occurred. These results were broadly in line with the views expressed by Mandler(1980) in that, for some famous faces, recall of the appropriate semantic and name information was fast and automatic. For other famous faces, however, subjects were only able to recall this information after engaging active search strategies using, as Mandler(1980) suggests, various contexts as a framework to guide searches. What is interesting for the sake of this discussion, are the reasons offered by subjects for reporting known faces as only vaguely familiar and, as a result, being unable to recall avaliable semantic information. Mandler(1980) proposed that such searches are instigated if the familiarity value, generated by comparing the FRU, is below some cut-off value. However, subjects in the Hay et al experiment provided a range of explanations which involve familiarity of viewing the face, in a number of different ways.

By far the most frequent explanation was that the photograph was a "bad likeness" of the celebrity involved. This lowered the familiarity level to such an extent as to prevent the recall of avaliable semantic information while still allowing subjects to state the face was familiar. Such responses were not dependent on particular photographs and happened in response to faces covering a wide range of post hoc estimates of familiarity. This highlights the the distinction that can be made between the familiarity of the person and the familiarity associated with a photograph of that person. In addition, it emphasizes the importance of the individual differences in the information stored in FRU's. Given the dynamic nature of the faces and the associated difficulties in storage and comparison, it is easy to understand why these factors are of minimal importance for words.

Another reason used by subjects in the Hay et al(in prep.) study as an explanation for some of their failures involved the concept of recency. This usually involved subjects stating that some faces which had been frequently encountered in the past, had not been "recently seen". This contrasted with the high recognition rates for tennis stars who were recognised better than expected as a result of media coverage of a major tennis tournament which coincided with the running of the experiment. Models, borrowed from the word recognition area, which view familiarity as equivalent to frequency have difficulty handling this aspect of the face data. It is interesting to note, however, that Mandler(1980) found it necessary to incorporate a similar concept when explaining familiarization effects. The distinction he proposed was between 'baseline' and 'effective' familiarity. The latter is a value reflecting the proportional increase, as measured against 'baseline' familiarity, caused by recent exposures. In this way more recent exposures are given a greater weighting.

Perhaps the most surprizing finding from the Hay et al study was that some failures were not the result of seeing these faces infrequently, but of not being interested in that person or class of person. For example, one subject reported a photograph of Kevin Keegan (an internationally famous soccer star) as being only slightly familiar, and was unable to recall any further information. Subsequent quizzing revealed that this subject knew both the name and the occupation and that the subject had been exposed to photographs and T.V. appearances involving this celebrity. Asked to explain his failure produced the reply that this subject was not interested in soccer. Although it could be argued that interest may, to some extent, influence exposure by individuals avoiding contact with individuals or groups, it is also possible, as in the case above, that frequently encountered faces are not attended to sufficiently. In addition it may be that the associated semantic information is not fully integrated into the person semantic network, as these individuals are not "salient" to the viewer. Thus it appears that the effects of frequency may be modified by the attitudes and interests of the viewer.

What seems to emerge from these studies is that familiarity cannot, as far as faces are concerned, be thought of as being equivalent to only frequency. This is obviously one factor in an equation which also involves time related factors. Unlike words, faces change with time and are also encountered more or less frequently in different time bands. It may be that the rate of encountering a face in a time band is a more appropriate measure. In addition, it seems necessary for the equation to give a larger weighting to more recent exposures and to take into account factors which reflect, not only stimulus characteristics, but observer factors.

1.2.Familiarity and FRU's

At a theoretical level the major difference between the recognition of familiar and novel faces centres round the concept of a recognition unit. These have successfully been used in theories of word recognition (Morton, 1969, 1979) and object recognition (Seymour, 1979) and have the great advantage of deliberately avoiding the processes involved in achieving recognition. Although helpful, the fact is that there is little or no empirical evidence to support the existence of these. One way of tackling this problem is to examine the properties of these units in an attempt to generate testable predictions.

FRU's can be thought of as having three basic properties:

(a) they store the structural information about known faces. This appears to include information about many views of the one face as indicated by the findings of the Bruce and Valentine (1985) study. They found an increase in recognition performance after subjects had been exposed to different photographs of famous faces although there was no correlation between the performance increase and the degree of similarity between the two photographs employed. Thus one effect of familiarity, at this level, is to increase the resolution of the stored representation making it less view dependent than the representations of faces seen only once.

(b) FRU's also compare the incoming stimulus face with this stored representation. Evidence has already been presented indicating the internal features are more salient when recognizing known faces (Ellis et al, 1979; Endo et al, 1984) again indicating enhanced storage which allows different comparison processes to operate. The original conception of FRU's involved the assumption that the comparison processes were qualitatively different from those employed in recognizing faces seen only once. This receives some support from the evidence indicating a change in processing strategy when handling familiar faces (Ross and Turkewitz, 1983; Sergent, 1982). The suggestion is that familiarity, by increasing the quality of the stored information allows qualitatively different forms of processing. These are faster and more efficient. Intuitively, familiar faces seem to capture attention as experienced by the automatic way in which familiar individuals are recognized in our everyday lives.

and (c) FRU's generate an index reflecting the degree of similarity between the incoming stimulus and the stored representation. This is a modification of the original conception of FRU's operating in an all or none fashion which was precipitated by the findings from the diary study of everyday slips and errors (Young et al, 1985), and the laboratory analogue (Hay et al, in prep.). Both studies indicated that subjects did not operate in a dichotomous fashion, but responded in a number of ways relating to how much the stimulus resembled the stored internal representation. Support has been found, however, for related property of FRU's as being able to be primed. At the simplest level this refers to the facilitation produced by a prior exposure of the same stimulus. These repetition effects are well documented in the field of word recognition (Haber and Hershenson, 1965; Jacoby and Dallas, 1981) and have recently been demonstrated to occur for faces. Bruce and Valentine (1985) found that recognition of a face as familiar was facilitated by an earlier presentation of the same photograph of the same person, and to a lesser extent by a different photograph of the same person, but not influenced by prior exposure to the name. They suggest that the facilitation for different photographs is mediated by residual activation in the FRU's. This repetition effect should not be observed for unfamiliar faces as the storage and comparison mechanisms are assummed to operate in a qualitatively different fashion.

One paradigm which allows these distinctions to be examined is that suggested by Shiffrin and Schneider (1977). In this, subjects are presented with a memory set containing 1, 2 or 4 elements. After an interstimulus interval, a target frame, again containing 1, 2 or 4 elements, is presented with subjects being required to decide whether or not any of the memory set appeared in the target frame. In their experiments two stimulus classes were employed (i.e. letters and digits). There were two conditions which, in the terminology used by Shiffrin and Schneider (1977), varied in the mapping of memory and target frames. In one condition the memory set was always drawn from one stimulus class while the target frame contained one element from the same class, called the target, and distractors drawn from the other class. This was termed the varied mapping condition and produced reaction time (RT) functions which did not vary with the size of the memory set nor with the number of elements in the target frame. In contrast, the consistent mapping condition, in which memory and target frame elements were draw from the same stimulus class, produced RT-functions which increased with both the size of the memory set and the number of elements in the target frame. Shiffrin and Schneider (1977) interpret these findings as reflecting processes that occur as a result of perceptual learning. That is, the features that discriminate between letters and digits are well learnt. This allows qualatatively different forms of processing to operate in the two experimental conditions. In the varied mapping condition the processes are automatic, as reflected by the zero slopes of the RT-functions, and demand no attentional resources. This is in contrast to more controlled forms of processing that take place in the consistent mapping condition. Here, more controlled forms of processing, requiring attentional resources, are required. The shift to more automatic forms of processing occurs only after considerably practice, and has at least two benefits. The first is that attention is captured by elements in the target frame which come from the same class as the memory set. That is, it is not necessary to engage in scanning the frame in order to find the target element. This is analagous to scanning the faces in a crowd and finding that familiar faces seems to stand out from the others. Second, this elemement, when found, can be compared quickly and efficiently with the members of the memory set as indicated by the RT-functions for the varied mapping condition being unaffected by the size of the memory set. This is similar to the idea of priming FRU's by repetition which allows recognition judgements to be made on the basis of residual activation.

The experiment detailed below is an attempt to examine the validity of the concept of FRU's by using familiar and unfamiliar faces in the Shiffrin and Schneider (1977) paradigm. More specifically, the paradigm allows a means of directly examining the proposals that qualitatively different processes underly the recognition of familiar faces.

2.METHOD

2.1.Subjects. Four males and four females acted as subjects. All had normal or corrected vision, were right-handed and were within the age range 22-37 years.

2.2.Stimuli & Design. The stimuli were black and white photographs of faces. All were, at least, 3/4 profile or full-frontal. Three groups of stimulus faces were used. The first was a pool of photographs of 120 famous faces provided by the Press Association. This included a range of celebrities drawn from a variety of occupational classes. These included; politicians, film stars, pop stars, T.V. celebrities, sportsmen and women etc. For each of the 120 celebrities two photographs were used, these being different poses of the same face. The second pool consisted of phototgraphs of 120 local individuals whose face had appeared in the Lancashire Evening Post. In this way comparible ranges of picture quality for famous and unfamiliar faces could be obtained. These two pools of photographs, which were also approximately matched for age range, and contained similar numbers of faces having beards, moustaches, glasses etc., represented the faces used as target stimuli. An additional pool of photographs of 100 unfamiliar faces in one pose only were used as distractor faces.

There were two basic conditions in the experiment. In the first subjects were faced with a frame containing 1, 2, or 4 famous faces presented along the horizonal midline. These faces were drawn at random with the proviso that the number of times any one face was used was kept to a minimum. Associated with each memory frame was a target frame which again contained 1, 2, or 4 faces. These could be presented in any of four positions situated at the corners of a square whose centre corresponded to the centre of the slide, with each corner representing the centre of the stimulus face. The distance from the centre of the slide to the centre of the stimulus subtended 7.5 degrees of visual arc. Each target frame was comprised of one photograph drawn from the pool of famous faces and the appropriate number of distractor faces. Half of the time the target face was a photograph of one of the memory frame faces, but this was of the celebrity in a different pose, and half the time it was a photograph of a celebrity not shown in the memory frame.The stimuli for the second condition were prepared in the same fashion except that the target faces were selected from the pool of unfamiliar faces .

Within the famous and unfamiliar face conditions there were thus, 9 conditions for which 40 pairs of memory-target frames were prepared. In half of these a memory face appeared in the target frame while in the remainder another face drawn from the appropriate pool was used.

2.3.Procedure. Subjects were run in groups of four, being asked to press one of two buttons - one for 'yes' judgements and the other for 'no' judgements - placed directly in front of them in their mid-line. They were positioned in an arc approximately 3 meters from a back-projection screen and separated by partitions. On each trial a memory frame was back-projected using a 3-field projection tachistoscope for a time dependent on the number of faces in the display. This was 1.5 seconds per face. Following this was a fixed interval of 2 seconds and then a target frame presented for 2.5 seconds. Subjects completed 3 of the 9 memory/target conditions in a session, each session being held on a separate day with at least 24 hours between sessions. Each session lasted approximately 1.5 to 2 hours with subjects given a 5 minute break between conditions. Presentation of the sessions, the conditions within a session, and the hand used to make 'yes' decisions were all counterbalanced. Subjects' times and error were automatically logged by a Commodore 4032 microcomputer. Trials on which errors occurred were repeated until the individual error rates were below 5% for each subject.

3.RESULTS

In each condition there were 20 'yes' and 20 'no' trials. The mean time for both type of decision were calculated for each subject using only those trials for which a correct response was avaliable. As the predictions involved arguments about the slopes of the RT-functions for famous and unknown faces two analyses were conducted. First the slopes of the RT-functions over frame size were calculated for each memory size for each subject, and data was submitted to Analysis of Variance. This revealed a significant memory set size x type of face interaction (F = 24.62; df = 2,14; p < 0.05) which is depicted in figure 1. Subsequent analyses, using

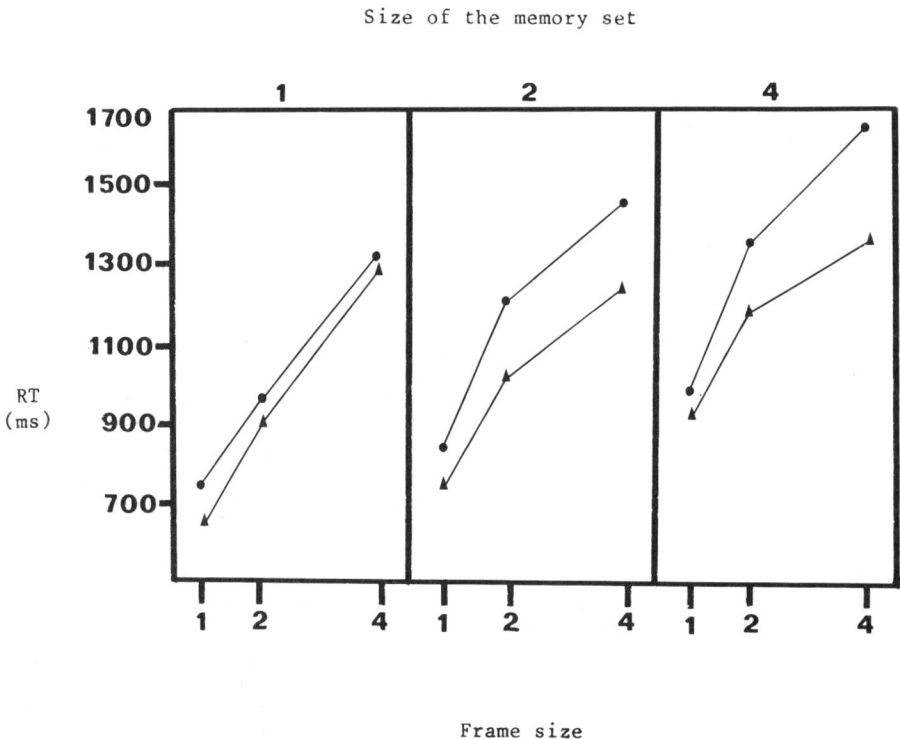

FIGURE 1. Mean RT-functions for each memory set obtained for famous (▲——▲) and unfamiliar faces (●——●).

the Tukey test (x = 0.05), indicated that for famous faces, the RT-functions decreased in slope, while for unknown faces the slopes increased. Second, a similar analysis was conducted on the slopes of the RT-functions for each frame size with variations in the size of the memory set. This also indicated a significant interaction between frame size x type of face interaction (F = 22.39; df = 2,14; p < 0.05). Tukey tests indicated that this resulted from a significant difference between the slopes of the RT-functions for the largest frame size. In this condition the slope of the function for famous faces was found to have zero slope, while that for unfamiliar faces increased as the memory load increased.

4.DISCUSSION

Although the RT-functions obtained for the conditions involving famous faces do not have zero slope, as did those for the varied mapping condition in the Shiffrin and Schneider (1977) study, the difference in function slope is consistent with a change in processing and is of a form predicted by Shiffrin and Schneider (1977). The increasing slopes of the RT-functions over target set size for unfamiliar faces is as expected, indicating that, as the load on the face processing system is increased the processing time increases, this being influenced by both the size of the memory and target frames. The decreasing slopes for the corresponding RT-functions for famous faces is predicted if it is assummed that a mixture of controlled and automatic processing is in fact taking place (c.f. Shiffrin and Schneider, 1977). Questioning of the subjects after they had taken part in the study revealed that many of the faces designated as famous were, in fact, either not known to individual subjects, or only vaguely known. In retrospect, the use of such a large pool of famous faces was almost certain to encounter this difficulty. Subjects, in addition to supporting the view that famous faces were processed using a variety of strategies, also commented that on many occasions when viewing target frames containing a famous face, this appeared to capture their attention, or as some subjects spontaneously suggested, "popped out". In this way the search strategies they utilized for examining frames involving only unfamiliar faces could be avoided. The decreasing slopes also indicate that, as memory and frame set size increases, comparing the famous face found in the target frame with those seen previously in the memory set, was also conducted more efficiently. This is particularly true when the memory set is at its maximum value of 4. Examination of figure 1 illustrates this point in that the mean RT's for the conditions in which there were four faces per frame, shows no evidence of an increasing slope as the number of faces in the memory set increases. This is similar to the zero slope functions observed by Shiffrin and Schneider (1977) and is predicted by the assumption that decisions are mediated by residual activation in the FRU's. This clearly does not happen for unfamiliar faces where the process employed to make inter-item memory set comparisons is a more controlled search through the memory set.

These results can be encompassed within the model of face processing presented earlier and highlight two of the possible ways in which increasing familiarity influences the processing of faces. The first, and perhaps most important, is the automatic processing of the highly familiar target frame faces. This can truely be described as automatic when the faces are highly familiar, since this type of processing is fast, mandatory (that is, cannot be interrupted) and does not demand attentional resources. It is proposed that this involves the activation of a permanent structural, view independent code; a process not avaliable to unfamiliar faces as no permanent internal representation of such faces exist. These must rely on other, as yet unspecified visual processes to construct a usable representation and to compare this with a second stimulus. Support was also found for the prediction that repetition effects vary with the familiarity of the face. This was only found to occur when the load on the system was at a maximum suggesting that the processes employed in making prior occurrence judgements varies with task parameters. This may, however, result from the large pool of famous faces employed in this study. As already stated, these contained a range of faces varying on familiarity. It may be that the most efficient strategy was to treat many of these as unfamiliar faces at low memory/frame loads, and to utilize the more efficient inter-item comparison process only when the task demands are high.

One criticism levelled at 'recognition unit' theories is that these do not explain how units are formed. It is tempting to believe that repeated presentation of a face is all that is required to produce the permanent internal representation. This is the argument forwarded by recent word recognition studies. For example, Salasoo, Shiffrin and Feustel (1985) have show that repeated presentations of non-words produce performance which is essentially the same as that exhibited for words. This process, which they call codification, appears similar to what is involved in setting up an FRU. However, subjects in the present experiment, as well as treating some famous faces as unfamiliar, commented that some of the unfamiliar faces could be treated as familiar after only one or two presentations. These faces were of unfamiliar people who were thought by individual subjects to be highly visually similar to either celebrities, friends or relatives. Since the unfamiliar faces were vetted by the authors in an attempt to avoid this possibility, this again indicates the individual differences that exist in the information stored in the FRU's, and also indicates a possible mechanism for creating FRU's which is less dependent on repeated presentations than suggested by theories of word recognition. Other frequency independent familiarization factors for faces have also recently been reported. Bartlett, Hurry and Thorley (1984) found that the familiarity of novel faces was related to their 'typicality'. They had subjects rate unfamiliar faces on both familiarity and 'typicality' (i.e. how typical or unusual a face seemed) and found that familiarity ratings were higher if the face was also rated as being typical. As these were novel faces this again highlights problems in viewing familiarity as equivalent to frequency of occurrence. They also found that, when these faces were used in a recognition task, pre-exposure to the whole collection of faces increased the familiarity values, but that the increments in familiarity were greater for faces rated as 'unusual'. As stressed earlier, how faces become familiar depends not only on on factors which expose the viewer to faces, but also include factors such as the saliency of the faces and how they relate to faces already known.

5. SOCIO-COGNITIVE FACTORS

LEVELS OF REPRESENTATION AND MEMORY FOR FACES

R.L. KLATZKY

1. INTRODUCTION

In this chapter, I intend, first, to describe some general ideas about visual representations, and second, to relate those ideas to face representation and recognition. My general assumption regarding visual representations is that such representations may exist at various levels of abstraction, and that to some extent at least, levels can be nested. When applied to faces, these ideas suggest that faces may be represented in human memory at different levels of abstraction, which in turn leads to implications for performance in memory tasks.

2. REPRESENTATIONS AS MAPPINGS

To begin, let me introduce the general concept of a representation as a mapping (Palmer, 1978; Klatzky, 1984) between the external visual world and an internal world. Both worlds consist of "objects", with relations between them. Some mapping function connects the objects and relations in the two worlds. In a psychological model, the mapping function is presumably embodied in some mental process or processes. Within this framework, we can call two representations different for several reasons: first, they may map different objects and/or relations from the represented world. I call this a "content" difference between representations. Second, the mapping itself — that is, the correspondences between worlds or the objects in the representing world — may be different, although the two representations preserve the same objects and relations from the represented world. I call this a "form" difference. Third, the psychological process that accomplishes the mapping may be different; I call this an "encoding" difference between representations.

Given these ideas about representations, we can relate them to another concept, that of levels of abstraction. The level of abstraction of some representation reflects the size of the set of objects in the external world that maps into a single object in the representing world. For example, the object in the representing world might be the general category of "spoon", into which are mapped many exemplars from the external world. By this yardstick, objects in the representing world differ in their level of abstraction. If Category A is a superordinate of Category B, A is clearly the more abstract, because it has at least as many objects as B mapping into it (i.e. all those in B plus any additional objects).

3. VISUAL REPRESENTATIONS

Now, let us turn from representations in general to visual representations. I shall describe below three types of visual representations that I think are reasonably distinct. Let me preface the descriptions by saying that as other chapters in this volume make clear, exposure to a visual stimulus initiates a cascade of processing operations. A memory representation can be viewed as the residue or trace of such operations. Since there are many operations, there are potentially many levels of representation. What I am seeking here, then, are cutpoints that differentiate conceptually distinct representations, and more important, representations that may function in a cognitively distinct manner. Table 1 indicates the proposed representations.

TABLE 1. Distinctions among visual representations

| | Type of Visual Representation | | |
	Pictoliteral	Visuoconceptual	Verbal
Form	analogue, depictive image	descriptive, conceptual, propositional	lexical or prelexical
Content	concrete, idiosyncratic detail	abstract, categorical	highly abstract, categorical
Encoding	visual perception and internal reperception	perception, categorisation, interpretation	perception, categorisation, interpretation, verbalisation

The first of these representations is probably what many would agree is a visual code. Psychologists have long tried to define some such uniquely visual type of representation, usually in contrast to verbal representation. Which of the criteria mentioned above do we use when we try to identify such a truly visual representation: content, form, or encoding process? As the table indicates, I would argue that all three of these bases for differentiating between mental representations have been used. That is, "pure" visual representations have been said to have a unique content, a unique form, and a unique encoding process. The content of these visual representations is thought to be highly concrete, not abstract. The form of these representations is sometimes said to be an analogue image, or a depictive form. And the encoding process is thought to be part of visual perception, not verbalisation or conceptual interpretation. I call this type of visual representation - a picture-like, perceptually processed, highly concrete image - "pictoliteral". It is one type of representation that we might have for the human face.

To relate the proposed pictoliteral representation to terminology used elsewhere in this volume, it is "viewer centred", in Marr's (1982) terms, but not necessarily at as low a level as the primal sketch. Possibly, Marr's 2½ D sketch might capture this notion. As for the spatial frequencies represented, presumably enough high frequency information exists so as to capture visual detail. However, the pictoliteral type of representation is not the only possible mapping from visual displays into human memory. We also have internal representations of visual objects that are abstract in content, not directly depictive, and not achieved solely by visual encoding processes. These are conceptually interpreted, categorical versions of visual stimuli.

It is not difficult to find empirical evidence of such representations in the psychological literature. Consider first evidence for representations with abstract visual content. Those representing categories of objects would be abstract, certainly. Do such mappings exist? Early work in Gestalt psychology emphasised the role of abstract idealisations of visual objects in remembering exemplars. More recent work has evoked a similar idea, for example, in describing schemas for scenes (e.g. Mandler & Parker, 1976; Tversky & Hemenway, 1983). Next, consider the evidence for visual representations that are not depictive, analogue images. The argument for this again evokes the literature on categorical visual representations. A categorical representation, by definition, conveys attributes that are common to or typical of its members. This excludes idiosyncratic attributes of objects such as their orientation, size, or colour (unless these are fixed by the category). Thus, such a representation is not a conventional image. Finally, consider the mapping process by which such abstract representations are achieved. This is not only low-level perceptual processing, but also conceptual interpretation and categorisation. In short, there appear to be internal structures that represent the appearance of external objects, but at an abstract, conceptually interpreted level. Yet, these convey information about the visual properties of the objects. I call such representations "visuoconceptual".

Finally, visual stimuli can have a representation in the verbal domain, that is, by means of words themselves or concepts that have direct lexical counterparts. Such an assumption is a basic premise of Paivio's (1971) dual-code model of imagery. Verbalisation constitutes a third type of representation of visual events.

4. FACE REPRESENTATIONS

Having introduced the general concept of representation and distinguished between types of visual representations, I am ready to turn to the main point of this chapter: faces. An obvious question to consider is whether the three types of representation I have described can be applied to faces. It seems reasonable, at the outset, to acknowledge two types of face representation - verbal description and some sort of visual code. We can verbalise a face by giving it a name or some other label of personal identity, or by characterising it by sex, race, or age, or even by labelling its features in a crude way. But few would argue that everything we know about faces is verbalisable; there must be a representation that conveys visual information that cannot readily be labelled.

But what type of visual code? Many people would probably say the visual representation of faces is pictoliteral; in fact, my initial interest in faces grew out of the assumption that they were an ideal stimulus with which to study pictoliteral coding. Think of what it means to recognise a face that we have seen previously only on a single occasion: we must have encoded details of an idiosyncratic member of what is a rather homogenous category. Knowledge of visual detail at this level suggests a pictoliteral representation. However, my own research suggests that the functional representation used in face recognition is more visuoconceptual than pictoliteral.

This research has considered the contribution of all three types of face representation to recognition performance. I am going to proceed by considering three general questions that these studies have addressed: (1) Is there a visuoconceptual representation for faces, that is, one which is abstract and interpreted? (2) Given such a representation, what is its role in face recognition, relative to the pictoliteral level? (3) What is the role of the abstract visual representation relative to the contribution of verbal coding of faces?

4.1. Evidence for a visuoconceptual face representation

My work that is most relevant to the first question concerns categorical representations of faces, where the categories are occupations. I began with the observation that we commonly hold stereotyped expectations of facial appearance for certain occupations: a rock star should be gaunt and hirsute; an undertaker should look lugubrious; a salesman should look a bit too friendly. With Gale Martin and Robbie Kane (Klatzky, Martin & Kane, 1982 and 1983), I demonstrated that people can readily assign faces to several occupational categories at above-chance levels on a forced-choice test. Note that affect seems to play a critical role in such stereotyping (e.g. a salesman must look friendly), suggesting that the category conveys more than purely visual information. The demonstration that such assignments of faces to occupations can be made does not necessarily imply that the occupations play a role in face processing. Further studies that we conducted do suggest a processing role for categorical representations, however. One relevant finding is that stereotyped faces produce better recognition performance. That is, the correlations between measures of facial sterotype and the d' measure of recognition are generally positive. I don't want to make too much of this, however, because I am not at all sure that it reflects some process that makes use of categorical information. It could simply reflect greater distinctiveness for stereotypeable faces.

A second, and less ambiguous way in which we have found stereotyped categories to function is to arouse facial expectancies. To demonstrate this, we used a priming task. On each of a series of trials, subjects saw either an occupational title like "athlete", or the word "blank". This was followed within as little as 350 msec by a face-like stimulus, consisting of two half-faces with a white line down the middle. The subject was to respond "yes" or "no", according to whether the two halves were from the same face. Response time was recorded. We used this particular task – deciding whether two half faces composed a true face – because it would appear to require a decision about the face at a physical level. Thus, evidence of effects of the occupational title would suggest interaction between physical judgements and knowledge about categories, which in turn would support the claim that the categorical knowledge is physical in nature.

Our principal question was whether the response time would be affected by the relationship between the occupational title and the face. If so, it would suggest that the occupation word activated information about facial appearance, and that this activation occurred quickly enough to affect the brief period between prime presentation and response generation. (The interval from prime onset to response was as little as 1.4s on average.) Our data did find priming effects. First, an incongruent occupation (preceding a salesman with "athlete", for example) produced a slower response time (by about 150 ms) than the word "blank". Second, although there was no overall facilitation due to priming with a congruent occupational title, some titles did lead to significantly faster positive responses when congruent – and those tended to be the same ones that produced the greatest negative effects when they were used as incongruent primes. It seems that at least some category names place strong constraints on facial appearance, and that these constraints can be activated very quickly.

In short, my research on facial stereotypes identifies a level of face representation that appears to convey visual information, but of a relatively abstract, categorical nature. There is another facial category that we might consider: that of familiar individuals. Our representation of familiar persons' faces must be abstract, because it is mapped into by a variety of poses, ages, expressions, and the like. The next studies I will discuss (Klatzky & Forrest, 1984) consider this type of facial abstraction in comparison to a mental representation of a particular facial image. Thus, these studies compare what I call the visuoconceptual and pictoliteral codes.

4.2. Contributions of visuoconceptual and pictoliteral representations to recognition

The studies I will describe demonstrate, first, that face recognition is better for faces that are associated with a familiar category, and second, that the superiority for such categorical faces does not reflect superior pictoliteral representation. The demonstration is very simple: I contrasted people's performance on two types of memory test, with two types of faces. The faces were either of famous individuals or nonfamous persons. The tests were either the usual episodic recogition memory, in which people indicated whether they had seen a face previously in the experiment, or a test of memory for particular details, such as the direction in which the face was pointing, hair length, or whether the mouth was open.

The first result concerns the proportion correct for famous and nonfamous faces in the episodic recognition test. Subjects were better at identifying previously presented famous faces, without any decrement in rejecting new famous faces. Thus, we see a memory superiority for faces that map into a known conceptual category, that of the famous individual.

But, now consider the tests of memory for detail. One such test asked subjects to identify in which direction a previously seen face had pointed. It showed: (1) a strong bias to say the test face was identical in direction to the original orientation, (2) an overall percentage correct near (but significantly above) chance, and (3) little difference in responses to famous and nonfamous faces. Other tests assessed subjects' ability to say whether the hair on a previously seen face covered the ears, and whether the mouth was open or closed. (In the test items, these details were masked.) The corresponding data for "new" faces (not previously presented in the experiment) established the guessing level. The percent correct for the faces that were previously presented, and recognised as such, was essentially the same as that guessing level - for both famous and nonfamous faces.

In essence, these tests show two things: (1) Memory for the details tested - pose, or particular facial features - was extremely poor, in fact, at chance for two of the tests. (2) There is no advantage for famous faces in such tests of detailed memory. Hence, we cannot attribute the better memory for famous faces to a superior pictoliteral code, at least to the extent that these memory-for-details tests are evaluating such a representation. (I also find little effect of mirror reversal or blocking out a feature on episodic recognition performance, further supporting the idea that matching such details is not critical to success.) I would argue, in contrast, that the observed superior recogition of familiar faces reflects the existence of a visuoconceptual representation.

4.3. Contributions of visuoconceptual and verbal representations to recognition

The argument that the famous-face effect resides in the visuoconceptual representation has one obvious flaw: people could remember famous faces better not because of an abstract visual code, but because of a verbal one. One version of this hypothesis holds that people have, stored in memory, nodes representing the famous person. These nodes might be conceptual or lexical; if the former, they could be easily converted to words. When people see a photograph of the famous face, they tag these person-identity nodes. Such tags then enhance performance in the episodic recognition task. The next experiment I will describe tested just this possibility, by asking whether a famous-face superiority would still be observed if people could not recognise the famous person from a brief description, including the name. If the only reason for superior memory for famous faces is encoding of the name or person concept, then we should find that when the person is not recognised by this brief description (and thus presumably has not been tagged), recognition of famous faces should descend to the level of nonfamous.

To test this prediction, I first presented subjects with faces of famous and nonfamous individuals, and then tested them on recognition by giving the name, along with a brief verbal description. For example, President Jimmy Carter was tested with, "Jimmy Carter, former US President". In a third stage of the study, the usual episodic recognition test on faces was given. The results were straightforward: the hit rate for faces of nonfamous people was about 75%. The hit rate for faces of famous people whose verbal descriptions were recognised was about 95% - but the hit rate on famous faces whose descriptions were not recognised was also about 95%. As one might expect, this latter hit rate was not significantly different from the overall hit rate for famous faces, and significantly greater than the hit rate for nonfamous. It does not seem that the famous-faces advantage can be attributed to memory for verbal labels; in fact, face recognition and name recognition appear to be independent. The proposed dissociation of names and faces is also supported by the findings that face recognition did not depend on subjects' being able to generate a name when first shown the picture, whereas name recognition did, and that even nonfamous faces were better recognised when they "looked famous" - although they could not be named.

4.4. Nature of the effective representation

In summary, my studies suggest that abstract categorical representations of faces do exist, that face recognition is facilitated by their existence, and that this effect is not simply due to tagging of a verbalisable representation. The effective code in recognising familiar faces, I would argue, is what I call "visuoconceptual". The precise mechanisms by which this visual code facilitates recognition are not specified by these data. The tagging model might be applied, but with this representation substituted for the verbal one. Alternatively, the structures that form the representation might be "primed" when the face is processed, and recognition might be based on perceptual fluency" at the time of reprocessing (Jacoby & Dallas, 1981). But in any case, episodic retention is aided when there are existing structures into which faces can be mapped. It does not seem to be the case that some exact copy of a familiar face is laid down in memory upon viewing and then re-evoked to effect recognition.

It might be argued that the data favouring a visuoconceptual basis for recognition pertain only to familiar faces. It is a much stronger inference to claim that episodic face recognition in general, whether of familiar or unfamiliar faces, is based on a relatively abstract representation. Yet, this inference does not seem unreasonable, in certain respects. For one thing, there is the low level of performance on the tests of memory for detail. This indicates a rather impoverished representation of a pictoliteral nature, one that would seem unlikely to support high levels of episodic recognition. Yet, robust recognition is observed for even unfamiliar faces. Further, it could be argued that whatever visual information makes familiar faces more memorable is likely to function in face recognition in general. The studies described here suggest that an important type of information underlying memory for faces is interpretive and not "pictoliteral".

5. GESTALT PROCESSING AND FACIAL ABSTRACTION

We might have been disposed to reject the pictoliteral theory at the outset, given existing evidence that configurational or Gestalt properties, rather than local details, are of greatest importance in face processing and memory. One interesting phenomenon along these lines arose in my experiments on facial priming. When subjects were exposed to two half-faces and required to judge whether they were the same person, error rates for some pilot stimuli were very high. For these stimuli, the two half-faces from different people merged effectively to form a coherent whole, despite strong cues to their different origins. We seem to build facial representations, in part, without reference to fine detail. This same point has been made with coarsely digitised faces, which can be recognised easily despite the filtering of specific featural information.

6. SUMMARY

To summarise this report, I have presented a three-level description that separates levels of face representations, according to the content, form, and encoding process of the mapping from visual world to memory. I have suggested that all three levels might be used to represent human faces, but that these representations differ in their contributions to episodic memory recognition. In particular, the effective representation in recognition may be a visual abstraction conveying properties of a face that remain constant over variations in viewing. Some of these properties may not be entirely "visual", but affective and interpretative conceptualisations.

FORMATION OF FACIAL PROTOTYPES

ROY S. MALPASS and KATHLEEN D. HUGHES

1. INTRODUCTION

Many researchers have suggested that schematic processes and prototype formation are important in face recognition (Goldstein & Chance, 1974; Malpass, 1975). A prototype is thought of as the "best" exemplar of a set or category of objects. Among it's properties is a high probability of being identified as a familiar entity in the context of the category it typifies. In the case of recognition, category prototypes have a high likelihood of being "recognized" as entities having been previously seen, even if they have actually not been previously seen. It is thought that this is because more than any other category member, they summarize, or represent, attributes of the category.

Two major models of facial prototype formation have been proposed. Neumann (1974) proposed the Attribute Frequency Model. Facial prototype formation following this model is accomplished by extracting from a set of faces the modal feature value for each dimension of feature variation. A face made up of that combination of feature values is said to be proto-typical. For example, on a feature dimension of noses, from narrow to broad, the modal Euro-American nose might be towards the narrow feature values, while the modal Afro-American nose might be towards the broad feature values. In both cases, the category prototype face would possess this modal nose. Posner et al. (1967) suggested an Averaging Model, in which prototypes are formed by extracting the mean value for each feature dimension.

Solso and McCarthy (1981) demonstrated that a previously unseen face, constructed from the most frequently seen features, was given a recog-nition confidence rating greater than faces which actually had been shown. Solso and McCarthy, however, did not evaluate alternative models of prototype formation against each other. If, in a set of faces, the feature values along the respective feature dimensions are distributed normally, the two models of prototype formation converge to predict the same face as the prototype of the set. However, other distributions of feature values can be constructed in which the two models identify different faces as prototypical.

To differentiate the predictions of the two models Neumann (1977) used a bimodal feature distribution in which the extreme values on each feature dimension were the most frequent while the middle values were least fre-quent. Neumann reasoned that if facial prototypes are formed by subjects "constructing" an image from their experience with a set of faces by extracting the most frequent exemplars of eyes, noses, etc., faces made up entirely of the extreme feature values will be the best recognized because they are the most frequently experienced. However, if the prototype is formed by extracting the average value of the distribution of feature values on each feature dimension and constructing a facial image made up of this combination of feature values, the infrequent but central (average) value on all feature dimensions will be that composing the "prototypical face" for that set of faces.

Neumann (1977) also varied the type of instructions which the subjects received prior to viewing the study set of facial images. Half of the subjects received instructions which included information concerning which features would vary, while the other subjects received instructions omitting feature variation information. The important comparisons in his study were the recognition confidence ratings of faces predicted to be prototypical on the basis of the averaging and attribute frequency models. The confidence ratings supported the attribute frequency model when subjects were given feature variation information, but otherwise the averaging model was supported. To account for these findings, Neumann proposed a third process, which he called the interval storage hypothesis.

The interval storage hypothesis proposes that a displayed feature value may represent to subjects an interval or range along the feature dimension. When a feature exemplar is presented not only will that specific value on the feature dimension be experienced, but adjacent feature values may also be experienced, with some probability. If the display of one feature value causes adjacent values to also be encoded, then an infrequently displayed value may be encoded with a higher frequency if it is adjacent to other displayed feature values. Thus, a non-displayed feature value located between two displayed values may be experienced. In this way an attribute frequency process may produce results which appear to result from an averaging process.

The bimodal distribution used by Neumann predicts one averaging prototype, but more than one attribute frequency prototype. There are some problems with using such a distribution of feature value frequencies. An important one is that it is not known what effect competing extremes have on prototype formation. Such a feature frequency distribution could be thought of as representing more than one category of faces. Thus Neumann's subjects were confronted with a set of faces that may have been treated as members of more than one category.

In summary, three different possibilities have been proposed to account for facial prototype formation. The averaging model suggests that it involves the averaging of feature values, the attribute frequency model suggests that it involves counting discrete features, and the interval storage hypothesis predicts experiential overlapping of features which are adjacent on the feature dimension, possibly resulting in prototype formation resembling that predicted by an averaging process.

Stimulus measurement and control are important problems in studying facial prototype formation. Attempts to work on this problem (Jones, et al., 1976) revealed that the measurement of the structural attributes of faces is extraordinarily complex. Achieving control over facial structures for experimental purposes is a problem requiring levels of information and technology quite beyond that presently available. While these problems are (hopefully) being solved, less complex techniques are in order. Following the lead of Solso, Neumann and others we have resorted to the Identikit model II as a facial image generator.

The facial images comprising the set used in the present study varied on 4 dimensions: eyes, nose, mouth and chin. Five discrete exemplars of each of these dimensions were utilized and can be combined to construct 625 individual faces. For each dimension the 5 exemplars were arrayed in order from the lightest/finest feature to the largest/most coarse. Based upon it's position in this array, each of the 5 exemplars were assigned a value from 1 to 5. Study sets of facial images were constructed based upon a series of feature value frequency distributions designed such that the three prototype formation models discussed above make contrasting predictions. The frequency distribution of feature values was the same for each feature, so all predictions focus on the relative recognition confidence ratings given by subjects to the five faces constructed of the same value on each feature. Thus the important comparisons for each experiment are among the mean confidence ratings of 5 critical faces: faces 1111 (that face composed of feature value 1 eyes, feature value 1 nose, feature value 1 mouth, and feature value 1 chin), 2222, 3333, 4444, and 5555.

2. METHOD

2.1. Subjects were White (Euro-American) students from various courses and curricula at the State University of New York College at Plattsburgh. At least 20 subjects were included in each of the experimental conditions.

2.2. Facial images were constructed using the Identikit model II. Two exemplars each of eyes, noses, mouths and chins were selected that marked the entire range of the respective features available in the Identikit with respect to the lightness / darkness, fineness / coarseness dimension. Three intermediate exemplar eyes, noses, mouths and chins were chosen which possesssed values between the two extremes so that the 5 specific eyes, etc. on each feature dimension were approximately equally spaced along that dimension. Facial images composed from the Identikit II overlays were made into black and white 35 mm transparencies by first making a negative image of the composite, and then making a positive image from this negative. Two sets of faces were constructed, one set of "white" (Euro-American) and one set of "Black" (Afro-American) faces. These are displayed in figure 1.

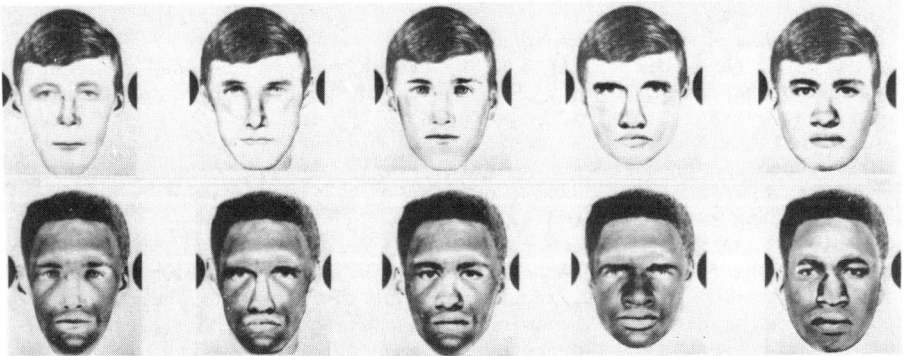

FIGURE 1. Black and White composite faces, 1111 to 5555, left to right.

2.3. Feature value distributions. Frequency distributions of feature values were constructed so that the placement of the mean and mode of the distributions would be useful in evaluating the prototype formation models under study. These will be described below. A number of additional criteria were used in the selection of faces for the study and recognition sets. An important criterion was that the frequency of association of any feature value with any other feature value was to be approximately equivalent across all combinations of features. Also, new faces added as distractors to the recognition set had approximately the same distribution of similarity to the predicted attribute frequency prototype as did the faces in the study set.

2.4. <u>Procedure</u>. Subjects received a brief description of what they were to be shown, and they were asked to "look closely at each face and try to memorize it." Following this, the facial images comprising the study set were projected on a screen, each for 10 seconds, with a 1 second inter-stimulus interval. This study set included either 12 or 16 facial images, depending upon the experimental condition. During the following 10 minute interval the subjects were asked to name the 50 United States in alpha-betical order. They were then presented with a set of recognition faces. Depending upon the experimental condition the recognition set included either 24 or 37 facial images: the study set faces, new faces, and the 5 critical faces. Each of these faces was displayed for 10 seconds each. Subjects were asked to rate each face on a 10 point scale according to their confidence that they had or had not seen it before.

Three experiments that evaluate the 3 prototype models in different ways are described below. For each experiment we will display the frequency distribution of feature values for any given feature, discuss the predictions made about subjects' recognition confidence ratings by the 3 models under these distributions, and present the resulting data. Both the frequency of the feature values and the resulting confidence ratings given to the 5 critical faces are plotted on the same figure, so that the relationship of recognition confidence ratings to the input feature frequency distributions is easily seen. The superimposed figures are plotted so that the entire range of the feature frequency scale and the recognition confidence rating scales are of equal extent in the figure. This is not intended to imply that comparison of the absolute levels of these two superimposed figures is important, but the respective ratios and configurations of the distributions are informative. Oneway ANOVA with Newman Keuls post hoc comparisons were applied to the confidence ratings of the 5 critical faces. As we report the ordering of the mean recognition confidence ratings an indication of a difference between means is based on at least a $p > .01$ criterion, unless specified otherwise.

2.5. <u>Experiment 1</u>. The distributions of feature values used in experiment 1 are shown in figures 2, 3, 4 & 5. This experiment was done primarily as a demonstration that prototype formation would occur with these particular sets of facial images. In symmetrical unimodal distributions such as these the attribute frequency and the averaging models are totally confounded, although the interval storage hypothesis does make predictions in this distribution not made by the other two models. Data from white and black faces are reported separately for the first distribution (figures 2 & 3) and second distribution (figures 4 & 5).

All three prototype formation models predict that face 3333 will be recognized with greater confidence than the other 4 critical faces. The interval storage hypothesis makes additional predictions: faces 2222 and 4444 should have mean confidence ratings at first approaching, and finally surpassing those of faces 1111 and 5555. The greater the probability of encoding adjacent values, the greater the mean recognition confidence ratings for faces 2222 and 4444.

2.5.1. <u>Results</u>. For white faces in both distributions and the black faces in the first distribution, the mean confidence rating of face 3333 is significantly greater than the mean confidence ratings of the other critical faces. For the black faces in distribution B the mean confidence rating for face 3333 was significantly greater than those for faces 2222, 4444, and 5555 but was not significantly different from the mean confidence rating of face 1111. In all cases, in contrast to predictions of the interval storage hypothesis, faces 2222 and 4444 had significantly smaller mean recognition confidence ratings than faces 1111 and 5555.

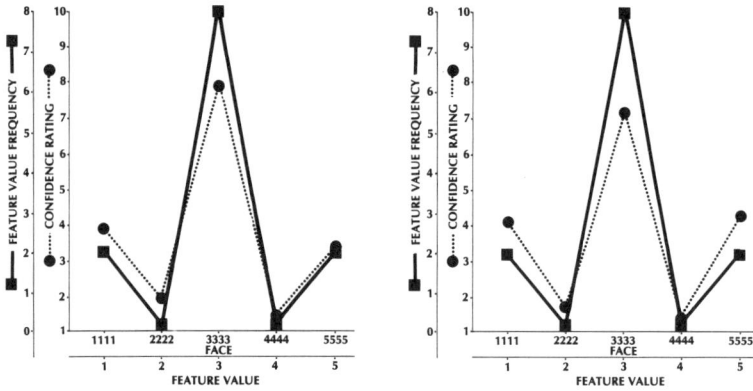

FIGURES 2 and 3. Feature value frequencies and mean confidence ratings for White and Black faces, respectively.

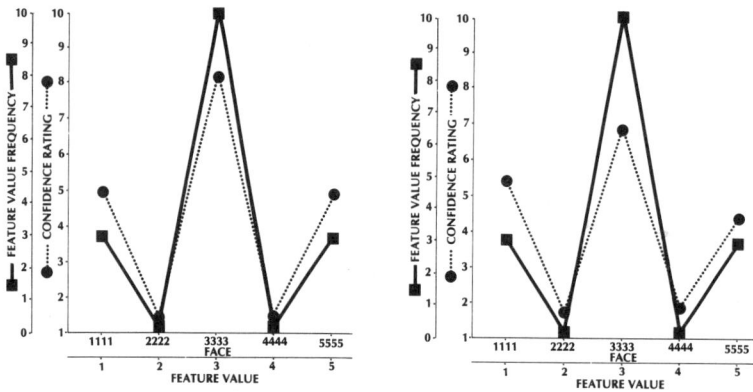

FIGURES 4 and 5. Feature value frequencies and mean confidence ratings for White and Black faces, respectively.

2.6. Experiment 2. The distributions of feature values used in experiment 2 are shown in figures 6 through 8. Two assymmetrical distributions were used, L and R, mirror images of each other, so that the form of the distribution could be unconfounded from the particular facial images used. For these distributions the attribute frequency and averaging models make con- trasting predictions. Again the data are presented separately for white faces (figures 6 & 7) and for black faces (figure 8).

The attribute frequency model predicts that the prototypical face will be composed of the modal feature value on each of the four feature dimensions (face 1111 in the L distribution, - figure 6; face 5555 in the R distribution, - figures 7 & 8), while the averaging model predicts that the prototypical face will be composed of the mean feature value on each of the four feature dimensions (face 2222 in the L distribution, figure 6; face 4444 in the R distribution, figures 7 & 8).

The interval storage hypothesis predicts that any given feature exemplar will be encoded with some probability when an adjacent exemplar is displayed. For instance, in the L distribution (figure 6) since feature value 2 is adjacent to frequently occuring feature values exemplars with this value should be encoded with a greater frequency than those with feature value 4, which are not adjacent to frequent feature values. Likewise, in the R distribution (figures 7 & 8) face 4444 should have a higher mean confidence rating than face 2222.

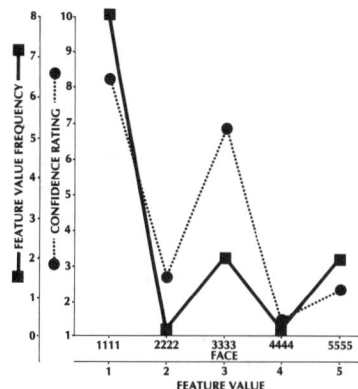

FIGURE 6. Feature value frequencies and mean confidence ratings for white faces in the L distribution.

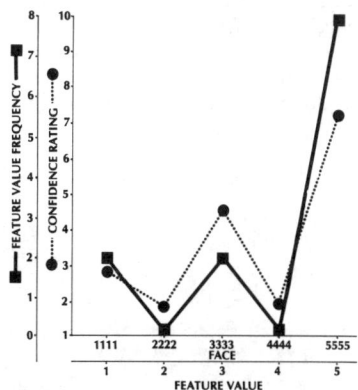

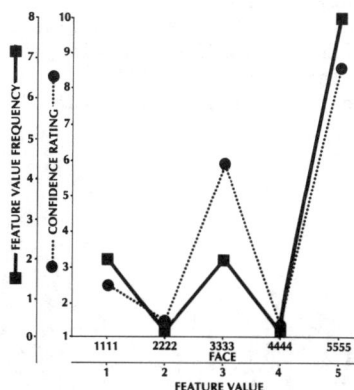

FIGURES 7 and 8. Feature value frequencies and mean confidence ratings for white faces and black faces, respectively, in the R distribution.

2.6.1. <u>Results.</u> The results for the L distribution (figure 6) showed face 1111 to have a higher mean confidence rating than the other critical faces. In support of the interval storage hypothesis, the mean confidence rating of face 2222 was greater than that of face 4444. The results for the R distribution (figures 7 & 8), show face 5555 to have a higher mean confidence rating than the other critical faces. However face 4444 was not significantly different from face 2222 for either white or black facial images providing no support for the interval storage hypothesis. In all cases 3333, with the second highest frequency of occurance, has higher mean confidence ratings than the critical faces composed of lower frequency feature values.

2.7. <u>Experiment 3</u>. The distributions of feature values used in experiment 3 are shown in figures 9 through 14. As with experiment 2, two mirror image asymmetric distributions, L and R were used. This experiment was designed to address a limitation of the previous feature value frequency distributions as tests of an averaging model and the interval storage hypothesis. Since certain feature values had zero frequency it can be argued that averaging to (or encoding) feature values that have not been displayed requires more information about the feature dimensions than may have been provided. Neumann (1977) claimed that when subjects were not given good information about these intermediate feature values an attribute frequency model was confirmed, whereas an averaging model appeared to be confirmed when subjects were given information about feature variation. Experiment 3, then, has feature value frequency distributions shaped similarly to the previous experiment, but assures that each value of each feature is displayed at least once. For the L distribution, there was one study set of white faces (figure 9) and two different study sets of black faces (figures 10 & 11, respectively). For the R distribution there were two different study sets of white faces (figures 12 & 13, respectively) and one study set of black faces (figure 14).

The attribute frequency model predicts that the prototypical face will be 1111 in the L distribution (figures 9, 10 & 11) and face 5555 in the R distribution (figures 12, 13 & 14), while the averaging model predicts that face 2222 will be prototypical in the L distribution and face 4444 in the R distribution. The interval storage hypothesis predicts that face 2222 should have a higher mean confidence rating than faces 4444 and 5555 in the L distribution while face 4444 should have a higher mean confidence rating than faces 1111 and 2222 in the R distribution. The secondary attribute frequency prediction is that 1111 > 3333 > 2222, 4444, 5555.

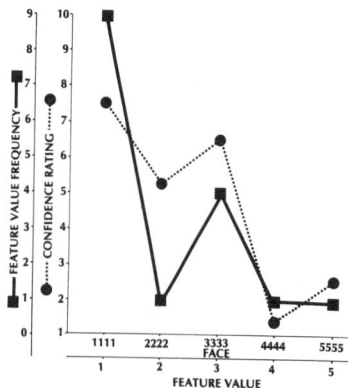

FIGURE 9 . Feature value frequencies and mean confidence ratings for white faces in the L distribution.

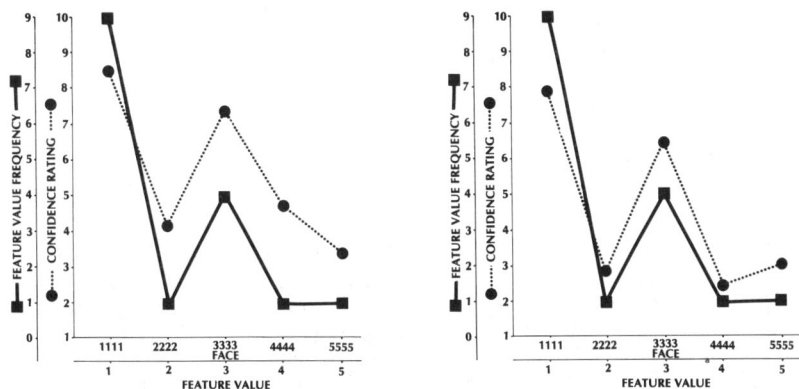

FIGURES 10 and 11. Feature value frequencies and mean confidence ratings for black faces in the L distribution.

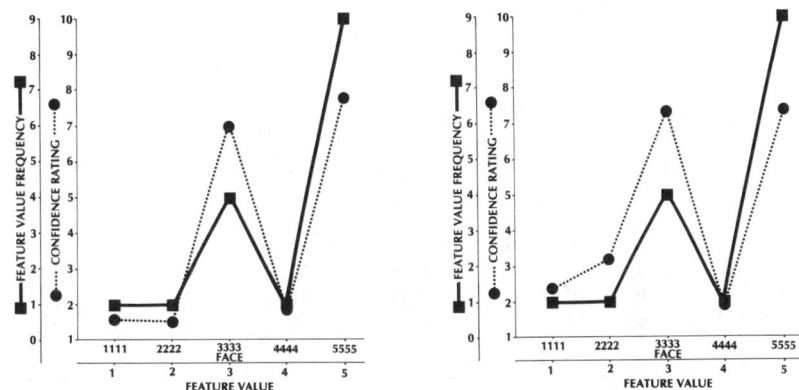

FIGURES 12 and 13. Feature value frequencies and mean confidence ratings for white faces in the R distribution.

2.7.1. <u>Results.</u> The results for the L distribution showed face 1111 to have a mean confidence rating greater than faces 2222, 4444, and 5555 but not significantly different from face 3333 for both the white faces (figure 9) and the first black study set (figure 10). For the second black study set (figure 11), the mean confidence rating of face 1111 was significantly greater than those of all the other faces.

In support of the interval storage hypothesis, for the white faces in the L distribution (figure 9) face 2222 had a mean confidence rating significantly greater than faces 4444 and 5555. However, the results from the two black study sets (figures 10 & 11) revealed no significant differences among the mean confidence ratings of faces 2222, 4444, and 5555.

The results for the R distribution (figures 12, 13 & 14) show face 5555 to have a mean confidence rating greater than faces 1111, 2222, and 4444, but not significantly different from face 3333. In contrast to the pre-

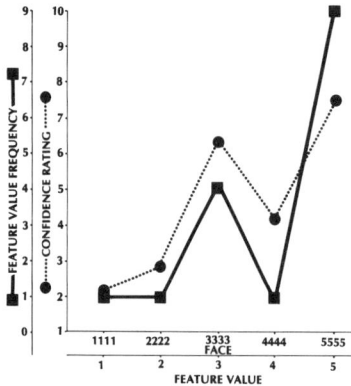

FIGURE 14. Feature value frequencies and mean confidence ratings for black faces in the R distribution.

dictions of the interval storage hypothesis, face 4444 was not significantly different from faces 2222 and 1111 in either study set of white faces (figures 12 and 13). However, the results for the black faces (figure 14) did show face 4444 to be significantly greater than faces 1111 and 2222. Finally, for both the L and R distributions, face 3333 always received greater mean confidence ratings than faces 2222, 4444 and 5555, a secondary prediction of the attribute frequency model.

3. DISCUSSION

Our data support the hypothesis that facial prototypes are formed utilizing the modal discrete exemplars on feature dimensions. No support was found for the averaging of feature values on feature dimensions. The interval storage hypothesis received some support, but most findings did not support its predictions.

One possible interpretation for this pattern of results, in which averaging processes appear to be unimportant, is that the feature dimensions used are not amenable to quantitative manipulation by subjects: i.e. that the input data for subjects is of merely nominal, not ordinal scaling. Both the averaging model and the interval encoding hypothesis assume that dimensionalization of at least ordinal level is present. If this is the case, then facial prototypes will nearly always be formed on the basis of an attribute frequency process, since faces and facial images outside of the manipulations possible with the Identikit rarely vary on simple quantitative dimensions.

How prevalent might we expect mistaken recognitions to be on the basis of attribute frequency processes in the natural social environment? We don't have an adequate basis for answering this question. However, in any environment where the range of variation on facial images is artificially constrained one might except attribute frequency prototype formation to occur. One context that comes to mind is the set of images displayed to witnesses, selected for their similarity to a verbal description of an offender's face.

STEREOTYPING AND FACE MEMORY

JOHN H. MUELLER and W. BURT THOMPSON

1. INTRODUCTION

We often hear it said that "I never forget a face," but those involved in face memory research know that there is variation in subjects' performance. Is there a way to identify people who are good face recognizers? This question has pragmatic significance to people sifting through eyewitness reports, for example, but it would be of theoretical value as well insofar as it helped identify the mechanisms involved in face processing.

One strategy in pursuit of an answer has been to identify people who are good or poor at recognizing other forms, then determine if that ability carries over to face memory (Woodhead & Baddeley, 1981), or perhaps conduct repeated face memory sessions to identify good performers (Chance & Goldstein, 1979). These classifications could then be followed by some effort to identify traits shared by good performers, working backward from performance differences to traits, in the spirit of the individual difference analysis suggested by Underwood (1975). A second strategy begins by selecting traits plausibly related to face processing, then relating scores on that dimension to face memory. For example, mental imagery ability (Courtois & Mueller, 1981; Phillips, 1978), repression-sensitization (Polans, 1985), field independence (Hoffman & Kagan, 1977), sex (cf. review by Shepherd, 1981), and many other traits have been considered in this way. Although some relationships periodically emerge, most reviews of these ventures have not identified a major connection between face processing and subject traits (cf. Ellis, 1975; Shepherd, Ellis, & Davies, 1982; Yarmey, 1979).

2. RATIONALE

Our approach has been of the second variety. It follows from work in verbal memory, specifically the Craik and Lockhart (1972) "depth" of processing analysis, but the main idea can be posed from other perspectives. The "levels" of processing analysis assumed that memory for a word was a function of which features were processed. If "deep" (i.e., semantic) content was processed, then retention would be better than if "shallow" or superficial features were processed (e.g., orthography). This basic notion has seen a number of elaborations and critiques, but when extended to face memory it produced an interesting result. Bower and Karlin (1974) initiated a line of research that showed face memory was improved by thinking about aspects of a stranger's personality (e.g., intelligence or honesty) as opposed to noting physical features of the face (e.g., gender). This outcome has been reported many times since, and may be understood by assuming that personality decisions require more processing and thus increase the likelihood of finding a truly distinctive feature (Courtois & Mueller, 1979; Winograd, 1981).

In the depth of processing tradition, different levels of processing have been considered in two ways. First, a specific level of processing can be constrained by using some orienting task during study, such as requiring synonym decision versus a rhyme decision. Alternatively, implicit spontaneous differences have been proposed to explain various phenomena. For example, it has been argued that the primacy-recency effect in immediate free recall and the "negative recency" effect in delayed recall can be understood in terms of deep processing at the early input positions and shallow processing at the end of the input sequence (e.g., Craik & Watkins, 1973). Likewise, the relative performance of various subject groups has been explained in terms of intrinsic differences in spontaneous depth of processing, such as children vs. young adults (Lorsbach & Mueller, 1979), elderly vs. young adults (Eysenck, 1974), anxious vs. nonanxious subjects (Mueller & Courtois, 1980), and so forth.

This last strategy provided the rationale for the present studies, as we tried to bridge the gap from constrained depth of processing in face memory to an analysis of differences in spontaneous depth of processing. Briefly, if constrained processing along deep, personality dimensions enhances face memory, do some subjects do that type of processing spontaneously? Are these subjects then the ones who do best at face memory "naturally"? If so, how can we identify them? We don't need to assume that these subjects do this deliberately or consciously, just that people differ in how they spontaneously "analyze" photographs of strangers, and that this carries with it an effect on encoding and retention comparable to the effect of an experimenter-imposed orienting task.

Lacking a better term to characterize this behavior, we refer to it as "stereotypy." However, when we asked colleagues about existing measures of stereotyping, we quickly found that the term has a very negative connotation, and the indices that were suggested had to do with dogmatism, prejudice, authoritarianism, rigidity, and so forth. These aspects seem to involve shallow processing, instead of the deep processing behavior we had in mind. As a result, we tried to develop an instrument that seemed more relevant to our interests.

3. EXPERIMENT 1

The instrument involved in the first experiment had subjects form as many subsets as possible of people having something in common from a larger set of well-known people, and explain the basis for the grouping. In fact, this was an adaptation of an Educational Testing Services subtest (French, Ekstrom, & Price, 1963) called "Making Groups (XU-3)," which requires things to be grouped. For example, given the set (a) trout, (b) robin, (c) frog, (d) car, (e) boat, (f) bat, (g) airplane, the subject might put B, F, and G together because they fly, D, E, G together because they are inanimate, and so forth.

In our case, we provided a set of well-known people, so for the set (a) Dan Rather, (b) O. J. Simpson, (c) Abraham Lincoln, (d) Howard Cosell, (e) Wilt Chamberlain, (f) Barbara Walters, (g) Richard Nixon, (h) Ben Franklin, the subject might group A, D, F as journalists; B, D, E as sports figures; C, G, H as political figures, B, E, G as retired, and so forth. The hypothesis was that subjects who are good at this task may be the subjects who spontaneously attend to the benefical deep traits associated with good face memory.

3.1. Procedure

The procedure for the 42 subjects involved an initial study phase for 40 black-and-white photographs (20 male and 20 female college students, none with unusual features such as glasses or facial hair). Each was shown for 5 seconds, and there was no cover task (i.e., subjects knew a memory test would follow). The study phase was followed by the Grouping People task. There were six groups of eight people each, and subjects had 3 minutes for each group, resulting in a study-test interval of about 30 minutes. The test phase involved the 40 old faces mixed with 40 new photos, presented singly at a 5 second rate for an old/new decision. (The two sets of 40 faces were counterbalanced as study and test sets.) After the experiment we also obtained the subjects' college entrance examination scores (School and College Aptitude Test). Groupings were scored by two experimenters, with any disagreements resolved by a third person ($\underline{M}$s = 17.9, $\underline{SD}$ = 7.3).

3.2. Results

The results were quite clear: there was no evidence that score on the grouping test was related to face memory, $\underline{r}$s (42) = .02, .06, and -.04, for hits, false alarms, and $\underline{d}'$, respectively. The grouping score was correlated with quantitative entrance score, but not verbal, $\underline{r}$s (42) = .41 and .15, respectively. (For the record, neither quantitative nor verbal scores correlated with any measures of face memory, $\underline{r}$s (42) < .18.)

4. EXPERIMENT 2

The outcome of Experiment 1 was disappointing, but having confidence in the general rationale we were inclined to fault the particular instrument developed to identify stereotypers. In a sense, the score obtained on the grouping test is a measure of ability instead of tendency. Although ability and tendency should be highly correlated, perhaps grouping people along the dimensions possible (e.g., occupation) doesn't relate directly to personality traits. It is also possible that finding similarities among several people is a process only indirectly related to analyzing an individual's personality. Therefore, we decided to try another technique, one that more directly probes trait knowledge on an individual level.

4.1. Procedure

In the second experiment, subjects had 60 seconds to write down as many traits as possible for each of 12 well-known personalities (Jane Fonda, Johnny Carson, Dan Rather, Barbara Walters, Ronald Reagan, etc.). For one group of subjects, this task was done after the face task, whereas for a second group it was done before the study phase. It was our belief that doing this task first would prime all subjects to analyze deep traits, thus wiping out most differences due to intrinsic stereotyping.

Two other questionnaires were used, partly as filler tasks, but also to relate their scores to the trait generation measure. One was the Category-Width questionnaire (Pettigrew, 1958, 1982) which identifies broad and narrow categorizers. It has 20 four-alternative items of the type "If the average speed of birds flying is 17 mile per hour, what do you think is the speed of the fastest bird? the slowest bird?" Messick and Damarin (1964) found narrow categorizers were better at face memory (though their data are actually hard to interpret because they combined hits and correct rejects in a single measure). It could be argued differently, but it seemed reasonable to expect broad categorizers to generate more traits overall, because narrow categorizers would be less inclined to attribute the same trait to many different people.

The other questionnaire was a Hemispheric Cognitive Style inventory, designed to identify subjects as either "right hemisphere" or "left hemisphere" thinkers (Zenhausern, 1978; Zenhausern & Repetti, 1979). Considerable interest has attached to the question of whether faces are processed best by the right hemisphere (e.g., Rhodes, 1985), and even whether hemisphericity is a meaningful concept (Beaumont, Young, & McManus, 1984). One study has found right-dominant scorers on the Hemispheric Style test did better than left-dominant scorers on some aspects of a face memory task (Thompson & Mueller, 1984). There also has been one effort to link category width to hemispheric laterality assessed by eye movements (Huang &

Byrne, 1978), but the inclusion of the Hemispheric Preference questionnaire was essentially exploratory here.

The face task was exactly as in Experiment 1. The sequence for the After group ($\underline{n}$ = 42) was Category-Width test, study 40 faces, Hemispheric Preference test, yes/no recognition test on 80 faces, Trait Generation task; for the Before group ($\underline{n}$ = 46) the sequence was Trait Generation task, study 40 faces, Hemispheric Preference test, test on 80 faces, Category-Width test. As before, we obtained college entrance scores after the experiment.

4.2. Results

A median split was performed on the trait generation scores ($\underline{M}$ = 66.6, $\underline{SD}$ = 19.4), and this resulted in a 2 X 2 factorial design for Group (before, after) and Trait (high, low). The recognition data are shown in Table 1. No effects were significant for hit-rate, $\underline{F}$s < 1.04. There was a significant main effect of trait level for false-alarm rate, $\underline{F}$ (1,84) = 4.16, but no group effect or Group X Trait interaction, $\underline{F}$s < 1.35. Trait generation and false alarms were inversely related, i.e., subjects who generated a large number of traits produced fewer false alarms than subjects who generated fewer traits ($\underline{M}$s = .13 vs. .17).

TABLE 1. Recognition performance by level of trait generation (high, low) and point of trait generation (before or after face task).

	Hit-Rate	False-Alarm Rate	$\underline{d}'$	Beta	Traits
After Face Task:					
High Traits	.73	.12	1.97	3.14	82.5
Low Traits	.75	.17	1.73	1.47	51.1
Before Face Task:					
High Traits	.74	.15	1.82	1.91	81.3
Low Traits	.76	.18	1.78	1.59	51.5

Signal detection analyses indicated no significant effects for $\underline{d}'$, $\underline{F}$s < 1.11. There was a marginally significant Group main effect for beta, $\underline{F}$ (1,84) = 3.02, $\underline{p}$ < .09, as subjects who generated traits before the face task adopted a lower criterion than those who generated traits at the end ($\underline{M}$s = 1.73 vs. 2.42). The Trait main effect was significant, $\underline{F}$ (1,84) = 5.80, as the criterion level was higher for those subjects generating more traits ($\underline{M}$s = 2.58 vs. 1.54). The Group X Trait interaction for beta was marginally significant, $\underline{F}$ (1,84) = 2.80, $\underline{p}$ < .10, with a more pronounced trait effect in the After condition.

Table 2 shows the intercorrelations among the various measures. The trait score was significantly correlated with the quantitative ability score and the right hemisphere cognitive style score, but those two measures were not significantly correlated with face memory.

The trait measure was not correlated with category width, nor did category width correlate significantly with the conventional measures of face memory, i.e., hit rate and false alarm rate. The data in Table 2 are for Pettigrew's Factor 1 of the category-width scale, but the same result was found for the full-scale category-width score. This result is at variance with the findings of Messick and Damarin (1964). At first, we thought this was because Messick and Damarin combined correct performance on old faces (hits) and new faces (correct rejects) into a single measure. However, when we created a single measure combining hits and rejections, "accuracy" in Table 2, we still found no significant relationship in our data. The correlation here is in the same direction, negative, with narrow categorizers (low scorers) being more accurate, but nonsignificant.

TABLE 2. Correlations between face memory performance and questionnaire scores (Trait = trait generation score, Hits = hit rate, FA = false alarm rate, CW = category width, RH = right hemisphere score, QES = quantitative entrance score, VES = verbal entrance score, ACC = accuracy; * p < .05).

	Hits	FA	CW	RH	QES	VES	ACC
Trait	-.16	-.25*	-.06	.34*	.26*	.20	.05
Hits		-.02	-.06	-.07	-.19	.04	.75*
FA			.11	-.13	.20	-.03	-.67*
CW				-.01	.15	-.10	-.11
RH					-.03	-.05	.03
QES						.35*	-.27*
VES							.05

The reason that this relationship was not significant here is not clear. The overall accuracy level was 73% in the Messick and Damarin study, compared to 79% here, both quite typical of face recognition research, and unlikely to involve ceiling effect constraints in either case. As usual, there were procedural differences between their study and ours, such as the size of the target set (20 vs. 40) and the composition of the photographs (mixed ages vs. all college students). Perhaps most importantly, their subjects studied the faces in an incidental learning arrangement, rendering age estimation judgments and resemblance to another person judgments during study, and then performing the age estimation task again during the test phase as well. It may be that "free" intentional learning is relatively unaffected by category width, and that its effect emerges only when situational "demand characteristics" render category-width processing salient (as when judging some dimension of the person in the photograph, such as age).

4.3. Discussion

One hypothesis was that generating traits before the face task would prime all subjects to analyze the study photographs in terms of deep traits, thus eliminating differences between high and low trait generators. This seemed to occur, as the signal detection differences between high and low trait generators were larger in the After group than in the Before group, but the Group X Trait interactions were not significant. The absolute number of traits generated did not differ significantly as a function of whether the traits were generated before or after the face task ($\underline{M}$s = 64.4 vs. 69.1).

The second hypothesis was that high trait generators would remember faces better (at least in the After group). High scorers did make fewer false alarms than low scorers, but there was no effect on hit rates. In another analysis, we considered only the top and bottom thirds of the trait-score distribution, but the pattern of significant effects was the same. Apparently high trait generators operated under a higher criterion, which enabled them to improve their performance on new faces but at the same time hindered them on the old faces: new faces looked newer, but old faces were not enhanced. This does indicate some effect due to trait generating ability (especially if trait generation does not precede the learning task), but it clearly is a more limited effect than we had anticipated, and most importantly it is not an effect on encoding as we had proposed.

5. CONCLUSIONS

Considering Experiments 1 and 2, the evidence for "high stereotypers" being better face recognizers is certainly modest, no more substantial than the relationship linking several other individual difference variables to face memory. Given our initial confidence in the hypothesis, why might this effect be so limited?

One possibility is that stereotypes do not work for face processing. However, this seems contradicted by the work of Klatzky (Klatzky, Martin, & Kane, 1982a, 1982b, and elsewhere in this volume), Goldstein, Chance and Gilbert (1984), Solso and McCarthy (1981), and others (e.g., Ellis, 1981), plus our ability to make judgments about such aspects as the typicality of the face. There seems ample evidence for the existence of prototypical faces, so it seems more a question of whether subjects do differ in their use of such schemata, whether we can identify those differences, and just when or where in the course of face processing such differences have their effect.

The assessments of stereotyping used here seem likely to be part of the problem. Although groupings and trait generation seem reasonable, the differences associated with these classifications were not very impressive. With the benefit of hindsight, we can now point out that both of these techniques used known figures as the targets for trait analysis, whereas the face task involved unfamiliar faces. One might reasonably expect that there would be some similarity in how we analyze familiar and unfamiliar people, but it also seems reasonable that there would be differences as well. Such problems, plus a potential discrepancy between the ability to generate and the tendency to seek traits, serve to underline the difficulties associated with assessing this rather easy-to-describe personality trait.

It may also be the case that the operation of stereotypes in face processing depends upon a certain degree of priming, or the appropriate demand characteristics in the situation. Criminal stereotypes seem to exist when cued either by an experimental question (e.g., Goldstein et al., 1984) or being in a police station to identify a suspect, and the effects observed by Klatzky et al. occurred when the photographs were preceded by a specific relevant or irrelevant occupational title. Given the individual differences orientation of the present research, such priming seemed to defeat our purposes. That is, although it was only a weak effect, the fact that the high-low trait difference in Table 1 was smaller for the Before condition would be consistent with the notion that this activity can be primed, but when unprimed (After condition) the contribution of stereotyping (as operationalized here) was minimal.

The differences we were seeking are very general tendencies to spontaneously use stereotypes. Furthermore, the faces we used here were not selected to be instances of particular stereotypes, unlike many other studies of stereotypes (e.g., Klatzky et al., 1982a, 1982b). It could be that differences in spontaneous stereotyping would emerge more clearly with faces that instantiate stereotypes (even in the absence of overt labels). That would be of some interest, but would indicate that this individual difference variable has a rather specific role in face memory instead of the more general role that we anticipated.

And it is also conceivable that stereotypes guide initial processing, but once a judgment has been made further processing ceases, mitigating any other benefits. This would be related to the in-group/out-group phenomenon in social psychology, where out-group members are viewed more simplistically, and it would be in accord with the common prejudicial connotation of the term stereotype. In other words, having pigeon-holed the target face as a case of stereotype X, the subject has actually encoded

it shallowly, quite in contrast to the thorough analysis we posited at the
outset. Even if some, rather than most, high trait generators were doing
this, it would reduce the difference between high and low generators unless
the "shallow stereotypers" could be identified and isolated from the data.

Two instruments that we originally eliminated because they seemed to
have less to do with face processing may turn out to be useful.   One of
these is the "need for cognition" scale (Cacioppo & Petty, 1982), which
assesses the extent to which an individual needs to structure situations,
to analyze and make the world reasonable. Although it is not specifically
directed to analyzing people, there may be sufficient generality to this
attribute for it to have the effect on face processing that we have
postulated. At first glance, it does have the characteristic of measuring
"amount of thinking" that we originally wanted, and could circumvent the
shallow stereotyper problem.   Secondly, there is an extensive body of
literature deriving from George Kelly's "Personal Construct Theory" (cf.
Adams-Webber & Mancusco, 1983). This again is not particularly connected
with face processing, but it might provide some useful insights.

At this point, the hypothesis still seems plausible to us, but the
effect is admittedly weak in our data. It may be weak because we have not
identified a robust assessment strategy, because the effect is limited to
but a single stage of face processing, or it may just be yet another
subject characteristic that simply has only a small effect.

THE INFLUENCE OF RACE ON FACE RECOGNITION

J.C. BRIGHAM

1. OPINIONS ABOUT AN "OWN-RACE BIAS" IN FACE RECOGNITION

Recalling or recognising the human face is a difficult task under the best of circumstances. The practical situation in which face recognition has received the most attention, the identification of criminal suspects in photographic or live lineups, often involves additional factors that would make such recognition even more difficult. These factors include stress at the time of the original incident, poor lighting, a relatively brief opportunity to observe the person, and attention being drawn to other aspects in the situation such as a weapon, escape opportunities, or the plight of the victim (if it is not the observer). All of these factors help make eyewitness identifications a very controversial class of evidence. Judge Nathan Sobel (1972, p.vi), for example, suggested that inaccurate eyewitness identifications have accounted for more miscarriages of justice in the U.S. criminal justice system than all other factors combined.

Race is still another factor which might make facial identification more difficult. For years scientists and laypersons alike have postulated the existence of an "own-race bias" or "differential recognition effect", wherein people can more accurately recognise persons of their own race than persons of a different race. Years ago Feingold (1914, p.50) proposed that it was "well known that, other things being equal, individuals of a given race are distinguishable from each other in proportion to our familiarity, to our contact with the race as a whole. Thus, to the uninitiated American, all Asiatics look alike, while to the Asiatic, all white men look alike". In a widely-read law textbook, Wall (1965) cited the situation where the witness and the perpetrator are of different races as one of 12 "danger signals" to be taken into account in evaluating eyewitness evidence. Loftus (1979, pp.136-137) suggested that "It seems to be a fact – it has been observed so many times – that people are better at recognising faces of persons of their own race than a different race". Yarmey & Jones (1983) found that 15 of 16 expert researchers in the area agreed with the existence of an own-race bias, as did 63% of legal professionals, 81% of law students, and 45% of student or citizen "jurors". In statewide surveys, prosecuting attorneys, defense attorneys, and law officers (police and sheriffs' department personnel) all supported the idea of an own-race bias, feeling that same-race identifications were more likely to be accurate than were other-race identifications (Brigham, 1981; Brigham & WolfsKeil, 1983). However, despite the popularity of this concept, race was not included among the factors which the U.S. Supreme Court cited as important in evaluating eyewitness evidence in important decisions (Neil v. Biggers, 1972; Manson v. Braithwaite, 1977).

2. RESEARCH FINDINGS ON THE OWN-RACE BIAS

2.1. Recognition accuracy

Despite the widespread acceptance of the idea of an own-race bias, there had been little research on its existence until the past 10 to 15 years. In a review of relevant studies, Lindsay & Wells (1983) identified 13 samples in which both own- and other-race identification accuracy was studied. Eleven of the 13 samples yielded significant interactions between race of perceiver and race of target. Six of the 11 significant interactions were "full crossover interactions" where, for both races, own-race identification was better than other-race identification. Lindsay & Wells (1983) criticised what they saw as oversimple interpretations of this research literature. Lindsay & Wells argued that (1) the research results were more inconsistent than previous observers had realised; (2) the race-related differences might be of small magnitude and of little importance; (3) research has been based on no firm theoretical understanding of the processes involved; and (4) the researchers often failed to ask "forensically relevant" questions.

Feeling that the Lindsay and Wells review painted a too-negative picture of the consistency and magnitude of the own-race bias, we (Bothwell, Brigham & Malpass, 1985) undertook a meta-analysis of the relevant studies. Usable data were available for only eight of the 13 samples reviewed by Lindsay and Wells, but we were able to obtain appropriate data from six additional studies, so that a total of 14 laboratory studies were analysed. These studies employed 693 black subjects and 752 white subjects, each of whom attempted to identify both black and white faces. Effect sizes (d) were derived by subtracting other-race accuracy scores from own-race accuracy scores in standard score form. Hence, a positive effect size indicates better recognition for own-race faces whereas a negative effective effect size would indicate better recognition of other-race faces. As Table 1 indicates we found comparable effect sizes for black perceivers and white perceivers (d = .71 for blacks and .69 for whites). These effect sizes are in the moderate-to-large range, according to the standards proposed by Cohen (1977), accounting for 11%-12% of the variance in the dependent variable. The standard deviation of the effect sizes was considerably greater for black perceivers than for white perceivers. Hence, while the 95% confidence interval for white perceivers did not include zero, ranging from .15 to 1.22, the 95% confidence interval for black perceivers did include zero, ranging from -.34 to 1.76.

We also reviewed two field studies (Brigham, Maas, Snyder & Spaulding, 1982; Hosch & Platz, 1984) which involved face identification in a more ecologically valid situation. Clerks in convenience stores were the subjects and they attempted to identify "customers" who had been in their store several hours earlier. Meta-analysis of these two studies indicated a strong cross-race effect for white clerks. The 95% confidence interval for whites was from 33 to 55% accuracy in identifying blacks, but 53 to 68% accuracy in identifying whites. Unfortunately there were too few minority subjects in the studies to allow computation of comparable confidence intervals for black subjects.

2.2. Response criteria

Race may affect not only recognition accuracy, but one's style of responding as well. Barkowitz & Brigham (1982) analysed the response criterion (Beta) used by subjects (cf., Schiffman, 1976), that is, the tendency to positively identify a face as "seen before", and found a strong interaction between race of subject and race of target, parallelling the interaction discussed above for recognition accuracy. Both blacks and whites tended to

TABLE 1. Own vs other effect sizes for Black$_b$ and White$_w$ subjects.

Meta-analysis of the influence of race on facial recognition (Bothwell, Brigham & Malpass, 1985)

	N_b	N_w	d_b	d_w
Barkowitz & Brigham, 1982 (Study 1)	81	174	- .190	.760
Barkowitz & Brigham, 1982 (Study 2)	58	43	.560	.450
*Brigham & Barkowitz, 1978	86	76	1.247	.757
Brigham & Williamson, 1979	27	14	1.986	.347
*Chance, Goldstein & McBride, 1975	48	48	.596	.685
Devine & Malpass, 1985	24	24	1.127	1.084
Ellis & Deregowski, 1981 (transformed faces)	48	48	1.575	.741
Ellis & Deregowski, 1981 (untransformed)	48	48	.556	.185
*Feinman & Entwisle, 1976	144	144	.436	.556
*Galper, 1973	16	14	1.317	1.245
*Malpass & Kravitz, 1969 (Illinois)	13	13	- .115	1.405
*Malpass & Kravitz, 1969 (Howard University)	7	7	- .107	1.343
*Malpass, Lavigueur & Weldon, 1973	61	67	.908	.364
*Shepherd, Deregowski & Ellis, 1974	32	32	.570	1.504

d_b = accuracy in recognising blacks minus accuracy in recognising whites (in standard score form).

d_w = accuracy in recognising whites minus accuracy in recognising blacks (in standard score form).

A positive effect size indicates .better recognition for own-race faces, whereas a negative effect size indicates better recognition of other-race faces.

N_b = number of black subjects, N_w = number of white subjects.

*: Studies included in the Lindsay & Wells (1983) review.

make more "seen before" responses to other-race faces than to own-race faces, yielding a false alarm rate on the average 22% higher for cross-race faces than for own-race faces. Hence, subjects used a stricter response criterion for their own race (Figure 1). This tendency was more pronounced among white perceivers than among black perceivers. It is the possibility of "false alarms", the positive identification of an innocent suspect, that has most concerned legal authorities.

2.3. The construction of fair lineups

If race affects both recognition accuracy and response criterion, it might also affect one's ability to construct a "fair" lineup, a lineup composed of foils who match the general appearance of the target person (suspect). It could be proposed that the own-race bias would cause people to discriminate

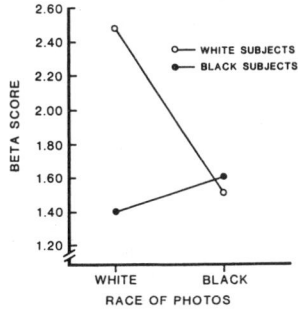

FIGURE 1. Response criteria as a function of race. Higher Beta score denotes a stricter criterion, fewer "seen before" responses. (From Barkowitz & Brigham, 1982).

more carefully among own-race faces than among other-race faces in selecting lineup foils. The result might be lineups which are fairer, i.e., have more similarity between target and foils, when the lineups are constructed by a person of the same race as the lineup members than when lineups are constructed by a person of a different race. To investigate this possibility we (Brigham & Ready, in press) attempted to approximate in the laboratory the way that photo lineups are constructed in criminal cases. We presented subjects with a male target photo and a stack of 80 same-race similar-age photos of males. Black subjects and white subjects were instructed to go through the stack of head and shoulder facial photos until they have selected five photos which were "reasonably similar in appearance" to the target photo or reached the end of the stack. Eight different target photos were used; each subject saw two target photos, one white and one black. Analysis of the number of photos chosen yielded significant interaction between race of subject and race of target. Subjects chose fewer own-race photos as similar to the target person than other-race photos. Apparently they were discriminating more carefully among own-race photos than among other-race photos. This tendency is likely to result in lineups which are fairer for own-race foils and targets.

In a follow-up study we (Ready & Brigham, in preparation) used a different sample of target photos, this time using both male and female photos. Once again a significant interaction between race of photo and race of subject occurred (Figure 2), with each race being more selective for own-race photos. However, the racial differences in selectivity showed no relationship to self-reported degree of cross-racial experience or to racial attitude, as measured by the MRAI (Brigham, Woodmansee & Cook, 1976).

Taken together, these studies suggest that the own-race bias is a moderately strong and consistent phenomenon which effects not only recognition accuracy but also response criterion and the care with which one discriminates among photos of faces.

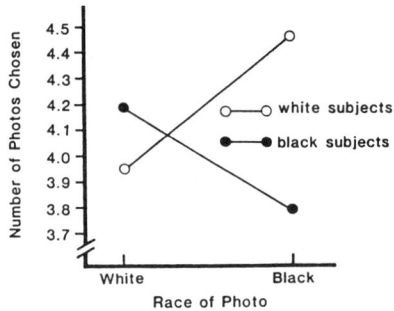

FIGURE 2. Number of photos chosen as "reasonably similar" to a target photo, male and female photos. N = 66 blacks and 66 whites. (From Ready & Brigham, in preparation)

3. WHY DOES THE DIFFERENTIAL RECOGNITION AFFECT OCCUR?

There has been little attention to the theoretical determinants of the own-race bias, as Lindsay & Wells (1983) correctly noted. There are several general principles which apply to intergroup perception which may shed some light on the origin of this effect. The illusion of outgroup homogeneity has been amply demonstrated for attitudinal intergroup perceptions (e.g., Linville, 1982; Park & Rothbart, 1982). People tend to assume that their own group is more heterogeneous in terms of attitude and personality than are members of an outgroup. This tendency seems to persist even within increased contact between the groups. One could propose that the own-race bias involves the application of this illusion of outgroup homogeneity to appearance as well as to personality. People also fail to learn or remember individuating information about outgroup members as well as they do about ingroup members (Rothbart, 1981; Park & Rothbart, 1982). Again one could propose that such differences in learning and memory might apply to distinctive facial information as well as to attitudinal, personality, and social information.

Turning more specifically to race, at least four hypotheses have been proposed for the own-race bias (Brigham & Malpass, 1985). The inherent difficulty hypothesis, the suggestion that some races are simply more difficult to identify than others, has not been supported by research findings (e.g., Goldstein, 1979a, 1979b; Goldstein & Chance, 1976; Shepherd & Dregowski, 1981). A second possibility is that difficulties in cross-racial identification are related to prejudicial attitudes. While our surveys indicated that many present-day attorneys share an assumption that more prejudiced persons will do more poorly on cross-race identification (Brigham & WolfsKeil, 1983), studies that have directly measured both interracial attitudes and face recognition have generally found no association between the two (e.g., Brigham & Barkowtiz, 1978; Lavrakas, Buri & Mayzner, 1976; Yarmey, 1979).

A third possibility is that people may spontaneously orient differently to own- and other-race faces. Chance & Goldstein (1981) suggested that people may orient in an inferential manner to own-race faces but in a more superficial manner to other-race faces. In laboratory studies, instructions orienting subjects to superficial orientations tend to lead to poorer subsequent recognition performance than does an inferential orientation (e.g., Bower & Karlin, 1974; Winograd, 1976, 1981). As compelling as this possibility seems, a recent study which manipulated subjects' orientation via face instructions and had them perform a lineup task (Devine & Malpass, 1985) found that orienting instructions had no impact on own-race effect. Devine and Malpass found a significant own-race bias under both superficial and inferential orientation conditions. In a similar vein, Barkowitz & Brigham (1982) found that giving a reward for accurate identification did not affect the magnitude of the own-race bias.

A final position, as implied in the Feingold (1914) quote above and endorsed by many attorneys and law officers (Brigham & WolfsKeil, 1983), suggests that different levels of experience (contact) with own- and other-race persons affects recognition ability. Many social scientists have argued that interracial contact under optimal conditions is likely to lead to decreases in prejudice and stereotyping and increase in interracial friendships and understanding (Allport, 1954, Amir, 1969; Cook, 1970). Reduction in prejudice is particularly likely when the equal status contact involves cooperative independence, a successful outcome, the potential for developing intimacy or friendship, when the authorities in the situation favour intergroup contact, and when the outgroup members encountered are of high status or at least do not embody the negative stereotypes held by prejudiced others. Rothbart & John (1985) have suggested that whereas the traditional view of prejudice reduction aims for a change in average evaluations in a positive direction, another beneficial result could be changes in the perceived homogeneity of the outgroup. That is, the realisation that the outgroup members are just as different from each other in appearance and personal characteristics as the ingroup members are. If the differential experience hypothesis is valid then the degree of contact should also improve people's ability to differentiate between members of another race.

However, despite the intuitive appeal of this notion, current research support for it is limited. Cross, Cross & Daly (1971) found that white children from segregated neighbourhoods showed more differential recognition than those from integrated neighbourhoods, but a similar difference was not evident in black children. Another study found that children in integrated schools showed a somewhat smaller own-race bias than those in segregated schools, but the findings were not entirely consistent (Feinman & Entwisle, 1976). Our convenience store field study (Brigham, Maas, Snyder & Spaulding, 1982) found a weak but statistically significant relationship (r = .28) between self reported degree of cross-race experience and cross-race recognition ability for white clerks. Other studies have found no relationship at all between self reported cross-race experience and recognition accuracy in the laboratory (Brigham & Barkowitz, 1978; Luce, 1974; Malpass & Kravitz, 1969).

As Brigham & Malpass (1985) have noted, although we cannot dismiss the possibility that interracial experience is not a significant factor in cross-race recognition, well-established principles on the role of experience on learning and remembering would seem to lead to the prediction that increased contact between groups should lead to greater ability to differentiate between the faces of outgroup members. Why is the research support so skimpy? Shepherd (1981) observed that either we are incorrect in these assumptions or we do not understand intergroup contact and experience sufficiently well to identify the important aspects of intergroup experience. Measures of contact and experience which more accurately assess the quality and depth of contact, as well as its frequency, may help us identify the relationship between experience and a cross-race effect if indeed one exists. We can speculate that more frequent intergroup contacts in positive interaction contexts would reduce the likelihood of differential recognition (Brigham & Malpass, 1985).

4. CAN THE OWN-RACE BIAS IN FACE RECOGNITION BE REDUCED OR ELIMINATED?

4.1. Special experience via occupational training

Several researchers have compared police with non-police to see if the special training in analysis of situations given to police improves their recognition accuracy. In general, results indicate little or no difference between police and non-police in recognition accuracy. Tickner & Poulton (1975) found that police detected slightly more thefts in a film than did the general public but were no better at recognising the faces seen in the film. Clifford & Richards (1977) found that with short exposure times police and non-police did not differ in accuracy of facial recognition but with longer exposure times police did better than non-police presumably because they had processing skills which could be employed during the long exposure interval. Marshall and Hanssen (reported in Clifford, 1976) found that police picked out more details from a film than did non-police but they also saw twice as many "incorrect facts". In a study done in Great Britain, Billig & Milner (1976) found no difference in the recognition of other-race faces between veteran policemen (who presumably had considerable degree of experience with other-race people) and younger policemen.

4.2. Training in face recognition

A number of studies have attempted to train people to do better in cross-race recognition accuracy. The results of these training attempts have generally not been very impressive. Elliot, Wills & Goldstein (1973) trained white subjects for recognition of white or Oriental faces. They found that the training on white faces did not increase recognition for white faces but training on Oriental faces did increase performance on Oriental faces somewhat immediately following training. Malpass, Lavigueur & Weldon (1973) worked with black and white subjects in a series of training tasks which included (a) describing faces so that another person could recognise the face from the description, (b) recognising faces from descriptions and (c) noting similarities and differences among triads of faces. None of these techniques significantly increased accuracy in facial recognition for own- or other-race faces. In a second study involving 100 faces in blocks of 20 faces each, Malpass et al. (1973) found that the own-race bias in white subjects was visible in the first and fourth training blocks but was no longer evident in the fifth block. Finally, Lavrakas, Buri & Mayzner (1976) used a conjunctive concept learning task and a simple concept learning task with their white subjects. Both concept learning tasks increased recognition performance for black faces on an immediate post-test but this difference disappeared one week later. Taken together these results seem to show that intensive training may lead to a temporary reduction in the own-race bias but that the change seems to be transitory.

Turning to training on own-race faces, the results are even more ambiguous. Woodhead, Baddeley & Simmonds (1979) conducted two studies, employing three days of instructions at an intensive level for white subjects and white faces. A recognition test four days later found no improvement in the first study, while in the second study performance was actually significantly worse after the training. In a similar vein, Malpass (1981a) used a series of 12 1-hour training sessions for each subject which involved either feature analysis training, global personality scoring, global facial judgements, or repeated face recognition tests. Training sessions were held two days a week for six weeks and the recognition test was given immediately after the last training session. The result of this intensive intervention was that the experimental subjects performed signifi-cantly more poorly on face recognition after the training than they had before the training.

Why have these studies found little or no improvement in face recognition despite intensive training procedures? Malpass (1981a) suggested that perhaps face recognition is overlearned and continually practiced, at least for own-race faces, and therefore significant improvement is unlikely due to a ceiling effect. A second possibility is that the training methods are unnatural and do not enhance the natural processes which people use in everyday face recognition situations.

There is one recent study which suggests that training on cross-race face recognition can have lasting results. Goldstein & Chance (1985) selected eight women who were normal in their recognition of white faces but very poor in recognising Oirental faces. The experimental group (n = 4) underwent eight training sessions to a quite difficult criterion. The recognition testing was done two days, one month, and five months after the last training session ended. They found significantly better recognition for Oriental faces (all faces in the testing situation were different from the ones utilised in training) for those subjects who had undergone the experimental training.

5. FUTURE DIRECTIONS FOR THEORY AND RESEARCH

The own-race bias in face recognition seems to be a well-established phenomenon in laboratory studies and preliminary evidence suggests its applicability to more ecologically valid field situations as well. We know, as yet, very little about the effect of other variables on the own-race bias. This includes situational variables such as observing conditions, arousal, stress, and retention interval, as well subject variables such as age, motivation, amount of equal status contact with outgroup members, and so forth. The social cognition/cognitive psychology literature suggests a number of promising concepts, but to date few have been applied to the area of face recognition.

Methodologically, the use of more forensically relevant situations and samples, such as event studies which mimic eyewitness identification situations, will add considerably to our knowledge. Such studies are not easy to carry out, as they require at a minimum two races of subjects and two races of target persons in order to investigate the own-race bias fully. Further research using as subjects people likely to serve as eyewitnesses, e.g., convenience store clerks, bank clerks, police officers, should also yield valuable information. The effect of race on lineup construction can be further investigated through calculations of the functional size (Wells, Leippe & Ostrom, 1979) and effective size (Malpass, 1981b) of lineups constructed. The own- and other-race lineups created can also be compared on other criteria such as police officers' ratings of fairness and target-foil similarity ratings made by experimental subjects.

Further investigation is obviously needed in possible ways of training people to be more accurate in recognition own- and other-race faces. Results of studies employing short- and long-term training procedures and laboratory face recognition assessment have yielded ambiguous results. It is even less clear what the impact of different types of training might be on face recognition in less artificial, more ecologically valid event situations.

FACES, PROTOTYPES, AND ADDITIVE TREE REPRESENTATIONS

H. ABDI

1. INTRODUCTION

The general purpose of this paper is to present a new method which particularly suits the typicality problem: the additive tree representations. These trees are used to represent objects as leaves on a tree so that the distance on the tree reflects the similarity between them. The problem of constructing these trees is well documented elsewhere, and will not be detailed here (cf. Sattah & Tversky, 1977; Abdi et al., 1984 to appear). If the data to be analyzed are in the form of a rectangular matrix (e.g. crossing objects and their features), the first step is to compute a distance between either the set of objects or the set of features. The additive tree representation is strongly linked with the well-known Tversky's (1977) contrast model, and is worth interpreting in this light. So, these links are first described, and then applied with an analysis of the data from the Goldstein et al. (1984) study of "bad guys and good guys".

2. TREE AND CONTRAST MODEL

In a famous paper, Tversky (1977) developed a general approach to similarity called the contrast model: each stimulus (say a, b...) is associated with a set of features (denoted A, B...). The similarity from a to b is defined as a function of 3 sets:

$$A \cap B, \quad B/A, \quad A/B.$$

Thus $s(a,b) = F(A \cap B, A/B, B/A)$.

If some additional conditions are imposed (namely: monotonicity, independence, and two "technical ones", (solvability and invariance), then the similarity between a and b can be expressed as:

$$S(a,b) = \theta \; f(A \cap B) - \; f(A/B) - \beta \; f(B/A)$$

with f an isotonic function, and α, β, θ 3 positive constants. When $=\alpha$, β and f additive (i.e. $f(A \cup B) = f(A)+f(B)-F(A \cap B)$), then, there exists a measure g such as:

$$S(a,b) = \lambda \; -g(A/B)-g(B/A) = \lambda \; -g(A \triangle B).$$

With λ a positive constant, and $A \triangle B$, symmetric difference between A and B.

Moreover, when the features follow a tree model (that is, if 3 stimuli can always be named a,b,c with $A \cap B = A \cap C \subseteq B \cap C$), this property allows a very convenient tree representation of the similarities. If the stimuli are leaves on the tree, and the edges of the tree appropriately valued, then the tree distance from a to b will be $d(a,b) = g(A/B)+g(B/A) = g(A \triangle B)$; which accumulates to define the distance in terms of distinctive features.

This expression of the distance on the tree in terms of distinctive features can be used to estimate the features composing the stimuli. To see how, it is convenient to introduce three notions: the median of a tree, the eccentricity of a vertex (eccentricity is to be taken here as "far from a centre"), and the intersection vertex of two vertices. The median of a tree is the vertex that minimised the sum of the distances to the set of the vertices. The eccentricity of vertex a, denoted e(a) is simply defined as the distance from a to the median of the tree. The intersection vertex of vertices a,b is the vertex, with minimal eccentricity, situated on the path from a to b; this appelation will become obvious later. Call a, b two vertices and x their intersection vertex, then the set components of the contrast model can be obtained as:

$g(A/B) = d(a,x) = e(a)-e(x)$; $g(B/A) = d(b,x) = e(b) - e(x)$; $g(A \cap B) = e(x)$.

Note, incidentally, $e(a) = g(A)$ can be seen as a measure of the overall salience of the stimulus a.

Thus the additive tree representation can be used as a tool to recover "a posteriori" the features (and their weights) composing a set of stimuli from a distance matrix (.e.g obtained by a sorting task, or any other scaling method), and can thus contribute to resolve the contention between wholistic and analytic similarity. In particular, a tree can give the number of distinctive features common to every pair of stimuli; and decompose each stimulus in (weighted) features so that the distance on the tree between stimuli is simply computed as a distance between (weighted) features (suffice to use the so-called city-block distance which can be interpreted as a generalization of the symmetric difference distance – for more details on this point, see Abdi, 1986). All these notions, it is hoped, then will be enlightened by an example.

3. GOOD GUYS AND BAD GUYS: A TREE ANALYSIS

In a recent paper, Goldstein et al. (1984) added a new contribution to the "implicit physiognomy" topic, i.e. the fact that observers find meaningful, and agree among themselves to attribute personality traits, intentions, occupations, etc. merely by looking at a face or photograph of a face. This fact has been repeatedly established in the literature (see, among others, Brunswick, 1945; Thornton, 1943; Secord, 1958; Shoemaker, 1973; Bull & Green, 1980). Although the basis for this attribution process is not always clear, due to possible confounding between descriptive variables such as attractiveness, beauty, uniqueness, typicality, etc. of faces (see, Cohen & Carr, 1975; Courtois & Mueller, 1981; Mueller et al., 1984), the attribution of character – or "semantic interpretation" – seems to influence the memory for faces, as well as being influenced by some characteristics of the stimuli (see, Bower & Karlin, 1974; Shepherd et al., 1978; Klatzky et al., 1982); and has been often suspected as a cause of systematic distortions in eyewitness testimony (see, Dion et al., 1972; Efran, 1974). In the Goldstein et al. study, subjects were presented with 5 arrays each composed of 20 white middle-aged men – photographs cut from a casting directory – and asked to find among the 20 portraits of each array 3 bad guys (mass murderer, armed robber, rapist) and 3 good guys (medical doctor, clergyman, engineer). The data were analyzed via 30 chi-square tests (one for each of the 6 "occupations" of the 5 arrays); as 27 of these 30 tests reached a significant level of .05, it was concluded that there was indeed a clear consensual agreement among the subjects. As an illustration, Goldstein et al. gave a contingency table corresponding to the results obtained from 58 subjects with array 3 (i.e. they gave the number of subjects that assigned a given occupation to each portrait). These results – recalled in Table 1 –

TABLE 1. Selection of faces in arrays 3 as exemplars of 6 "Occupations" (Data from Goldstein et al., 1984)

	A	B	C	D	E	F	G	H	I	J	K	L	M	N	O	P	Q	R	S	T
Mass Murderer	11	6	3	2	0	0	0	18	2	6	5	1	1	0	0	1	1	0	0	1
Armed Robber	3	4	0	4	0	4	0	13	0	6	4	1	7	1	0	3	0	5	2	1
Rapist	5	2	1	7	4	5	0	4	1	18	0	0	1	1	0	8	0	1	0	0
Medical Doctor	0	1	2	0	2	1	12	1	0	0	6	8	0	2	4	2	5	2	4	6
Clergyman	0	1	5	0	1	1	6	0	2	0	4	1	1	0	6	2	20	1	3	4
Engineer	0	1	1	0	1	3	6	0	1	0	1	5	3	4	6	5	6	2	4	9

are used as an example of a tree-analysis. The analysis proceeds in two steps: first the analysis of the occupations, second the analysis of the set of faces.

3.1. Occupations

The strong connection, already mentioned, between the tree distance and the city block metric justifies its use to compute distance between occupations. To be precise, if k_{ij} denotes the number of subjects that assigned the face i to the occupation j, then the distance between two occupations j, j' is computed by: $d_{jj'} = \Sigma \left| k_{ij} - k_{ij'} \right|$

Table 2 gives the city block distance matrix, Table 3 the tree-distance matrix and Figure 1 the tree. The squared correlation between the original matrix and the tree-distance matrice (.972) denoted by r is to be taken as an index of goodness of fit, and indicates, obviously, a fairly good fit between the data and a tree-model.

TABLE 2. City block distance from Table 1

	Doctor	Engineer	Clergyman	Murderer	Robber	Rapist
Doctor	–	34	46	90	84	96
Engineer	34	–	44	98	80	86
Clergyman	46	44	–	86	88	98
Murderer	90	98	84	–	44	70
Robber	84	80	88	44	–	58
Rapist	96	86	98	70	58	–

TABLE 3 - Tree distance approximation of distance of Table 2

	Doctor	Engineer	Clergyman	Murderer	Robber	Rapist
Doctor	–	34	46	91.25	82.75	94
Engineer	34	–	44	89.25	80.75	92
Clergyman	46	44	–	93.25	84.75	96
Murderer	91.25	89.25	93.25	–	44	68.25
Robber	82.75	80.75	84.75	44	–	59.75
Rapist	94	92	96	68.25	59.75	–
Sum:	348	364	340	386	352	410

TABLE 4 - Tree-reconstitution of the specific and common features

	Doctor	Engineer	Clergyman	Murderer	Robber	Rapist
Doctor	18					
Engineer		16				
Clergyman			24			
Murderer				26.25		
Robber					17.75	
Rapist						35.5
Engineer & Doctor	4	4				
Engineer & Doctor & Clergyman	18.25	18.25	18.25			
Murderer & Robber				6.5	6.5	
Murderer & Robber & Rapist				18.25	18.15	18.25
Sum = eccentricity	40.25	38.25	42.25	51	42.5	53.73

TABLE 5 - Tree reconstitution of the common features

	Doctor	Engineer	Clergyman	Murderer	Robber	Rapist
Doctor	–	22.25	18.25	0	0	0
Engineer	22.25	–	18.25	0	0	0
Clergyman	18.25	18.25	–	0	0	0
Murderer	0	0	0	–	24.75	18.25
Robber	0	0	0	24.75	–	18.25
Rapist	0	0	0	18.25	18.25	–
Sum:	40.5	40.5	36.5	43	43	36.5

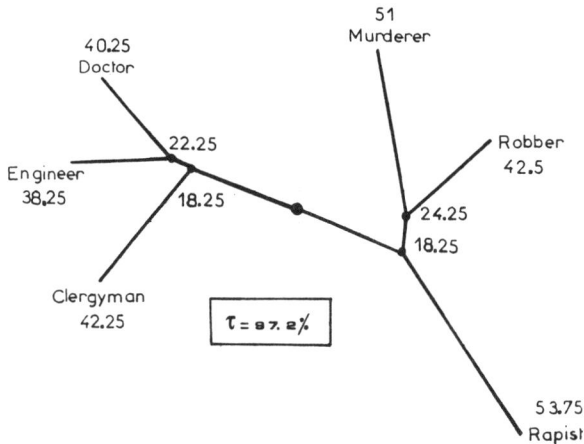

FIGURE 1. Additive tree representation of the "occupations" distance matrix from Table 2 the number near each vertex is the eccentricity of this vertex

The tree shows that the subjects separated clearly the "bad guys" from the "good guys". Moreover, the stereotypes of the "good guys" are less differentiated than the stereotypes of the "bad guys"; that is, the subjects do not distinguish between the "good guys", but do between the "bad guys". In particular, the rapist is the most stereotyped occupation, the engineer the least, and among the "good guys", the clergyman is the most stereotyped. These conclusions are supported by Table 5 where the eccentricity of the occupations is decomposed in specific and common weighted features (and so, the tree analysis can be seen as a variety of the classical factorial analysis). As pointed out previously, this "canonical weighted features matrix" is equivalent to the tree-distance matrix when the computed distance is the city block. Note that the features are labelled in agreement with the contrast model interpretation of the tree.

This small set of data can be used to raise a problem that will take its full sense (in terms of typicality and distinctiveness) with the analysis of the faces: the choice of the leaf representative of the set of leaves. To do so, we can adopt either of two criteria: select the median leaf (i.e. the leaf closer to the other leaves), or the leaf with the greatest number of common features. As can be seen in Table 2 and Table 5, the first approach leads to the choice of clergyman, the second to murderer and robber. Thus, the problem of choosing a best representative on a tree (or more generally from a similarity matrix) is not an obvious one.

3.2. Faces

The faces are analyzed with the same method as the occupations. The tree in Figure 2 reveals 3 clusters in the faces: the first composed of the "bad guys" faces (in order of specificity: H, J, D, A, B), the second of the "good guys" (Q, G, T, O, C, S), and the third of "misters average". This configuration is worth relating to the "typicality" (or distinctiveness, or similarity, etc.) problem which has received some attention in the face literature recently (cf. Courtois & Mueller, 1979; Davies et al., 1979; Light et al., 1979; Winograd, 1981; Bartlett et al., 1984). The general topic of this discussion can be subsumed under a main slogan "typical? yes! but of what?". If typicality is defined as representativeness (as contrasted with distinctiveness), then, as previously mentioned, two such kinds of representatives exist: the median leaf (here S), and the "greatest number of common features" leaf (here Q, G, T, or O). And, so there are, at least, two sets of criteria for the (proto)typicality within a whole category. However, when the category has an internal structure (as depicted here), the typicality has to be restricted to each cluster (although the contrasted clusters have to be taken in account). Then, the additive tree represents the distinctiveness of each face within its cluster by its eccentricity, which is one of the characteristics of the additive tree (contrary to other scaling methods: e.g. Euclidean representation, ultrametric tree, etc.). For example, the more typical (now in the sense of more distinctive) faces for the "bad guys" are H and J, for the "good guys" G and Q. Conversely the more typical "mister average" (and so the least distinctive) is E or even K. To conclude, it is hoped that the tree analysis can contribute to pinpoint the different (and sometimes contradictory) criteria for the notion of (proto)typicality, and to emphasize the necessity of taking in account the structure of categories when talking of models of typicality.

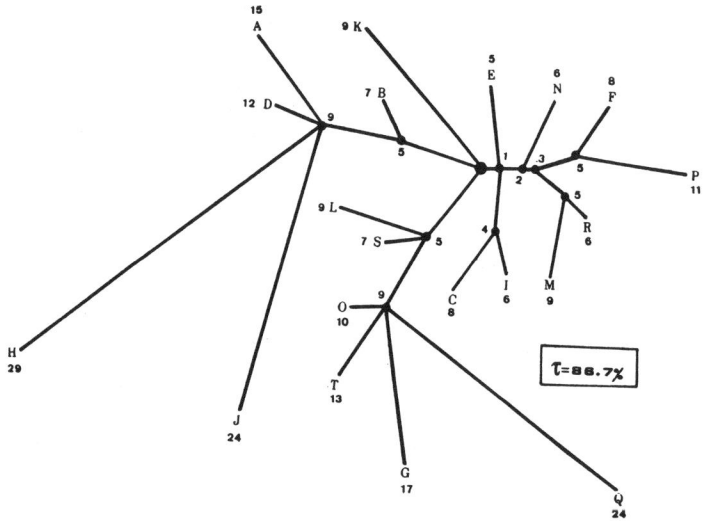

FIGURE 2 – Additive tree representation of the faces distance computed from Table 1 the number near each vertex is the eccentricity (in rounded figures)

ACKNOWLEDGEMENT

  The author is grateful to A.J. O'Toole for comments and discussions about this paper)

6. CORTICAL SPECIALISATION

FUNCTIONAL ORGANIZATION OF VISUAL NEURONES PROCESSING FACE IDENTITY

PERRETT, D.I., MISTLIN, A.J., POTTER, D.D., SMITH, P.A.J., HEAD, A.S., CHITTY, A.J., BROENNIMANN, R., MILNER, A.D. AND JEEVES, M.A.J.

1. ABSTRACT

We have found five different types of cell in the macaque temporal cortex each selective for one prototypical view of the head (face, profile, back of head, head up and head down). Neuronal analysis of these different head views is performed in anatomically discrete "columns" or patches of temporal cortex. In each of the five classes we have found cells sensitive to identity. Such cells respond selectively to one view of a particular individual and generalize across facial expression, viewing distance and changes in lighting or orientation (upright, inverted). A further class of cells responsive to all views of the head also contains cells selective for identity. We propose that sensitivity in this class to identity, independent of view (person recognition), is established by pooling the outputs of cells sensitive to identity for each prototypical view. This hierarchical scheme corresponds to computing view-independent (object centred) descriptions from high level view-dependent descriptions.

2. INTRODUCTION

In this paper we will review findings from our studies of single neurones in the temporal cortex of the monkey brain, that respond when the monkey looks at faces. In particular we will discuss how processing manifest in the responses of these cells may be organized to permit the recognition of individual faces. To this end we will describe a simplified model of visual processing that begins with early cortical processing and culminates with the successful visual identification of individuals and an input into the semantic stages of contemporary psychological models of face recognition.

2.1 Early Visual Processing

Consideration of the early stages of visual processing serves to emphasise the complexity of the task of recognizing individual faces. In the early stages of visual processing as witnessed in the electrophysiological recordings of Hubel and Wiesel [6,7] and in the computational model of Marr [9], the image is "broken up" into an extensive data array where the orientation, contrast and position of small elements of the image are specified. Marr labelled this early stage as the raw "primal sketch" - the two depictions at the top of Fig. 1 give a representation of a primal sketch of images of the face and profile of one person. These images are composed of many individual line elements each representing the resolved orientation at different points in the image. In reality the primal sketch or neural encoding of such images would be more complicated and would contain elements of many sizes.

Marr proposed that the operation of grouping principles (which essentially follow the laws of Gestalt psychologists) could label certain areas of the image as "belonging together" on the basis of the proximity, similarity etc. of the component elements within those areas. One can envisage the operation of grouping principles on the images in Fig. 1 separately labelling the areas of the image containing vertically oriented fine elongated elements; or a pair of horizontally oriented dark concentric circles, or four close blobs with a vertically symmetrical arrangement.

The grouping principles might in this way label regions of the image which should be treated together for further processing, but they would not make explicit what these regions were.

At the time Marr was developing his computational model of vision there was little physiological data for stages of visual processing beyond the early encoding in primary cortex. Indeed there still is a remarkable paucity of physiological data which can provide guidelines or constraints for computational models of recognition. Over the past five years several reports have emerged concerning the properties of visual cells in the temporal lobe of monkeys [1,2,13-18]. These reports do, we think, provide guidelines for formulation of a model of higher stages of processing of visual information for face recognition.

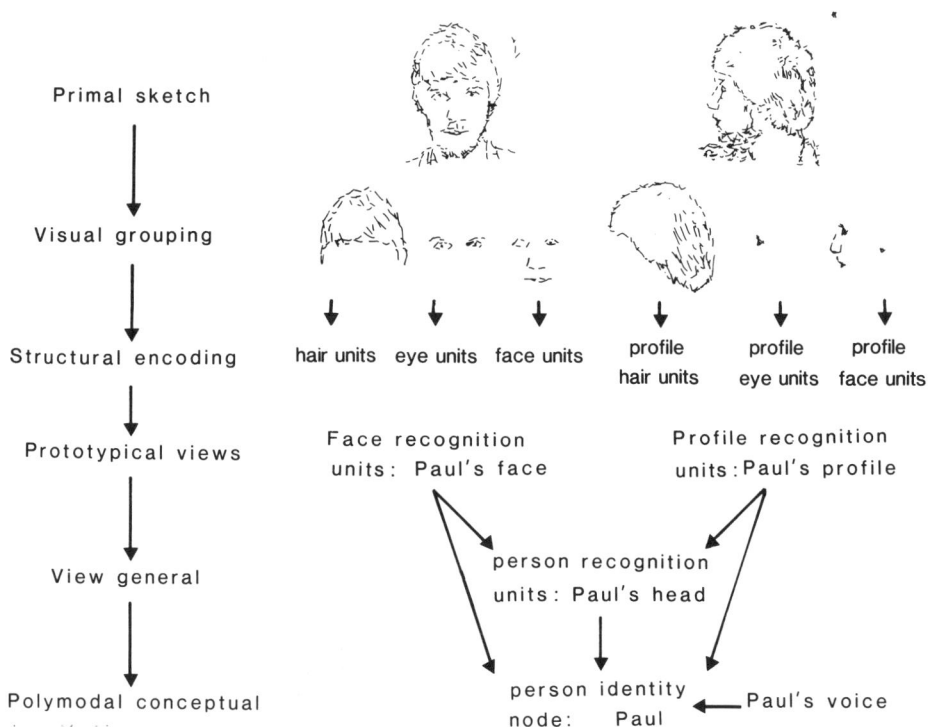

Figure 1. Flow of information processing leading to face recognition. The left hand column gives the computational stage of processing and the right hand side illustrates examples of the type of information available at each stage (for details see text).

2.2 Cells Sensitive to the General Characteristics of Faces

Substantial numbers of cells in the temporal cortex have now been studied which respond selectively to the sight of faces - or particular facial features [1,2,13-16]. In the main these cells are responsive to the general characteristics of the face since they respond equally to faces of differing identity and species (e.g. human and monkey). These cells are remarkable in their visual selectivity in that they do not respond to the sight of a great variety of simple geometrical stimuli (bars and edges) or to more complex 3-dimensional junk objects (such as an alarm clock) [1,2,13]. Furthermore the cells are unresponsive to a variety of arousing stimuli (such as loud noises, the sight of the body of a snake or a banana) [13]. Thus the responses to faces are not due to the arousal which might be evoked by the sight of a face.

In addition to the specificity in response to faces as opposed to other stimuli, the cells also show a capacity to generalize across many different examples or instances of this class of stimuli. The cells are capable of responding to the presence of a face despite changes in its position within the visual field, [1,2] changes in viewing distance and hence retinal size of the face[13,16], changes in face orientation (upright, horizontal, inverted) [3,13,14], and changes in the strength and direction of illumination [15]. (While responses do generalize to such unusual views generalization is not perfect since cell responses to unusual views are often slightly decreased in magnitude and are increased in latency to particular unusual views [15]).

These cells then display considerably more complexity in the trigger features required for activation compared to neurones in early visual cortex. The cells also generalize across variables (such as position and illumination level) which are made explicit during early encoding [6,7]. Considering this, the cells in the temporal cortex represent a considerable leap in processing from the primal sketch. But just what information has been extracted in the processing subsequent to the primal sketch? This can be answered in part by considering the visual basis of responses.

2.3 Structural Encoding

2.3.1 Features. The initial investigations of cells responsive to faces revealed that different cells were responsive to different parts of the face [1,13,14,15]. For many cells the eyes proved to be essential for responses to the entire face since covering the eyes of a face reduced responses to the level of spontaneous activity. Reciprocally, presenting the eyes in isolation produced responses equivalent to those evoked by the entire face. More recently we have studied a patch of cells for which the mouth region is a necessary and sufficient part of the face for producing responses. In this way we have found that many cells encode the presence of particular facial features, but do not appear to utilize visual information about other facial features [15,16].

2.3.2 Configuration. Faces are characterized by more than the presence of features. The features have a specific (normal) arrangement. We have studied sensitivity to configuration of facial features by comparing responses to pictures and 3-D models of monkey faces in which the individual features either have a normal or a jumbled arrangement. As reported in earlier work with 2-D jumbles we have found that some (but not all) cells responsive to the face require the normal organization of features for maximal response [2,13,14].

Studies of the visual basis of cells responsive to faces have revealed that the structural encoding of facial information is not a unitary process. Instead there appear to be several encoding processes proceeding in parallel. This is schematically illustrated in Fig. 1. Structural encoding of visual information about eyes leading to activation of "eye units", appears to be executed separately from encoding of information about the presence of hair. Cells sensitive to the configuration of facial features ("face units") may utilize information from several different encoded facial features but must also require information about the relative spatial distribution of major features in the face. This latter configurational information is presumably derived directly from earlier processing since cells within the temporal cortex generalize for position of preferred stimuli. Obviously the processing between the operation of grouping processes and the explicit labelling of structural entities such as eyes is the largest gap in our understanding of vision. The arrows corresponding to this stage in Fig. 1 are equivalent to "and then a miracle occurs".

2.4 Prototypical Views

Before considering the encoding of identity it is important to consider the different views in which a face (head) can be presented. The face can be turned away from the observer to profile or further to present the back of the head; the head can also be inclined towards the floor or the chin raised to the ceiling.

It is equally important to emphasise the distinction between changes in perspective or view of an object and changes in the illumination, size or orientation (upright, inverted) of a particular view. We have already noted that cells responsive to the general characteristics of a face respond to the many different examples or instances of one view of the head. At St Andrews we have sought to define the tolerance of cells' responses to changes in the view of the head in addition to the tolerance of different instances of each view [15].

For the majority of cells responsive to faces, but not to control objects, we found that responses declined as the head was rotated away from the observing monkey. Turning the face 45° away to profile or rotating up or down by the same amount reduced responses by about half. Turning the face 90° away effectively abolished responses. Thus it became clear that while cells were able to respond to many different examples of faces, the cells were nevertheless able to cope only with limited perspective transformations.

Studies of different views of the head, however, revealed in total five types of cell in the STS each maximally responsive to one view of the head. The five types of cell were separately tuned for full face, profile, back of the head, head up, and head down.

For each of these views the analysis of visual information seems to proceed in the same way as that already described for faces. For example, cells maximally responsive to the profile face were able to respond to many different examples of left or right profile faces, with changing orientation (upright/inverted), lighting and size. Moreover as indicated in Fig. 1 different cells responsive to the profile face depend on different facial features or combination of features. For particular cells the profile eye was a necessary and sufficient feature for responses to the profile face. For other cells the important feature was the profile mouth and for others the combination or configuration of profile features was important.

It is perhaps most significant that we did not find a greater variety of cell types. We found no cells tuned to views intermediate between those mentioned; for example, no cell was found maximally responsive to a half profile face turned 45° from the observer, yet all cells were tested with this view.

Of course because of the limited capacity for generalization over perspective change, the half profile face would be handled equally by cells tuned for the full face and cells tuned for the profile, each of these two cell populations being activated to half the rate produced by the preferred prototypical view.

The views for which we have found separate encoding we have referred to as "prototypical" views and they correspond to those which are maximally distinct. This is clearest in the horizontal plane since the full face, profile and back of the head, are orthogonal views. In the vertical plane it is still not clear whether coding is for distinct views or for distinct postures relative to gravity for which there are a variety of appropriate views (e.g. face head up, profile head up, back of the head up). Evidence so far is consistent with both alternatives with head posture being established through initial encoding of head view.

The reason for placing the encoding of prototypical views of the head at a level subsequent to the structural encoding of facial features comes from studies of sensitivity to different regions of the face. For cells responsive to the full face we find that the cells respond to eye contact but not to a face with averted gaze. Yet when the eyes are covered we still find a greater response to the face view than the profile view.

For cells responsive to the profile view we find the opposite situation. These cells respond selectively to averted eye gaze, and when the eyes are covered they respond to other regions of the profile face, but not to the same regions of the full face. Such findings demonstrate an appropriate convergence of information about the appearance of different facial features that are characteristic of one view of the head.

Summarizing so far it would seem that five distinct (orthogonal or prototypical) views of the head are subjected to a separate and parallel analyses. Each population of neurones handling information about a particular view is able to process virtually all possible examples of that view.

2.5 Sensitivity to Identity

All the above remarks have been made about cells responsive to the general characteristics of the face (or other view of the head). These cells respond to the faces of different individuals, different species and sometimes even to impoverished line drawn faces. During our studies we became aware of cells that apparently responded more to one individual (experimenter) than to others. On such occasions we have explored responses to different examples and views of preferred and non-preferred faces to determine the extent to which cell responses could signal information about identity [16].

Fig. 2 gives the responses of one cell to different examples of two faces (Paul Smith and David Perrett). The cell gave larger responses to Paul's face over all the different examples despite changes in the orientation, size, colour and expression of the faces. The cell was however unresponsive to the profile of PS. About 10% of cells responsive to faces show sensitivity to identity in this way.

We have found evidence for sensitivity to identity amongst each of the five classes of cell tuned to one head view. Thus (as depicted in Fig. 1) we found one set of cells most responsive to Paul's face, and another set most responsive to Paul's profile, yet other sets of cells are most responsive to particular views of other individuals familiar to the monkey. In this way we believe that the recognition of each individual known to an observer proceeds by the analysis of a small set of prototypical views of that individual. For each known person there would be a set of "face

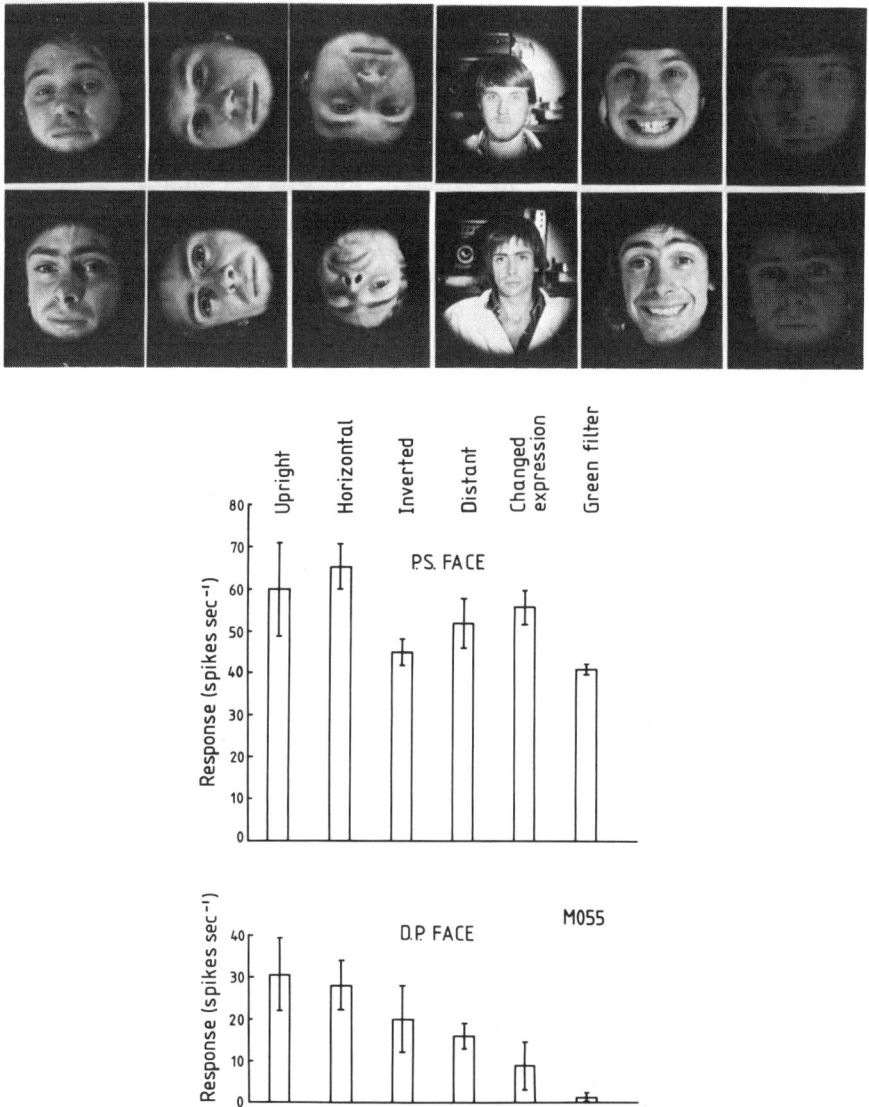

Figure 2. Effects of face identity. (a) Examples of the different views of the faces of the two experimenters PS (upper row) and DP (lower row). (b) The mean and standard error of response are illustrated for cell M055 to these views. Upper: the cell responds to the face of PS under a variety of viewing conditions: as his face was presented upright, horizontal, inverted, at an increased distance, with changed expression or through a green filter. Lower: comparable views of the face of DP produced less response.

recognition units" and a set of "profile recognition units" etc.

To explore the visual basis of such sensitivity to identity we examined responses to three different regions of preferred and non-preferred faces (hair and forehead; eyes; nose, mouth and lower face). We found that sensitivity to identity can arise in at least two ways: either by cells responding to particular characteristic features of the preferred individual, or by sensitivity to some combination (or configuration) of pictures which typify that individual.

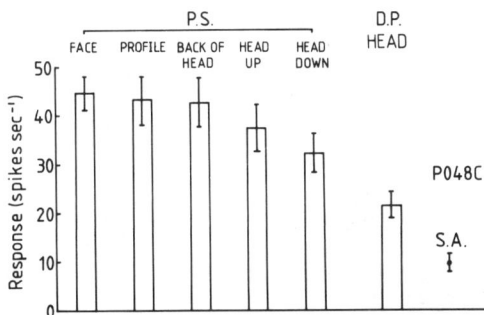

Figure 3. Sensitivity to identity over different views of the head. The mean and standard error of response are illustrated for cell P048. The cell responds to the different views of PS's head including the full face, profile, back of head, head up (face raised 45 degrees) and head down (face lowered 45 degrees). Comparable views of the head of DP produced less response.

The model of recognition we envisage does not stop at the level of prototypical views. We have studied large numbers of cells that are responsive to many or all views of the head but yet are unresponsive to the sight of control objects. We have suggested that such "view general" cells can be "wired up" by pooling the outputs of cells tuned to prototypical views. Again 10% of the cells responsive to all views of the head exhibit additional selectivity for identity. Thus the cell illustrated in Fig. 3 responds well to many different examples of Paul's face and in addition it responds well to the other views of Paul (profile, back of head, head up, head down). Corresponding examples and views of a second face produce reduced responses (though these are above the spontaneous activity). In our model such a cell corresponds to a "person recognition unit" which signals the presence of one particular person from any view [c.f. 18]. Note that the existence of many such units would be likely for each known person to the observer.

2.6 Facial Expression

So far we have made only a few observations which we can be sure have direct relevance to the encoding of expression. The first observation is a negative one: cells that we have studied that appear sensitive to identity seem to ignore expression. That is they respond equally to a preferred individual with different expressions. Where we have studied cells sensitive to expression we have found them generally insensitive to identity, responding equally to the equivalent expression of humans and of monkeys [16]. These two observations suggest that the neural mechanisms responsible for processing identity and expression information are to some extent separate [5].

Recently we have had the opportunity to study a group of cells sensitive to mouth configuration. Several of these cells have been selective for very wide open mouths without teeth visible, that is characteristic of open mouth threat expressions. These cells were insensitive to other dark circular control stimuli, and were more responsive to the full-face view with open mouth than to the profile view. Other neighbouring cells required the visibility of teeth within an open square mouth (common to grimaces and teeth chattering expressions). The cells sensitive to teeth, however did not discriminate between humans simulating teeth chattering expressions and human faces biting a food item with similar mouth posture.

Without additional evidence for response sensitivity to other facial attributes characteristic of expression for the same cells it is parsimonious to propose that such cells represent a structural encoding stage for mouth configuration. For cells to be labelled "tuned for open mouth threat expression" it would be necessary to show simultaneous tuning for several characteristics of this expression (e.g. open mouth configuration, and raised eyebrows, and/or slightly lowered head posture.) We postulate that the use of information from several regions of the face - and contextual information (e.g. presence of food near the mouth) may converge at a subsequent stage of processing to disambiguate true expressions from incidental facial actions.

3. Speculations on the Role of Experience in the Formation of "Person Recognition Units"

One of the most intriguing questions which arises from the discovery of units with an apparent selectivity for face identity (and from the postulated existence of "face recognition units" in models of face recognition) is "How do they get there?" There are two major theoretical alternatives. The first follows the suggestion of Konorski [8] that at birth there would be recognition units tuned only to general facial characteristics. These would be wired up genetically and would be capable initially of detecting the presence of eyes or faces per se. During early life they would function in this role only, allowing the infant the ability to orient to faces and perhaps mimic facial gestures of care-givers [10]. As the infant becomes familiar with particular care-givers a few cells would become tuned to the distinctive face features of these individuals. In short there would be a genetic programming of cells sensitive to coarse facial features and an experience-dependent commitment of some such cells to the detection of individuals important to the observer. The number of cells committed to one person would be proportional to their importance to the observer. This proposition does not account for the actual process of commitment or provide a mechanism for discriminating unfamiliar individuals.

The second alternative is that an extensive catalogue of cells selective for possible types of facial features and for possible configurations of features is set up under genetic influence, much as the genetic programming of the immune system sets up millions of clones of cells each selective for one type of potential antigenic protein. This alternative seems less plausible but the analogy should make it clear that it is by no means impossible. Under this second scheme individuals that an observer becomes familiar with just happen to activate particular subsets of cells or catalogue entries. Experience would only then come into play, simply to establish connections between such cells and semantic information related to the now familiar individual (Final Stage in Fig. 1).

It is difficult to conceive of experimental data which could clearly rule out the second intuitively less plausible alternative. Considerations of probability tend to favour an experience dependent process. Cells such as that in Fig. 3 can respond to several views of one individual yet less well to corresponding views of a second individual. Moreover "person recognition units" often respond to internal parts of a preferred face in addition to external features such as the hair. But apart from information about hair there are no visual cues to specify that the back and front view of one person's head actually belong to the same person. The probability that 5 views of one person will match the selectivity of a genetically prewired cell and 5 corresponding views of a second person (with similar hair) will not match is remote (p = $1/2^5$ = 0.03). Again studies of "face recognition units" have revealed that they are often sensitive to several visually distinct yet characteristic regions of a preferred face [16]. It thus becomes increasingly improbable that such an appropriate combination of information about different parts of a face or different views of a face can be established through fortuitous genetic wiring.

3.1 Limitations to Effects of Experience

It is also interesting to note that if experience does account for the selective responses to a particular individual, experience does not result in these cells becoming sensitive to all the information that is pertinent to the identification of that individual. Thus while particular cells may be responsive to two regions of the face of one individual (the mouth and eyes) such cells may be unresponsive to the hair of the same individual [16].

3.2 Experience-Dependent Wiring of Face Recognition Units

The organization of information processing for discriminating identity could depend on the cells accepting inputs from particular characteristic facial features (in an OR gate fashion), or combinations of facial features (in an AND gate fashion). Far more information processing may, however, be executed that is not apparent from an inspection of cells' responses to separate facial features. This can occur if cells possess connections that deny activation - in an AND NOT (NAND) gate fashion. Thus a cell might appear unable to use information about one preferred individual's characteristic hair but may nonetheless be inhibited by the sight of hair of other individuals or a wig of hair worn by the preferred individual.

One cell studied responded well to the eye and mouth region of one person's face but was unresponsive to the hair of that person. When that person's face was now presented with a wig the cell was now totally unresponsive. This indicates a mechanism by which disguise can operate. Thus while the cell appears to be unable to use hair information in any positive way it nevertheless can use it in a negative way. Incorrect hair denies the cell activation by other correct facial features.

Studies of the importance of different facial features in discriminating among faces (e.g. see Haig [3,4]) can be limited by the size of the set of faces to be discriminated. For instance while the mouth region may be generally unimportant for distinguishing any one of four faces from the other three, the mouth region may become critical for distinctions between these faces and a fifth which may have a distinctively large mouth. Simply updating descriptions of the original set of four faces with information, "and not large mouth" presents an efficient way of tightening up the selectivity of face recognition units when faced with new individuals to be discriminated from those that are already familiar.

It is always possible that a cell which appears selective for Paul when tested against a second face or even 10 others, may actually be equally responsive to a second individual (such as Paul's brother). Paul and his brother may share some facial characteristics but may differ in others. Should the discrimination between Paul and his brother become pertinent to some observer then presumably cells tuned to Paul may "learn" to stop responding to particular characteristics possessed by his brother.

4. Relation to Computational Models of Recognition

The initial stages of visual processing and the view-general stage of processing in the scheme of Fig. 1 have a direct correspondence to the start and goal of Marr and Nishihara's computational theory of visual recognition. Their theory progressed from a basic description of surfaces present in the image directly to descriptions of objects that allowed generalization over different views. Thus Marr and Nishihara's theory lacked what we see as a useful intermediate stage of processing, the separate analysis of prototypical views of an object. Our recent studies indicate that the encoding of prototypical views does not only happen for the face: it would also appear to be true for other parts of the body such as the hands. Indeed on logical grounds an independent analyses of the distinct views of an object would seem necessary. For the majority of objects only learning can specify that the back and front views of an object belong to the same object.

Associative networks have a prominent position in current computational models of human memory. This position may be well justified since such networks do show many properties analogous to human memory. The only deficiency presented by the proposition that the human brain uses an associative network is that there are no guidelines as to the nature of inputs to be used by the associative network. To take the most basic position: in principle it should be possible to use photoreceptors (or individual pixels in the case of a computer simulation of human memory) as inputs to a huge associative network with outputs to an array of motor fibres. Indeed, the WISARD, a hardwired electronic recognition system, uses small sets of (five) randomly chosen pixels as an input to memory [19]. An associative network should however perform more efficiently if the information fed along input lines is pertinent to the distinction to be made with memory. The WISARD can be seen as a remarkable automated recognition device but it would be unwise to assume that it is an adequate model for understanding the human facial recognition system.

Millward and O'Toole [11] report in a simulation of human face recognition using associative memory, that the recognition process bears greater similarity to human performance when zero crossings (contour boundary positions) are used as inputs rather than raw pixel information. Further gains in efficiency or similarity to human face memory would seem likely if highly processed information about facial features and feature configurations could be used instead of zero crossings. Network modelling may have contributed to the understanding of memory functions but as yet it has contributed little to the understanding of the visual processes themselves which may input into memory systems.

5. Anatomical Organization

Fig. 1 presents only a functional scheme of organization. The figure is not meant to imply a structural scheme whereby discrete cortical areas are involved in processing of information at one of the vertical levels in the model. Indeed we have found that three levels of processing (structural

encoding of facial features, prototypical views and view-general
descriptions) are all executed within one cytoarchitectonic region of the
STS.

Our studies of the superior temporal sulcus over the past five years have
not only revealed an increasing diversity in cell types sensitive to facial
information but they have also revealed an increasing number of cell types
handling static and dynamic visual information about other parts of the
body. Thus the brain area containing cells responsive to faces is not face
specific, rather it processes a variety of visual information pertaining to
the face and to the rest of the body (in addition to somatosensory,
auditory information and particular types of visual movement). How then is
processing organized? A random organization of cell types would indicate

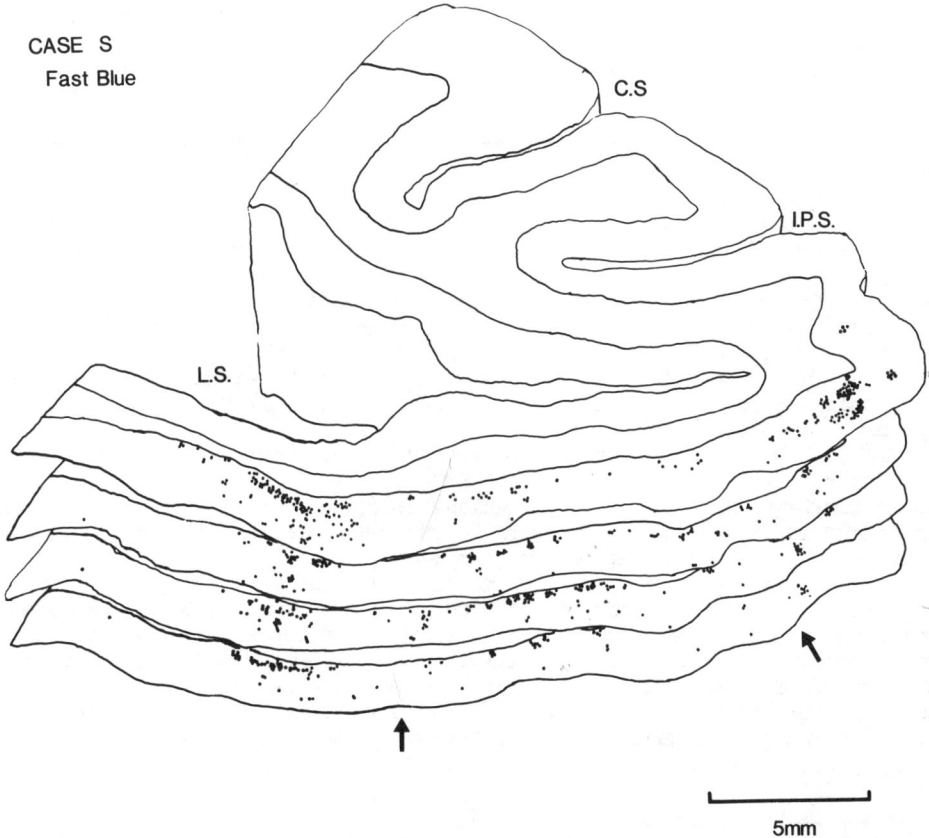

Figure 4. Illustrates the distribution of cells within the cortex of the
upper bank of STS labelled after injection of fluorescent dye fast blue
into inferior parietal cortex (caudal area PG). The four serial sections
were cut saggitally at intervals of 0.25 mm. C.S., central sulcus; I.P.S.,
inferior parietal sulcus; L.S., lunate sulcus. The distribution of
labelled cells divides STS into 3 regions, caudal, middle and rostral.
Within the middle region (between the arrows) labelled cells show a
periodic distribution of small clumps in lower cortical layers. Neurones
responsive to faces are found in this middle region.

that the brain area had some general visual function. The presence of large numbers of cells processing faces with this area would only indicate an allocation of part of this general mechanism, in proportion to the importance of this class of stimuli.

Reconstructions of the positions of all recorded cells and mathematical analyses of the proximity of cells of a given type indicates two levels of anatomical organization. Cell types are grouped together both vertically through the thickness of the cortex and horizontally in clumps or "columns" which extend laterally across the surface of the cortex [15, 16, 17].

The exact geometry and dimensions of the clumps are not yet clear but the data obtained so far lead us to suspect that the functional organization of the temporal cortex may follow the same anatomical principles as the columnar organization that has been extensively described for early sensory cortex [6,7,12,20].

The very existence of a clumped distribution of the cells responsive to particular views of faces indicates that there is a distinct specific anatomical substrate for face processing. But at the same time the existence of clumps of cells processing other types of information within the same brain area indicates that this brain area should not be regarded as face-specific.

The clumping of cells processing particular types of information may be the result of patches of cortex having distinct patterns of input and output connections. Thus processing within this region of STS may be organized in a system of columns which can be defined anatomically in a similar manner to primary and secondary visual cortices. We have evidence that at least one of the outputs of STS is arranged in a patchy fashion. Fig. 4 shows the distribution of labelled cells within STS after an injection of the retrograde fluorescent tracer Fast Blue into inferior parietal cortex. Labelled cells represent neurones within the upper bank of STS cortex which project into posterior parietal cortex. It can be seen that in the middle regions of STS cortex (between the 2 arrows) corresponding to the area in which face selective cells have been encountered, labelled cells occur in discrete patches in lower cortical layers. These patches appear to possess some periodicity. Thus at least one of the afferent connections of this area is arranged on a columnar basis. This is not to say that the cells labelled may actually correspond to a part of the face processing system; they may represent clumps of cells processing some other visual dimension. We can at present only offer the anatomical demonstration of an instance of columnar organization within this brain region to support our physiological evidence that face processing may be organized in a system of columns.

HEMISPHERIC ASYMMETRY IN FACE PROCESSING IN INFANCY

S. de SCHONEN, M. GIL DE DIAZ, E. MATHIVET

1. INTRODUCTION

Besides the interest for the development per se of face processing, developmental studies can be considered as offering the opportunity to get access to basic questions involved in face processing that may be masked, but not suppressed, in the adult by the occurrence of other kinds of processing. The absence, for instance of operational language, of cultural knowledge and habits, may in some way simplify the question. Infants constitute from this point of view a simpler model than adults. Of course this claim relies on the assumption that the processes at work in infancy are still at work in adulthood but that they are merely more difficult to disentangle from processes that have developed later on. This assumption is plausible. It is known that some behaviour as well as some organs disappear totally in the course of development. However the behaviour or organs that have been observed as disappearing serve functions that also disappear during ontogeny (such as behaviour exhibited during hatching for instance). Since face and physiognomy processing correspond to a set of functions that are, on the contrary, to be developed and used throughout life, it is sensible to believe that face processing in infancy is somehow related to the same processes in adults.

However developmental studies on face processing in infancy have never considered seriously the possibility that infants may not process faces in the same way in each hemisphere or that the functions of face processing may be not the same in each hemisphere. Contrary to adult experimental tasks, the experimental situations in which infant competences are studied, are not very constraining and the infant is free in some way to define his/her own task or own interest; that is, an infant is not asked to discriminate as accurately as possible which is the new and which is the familiar stimulus, he/she is merely presented with a familiar and a new stimulus. In paradigm such as preferential looking or as habituation/dishabituation with or without conditioning, the infant is free to direct his attention and processing to whatever he likes. This has important consequences if one considers the fact that nothing is known concerning the possibility of an interhemispheric coordination or transfer, or concerning rules of dominance or precedence of one hemisphere over the other in infancy. Suppose, as a very trivial instance, a habituation/dishabituation experiment where infants are habituated first with a physiognomy A with different emotional expressions and then with a physiognomy B, also with different expressions. Suppose now that one hemisphere reacts preferentially to physiognomy identity, and the other hemisphere to positive or communicative expressions. If half of the infants work with one hemisphere and half with the other the conclusion will be that there is no identity discrimination. The same if a same infant reacts sometimes with one hemisphere and sometimes with the other. If one hemisphere is dominant over the other for reasons that are not directly related to the discrimination under study, the experiment will measure the competence or incompetence of this dominant hemisphere and will not tell whether at some other time or at the same time the other hemisphere may be efficient.

That is why we thought of developing a technique to test face and physiognomy processing in infancy in each hemisphere separately and also to test inter-hemispheric transfer and coordination. Such studies should also shed some light on how each hemisphere develops its own way of processing: is face processing similar in the two hemispheres during the first months of life or already different ? In the latter case is the difference a mere question of a "gap" between maturation of the two hemispheres or not ? When do coordination and information "transfer" between the two hemispheres develop ?

Our first aim was to check whether the hemispheres react spontaneously in the same way when presented with a familiar face and a non-familiar face. This paper will focus on this question.

2. EXPERIMENT I : MOTHER/STRANGER DISCRIMINATION

2.1. Method. The method principle is the same as that used in adult studies where tachistoscopic presentations in each visual hemifield at a time permit to control which hemisphere is stimulated first. However, different from adult studies, the response used here as the dependent variable is the latency of the ocular saccade in response to the stimulus onset.

2.1.1. Apparatus. The stimuli were rear-projected by a Kodak Carrousel projector on one of two translucent screens (140 x 107 mm each) situated to the right and the left of a red luminous light (2 mm square): this light served as the central fixation point. The innermost boundary of the stimulus was situated at 2° to the right or the left of the fixation point. The exposure duration was controlled by an electronic shutter (Compur Electr. 5FS) installed on the projector. The shutter's rise time from fully closed to fully open was 7 ms ensuring a relatively squarewave onset and offset.

Subjects sat in front of the screen with their eyes at the level of the fixation point at about 50 cm from the screen. They were seated on their mother's laps. The mother was seated on a chair in a kind of cage that restrained her lateral and antero-posterior movements. She was asked not to talk, move, and to keep the infant's back against her.

A video I.R. camera situated under the level of the stimuli, and at the vertical of the central point, recorded the subject's face and eyes on a video tape recorder (Sony VO 5850 P). An experimenter watched the position of the subject's head and eye fixation on a video screen; the eye fixation was assessed by means of the corneal reflections of the central point of fixation and of 2 sets of 4 reference I.R. sources situated on each side of the infant's head at about 15 cm from its eyes and projecting on the border line between the iris and the sclera. A stimulus was projected when and only when the infant fixated the fixation point with the head in the proper position and at a proper distance from the screen (variations in distance between the subject's head and the screen were detected by both the size of the face and the blur of the video picture).

The subject's face and eyes were recorded throughout the experiment. A video timer (1/100 s) was simultaneously recorded as well as the signals of onset and offset of the stimuli. The tapes were analyzed following experimentation in order to measure the latencies of the ocular saccades directed toward the stimulus (see below).

2.1.2. Stimuli. The stimuli were colour slides of female faces. Each subject was presented with two physiognomies: its mother's physiognomy and the physiognomy of another subject's mother (a "stranger"). Each face was photographed with a neutral expression while facing the camera, against a common black background in the same condition of luminance. The women wore a black bathing cap and a black scarf in order to suppress variations in hair dressing, in hair-face separation, ear and neck shape. Make up and spectacles were excluded. All the faces were photographed in such a way that the greater horizontal axis of each face occupied the same width on the display. Photographs were mounted in such a way that the upper limit of the inferior eyelids be horizontally aligned with the fixation point when projected.

A stranger's face was paired with the mother's face with the following criteria: the complexion colour and the outer contour shape of the faces should be very similar; the vertical axis size of the two faces should be equal (chin to forehead/bathing cap line) and finally the amount of light transmitted by the two slides should be approximately equal (as measured by a luxmetre to 1/10 L). Each mother was also used as a stranger for another infant.

Each face of a pair was reproduced in 20 copies making 40 stimuli or trials with 10 mother and 10 stranger stimuli presented in each visual field. The exposure duration was 250 ms for subjects aged 7 to 9 months and 350 ms for subjects aged 4 to 6 months. These durations were chosen following the results of a pilot study as the shortest durations at which given aged infant reacts with an ocular saccade at all presentations in the hemi-visual fields when presented with a long sequence of trials.

2.1.3. Procedure. Once the infant was seated correctly, the lights were switched off and the central point of fixation was switched on. When the infant fixated the fixation point, a stimulus was delivered and the fixation point was switched off. The stimuli were presented alternately in the right visual field (RVF) and the left visual field (LVF). This procedure minimized uncertainty on the location of presentations while keeping constant the subject's state for comparison between the two visual field performances. Stranger and mother stimuli were presented in a pre-arranged random order. The 20 first trials consisted in 5 mother and 5 stranger stimuli in each visual field; the same applied for the last 20 trials. Half of the Ss of each age group began with a right field presentation and half with a left field presentation but the first stimulus was always a mother stimulus.

Every 5 trials, a female face, totally different from the other two faces was presented for 4 s in order to quiet the infants and keep them attentive. These 8 supplementary trials are not considered in the results.

The intertrial delay between the response to a stimulus and the presentation of the next stimulus depended on the subject (varying between 3 and 10 s). Subjects quickly learned to fixate the central point as soon as it lit up.

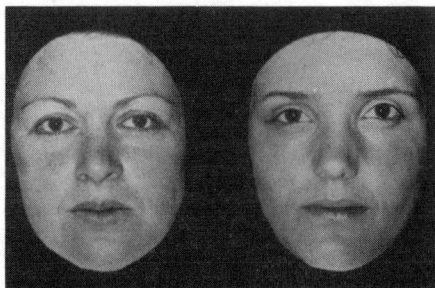

FIGURE 1. Experiment 1: An example of a pair of faces used in the mother/stranger discrimination task.

2.1.4. <u>Subjects</u>. 40 males, 20 per age group: 4 to 6 months (mean: 5 mo.) and 7 to 9 months (mean: 7 mo.).

2.1.5. <u>Analysis of responses</u>. The latency of the ocular saccade in response to the onset of each stimulus presentation was measured on the video recording, with a frame by frame analysis performed by a scorer who did not know where (right or left) and what (mother or stranger) was the stimulus. Each trial was first examined at a normal speed in order to determine the approximate time zone of the saccade. Then, the first frame on which the corneal reflections of the 2 sets of 4 reference IR lights appear to move relative to the border line between the iris and the sclera were considered as the beginning of the saccade. If lid closure occurred at a stimulus onset or if a latency was shorter than 160 ms or longer than 1 s, the trial was discarded. If the measure of the latency of a saccade could not be replicated in a second examination of the tape the trial was also discarded. All these discarded trials, together with those with no response and those where the ocular saccade was in the wrong direction, left the mean number of reliable trials at 7.8 per subject out of 10 trials for each category of stimuli in each visual field, with no difference in the occurrence of discarded trials as a function of visual field, category of stimuli and place in the experimental sequence.

2.2. Results

The 40 trials were divided in two successive series of 20 trials, phase 1 and 2, in order to check for a possible differential effect related to stimulation repetition. It must be remembered that infants do not receive any consigne and thus the task they perform during the experiment may change with repetition of trials. Since there were no differences related to the slides of presentation of the first trial under all conditions, the data of both groups of Ss were combined. A 2(Age) x 2(Phase) x 2(Familiarity) x 2(Visual Field) factorial analysis of variance reveals that the following effects are significant: Phase ($F(1,38) = 20.70$, $p < .001$), Familiarity ($F(1,38) = 11.387$, $p < .005$), Phase x Familiarity ($F(1,38) = 7.51$, $p < .01$), Phase x Visual Field ($F(1,38) = 7.17$, $p < .025$), the Phase x Visual Field x Familiarity interaction approached significance ($F(1,38) = 3.19$, $.05 < p < .10$) (fig. 2). There was no significant effect of age, nor significant interaction with this variable.

The first question concerns discrimination between mother and stranger stimuli: do infants recognize their mother, are latencies differentially related to the two physiognomies ? Ss significantly decrease their latencies of response from phase 1 to phase 2 (406 ms to 368 ms); they react significantly faster to their mother than to the stranger (378 ms/396 ms). Analysis of the significant interaction between Phase and Familiarity

FIGURE 2. Experiment 1: mean latencies of the ocular saccades (ms) as a function of Stimuli, Visual hemi-fields and Phases

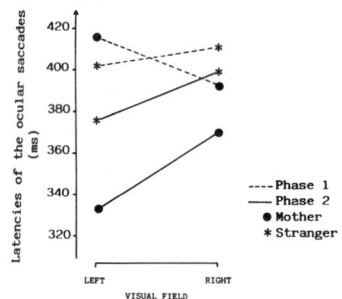

shows that the Familiarity effect is significant in phase 2 only (F(1,38) = 16.43, p < .005) and the decrease of latencies between the two phases is greater for the mother (F(1,38) = 30.14, p < .005) than for the stranger stimuli (F(1,38) = 3.33, .05 < p < .10). The systematic difference in latencies of responses between mother and stranger stimuli implies that infants recognize their mother.

The next question concerns the comparison between visual field performances. The analysis of the significant interaction between Phase and Visual Field effects shows that Ss decrease their latencies from phase 1 to phase 2 in the LVF (F(1,38) = 26.15, p < .001) and not in the RVF. The three factor interaction (Phase x Familiarity x Visual Field) sufficiently approaches significance to be analysed. Analysis of this interaction shows that the decrease of latencies in the LVF from phase 1 to phase 2 is significant for the mother stimuli (F(1,38) = 14.57, p < .005) and not for the stranger stimuli. The decrease of latencies from phase 1 to phase 2 for the mother stimuli is greater in the LVF (F(1,38) = 41.24, p < .001) than it is in the RVF (F(1,38) = 4.39, p < .05) whereas no significant decrease from phase 1 to phase 2 is observed for the stranger stimuli in either VF. The asymmetry of responses between the two visual fields is inversed from phase 1 to phase 2: a) in phase 1, the interaction between Visual Field and Familiarity (F(1,38) = 5.35, p < .05) comes from a non-significant tendency to respond in the RVF faster to the mother than to the stranger (F(1,38) = 3.09, .05 < p < .10), whereas no effect approaches significance in the LVF; and also from a non-significant tendency (F(1,38) = 4.07, .05 < p < .10) of the RVF to respond to the mother faster than the LVF, whereas the difference between visual fields for the stranger stimuli does not approach significance; b) in phase 2 this RVF advantage for the mother is replaced by a LVF advantage. Ss now respond faster in the LVF than in the RVF (F(1,38) = 5.54, p < .025); the difference in latencies between mother and stranger is more systematic in the LVF (F(1,38) = 15.27, p < .001) than in the RVF (F(1,38) = 4.79, p < .05); Ss respond to their mother faster in the LVF than in the RVF (F(1,38) = 11.41, p < .005), whereas no significant difference between visual fields is found for the stranger.

The Familiarity effect in phase 2 is greater in the LVF than in the RVF suggesting that faster responding to mother is not so systematic in the RVF as in the LVF. However the Familiarity x Visual Field interaction is not significant and it may be the case that the only difference between the two visual fields in phase 2 is that the LVF reacts faster than the RVF but that both tended to react in the same way, that is faster to the mother stimuli. One way to check this point is to consider the fact that in phase 2 there were 32 Ss out of 40 responding in the LVF faster to their mother than to the stranger while the remaining 8 Ss responded faster to the stranger than to the mother. Now, if indeed the two hemispheres were reacting similarly relative to the discrimination between mother and stranger, considering these two groups of subjects separately, should increase the probability of finding such a parallel discriminative performance between the two hemispheres. If within each of these two groups, selected on the basis of their discriminative responses in the LVF of phase 2, the interaction between Visual Field and Familiarity in phase 2 is increased relative to the interaction found in the whole group, we would be inclined to reject the null hypothesis of a parallelism in the discriminative performance of the two hemispheres. An analysis of variance 2(Groups) x 2(Phase) x 2(Familiarity) x 2(Visual Field) shows that the three- factor interaction is now stronger in the group of 32 Ss (F(1,31) = 8.83, p < .01). In phase 2 the Familiarity x Visual Field interaction has increased relative to that observed in the whole group $(F(1,31) = 3.99, .05 < p < .10$. These Ss which responded faster to the mother than to the stranger in the LVF in phase 2, exhibit no significant difference between mother and stranger in the RVF $(F(1,31) = 2.03, p > .10)$; whereas in phase 2, they respond to the mother faster in the LVF than in the RVF $(F(1,31) = 16.41, p < .005)$, no asymmetry is found for the stranger stimuli $(F(1,31) < 1)$. The interaction between Familiarity and Visual Field has also increased in phase 1 $(F(1,31) = 8.87, p < .01$, and the direction of the effect is inverse of that found in phase 2 with a tendency for the RVF to be faster than the LVF for the mother stimuli $(F(1,31) = 3.99, .05 < p < .10)$ but not for the stranger stimuli, as well as a tendency for the mother stimuli to be responded to faster than the stranger stimuli in the RVF $(F(1,31) = 3.18, .05 < p < .10)$ and not in the LVF.

In the other group of Ss the interaction between Visual Field and Familiarity in phase 2 is also increased relative to the whole group $(F(1,7) = 15.06, p < .01)$. Those Ss which responded faster to the stranger than to the mother in the LVF in phase 2 tended to do the opposite (faster to mother) in the RVF $(F(1,7) = 5.27, .05 < p < .10)$. Whereas their responses to the stranger are faster in the LVF than in the RVF $(F(1,7) = 11.11, p < .025)$ no asymmetry is found for the mother stimuli $(F(1,7) = 1.40, p > .10)$. Thus instead of increasing the parallelism between the two hemisphere performances, the separation of the Ss into two groups on the basis of mother and stranger response in the LVF, has decreased the plausibility of parallel performances between the two hemispheres in phase 2 of the experiment.

In summary, the two hemispheres do not react in the same way to the presentation of the two categories of stimuli and to the repetition of the trials. At the beginning of the experiment the RVF-LH seems to exhibit an advantage relative to discrimination between mother and stranger; thereafter the LVF-RH reacts faster than the RVF-LH and also reacts faster to the mother more systematically than the RVF-LH.

The data exhibit two kinds of asymmetries that may or not be related: a) one which is clearly assessed, in the latencies of responses which become faster in the LVF than in the RVF during the experiment; we shall discuss below whether this asymmetry can be related to other processes than to a difference in information processing between the two hemispheres; b) the second kind of asymmetry, which is less clearly assessed but which has strong arguments in its favour, is found in the discriminative responses which seem initially to concern the RVF more than the LVF, and thereafter concerns the LVF more than the RVF.

2.3. Discussion

Is the difference in the speed of responses between the two hemispheres related to information processing or to other processes? It could be argued that a motoric bias is responsible for the greater speed of response of the LVF in phase 2 if it is assumed that a motoric bias may be seen in latencies of responses if and only if these are as fast as possible, that is if latencies are considered as reaction times. Infants may take the same time to process the stimuli in the two visual fields and then try to react as fast as possible. The RH would have a motoric advantage in the command of the saccade. This explanation could account for the faster LVF response. One way to know whether this explanation is plausible is to find a situation where the fastest set of responses is not at the same time the most asymmetric set, or a situation where the fastest set of responses exhibits an inverse asymmetry. We shall see below (Experiment 2) such situations where the fastest set of ocular saccades is either not asymmetrical, or presents an inverse asymmetry. It is worth noting here that in experiments measuring the latencies of the ocular saccade in response to visual peripheral stimuli (static or mobile) no asymmetry in latencies between the visual fields was found in infants aged from 2 to 6 months (Aslin and Salapatek, 1975; de Schonen, McKenzie, Bresson and Maury, 1978).

Another possible explanation of the faster responses of one hemisphere over the other comes from a possible difference in acuity between the two eyes together with a difference in maturation between the nasal and temporal part of the fovea and perifovea. However Birch (1985) has not found any oriented difference between the acuity of the two eyes from birth to 11 months. Moreover he found that interocular acuity differences decreased as the infant matures during this period. This would result, if such an explanation of our data was right, in a difference in response pattern between our two age groups which is not the case.

A third possible interpretation relies on the assumption that the Right Hemisphere has a general advantage in attention directing. This should result in a LVF advantage in our experiment. The interaction between Familiarity and Visual Field and the direction of the asymmetry found in phase 1 do not fit with this. Moreover the data of experiment 2 (see below) do not support this interpretation.

Thus it is sensible to conclude that the faster responses of one hemisphere over the other in our experiment is related, in phase 2 as in phase 1, to information processing or to the cognitive process related to the response. The next question concerns the nature of this information: are the asymmetries found in our data related to visuo-spatial processing in general, or to face processing, or to the emotional aspects involved in presentation of the mother's physiognomy. Data coming from an experiment (Gil de Diaz, 1983) comparing physiognomy processing to geometrical shape processing may partially answer these questions

3. EXPERIMENT 2
3.1. Technique

The technique used was the same as in experiment 1 except for the following points. There were two groups of subjects. One group was tested on a discrimination between physiognomies, the other on a discrimination between geometrical shapes. Except for the stimuli, the two groups were presented with the same situation. In the physiognomy situation there was a set of 7 smiling female faces photographed as in experiment 1. The women were unknown to the subjects. For the geometrical shapes there were 7 different simple geometrical symmetrical shapes, completely red; the greatest horizontal and vertical dimensions of each shape were equal to the corresponding dimensions of the faces. In both situations, one of the 7 stimuli served as a stimulus to be familiarized (it will be called the Familiar stimulus), the remaining 6 stimuli constituted the New stimuli. Familiarization with a stimulus was not performed before testing of the hemi-visual fields but during the testing itself by presenting this stimulus for delays of 5 s (instead of 250 or 350 ms). The 6 other stimuli were presented for 250 or 350 ms (to 7-11 month olds and 4-6 month olds respectively). The Familiar stimulus was presented 12 times in each visual field (24 trials) and each of the 6 New stimuli were presented twice in each visual field (24 trials) making a total of 48 trials. Presentations alternated in the RVF and LVF and the order of presentation of Familiar and New stimuli was random with the same number of each category of stimuli in each visual field in the first 24 trials as in the last 24 trials. The visual angle of presentation was 3°8 instead of 2°. All other techniques and procedures were as in Experiment 1.

3.2. Subjects

12 males in each situation, with 4 aged from 4 to 6 months (mean age: 5 mo.), and 8 aged 7 to 11 mo. (mean age: 9 mo.).

3.3. Results

The results will only be summarized (Table 1). 1) As in experiment 1 the 48 trials were divided into two successive series of 24 trials: phase 1 and 2. The discrimination between Familiar and New stimuli was expected to be found in phase 2, that is after some familiarization. Two analysis of variance 2(Phase) x 2(Familiarity) x 2(Visual Field) performed on the 2 situations separately show that, as expected, the latencies of the ocular saccades differentiate between Familiar and New stimuli in phase 2 only. However in the case of physiognomies, infants reacted significantly faster to the Familiarized stimuli than to the new stimuli ($F(1,11) = 13.45$, $p < .01$), whereas in the case of geometrical shapes subjects responded faster to the new stimuli than to the familiarized ($F(1,11) = 8.96$, $p < .05$). 2) In the Physiognomy situation the discrimination was significant in the LVF only ($F(1,11) = 12.17$, $p < .01$), but the interaction between Familiarity and Visual field was not significant. The tendency was thus the same as in experiment 1: discriminative responding could be assessed for the LVF but not for the RVF. On the contrary, in the Shape situation, the discrimination was significant in the RVF ($F(1,11) = 13.29$, $p < .01$) and not in the LVF. 3) In the Physiognomy situation, the RVF responded faster than the LVF, in phase 2 ($F(1,11) = 10.40$, $p < .05$) but not in phase 1, the effect being due to both familiar and new stimuli. In the Shape situation there was no difference in the latencies between RVF and LVF and no interaction between Visual Field and Familiarity effects.

TABLE 1. Experiment 2: mean latencies of the ocular saccades (ms) as a function of Stimuli, Visual hemi-field and Phase in the Physiognomy situation and in the Shape situation.

Stimuli	Physiognomies						Shapes					
	Phase 1			Phase 2			Phase 1			Phase 2		
	LVF	RVF	Total	LVF	RVF	Total	LVF	RVF	Total	LVF	RVF	Total
Familiar	387	354	371	351	319	335	390	372	381	379	380	380
New	391	373	382	408	343	376	399	386	393	377	340	359
Total	389	364		380	331		394	379		378	360	

The discrimination performances in phase 2 between New and Familiar stimuli could be considered as due to the difference in exposition durations and not to familiarization. However if the exposition durations were efficient per se Ss should respond faster in both situations to the shortest durations (or to the longest duration), which is not the case. On the other hand if Ss were responding to the offset of the short duration stimuli, this would result in latencies of response of about 106 ms for the 4-month olds and of 118 ms for 7-11-month olds in the Physiognomy situation, and of about 50 ms for the 4-month olds and 102 ms for the 7-11-month olds in the Shape situation. These latencies are too short to be latencies of response. In adults, reaction time of the ocular saccade to a stimulus with a high probability location is between 130 and 140 ms for 3° and 15° of excentricity (Gorea, Findlay, Levy-Schoen, 1980; Findlay, 1985). Thus the difference in latencies of response between Familiar and New stimuli is related to the familiarization effect and not to the exposition durations.

In the Physiognomy situation, it could be argued that it is not known whether infants were processing the stimuli as faces or as non-face complex visual patterns. However it is most plausible that Ss processed the stimuli as faces since Experiment 1 showed that infants can recognize their mother at short delays of presentation; this implies that Ss were processing the physiognomical aspects of the stimuli. Thus it is most probable that in Experiment 2 also Ss were processing the stimuli as faces.

4. GENERAL DISCUSSION

These results suggest the following conclusions: 1) The hypothesis of a motoric bias advantaging the LVF (see Experiment 1) seems to be ruled out by the fact that the fastest set of latencies does not exhibit any systematic asymmetry in the Shape situation and exhibits a RVF-LH preferential advantage in the Physiognomy situation. 2) Similarly the interpretation in terms of a general attentional bias advantaging the LVF is ruled out for the same reasons. It seems sensible to conclude that the two kinds of asymmetry found in Experiment 1 (a more systematic discrimination in one visual field than the other and a faster responding in one hemifield than the other) are related to information processing. 3) The LVF-RH advantage found in Experiment 1 in the discriminative performances in phase 2 are not exclusively related to the emotional aspects involved in mother stimuli since it is also found with a briefly familiarized physiognomy (Experiment 2). 4) The LVF-RH advantage in the discriminative performances may not either be related to visuo-spatial processing in general, since the asymmetry found in the Shape situation of Experiment 2 differs from the one found in the Physiognomy situation and in Experiment 1.

Many other points remained in question. First, why in the Physiognomy situation of Experiment 2 does the RVF-LH react faster than the LVF-RH while no systematic discrimination is present? It must be recalled that there is no reason to assume that the two hemispheres perform the same task. Discriminative performances may differ from one visual field to the other because of a difference in accuracy and speed, but also because one hemisphere may be less constrained in responding faster to a particular category of stimuli or because one hemisphere may be responsive to one aspect of the stimuli, identity for instance, while the other is more responsive to another aspect. It may be the case that in Experiment 2, the RVF-LH exhibits responsivity to the positive smiling expression of the physiognomies with or without interaction with the identity of the physiognomies. Similarly, in Experiment 1, the differential responding of the two hemispheres in phase 1 and in phase 2, may not be related to the same aspects of the mother identity. It may be the case that in phase 1 the tendency to respond faster to the mother in the RVF-LH was related to some aspect of the mother's function such as communication, or to the strangeness of the mother's apparition at that place with a bi-dimensional pattern, or with that size, and so on; whereas in phase 2, infants may react to other aspects or other functions of the identification of the mother. The hypothesis that the two hemispheres may react to different aspects of stimuli during a task is also suggested by data from a pilot study where different physiognomies, each with three different expressions and three levels of luminance were presented to infants 4 to 11 months of age in each visual field with the same technique as in Experiment 1. In the RVF, infants responded faster to smiling faces than to the other facial expressions whereas in the LVF they responded faster to surprised faces than to neutral and smiling faces. The level of luminance had no effect showing that the differentiation of expressions was not related to the fact that variations of expressions are always accompanied by variations of luminance.

The asymmetries observed in our data may be related to an asymmetry in spatial frequency processing (see Sergent, this volume). This interpretation predicts a LVF-RH advantage in processing low spatial frequencies. However in Experiment 2, the shapes which were a good candidate for low spatial frequency processing were discriminated systematically in the RVF and not in the LVF. Nevertheless, since it cannot be excluded that discrimination may have also been performed in the LVF (with some SS responding faster to New stimuli and some to Familiar), the argument is not very strong and needs more direct testing.

Another question is worth mentioning. Discrimination between shapes was systematic in the RVF and not in the LVF contrary to discrimination between physiognomies, but responses were faster to New stimuli than to Familiar in the case of shapes contrary to the case of faces. Bradshaw, Gates and Patterson (1976) suggested that in adults the RH is superior at perceiving the relationships between component parts and the whole configuration in making rapid identity matches, while the LH is concerned with isolating discrete features or elements within the entire configuration and possibly difference detection. This fits well with a part of our data. It is not impossible that infants preferentially process differences between bi-dimensional geometrical shapes within an analytic framework whereas at the same age either they are able to process differences between physiognomies both in an holistic and an analytic way or they preferentially process faces in a holistic way. If this were true it would suggest that, from a visual processing point of view (and not only from a social point of view), faces are specific objects for infants. This point needs to be tested with techniques that constrain the infant more to performing particular discriminative tasks than the techniques used here which test spontaneous responses. An experiment is now in process using discriminative conditioning in each visual field separately in order to test what kind of discrimination is possible in each visual field and whether there is transfer of information built up by one hemisphere to the other hemisphere.

Our final point concerns the ontogeny of the observed asymmetries. If the differences of reactions between the two hemispheres were due to a delay of maturation of certain structures of one hemisphere relative to the other, it would involve this delay could last for 5 months since, for mother recognition at least, the observed asymmetries remain identical from 4 months to 9 months of age. The difference in rate of maturation of two identical neuronal structures of the hemispheres should thus be of at least 5 months which is a very implausible delay. It is more plausible that the asymmetries observed in our data refer to a differential specialization of the hemispheres.

5. CONCLUSION

Our data show 1) that male infants aged 4 to 11 months can discriminate visual stimuli presented for very brief durations in each visual field. These infants recognize their mother on the basis of the physiognomic internal features of the face. They also discriminate a physiognomy with which they are much less familiar than the mother's. These data bring some precisions to Bushnell's data (1982) who showed that in an habituation/dishabituation paradigm with normal visual presentations, infants aged about 5 months can discriminate the mother's face from a stranger's face even when the hair is standardized but that the hair face outline is still important information at about 5 months of age. Our data show that even with brief hemi-visual field presentations, standardization of hair, forehead line and ear/face line does not prevent mother recognition. Alteration in this part of the face may result in perturbation of discrimination between physiognomies when the infant is provided with a long exploration time. But such alteration does not matter for the recognition process that takes place during the first hundred ms. This suggests that brief exposition durations should be used in infants in order to differentiate between the features that are processed at the very beginning of the visual process and the features that are processed later on. Habituation/dishabituation experiments may give different results than brief duration expositions experiment because complex cognitive operations may occur during long period of visual examination. 2) The latencies of the responses show that in our situations the information processing in infants can be faster than the 2 sec found by Lasky (1980) with presentations in the whole visual field. 3) The asymmetry found between visual fields is related to difference in information processing or cognitive response elaboration of each hemisphere. 4) Both hemispheres perform spontaneously (without instruction or constraint) a discrimination between mother and stranger but this discrimination does not occur at the same moment in the experiment for both hemispheres. Moreover recognition of the mother's physiognomy that occurs in the LVF-RH after occurrence of the recognition trend in the RVF-LH, is performed faster than the RVF-LH recognition responses. This fits well with adult data on the RH advantage for recognition of familiar physiognomies (see this volume). The pattern of results of Experiment 2, where a systematic advantage of responses to a recently familiarized physiognomy is found in the LVF only, also supports this suggestion. 5) Spontaneous reactions of each hemisphere differ also as a function of the nature of the stimuli, faces vs geometrical shapes, suggesting that hemispheric asymmetries in infants are not only attributable to an advantage of the RH for visuo-spatial processing. 6) It is most plausible that the observed asymmetries correspond to an early hemispheric specialization in different kinds of information processing or in different kinds of behavioural functions in response to stimuli.

MODELS OF LATERALITY EFFECTS IN FACE PERCEPTION

C. UMILTA'

1. INTRODUCTION

The so-called divided-visual-field procedure for studying hemispheric specialisation in normal people capitalises on the fact that each visual field (VF) projects initially to the contralateral hemisphere and thus, provided certain variables are controlled, the differences in speed and/or accuracy between the two VFs can be attributed to the underlying different specialisations of the two hemispheres (see, e.g., Beaumont, 1982).

The first divided-visual-field studies that employed face stimuli (Geffen, Bradshaw & Wallace, 1971; Rizzolatti, Umilta & Berlucchi, 1971) were aimed at demonstrating a left visual field-right hemisphere (LVF-RH) superiority comparable to the right visual field-left hemisphere (RVF-LH) superiority that had already been found with verbal material. Based on previous clinical findings (see, reviews in Benton, 1980; Hecaen & Albert, 1978), it was thought, correctly, that faces were the kind of stimulus material for which an RH specialisation could be found. Subsequently, it became apparent that several variables influenced hemispheric competence for processing faces, resulting in laterality differences in favour of the LVF-RH, of the RVF-LH, or in no laterality asymmetry (see reviews in Sergent, 1982; Sergent & Bindra, 1981).

Such findings were instrumental in shifting the emphasis from the notion of hemispheric specialisation for type of stimulus material to that of hemispheric specialisation for type of processing mode. The latter is usually considered in terms of a number of dichotomies, which assign serial, sequential, temporal, analytic, or high spatial frequencies processing to the LH, and parallel, holistic, gestalt, simultaneous, or low spatial frequencies processing to the RH (see, e.g., reviews in Bradshaw & Nettleton, 1981, 1983). Within this framework, faces are no doubt a very suitable kind of stimulus material, because they can be processed on the basis of either their component features or their configurational properties (see, e.g., Davies, Ellis & Shepherd, 1981). Hence the growing number of studies of hemispheric specialisation which employ face stimuli for testing the processing modes of the hemispheres.

Most of these studies take for granted, often implicitly though, a model of laterality effects that, as will be argued in the present paper, is likely false.

The model assumes that whichever hemisphere receives the stimulus through the contralateral VF, processes it without recourse to transfer along the forebrain commissures. If this is true, then it is apparent that one can investigate the way each hemisphere processes information by presenting the stimuli to the two VFs: when the stimuli are presented to the RVF, the mode of processing of the LH is tested, whereas the mode of processing of the RH is tested through stimulation of the LVF. However, laterality effects can also be explained by assuming that when information reaches the specialised hemisphere it is immediately processed, whereas from the non-specialised hemisphere it is relayed to the other side for processing. If this is true, it must be concluded that the processing mode of specialised hemisphere only can be tested, either directly through the contralateral VF or indirectly through the ipsilateral VF and the forebrain commisures.

Interestingly enough, of the first two studies that dealt with laterality effects for faces, one (Rizzolatti et al., 1971) espoused the latter model, whereas the other (Geffen et al., 1971) favoured the former. In the present paper it will be shown that neither model fares well if submitted to empirical testing and it will be argued that a third model should instead be adopted. Such new model is largely based on a series of experiments by Umilta, Rizzolatti, Anzola, Luppino & Porro (1985), while the discussion of the other two models is based also on theoretical papers by Cohen (1982), Moscovitch (1985), Nettleton (1983) and Zaidel (1983).

2. THE INTERHEMISPHERIC TRANSMISSION (IT) MODEL

This is the model proposed by Rizzolatti et al. (1971) to explain the LVF-RH superiority for discriminating faces found in a reaction time (RT) task. It assumes that: a) only the RH can process faces; b) speed of response is faster when the stimuli are channelled directly to that hemisphere through the LVF; and c) the difference in response latency between the VFs is attributable to the delay and loss of information that occur when the stimuli shown in the RVF must be transmitted to the other hemisphere (Rizzolatti, 1979).

These points can be made more explicit. For simplicity, let Pr represent the time taken by all the processing stages, from stimulus encoding to response emission, which take place in the RH and T represent the transmission time from the LH to the RH. It is apparent that the response latency to stimuli shown in the LVF has only one component, namely Pr, whereas response latency to RVF stimuli has two, namely, T+Pr. There can also be little doubt that Pr (Pr+T). Hence, RT is faster in the LVF and the difference is entirely due to T. In sum, the IT model maintains that the RH always processes the input and that stimulus presentation to the RVF simply results in information transfer, which in turn causes the slower RT. Admittedly, it is not entirely clear at which stage of processing the transfer of information from the LH to the RH occurs (Rizzolatti, 1979), but this does not matter, provided the transfer is necessary for the processing sequence to be completed. A more serious difficulty arises from those experiments which demonstrate that information is processed differently in the two VFs. That would seem strong evidence of independent processing in the two hemispheres. However, it is conceivable that the processing mode changes when the stimulus quality is degraded by the interhemispheric transfer. Not even the obvious criticism that no experimental task comprises only processing stages uniquely lateralised to one hemisphere is fully convincing. In fact, as Moscovitch (1985) aptly points out, the IT model applies whenever one single component of the processing sequence is localised to one hemisphere only. The reason is that all input to the subsequent stages must be relayed through it and thus requires interhemispheric transfer. Therefore, any processing bias introduced after the first lateralised stage has no effect on the magnitude or direction of perceptual asymmetry.

The true weakness of the model is the assumption that at least one component of the processing sequence for faces is uniquely lateralised to the RH. This runs counter to a number of studies in normals, which have shown that the RH superiority for processing faces can be eliminated or reversed (see reviews in Bradshaw & Nettleton, 1983; Davidoff, 1982; Sergent & Bindra, 1981), and to clinical evidence that only bilateral lesions produce prosopagnosia (see reviews in Benton, 1980; Hecaen & Albert, 1978).

Still more importantly, the predictions of the IT model were tested by Umilta et al. (1985) and proved inaccurate. In that study, which was based on a dual-task procedure suggested by Geffen, Bradshaw & Nettleton (1973), there were three experimental conditions. In one the subject had to perform a face discrimination task alone, whereas in the other two this primary task was coupled with either an ordered tapping task, which was known to yield an LH interference, or a finger flexion task, which was known to yield an RH interference. The logic for testing the IT model was as follows.

If D indicates the delay caused by the interfering task, then when it is the RH to be affected, the components of RT in the LVF are Pr+D and those in the RVF are T+Pr+D. As happens for the primary task alone, RT should be faster in the LVF because (Pr+D) (T+Pr+D) and the difference should be due to T. In other words, the model predicts a lengthening of overall RT but no change in the asymmetry in favour of the LVF. In the case of the secondary task that interferes with the LH, the situation is even simpler because the RT components should be the same as in the primary task in isolation: Pr in the LVF and T+Pr in the RVF. This is because the secondary task affects only the LH, which is not involved in processing faces. In brief, since there is no reason why the secondary task should influence interhemispheric transmission time, the IT model predicts that the difference in RT favouring the LVF found with the primary task, should remain unchanged regardless of the type of secondary task. The results showed significant advantages of 21 and 13 ms (a nonsignificant difference) for face discrimination alone and with the LH interference, respectively. In contrast, the LVF advantage for face discrimination decreased to a nonsignificant 4 ms when the RH interference was added. Therefore, the IT model was disproved because it cannot explain why the LVF advantage vanishes when the secondary task affects the RH.

3. THE DIFFERENTIAL PROCESSING SPEED (DPS) MODEL

Geffen et al. (1971) were the first to adopt this model to explain the LVF-RH superiority for processing faces in an RT task. It assumes that: a) no component stage in the processing sequence for faces is exclusively lateralised to the RH; b) stimuli are always processed by the hemisphere directly accessed through the contralateral VF; c) RT is faster in the LVF because of the faster processing that occurs in the RH; and d) with respect to the LH, the RH is characterised by a different and more efficient processing mode or by a more efficient use of the same processing mode. The crucial assumption is that hemispheric specialisation for faces is a matter of degree and there is no uniquely RH component. In other words, hemispheric specialisation for faces is assumed to be relative rather than absolute. As already pointed out, this is supported by the empirical evidence available. It is also clear that, at variance with the IT model, the DPS model denies any role of interhemispheric transmission in bringing about laterality effects. This is its main weakness because there can be little doubt that when information reaches one hemisphere, it is immediately and automatically relayed to the other side along the forebrain commisures. In other words, in the intact human brain there is no way for the input to be confined within one single hemisphere. Hence, the RH always starts processing face stimuli through either a direct or a commissural input. (Note that this is no doubt true of the LH also). Therefore, the advocates of the DPS model are forced to assume, only implicitly though, that the difference in speed of processing in favour of the RH is smaller than interhemispheric transmission time. In fact, if it were larger, then the LVF advantage could well be attributed to the latter in spite of the fact that hemispheric specialisation for faces is relative.

The results of the experiment by Umilta et al. (1985) can be used to test also the DPS model. According to it, with the primary task alone, RT in the LVF is due to Pr and in the RVF is due to P1, where Pr and P1 represent the time needed for the processing of faces, again from stimulus encoding to response emission, in the RH and LH, respectively. Since RT is faster in the LVF, it follows that Pr   P1, and the difference (21 ms, in the experiment) can be represented by Pd. Note that the model does not imply that every stage of processing is faster in the RH, it simply implies that the sum of the times taken by the whole sequence is smaller in the RH. When the RH interfering task is added, RT in the RVF is still attributable to P1, whereas in the LVF it increases due to the delay caused by the secondary task and becomes Pr+D. Now the difference in RT between the VFs must be smaller than Pd, namely Pd–D. Therefore, there should be a decrease, and possibly even a reversal, of the LVF superiority. The results supported this prediction by showing a much smaller, and nonsignificant, LVF advantage (4 vs 21 ms). In contrast, the LVF superiority should be enhanced when the secondary task affects the LH. This is because Pr still accounts for RT in the LVF, whereas RT in the RVF should be due to P1+D, hence the difference in favour of the LVF becomes Pd+D. This second prediction was not borne out by the data, which in fact showed a small decrease in the LVF advantage (13 vs 21 ms, a nonsignificant difference at any rate). In conclusion, the DPS model does not hold true for face discrimination.

It is important to point out that these findings disproved also those models that attribute laterality effects to hemispheric differences in allocation of attentional and processing resources (see, e.g., Friedman & Campbell Polson, 1981; Kinsbourne, 1975). Such models assume, in accordance with the DPS model, that input is always processed by the hemisphere of entry and the difference in RT between the VFs reflects the advantage in processing efficiency enjoyed by the RH. Therefore, although the different-ial speed of processing is attributed, at variance with the DPS model, to a bias in availability of processing resources, the predictions are the same as those of the latter model.

4. THE CONDITIONAL INTERHEMISPHERIC TRANSFER (CIT) MODEL

This is the model proposed by Umilta et al. (1985) to account for the results of their experiments (but see also Moscovitch, 1985, for a similar view). The two models discussed so far, besides not being supported by empirical evidence, meet with logical difficulties because are based on assumptions which are almost certainly false. The IT model assumes that hemispheric specialisation for faces is absolute and hence only the RH can process them. The DPS model assumes that the automatic transmission of information along the forebrain commisures is immaterial and hence process-ing is confined within the hemisphere of entry. There can be little doubt that a tenable model should not resort to such unlikely assumptions. In some sense, what is needed is a mixed model that takes into account both r·lative specialisation and interhemispheric transmission. Accordingly the C IT model maintains that a) face processing occurs in both hemispheres regardless of the VF where the stimuli are shown; b) the sum of interhemisph-cric transmission time plus RH processing time is usually shorter than the processing time of the LH; and c) normally interhemispheric transfer is the cause of the LVF advantage, unless the difference in speed of processing between the hemispheres becomes smaller than the transmission time. As usual, these assumptions can be clarified by expliciting the components of RT in the two VFs. When the stimulus is presented to the LVF, two processing sequences begin. One takes place in the RH and is completed in a time Pr, that is the overall time attributable to the component operations in that hemisphere. The other takes place in the LH and is completed in a time T+P1, that is the transmission delay plus the overall time of the component operations in that hemisphere. Undoubtedly, Pr (T+P1), hence RT in the LVF is due to Pr. When the stimulus is presented to the RVF, the processing sequence in the LH is completed in a time P1, whereas that in the RH takes a time T+Pr, and it is not known which one is faster. Of course, this is the crucial point because if P1 (T+Pr), then the RT advantage for the LVF is attributable to Pd, that is the difference in processing speed between the hemispheres. Conversely, if P1 (T+Pr), then the laterality effect must be attributed to T.

The CIT model has no difficulties in explaining the results of the experiment by Umilta et al. (1985). When there was only the primary task, as well as when the secondary task affected the LH, the LVF advantage was caused by the interhemispheric transfer and its magnitude was the same in the two conditions (21 vs 13 ms, a nonsignificant difference). This is because in the LVF RT is always due to Pr (note that with the LH interference the other processing sequence has a duration of T+P1+D instead of T+P1 as with the primary task alone), whereas in the RVF RT is always due to T+Pr because (T+Pr) P1 and, of course, (T+Pr) (P1+D), where D is the delay caused by the LH interference.

In contrast, when the secondary task interfered with the RH, the difference in processing speed between the hemispheres tended to disappear and, being shorter than the transmission time, brought about a very small laterality effect (a nonsignificant difference of 4 ms). Note that the two processing sequences that arise from the RVF have durations of P1 in the LH and T+Pr+D in the RH, and apparently one of them is nearly as fast as the faster of the two that originate from the LVF, namely Pr+D in the RH and T+P1 in the LH.

In sum, the CIT model is not predictive as to whether response latency in the RVF is to be attributed to P1 or T+Pr. It simply maintains that the shorter one determines RT and the time courses of the two parallel processing sequences can be influenced by experimental manipulations. Remember that, in contrast, the other two models make very precise predictions. The IT model maintains that RT in the RVF is to be attributed to T+Pr, whereas for the DPS model P1 is the only relevant component. Of course, the three models concur in ascribing to Pr response latency in the LVF. Such lack of predictivity enables the CIT model to accommodate the results of the Umilta et al.'s (1985) study and many other results. This is because whether laterality effects depend on interhemispheric transmission time or on the difference in processing speed between the hemispheres is considered to be an empirical question to be answered for each experiment independently. That renders the model very hard, perhaps even impossible, to falsify, which, admittedly, is not a desirable feature. However, there seems to be no better alternative if one admits that hemispheric specialisation for faces is relative and the forebrain commisures transmit information to the other side automatically. Of course, if hemispheric specialisation were absolute, in the sense that at least one necessary component of the processing of faces were located in the RH only, then the IT model would apply. This is likely what happens in the case of phonetic processing, for which the LH is uniquely specialised. Conversely, when commissural input is lacking, as in the case of split-brain patients, the DPS model applies, provided hemispheric specialisation is relative.

HEMISPHERIC ASYMMETRIES IN FACE RECOGNITION AND NAMING: EFFECTS OF PRIOR STIMULUS EXPOSURE

C.A. MARZI, P.E. TRESSOLDI, C. BARRY AND G. TASSINARI

1. INTRODUCTION

Detailed models of the cognitive operations subserving performance in a number of processing domains such as reading, spelling and object recognition have become increasingly prevalent in both cognitive psychology and neuropsychology. Such models attempt to distinguish between functionally separable components of processing, and to describe their organisation and operation. The study of face recognition has recently been the subject of the development of such models, and in the last three or four years at least four models have been offered (Bruce, 1983; Ellis, 1983; Hay & Young, 1982; Rhodes, 1985). These models are similar in that they distinguish between the following processing components (or stages) in face recognition: 1) visual-spatial processing; 2) a face representational system which permits recognition of known or familiar faces; 3) semantic information; and 4) naming. The precise details of the model differ, however, in many respects and in particular in the characterisation of how the system which permits the recognition of a face as a known or familiar face (without necessarily fully accessing semantic and name information) is assumed to operate. Ellis' (1983) model posits a "familiarity check", whereas Bruce's (1983) model would suggest that the "structural code" would be accessed, and in Hay & Young's model known faces may be classified as such when they gain access to "face recognition units" which may be seen as being face analogs of input logogens in Morton's (1979) model of visual word recognition. Finally, Rhodes' (1985) model would appear to involve the accessing of her posited processing stage labelled "view-independent topographical representation".

We have used such models (or rather the features common to them all) to investigate hemispheric asymmetry at different functionally defined components of processing. In a previous study (Marzi et al., 1985) carried out using a divided visual field technique (see Young, 1982) we employed the same set of stimulus faces in three experiments which varied the nature of the binary decision necessary to master the task. Experiment 1 required subjects to decide if a face was of a male or of a female person, and found no significant hemispheric asymmetries in either male or female subjects. Experiment 2 required subjects to decide if the face was of a known or an unknown person, and found a significant right hemisphere (RH) advantage, as has also been found by Young et al. (1985). Experiment 3 required subjects to name famous faces (and to respond "unknown" to unknown faces), and no significant hemispheric differences were found.

The three experiments would appear to have called for progressively more complex levels of cognitive processing as there was a clear increase in overall response time (RT) in each experiment (note that all experiments used a vocal response).

In terms of the models cited above, the male/female discrimination task would be performed by relatively early representational and/or visual processes (Hay & Young's model), and the result of Experiment 1 would suggest that such components are not lateralised. Such a conclusion has also been suggested by Ellis but not by Rhodes whose model suggests that visuo-spatial processing is "localised" in the RH. The earliest point in Hay & Young's model where known/unknown discriminations could be made is at the face recognition units level, as accessing a representation here would be sufficient for a "known" response to be made. The results of Experiment 2 (and of Young et al., 1985) would suggest that the RH is specialised for the accessing or the possession of such units, or both. According to Hay & Young's model, naming faces could be achieved only after a relatively long and complex chain of processing: representational processes then face recognition units then person information and only then naming. A similar chain of stages is also required by Ellis' and Rhodes' models which further suggest that naming is a left hemisphere (LH) function.

Experiment 3 failed to find any reliable hemispheric asymmetry in time taken to name famous faces. One possibility is that there was a LH advantage for this task, but that it was effectively cancelled by the RH advantage for the known/unknown task (see Marzi et al., 1985). Another, not completely unrelated possibility, is that the prior exposure of the faces before the laterality tests began might have interfered with a LH advantage. Such a possibility is suggested by the results of Marzi & Berlucchi (1977) who found a LH advantage in accuracy of naming famous faces which were not pre-exposed before laterality testing. In the three experiments mentioned so far, the subjects were given prior exposure in central vision of all the faces used in the experiment. This was done in order to familiarise the subjects with the set of stimuli to be used (80 in all, 40 famous and 40 unknown faces) in an attempt to reduce variability due to uncertainty and perceptual difficulty, but it also served the purpose of being able to assess which of the famous faces each subject was in fact able to recognise. With this procedure only those faces of famous people actually known by each individual subject were classified as being known.

We shall now report two further experiments aimed at assessing the role played by stimulus pre-exposure on the emergence and/or the direction of hemispheric asymmetries. In these experiments, which were identical under all other respects to those of Marzi et al., 1985, the stimulus faces were not shown prior to the laterality testing but were presented at the end of the experiment in order to adjust the data according to the reported recognition levels of each individual subject.

2. EXPERIMENT 1
2.1. Method

Eight male and eight female right-handed university students served as subjects. The stimuli were 80 photographs of faces. Half of the photographs represented faces of famous celebrities (actors, politicians, and so on) and the other half represented faces of unknown persons matched for sex, age and expression. Most non-facial cues were removed and the background was rendered identical for all photographs. During stimulus presentation, both famous/unknown and male/female faces were randomly intermingled. The stimuli were back-projected onto a translucid tangent screen by means of a Kodak Carousel slide projector supplemented with an electronic shutter. Stimulus exposure duration was 150 msec and its average luminance was 40 foot lamberts. The centre of the face stimulus was distant 2.2° from the fixation point and the whole face subtended a visual angle of about 4°.

The activation of a microphone placed in front of the subject's mouth stopped an electronic clock that yielded vocal RT to the nearest msec. RT data were fed into a microcomputer (Commodore) that calculated arithmetic and harmonic means as well as RT medians for each session and each type of response ("famous" or "unknown"). The advancement of the slides and the opening of the shutter were performed automatically by the computer. Eye positions before and during stimulus presentation were controlled by means of a TV system.

The subjects were briefly pre-trained with a set of faces different from those used for subsequent formal testing. Following an acoustic warning signal (the time interval between warning signal and stimulus appearance was randomized within a 3-sec maximum delay) a slide was projected either to the right or to the left of the fixation point according to a blocked sequence. Each subject saw a given slide only once and the relation between slide sequence and alternation of the visual fields was balanced across subjects. Reaction times faster than 250 msec were considered as anticipations and discarded together with those exceeding 1500 msec that were considered as no responses.

In this experiment (as in experiment 2 of Marzi et al., 1985) the subject's task was to decide as soon as possible following stimulus presentation whether he saw a famous or an unknown face. The vocal response was identical for all subjects and consisted in uttering the Italian word "famoso" for famous faces and the word "sconosciuto" for unknown faces.

At the end of the lateralised presentations, all the faces were again shown to the subject in central vision and with a long exposure duration. The famous faces that a subject could not recognise were considered as unknown for that subject and his/her data were adjusted accordingly.

2.2. Results and Discussion

Table 1 shows the mean correct RTs for Sex of the Subject, Type of Stimulus (famous/unknown) and Visual Hemifield of stimulus presentation.

An analysis of variance with one between-subject factor (Sex) and two within-subject factors (Hemifield and Type of Stimulus) revealed only one significant main effect, namely Type of Stimulus ($F = 14.7$; df = 1,14; $p < 0.005$), with the famous faces being responded to faster than the unknown faces by 74 msec. Another significant effect concerned the interaction Sex x Stimulus ($F = 18.08$; df = 1,14; $p < 0.001$). Two separate t-tests showed that the response "famous" was significantly faster than the response "unknown" in females but not in males.

As to the main thrust of this experiment, namely laterality effects, there was no reliable visual field effect but only a trend toward a right visual field-left hemisphere advantage (RVF/LH = 1074 msec) over the left visual field/right hemisphere (LVFQ/RH = 1103 msec). Such a difference, however, was statistically insignificant.

A second analysis was carried out on the percentage of errors (arc-sine transformations). The only significant effect was an interaction between Visual Hemifield and Type of Stimulus ($F = 7.2$; df = 1,14; $p < 0.05$). A t-test showed that for the "famous" stimuli accuracy was higher in the LVF/RH (25.3% errors) than in the RVF/LH (29.5%). On the contrary, for the "unknown" stimuli there was an advantage of the RVF/LH (26.7%) over the LVF/RH (32.5%). However, neither difference reached statistical significance when separately analysed by post-hoc t-tests.

The main results of this experiment are represented by the lack of hemispheric differences in RT as well as by a trend toward a RH advantage in accuracy of response to the famous faces and toward a LH advantage in accuracy of response to the unknown faces. These results need to be reconciled with those of Young et al. (1985) who found a significant RH advantage for a similar familiarity decision task with faces.

TABLE 1. Mean RTs (in msec) for Stimulus Material, Sex of the Subjects and Visual Hemifield in the familiarity decision task.

Stimulus	Males		Females		$\bar{X}$
	RVF	LVF	RVF	LVF	
"Famous"	1050	1031	957	964	1000
"Unknown"	1045	1074	1070	1099	1072
$\bar{X}$	1047	1052	1013	1031	

There are a number of differences in procedure which may explain the different pattern of results between the two experiments. First, the present experiment used a vocal rather than a manual response, and presented each face only once. Second, the degree of familiarity might have been different in the two experiments. Our procedure has been to remove all responses to faces that in the final control in central vision turned out to be unknown to a given subject. In Young et al.'s study, instead, there was no such adjustment and the familiarity of the faces was rated by independent judges before the experiment began. This procedural difference might explain the lack of asymmetries in accuracy of performance in Young et al.'s experiment where the error rate included "false" errors of particular subjects not knowing some of the famous faces and this might have increased the variability of the scores and lowered the probability of obtaining a reliable hemispheric effect.

Finally, the results of the present experiment are at odds with Experiment 2 of Marzi et al. (1985) which was carried out with identical stimuli and procedure but in which there was a prior exposure of the faces in central vision. A RH advantage was found in the latter study, while no RT asymmetries could be obtained in the former. Such a discrepancy suggests, as will be discussed below, that stimulus prior exposure is an important factor for the emergence and the direction of hemispheric effects.

3. EXPERIMENT 2
3.1. Method
The only difference with the previous experiment is that in experiment 2 the famous faces had to be correctly named. Except for stimulus exposure duration that was increased to 250 msec in consideration of the greater difficulty of the task, method and procedure were the same as in the preceding experiment. Eight male and eight female subjects different from those of the previous study were recruited. As previously, if a famous face turned out to be unknown to a particular subject in the final control carried out in central vision, it was included among the unknown faces and scored accordingly.

The subject's task was to pronounce as fast as possible following stimulus appearance the Italian word "sconosciuto" for unknown faces and the appropriate name for the famous faces.

3.2. Results and Discussion

As a result of the greater difficulty of this task in comparison with that of the preceding experiment and in keeping with the cognitive models of face processing discussed above, overall RT was slower than in experiment 1 by about 300 msec. Table 2 shows mean RTs for Sex, Type of Stimuli and Visual Hemifield.

TABLE 2. Mean RTs (in msec) for Stimulus Material, Sex of the Subjects and Visual Hemifield in the naming task.

Stimulus	Males		Females		$\bar{X}$
	RVF	LVF	RVF	LVF	
"Name"	1367	1482	1525	1473	1461
"Unknown"	1257	1292	1164	1120	1208
$\bar{X}$	1312	1387	1344	1296	

An analysis of variance showed that the only significant main effect was Type of Stimulus material (F = 27.9; df = 1,14; p < 0.0005) with an advantage in RT speed of the "unknown" stimuli over the name stimuli (1208 msec vs 1461 msec).

Such a result is not unexpected and is in keeping with the model of Hay & Young (1982) where the naming component is after the face recognition units and failure to access a representation in the latter is sufficient to make an "unknown" response. Furthermore, there were two significant inter-actions: Sex x Stimuli (the advantage of the "unknown" stimuli over the "known" stimuli being larger in female subjects) and, more importantly, Sex x Visual hemifield (F = 4.3; df = 1,14; p < 0.05). The latter results from an opposite visual field effect in the two sexes. Post-hoc t-tests revealed that in males there was a significant RVF/LH advantage, whereas, in females there was a non-significant LVF/RH advantage.

The LH superiority in male subjects is in complete agreement with the results obtained by Marzi & Berlucchi (1977), who used only male subjects, in a task of verbal identification of famous faces.

At variance with the previous experiment, accuracy of performance did not yield any significant main effects or interactions.

Finally, the present results are in contrast with those of Marzi et al.'s experiment 3 in which no hemispheric effect was found. Since the two experiments differed only in the presence of a prior stimulus exposure (which was present in Marzi et al.'s Experiment 3), it follows that such a factor must be of great importance for the presence and/or the direction of hemispheric differences in a naming task (as well as in a familiarity decision task). The next section provides experimental evidence and a general discussion on the role of advance visual information in laterality effects.

4. EFFECTS OF ADVANCE STIMULUS EXPOSURE

In the two experiments reported above we have found that, without prior exposure of the faces, the familiarity decision task yields no hemispheric effects in RT while in the naming task there is a LH advantage (but for male subjects only).

In two previous experiments carried out with the same stimuli and procedure but <u>with</u> prior face exposure, the familiarity decision task resulted in a RH advantage in response speed while there was no hemispheric asymmetry in RT for the naming task. Table 3 shows an integrated summary of both Marzi et al.'s and the present findings.

TABLE 3. Summary of hemispheric asymmetries in RT at three cognitive stages of face processing (data from Marzi et al., 1985 and present article).

	Stage 1	Stage 2	Stage 3
Decision	Female or Male ?	Known or Unknown ?	Name ? or Unknown
Pre-viewing	Yes	Yes – No	Yes – No
Overall RT msec	649	945 – 1036	1057 – 1334
Dominant Hemisphere	None	RH – None	None – LH

It is clear from Table 3 that overall RT increases progressively as one goes from the relatively simple stage of male/female face discrimination to the familiarity decision and finally to naming. Furthermore, pre-viewing results in a marked decrease in RT for both the familiarity decision (91 msec) and the naming task (277 msec). This result has also been found in a recent study by Bruce & Valentine (1985). Using central presentation of faces, they found a facilitatory effect of the pre-exposure of familiar faces in both a familiarity task and in naming recognition accuracy.

Hemispheric differences are absent at stage 1, while at stage 2 there is a RH dominance in the pre-viewing experiment and at stage 3 there is a LH advantage in the experiment without pre-viewing (but only in male subjects). From this pattern of results it appears that pre-viewing has different effects in the two hemispheres and at the two different cognitive stages. In order to substantiate such an impression we carried out two analysis of variance (one for each cognitive task) in which we put together the data of the subjects who received pre-viewing and those of the subjects who did not receive advance information.

In the familiarity decision task, there was a significant effect of Pre-Exposure ($F = 6.5$; df = 1,32; $p < 0.05$) which resulted in a 8.8% overall decrease in RT. Another interesting finding was a significant interaction Exposure x Stimuli ($F = 13.6$; df = 1,32; $p < 0.001$). A t-test showed that the facilitatory effect of pre-exposure was more marked for the famous faces (131 msec reduction in RT) than for unknown faces (51 msec reduction in RT), a finding which suggests that the priming of pre-established face recognition units produces a larger effect than the initial establishment of new units for the unknown faces. Importantly, the interaction Exposure x Visual hemifield was significant (F = 4.0; df = 1,32; p = 0.054). A t-test showed that the advantage of a face receiving previous exposure was more marked in the LVF/RH (112 msec reduction in RT) than in the RVF/LH (71 msec). Finally, a significant three-way interaction Exposure x Stimulus x Visual hemifield and subsequent post-hoc tests revealed that the LVF/RH showed a facilitatory effect in making use of advance facial information which was slightly larger for famous than for unknown faces (138 msec vs 86 msec). However, the RVF/LH showed both small effects, and a much larger difference between famous and unknown faces (125 msec vs 17 msec). No clear pattern of results emerged from an analysis of errors probably because of a rather large inter-subject variability.

As for the familiarity task, also in the naming task an analysis of variance showed a highly significant main effect of Exposure (F = 35.5; df = 1,32; p < 0.00001): previous exposure of the faces yielded an overall shortening of RT of 20.8%.

In accord with the results of the familiarity decision task, there was a significant Exposure x Stimulus interaction and again the famous faces had more benefit from previous exposure (407 msec decrease in RT) than unknown faces (150 msec). However, as far as hemispheric asymmetries in the use of advance information are concerned, there was no significant interaction involving visual hemifield. Thus, at variance with the familiarity decision task, face naming shows an equally large benefit from stimulus pre-exposure in both hemispheres. As in the previous analysis, no reliable effects were obtained in accuracy of performance.

5. CONCLUSIONS

The novel finding of these series of experiments is represented by the differential effect of advance visual information on hemispheric processing at two cognitive stages of face perception. At the stage of familiarity decision there is a clear hemispheric asymmetry in the use of stimulus pre-exposure with the RH showing a larger facilitatory (or priming) effect than the LH.

What is the meaning of such an asymmetry in terms of the models of face recognition mentioned in the introduction?

If we permit some analogies to the research on priming in word recognition within the logogen model (Morton, 1979) then we may explain our results on the basis of Hay & Young's model which is explicitly homologous to the overall organisation of Morton's word recognitgion model.

The prior presentation of faces would have at least two possible loci of priming effect. First, there will be priming at the locus of the face recognition units where known faces will activate existing units and unknown faces will create new recognition units. Second, the presentation of the famous faces will permit person information to be accessed which may permit the full activation of semantic information concerning a person, and may also include the name to be retrieved. Such activation may then remain in the system and serve to prime face recognition units at a later time.

The lack of hemispheric asymmetries in experiment 1 of the present study suggests that accessing face recognition units may be a process equally subserved by both hemispheres in the absence of priming. However, in the presence of advance information, a RH advantage arises because priming of recognition units is more efficiently carried out by this hemisphere. Which hemisphere is more involved in priming, however, may depend on the nature of the stimulus and in the case of our familiarity decision task the visual nature of the prime may explain the selective RH involvement.

The LH advantage in experiment 2 of the present study in which no prior stimulus exposure was provided suggests, and this is corroborated both theoretically by the models of Ellis (1983) and Rhodes (1985) and experimentally by the results of Marzi & Berlucchi (1977), that verbal identification of a face is a LH function. If, however, as in the naming task of Marzi et al. (1985), face recognition units are primed, the resulting large bihemispheric increase in processing speed (and accuracy) tends to cancel the LH superiority in accessing the name of the face. Further experiments are obviously needed to clarify the nature of the RH selective involvement in the use of advance facial information and why such an advantage is not present in the face-naming task. In particular, it would be interesting to pursue the Bruce & Valentine (1985) finding that the prior reading of a celebrity's name facilitates the subsequent naming accuracy of the person's face, but not response to that face in the familiarity task. Another, important point is whether the RH is more involved than the LH in priming in general or its role is restricted to face processing and visual primes. Perhaps a RH advantage in priming is also present for verbal information since Young & Bion (1983) have found a RH advantage in naming faces only when a list containing the names of the face stimuli was given to the subjects prior to the laterality experiment.

Taken together our experiments provide confirming evidence for some general features of the models of hemispheric processing of faces proposed by Ellis (1983) and by Rhodes (1985). In agreement with Ellis' "familiarity check" stage is probably common to both hemispheres unless there is priming of the faces to be recognized. Finally, in agreement with both Ellis' and Rhodes' models, the naming stage is clearly lateralised in the LH unless the presence of a face prime speeding up naming in both hemispheres does not cancel such a LH advantage.

PATTERNS OF CEREBRAL DOMINANCE IN WHOLISTIC AND FEATURAL STAGES   OF   FACIAL
PROCESSING

ALAN J. PARKIN and PAMELA WILLIAMSON

1. INTRODUCTION

Ellis (1983) has proposed that an initial stage of face processing is
"classification" whereby a face is categorised as such in order for it to
undergo further face-related processing. This involves an overall assessment that the stimulus configuration is consistent with the organisation of
a face. It is therefore 'wholistic'; being principally concerned with the
relationships between stimulus elements rather than the identity of
specific features. A right hemisphere superiority in wholistic processing
is generally assumed (e.g. Nebes, 1978) thus one would expect facial classification to be right lateralised.   This prediction is supported by
Newcombe (1974) who found that patients with right hemisphere damage had
difficulty in performing successful closures on Mooney (1957) Faces (see
Figure 1).   Effective closure is assumed to depend on a process analogous

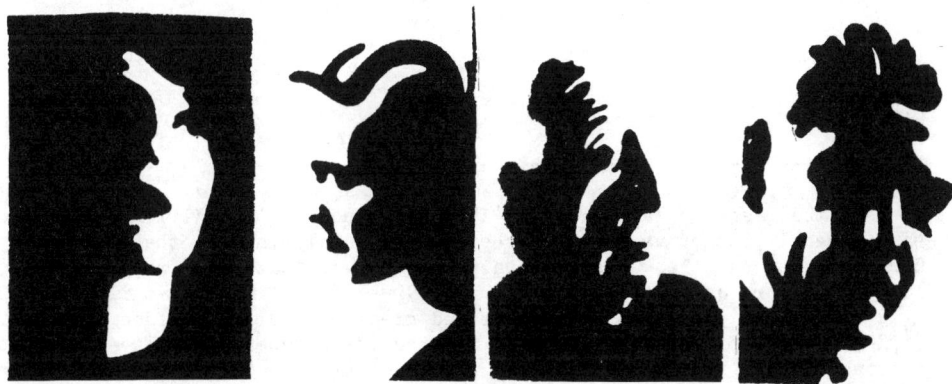

FIGURE 1. Examples of Mooney faces used in Experiment 1.

to Ellis's classification stage. Using normal subjects Hay (1981)
presented either real faces or faces with jumbled features to either the
right or left visual field. Subjects classified the stimuli as either
'face' or 'nonface' and a left visual field advantage was obtained. These
data were interpreted as showing a right hemisphere superiority for "syn-
thesising facial percepts".

2. EXPERIMENT 1

This experiment further examined whether there is a right hemisphere superiority in tasks involving facial classification. It utilised the split field technique: Subjects were presented, tachistopically, with a stimulus to either the right or left visual field (RVF/LVF). They were required to judge whether each stimulus was a face or not. Both accuracy and response time (in msec) were measured. The face stimuli were Mooney Faces (see Figure 1) and the non-face stimuli were the same materials presented upside down.

2.1. Method

The subjects were 30 confirmed right handers between 18 and 24 years old. The stimuli were prepared on cards and presented using an automatic tachistoscope. Each trial involved presentation of a fixation point (1 sec) followed by presentation of the stimulus (150 msec). There were 40 experimental trials in a random sequence. Face and non-face trials occurred an equal number of times in the LVF and RVF.

2.2. Results

The results are shown in Table 1. Tests for homogeneity of variance

TABLE 1. Mean response latencies, in msec, Experiment 1 as a function of visual hemifield and response type.

	LVF		RVF	
	"face"	"non-face"	"face"	"non-face"
	981	1287	1064	1267
S.D.	220	337	276	434
errors	2.0	4.6	2.7	3.1

across the response latencies in 'face' and 'nonface' conditions indicated significantly larger variance in the latter. Analysis was therefore only carried out on the 'face' data. This showed that faces were correctly identified more quickly in the LVF, $t(28) = 2.3$ $p < .05$ (two-tailed). A 2 x 2 ANOVA of the error data revealed greater accuracy on face trials, $F(1,29) = 12.16$ $p < .01$. However an interaction between visual field and response type, $F(1,29) = 12.5$ $p < .01$, indicated that greater accuracy on face trials only occurred with LVF presentation.

2.3. Discussion

The data confirmed the predictions from the Newcombe (1974) and Hay (1981) studies. A right hemisphere superiority was found in a task requiring the classification of stimuli as face-like or not. Thus Ellis's contention that facial classification is right lateralised receives further support.

In Ellis's model, classification is followed by the process of physical analysis. This involves the extraction of information about the individual features of a face. Thus information about nose-shape, eye colour, etc. would be produced by this process. This stage would also detect the presence of any featural anomaly and it is this assumption that underlies the logic of Experiment 2.

3. EXPERIMENT 2

This experiment examined the lateralisation of the physical analysis stage of facial processing.   Ellis is non-committal on this issue but one might expect this stage to exhibit the general pattern of right hemisphere superiority in facial processing.   The experiment again employed the split-field technique using the same apparatus as Experiment 1.   Subjects were presented with a face and asked to decide whether all the features of the face were correct.   The stimuli are shown in Figure 2 and it can be

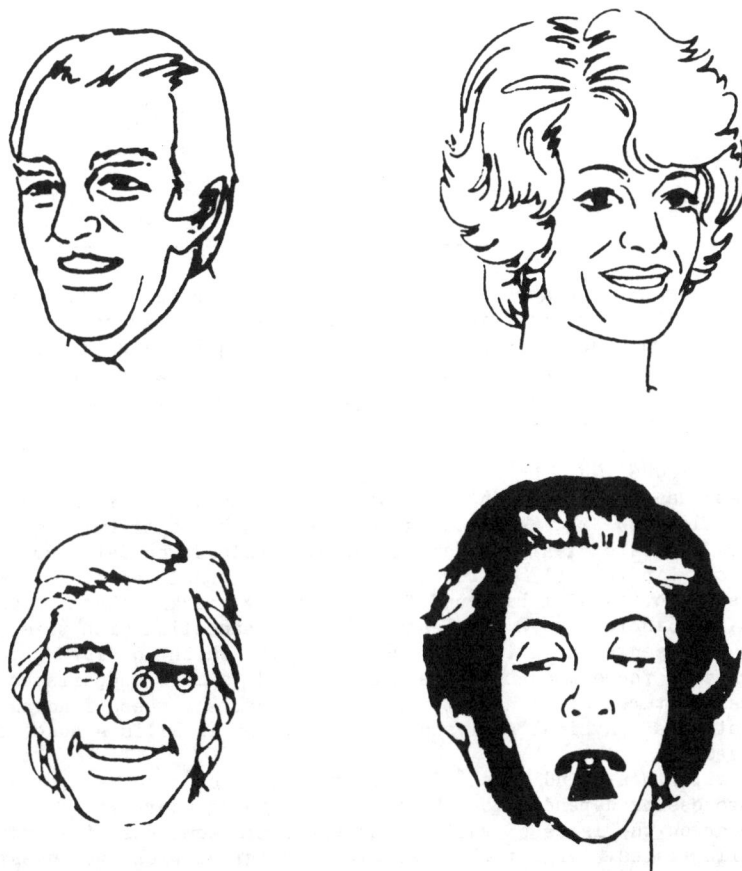

FIGURE 2. Examples of Facial stimuli used in Experiment 2.

seen that "incorrect" faces were devised by replacing one feature with an inappropriate symbol. However, care was taken to preserve the featural configuration of a face. It was assumed that the detection of anomalies is reliant on the physical analysis stage; thus the pattern hemifield superiority of this task would reflect the lateralisation of the physical analysis stage itself.

3.1. Method

Thirty subjects took part, all but one of whom had also served in Experiment 1. Except for the response required - "features correct or incorrect", the procedure was identical to Experiment 1.

3.2. Results

The results are shown in Table 2. Tests for homogeneity of variance

TABLE 2. Mean response latencies, in msec, Experiment 2 as a function of visual hemifield and response type.

	LVF		RVF	
	"Correct"	"Incorrect"	"Correct"	"Incorrect"
	1259	1125	1294	1026
S.D.	338	286	339	214
errors	3.5	2.0	3.1	2.0

---

revealed larger variance in the "features correct" response times. Analysis was therefore restricted to the "features incorrect" and this showed that this decision was carried out more quickly with RVF presentation, t (28) = 2.6 p < .025. ANOVA revealed a higher error rate on correct faces F (1,29) = 10.79 p < .01 but there was no interaction with hemifield.

4. GENERAL DISCUSSION

The task used in Experiment 2 is unlikely to have been amenable to verbal mediation so the LVF advantage cannot be attributed to the left hemisphere's greater language capabilities. Instead the data concur with Sergent and Bindra's (1982) recent review which concluded that a left hemisphere superiority will be found for processing tasks that require the analysis of discrete physical features. In connnection with this, Sergent (1982) has presented a series of experiments in which a left hemisphere superiority is found when subjects are required to make comparisons between individual features of identikit faces. Collectively these findings indicate that the physical analysis stage proposed in Ellis's model is left-lateralised.

These experiments indicate a different pattern of cerebral dominance for facial processing dependent on the stage processing addressed. The results do not bear on the issue of whether the brain has some specific adaptation for handling faces. Whilst there are methodological problems in establishing this fact (e.g. Anderson & Parkin, 1985) it can be argued that the basic question "are faces special?" may not be worth asking. If we could play "20 questions" with nature and win (c.f. Newell 1972), and discovered that the answer to the question "is the brain specifically adapted for faces?" was "yes", where would this get us?

First, attemps to demonstrate qualitative differences in the memory and perception of faces compared with other classes of stimuli per se would no longer be necessary. Another issue would be the relevance of prosopagnosia. Psychological interest in this syndrome centres on whether or not it is face-specific. If we knew the answer to this question what additional value would the phenomenon of prosopagnosia have? Would it, for example, force us to hold a view about the organisation of facial processing that we would otherwise reject? Neuropsychology has a habit of finding patients to fit models rather than vice versa. If this extremely rare syndrome is to be of maximum interest it should enlighten us on the nature of facial processing rather than confirm our ideas about it.

Knowing that faces were special would force us to ask more detailed questions such as "how is face specificity manifest in the system?" Three possibiities can be immediately considered and there are probably many more. 1. That we are peculiarly sensitive to the particular configuration of elements that constitute a face. 2. That we are 'tuned' perceptually to the precise physical characteristics of facial features. 3. That we possess a series of memory vectors specifically developed to enable the accurate storage of many highly similar faces. My contention is that issues like these are worthy of consideration even if we don't know the answer to the basic question of face specificity.

HEMISPHERIC DIFFERENCES IN THE EVOKED POTENTIAL TO FACE STIMULI.

MARIAN SMALL

INTRODUCTION

Investigation of patients with cerebral lesions and tachistoscopic studies in both normal subjects and commissurectomised patients clearly indicate that the right hemisphere has a distinctive role in the processing of faces. Given these indications of a cerebral asymmetry, the possibility that such specialization might be mirrored electrophysiologically seemed worthy of investigation. Schulman-Galambos and Galambos (1978) and Neville et al (1982), recording evoked potentials in response to coloured slides of scenes and people, have reported a late wave, P300, which seems to reflect cognitive events.

The aim of the present study, therefore, was to investigate whether evoked potentials could be recorded in response to slides of faces, and if so, whether a hemisphere asymmetry would be apparent particularly in respect to P300. A group of right handed controls was examined initially. Both known and unknown faces were presented to observe the effects of recognition, and two control series of non-verbal stimuli were included to provide (i) complex stimuli other than faces and (ii) a physical stimulus without cognitive content. The effect of inversion of face slides on the evoked potential was also studied.

Subsequently, a group of left handers was investigated because, while the association between the right hemisphere and non-linguistic functions seems definite for dextrals, it is less clear for left handers. In theory, the latter group should have a higher proportion of right hemisphere speech and left hemisphere non-verbal function and should therefore show less evidence of cerebral evoked potential asymmetry.

PROCEDURE

Recording electrodes. Silver/silver chlorided discs were placed symmetrically over right and left posterior temporal, parietal and occipital regions (namely T6, T5, P4, P3, O2 and O1 of the 10/20 system) all referred to a frontal, midline electrode, Fz. Resistances were below 5 Kohms.

Apparatus. The amplifier frequency response was 0.1 - 250 Hz (-3 dB points). Responses were summated in a digital averager. The sweep, triggered simultaneously with the shutter release of the slide projector lasted 1000 ms with a sampling rate of 256 points/sec. 42 or 64 responses were summated for each condition.

Subjects. Group 1: Thirty right handed normal controls participated, 15 males and 15 females with ages ranging from 14 to 60 years, mean age 30.5 years. Visual acuity was 6/9 or better.
Group 2: There were twenty two left handed normal controls, 15 males and 7 females with ages ranging from 14 to 62 years, mean age 33 years. Visual acuity was 6/9 or better with one exception (6/18 corrected).

Stimuli. All slides were presented for 2 seconds at random intervals and subjects were requested to fixate centrally.
Upright known faces: 42 monochromatic slides of well known faces, e.g. the Royal Family, political leaders and celebrities.

Upright unknown faces: 64 monochromatic slides of faces of members of the Armed Forces, all unknown to the subjects.

Geometric designs: 64 monochromatic slides of complex shapes and designs.

Pattern reversal: A black and white checker board pattern back projected on to a screen in front of the subject, subtending an angle of 22 degrees at the subject's eye. The pattern moved horizontally the width of 1 square every 1.5 seconds. The start of the sweep coincided with the onset of the pattern displacement.

Inverted faces: The slides consisted of the same two sets of faces previously presented; they were merely placed upside down in the projector for presentation.

RESULTS

Evoked potentials were consistently recorded from every subject under all conditions and from each electrode position. The typical response (Fig.1) consisted of an initial positivity between 80 and 120 ms (P100) and an upgoing negativity followed by a positive wave around 260 to 300 ms (P300).

Fig.1

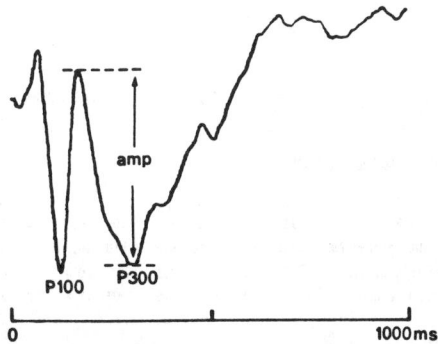

Tables A and B show the latencies and the mean peak to peak amplitudes of P100 and P300 under each condition for right and left handed subjects respectively.

TABLE A RIGHT HANDED SUBJECTS

P100 LATENCY AND AMPLITUDE

	T6		P4		O2		T5		P3		O1	
	lat	amp	lat	amp	lat	amp	lat	amp	lat	amp	lat	amp
Upright known faces	117	7.9	118	7.6	116	11.7	114	7.2	115	7.1	115	11.0
Upright unkown faces	116	8.3	117	7.9	115	12.7	117	7.1	116	6.5	116	11.6
Geometric designs	93	8.4	92	8.5	91	12.2	90	7.2	89	6.6	90	11.4
Pattern reversal	96	6.5	93	6.2	92	13.3	93	5.6	92	4.9	91	12.5
Inverted known faces	113	7.3	111	6.4	110	9.0	110	6.5	109	5.5	109	8.7
Inverted unknown faces	116	7.3	115	7.2	116	9.1	114	6.4	114	6.4	114	8.7

P300 LATENCY AND AMPLITUDE

	T6		P4		O2		T5		P3		O1	
	lat	amp	lat	amp	lat	amp	lat	amp	lat	amp	lat	amp
Upright known faces	293	20.6	291	15.2	292	22.1	291	17.4	291	12.8	293	19.1
Upright unknown faces	295	20.1	294	15.0	293	21.5	292	17.8	291	13.2	293	18.5
Geometric designs	279	14.5	278	12.5	268	15.1	277	13.2	273	11.3	267	14.6
Pattern reversal	275	7.8	270	7.7	267	9.2	272	6.5	269	6.0	265	8.9
Inverted known faces	288	13.3	288	10.7	290	13.8	284	12.8	285	9.2	287	12.8
Inverted unknown faces	294	12.4	291	9.5	292	12.2	291	12.1	295	8.3	290	11.2

TABLE B LEFT HANDED SUBJECTS

P100 LATENCY AND AMPLITUDE

	T6		P4		O2		T5		P3		O1	
	lat	amp	lat	amp	lat	amp	lat	amp	lat	amp	lat	amp
Upright known faces	110	9.7	108	8.5	109	14.2	108	8.5	107	7.0	109	13.7
Upright unknown faces	110	9.5	108	8.6	110	14.7	108	8.6	105	7.6	109	14.3
Geometric designs	95	7.9	94	7.9	94	10.4	93	7.4	94	6.6	93	11.0
Pattern reversal	95	5.5	93	5.0	93	11.8	95	5.6	93	4.7	93	12.3

P300 LATENCY AND AMPLITUDE

	lat	amp	lat	amp	lat	amp	lat	amp	lat	amp	lat	amp
Upright known faces	286	15.3	287	10.4	285	15.5	284	15.1	282	10.0	285	15.0
Upright unknown faces	278	16.2	278	10.3	273	15.2	277	15.4	277	9.5	276	13.7
Geometric designs	282	11.2	277	8.6	275	11.2	280	10.8	275	7.6	273	10.2
Pattern reversal	286	6.4	287	7.0	285	8.4	285	7.1	286	6.3	282	8.2

Analysis of Variance (ANOVA) was performed separately on each of the four dependent variables, namely P100 amplitude, P100 latency, P300 amplitude and P300 latency for (1) the right handed group: upright known faces, upright unknown faces, geometric designs and pattern reversal; (2) the right handed group: inverted known faces and inverted unknown faces and (3) the left handed group: upright known and unknown faces, geometric designs and pattern reversal. The reported results were all significant at the p<0.05 level or greater.

ANOVA (1) Right handed subjects. Upright known and unknown faces, geometric designs and pattern reversal.

P100 was of maximum amplitude in occipital regions. It occurred generally of higher amplitude (by 0.9 µV) over the right hemisphere compared to the left, but equally so for all four conditions. The latency of P100 was 25 ms earlier with geometric shapes and pattern reversal (90-96 ms) than with upright known and unknown faces (114-118 ms). It occurred significantly later by 1.4 ms in the right hemisphere.

P300 was of maximum amplitude in occipital and temporal regions. It appeared with a right greater than left amplitude asymmetry during all four conditions but the mean right/left sided difference of 2.3 µV for face stimuli was significantly greater (p <0.001) than the right/left difference (0.9 µV) found with geometric designs and pattern reversal (Fig.2). This right hemisphere superiority was reflected equally at all electrodes. There was no difference in amplitude between known and un-known faces. P300 occurred approximately 20 ms earlier with geometric designs and pattern reversal than with slides of faces. There was no difference in latency between right and left hemispheres.

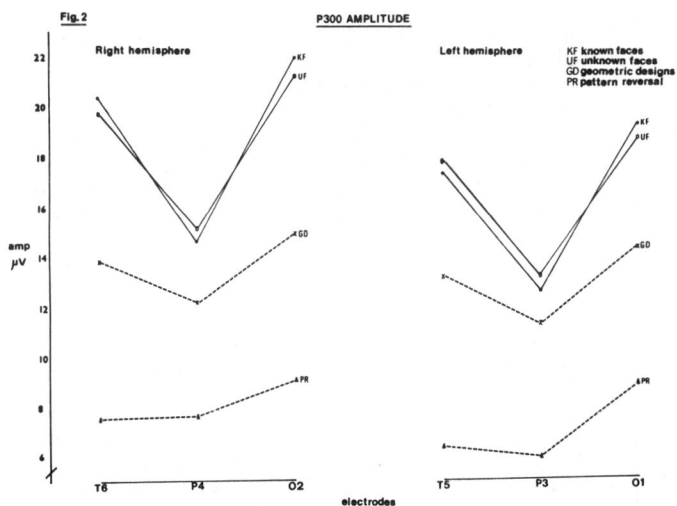

Fig.2   P300 AMPLITUDE

ANOVA (2) Right handed subjects. Inverted known and unknown faces.

The amplitude and latency of P100 were essentially the same as those reported with upright known and unknown faces. P300 amplitude was generally slightly higher over the right hemisphere (12.0 µV) compared to the left (11.1 µV) but this difference between the hemispheres did not prove significant (Fig.3). With both inverted known and unknown faces P300 was of much lower amplitude (at all electrode sites) than that found in response to upright known and unknown faces.

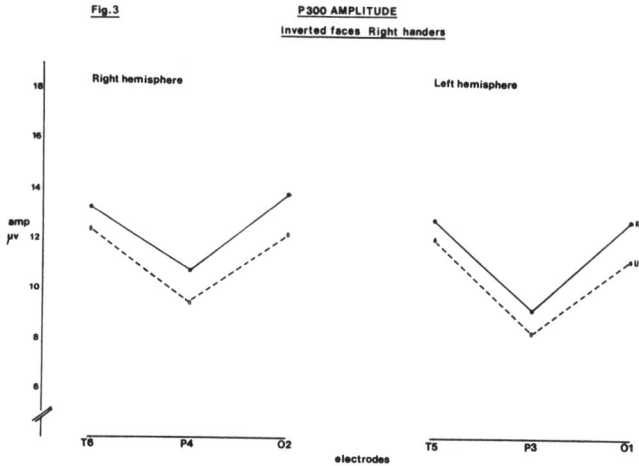

Fig.3

P300 AMPLITUDE

Inverted faces Right handers

Right hemisphere   Left hemisphere

amp
μV

electrodes

T6   P4   O2   T5   P3   O1

ANOVA (3) Left handed subjects. Upright known and unknown faces, geometric designs and pattern reversal.

The amplitude of P100 was again maximal occipitally and occurred with a slight right greater than left amplitude asymmetry in temporal and parietal areas. Geometric designs and pattern reversal produced earlier P100 latencies (by 14 ms) than both known and unknown face conditions.

Left handed subjects showed no difference in P300 amplitude between right and left hemispheres, either generally or during separate conditions (Fig.4).

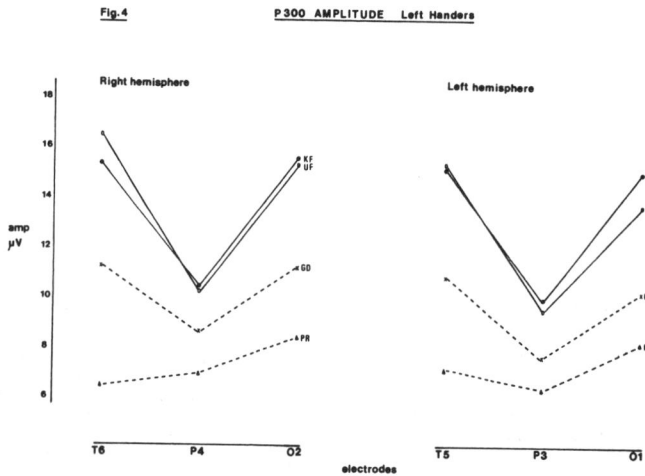

Fig.4

P300 AMPLITUDE Left Handers

Right hemisphere   Left hemisphere

amp
μV

electrodes

T6   P4   O2   T5   P3   O1

SUMMARY

The first experiment shows, that in respect to P300, the right hemisphere is more involved than the left in the processing of faces (in right handed individuals) compared to other complex visual stimuli, with the right occipitotemporal region showing maximal responses (Small, 1983). No difference was found between known and unknown slides of faces.

The clear right greater than left P300 amplitude asymmetry was not apparent with inversion, providing evidence that the right hemisphere superiority with upright faces is specific to vertical orientation. There was a general P300 amplitude reduction over both hemispheres with inverted faces (compared to upright faces), the values being similar to those found in response to geometric designs.

The results of the left handed subjects were very similar to those of the right handed group. However, the left handers did not show a significant P300 amplitude asymmetry in response to face stimuli, a finding which suggests that the previously reported hemisphere difference does indeed reflect organisation of cerebral function.

CEREBRAL AND BEHAVIOURAL ASYMMETRIES IN THE PROCESSING OF "UNUSUAL" FACES:
A REVIEW

R. BRUYER

1. INTRODUCTION
This paper presents one very particular aspect of face processing in neuropsychology, which reveals behavioural asymmetries that probably result from brain asymmetry. This kind of data, it is hoped, can increase our knowledge of both the cerebral mode of functioning and the cognitive operations underlying the processing of faces.
Like all experimental material, the faces used in laboratories are always ecologically unusual in a broad sense, because of the absence of motion or colour, the exposure duration, the location in the visual field, and other experimental parameters. However, there are designs in which the faces used are intentionally unusual: line drawings, upside-down presentations, symmetrical face composites, blurred faces, faces with exaggerated shadows and highlights, and so on. These particular stimuli have been used to study the mode of processing more natural faces. I have no precise criterion for identifying this "unusualness", and the various topics reviewed here have been selected for reasons of general relevance. In each case, data furnished by brain-damaged, by split-brain, and by normal subjects will be considered when available. Five topics will be examined, and a sixth point will concern studies involving more than one kind of unusualness.

2. INVERTED FACES
2.1.
A first kind of unusualness was studied by Yin (1970) in a famous paper. By using a recognition paradigm, he observed the well-known defect of right-brain damaged subjects with a posterior lesion for faces but not for other stimuli; moreover, this pattern of data disappeared when the material was inverted and presented upside-down. In a similar study, Bruyer and Velge (1981) were unable to reproduce such a group-by-orientation-by-stimuli interaction, but this could have been because we used a perceptual matching task while Yin used a recognition task. Grusser and Kirchoff (1982) did not observe this phenomenon, but they were studying long-term memory (delays of one hour and one week between the inspection and the recognition).

2.2.
However, Yin's effect has been observed in various studies with normal subjects being presented laterally displayed stimuli (Leehey, Carey, Diamond & Cahn, 1978; Rapaczynski & Ehrlichman, 1979) and even with children (Young & Bion, 1980 & 1981) in recognition tasks (but see Bradshaw, Taylor, Patterson & Nettleton, 1980). Ellis and Shepherd (1975) did not observe this effect, but this may have been for methodological reasons: they used a very short exposure duration (15 msec) and a perceptual same-different kind of task. Finally, the effect was observed with a task involving the identification of famous faces (Young, 1984).

2.3.

In short, in brain-damaged as well as in normal subjects, the right-hemisphere superiority "classically" observed in the processing of faces disappears when inverted faces are displayed, at least for short-term recognition tasks. It seems that this modification does not apply for tasks not requiring short-term memory operations or for tasks involving a very long duration of retention.

3. FACE DRAWINGS

Another type of unusualness involves simplified or realistic line drawings of faces. This kind of material has often been employed for specific purposes: indeed, it allows the researchers to control the type and the number of facial features that differ from one face to another.

3.1.

Studies have also been done in which the features are not experimentally manipulated. Concerning the performance of brain-damaged subjects, the usual deficit of right-damaged subjects has been reproduced with face drawings, both in recognition tasks and in same-different judgement tasks with pairs of simultaneously displayed faces (Bruyer & Velge, 1980; Murri, Arena, Siciliano, Mazzotta & Muratorio, 1984; Tzavaras, Hecaen & Lebras, 1970). It was not observed when the subjects had to match a target face with a copy on a multiple-choice board (Bruyer & Velge, 1980), but it was when accessories were added (Tzavaras et al., 1970). Finally, Wayland and Taplin (1982) noted a selective defect of fluent aphasic subjects in a categorisation task, but there is no equivalent study available with photographs of faces.

As regards normal subjects and laterally displayed stimuli, the studies generally used a same-different task upon pairs of successive drawings and evidenced a left-field advantage (Buffery, 1974; Geffen, Bradshaw & Wallace, 1971; Ley & Bryden, 1979; Moscovitch, Scullion & Christie, 1976; Patterson & Bradshaw, 1975), at least when a manual response was required. However, this was not observed by Sergent (1982); I will return to this qualification later. This asymmetry was not observed by Bradshaw, Nettleton and Patterson (1973), but their stimuli were profile views of faces. Asymmetry was noted, however, when the task was the recognition of a memorised target (Geffen et al., 1971, exp. 5; Moscovitch et al., 1976, exp. 2; Patterson & Bradshaw, 1975, exp. 2 & 3).

3.2.

As in same-different studies with photographs of faces, line drawings have been used to examine asymmetry in function of the kind of pairs (same versus different). In the study of Bruyer and Velge (1980), the deficit of the right-damaged subjects was particularly apparent in "same" judgements. These subjects, like the children examined in another study (Bruyer & Gadisseux, 1980), produced more errors when the stimuli were identical, which was not observed with normal or left-damaged adults.

In tachistoscopic studies with normals, the results vary as a function of some experimental factors. Patterson and Bradshaw (1975) reported a left-field superiority particularly for "same" judgements; Sergent (1982) reported no interaction between the visual hemifield and the kind of pairs; Bradshaw and Sherlock (1982) found no asymmetry for non-targets, and the direction of asymmetries for targets depended on manipulations of the features.

3.3.

Facial features can be studied by using drawings of faces. More precisely, it permits us to analyze both the effect of the number of features and the differential effect of facial areas.

In the study of Bruyer and Velge (1980), the "different" judgements of the normal and left-brain damaged subjects were affected by the number of different features, as we expected, but the right-damaged subjects remained globally unaffected by this number.

The study of normals by means of laterally displayed stimuli (Bradshaw & Sherlock, 1982; Buffery, 1974; Fairweather, Brizzolara, Tabossi & Umilta, 1982; Patterson & Bradshaw, 1975; Sergent, 1982, exp. 1 & 3, 1984) leads to the following conclusions. First, lateral differences for judgements of dissimilarity depend on the number of different facial features: with the exception of the paper by Buffery (1974), a right-field superiority is noted for pairs in which only one feature is critical, and an increase in the number of critical features leads to a reduction of this asymmetry and, sometimes, to a left-field advantage. Second, the features especially involved in these asymmetries seem to be the upper ones, like the eyes or the hair: the data suggest a feature-by-feature, top-to-bottom processing of faces, such processing being specific to stimuli displayed in the right field (Sergent, 1982). Third, nevertheless, it appears that stimuli are best described by a Euclidian model that suggests comparisons based on the overall similarity of faces (Sergent, 1982). Finally a right-field advantage is noted when one feature is critical, a left one when the general organization of the features is involved.

3.4.

In short, the use of face drawings has confirmed data collected by means of photographs. It also has expanded our knowledge of face processing, by showing that the asymmetries seem to depend on the number of different features and on the differential status of the features. These conclusions now have to be tested on more natural faces. In this line, I mention the study of Young (1984) in which famous faces were identified from incomplete photographs from which internal or external features had been removed: in both cases, a left-field superiority was noted.

4. COMPLETE UNUSUAL FACES

I now want to consider those studies in which complete photographs are modified to induce physically unusual viewing conditions. These are experiments in which shadows and highlights are exaggerated, in which unusual lighting conditions are used, or in which the stimuli are out of focus.

4.1.

The test of Benton and Van Allen (1968) is well known among those who work with brain-damaged people. The third part of this test concerns faces with various types of lighting; unfortunately, the publications generally do not present separate scores for the three parts. Therefore, even if defects of right-damaged subjects are generally observed in this multiple-choice task or in the short form of the test devised by Levin, Hamsher and Benton (1975), we are unable to evaluate the scores for the three parts separately (Benton & Gordon, 1979; Benton & Van Allen, 1968; Blunck, 1982; Hamsher, Levin & Benton, 1979; Jones, 1969; Poizner, Kaplan, Bellugi & Padden, 1984; Wassterstein, Zappulla, Rosen & Thompson, 1983; see also Wasserstein, Zappulla, Rosen & Gerstman, 1984). The same applies for the paired comparison test of Jones (1969) in which two parts of four involve photographs taken under reduced lighting conditions. Newcombe and Russell

(1969) showed faces with exaggerated highlights and shadows: a defect of the right-damaged subjects was observed in a categorisation task (male-female and old-young). In the study of Bruyer (1980a), the subjects pointed to the copy of a target on a multiple-choice board; the target was always clear, but six levels of defocusing were applied to the board. An impairment of the right-damaged subjects appeared, that was limited to the lowest levels of defocusing. If we assume that blurred faces are stimuli in which the highest spatial frequencies are removed, two interpretations are possible. First, if the subjects process the task with their undamaged hemisphere, then the results suggest that there is no asymmetry for the low frequencies and an advantage of the right hemisphere when the high frequencies are added. Such a conclusion could run against Sergent's hypothesis (see Sergent, 1983). The second interetation could be that the classical defect of the right-damaged subjects in the processing of clear faces is reduced by offering to the damaged right hemisphere the material for which it is specialised. Such a conclusion could agree with the Sergent's propositions.

4.2.
In a similar line, Gazzaniga and Smylie (1983) administered split-brain subjects a recognition task for laterally displayed faces. The left-field superiority observed with normal faces was modified neither by defocusing, which stresses low frequencies, nor by a reduction of size, which stresses high frequencies.

4.3.
Three studies with normal subjects were made in which the spatial frequencies were directly manipulated. Keegan (1981) asked his subjects to make same-different judgements on pairs of filtered photographs of faces. For the "same" responses, an advantage of the left field appeared for faces from which the highest frequencies had been removed, with no asymmetry for faces from which the lowest frequencies had been removed. Using various tasks, Sergent and Switkes (1984; see also Sergent, this book) observed an advantage of the left field for stimuli modified by a low pass; when a broad pass was used, the asymmetries were the same as with normal photographs. Thus, there is reason to suppose that the right hemisphere is particularly able to process low frequencies, as has been suggested by experiments in which frequencies were manipulated indirectly (by controlling the intensity, duration, size, or eccentricity of the material) (see also Parkin, this book).

5. "STRANGE" FACES
I would like to mention in passing two studies in which "strange" faces were shown to normal subjects, the first one concerning the processing of faces from another racial group (Bruyer & Dussart, 1985). In experimental psychology, the race effect refers to difficulty in recognising faces of people not belonging to the same race as that of the subject. Belgian and African subjects were enrolled in a recognition taks of Caucasian and African male faces laterally displayed. This preliminary study showed, for the Belgian subjects, that the race effect appeared only for stimuli displayed in the right field. Additional experiments are necessary to clarify these initial results.

The second research concerns the processing of laterally displayed photographs of puppets' heads. Bruyer and Stroot (1984) noted an advantage of the right field in a recognition-identification task and an advantage of the left field for "same" responses only in a same-different discrimination task.

6. "QUASI-FACES"

We now come to the use of "quasi-faces". I am thinking of two particular types of material: first, face-composites made by juxtaposing two hemifaces issuing from different faces or by a hemiface and its own mirror-image, and, second, isolated parts of faces.

6.1.

In the study published by De Renzi, Faglioni and Spinnler (1968), the brain-damaged subjects searched in a field of 12 complete faces for the face corresponding to a target. In two conditions, this target was a fragment of the face: the eyes or the mouth. No difference appeared between the left- and right-damaged subjects for these conditions. In the third condition, the target was a lateral hemiface, and a significant deficit of the right-damaged subjects appeared. When brain-damaged subjects were asked to choose which one of two symmetrical face composites was the most similar to the normal face (Kolb, Milner & Taylor, 1983), a bias appeared favouring the hemiface seen in the left part of the field; however, this bias was not observed for subjects with a lesion in the posterior part of the right hemisphere.

6.2.

The display of asymmetrical face composites has shown a preference for the left part of the stimulus in split-brain subjects, at least with a non-verbal mode of response (Levy, Trevarthen & Sperry, 1972).

6.3.

In normals, most of the studies using face composites have been designed to examine facial asymmetry as well as the asymmetry of emotional facial expressions; I will not discuss these topics here. The remaining publications can be classified into three categories. First, a left-field superiority appears when complete faces have to be recognized on laterally displayed hemifaces (Finlay & French, 1978; Rhodes, 1985, exp. 4). Second, an advantage of the hemiface perceived in the left field appears when asymmetrical face composites have to be recognized on complete faces (Milner & Dunne, 1977; Schwartz & Smith, 1980; but see Rhodes, 1985, exp. 2 & 3). Finally, studies using symmetrical face composites reveal a preference for the hemiface perceived in the left part of the visual field in recognition, at least in male, right-handed subjects with a normal hand position for writing (Gilbert & Bakan, 1973; Lawson, 1978; Oltman, Ehrlichman & Cox, 1977; Rhodes, 1985, exp. 1); an advantage of the right field for "same" responses in same-different judgements on pairs of faces and composites (Bruyer & Craps, 1985, exp. 3); and an advantage of the right field for composites in a facial decision task on faces and composites (Bruyer & Craps, 1985, exp. 4).

7. SEVERAL SIMULTANEOUS KINDS OF UNUSUALNESS

Finally, there are those studies in which two kinds of unusualness are simultaneously used.

7.1.

First, there are experiments where realistic drawings of "quasi-faces" are used for facial decision tasks on laterally displayed stimuli (normal subjects) (Christen, Davidoff, Landis & Regard, 1985; Hay, 1981; Young, Hay & McWeeny, 1985). The "quasi-faces" are made by modifying the position of the features. A left-field superiority appeared only when the stimuli were moderately scrambled, which could indicate a right-hemisphere dominance in the construction of facial representations and no asymetry for the classification of stimuli as faces. On the other hand, a right-field superiority appeared for "non-face" decisions when a short exposition was used. Nevertheless, Buffery (1974), in a study with highly scrambled faces, observed an advantage in the condition where the second stimuli appeared in the left field for same-different judgements.

7.2.
Second, studies using drawings of fragments of faces revealed that the defect of the right-brain-damaged subjects in same-different tasks was limited to the internal facial features (Bruyer, 1980b), and that the right-damaged subjects systematically avoided lateral hemifaces when invited to choose among upper, lower, left, and right hemifaces (Bruyer, 1980c). On the other hand, same-different judgements on laterally displayed isolated features (normal subjects) (Sergent, 1982, exp. 2) revealed neither an effect of the visual field nor a visual-field-by-feature interaction. Nevertheless, it appeared that performance on laterally displayed complete faces depends on the discriminability of the features, in the left field only.

7.3.
In a third category of studies, drawings of faces are displayed in an inverted, upside-down presentation (normal subjects). In a same-different task on successive stimuli, Buffery (1974) noted a superiority of the conditions in which the second stimulus was displayed in the left field, this asymmetry being limited to the right-handed subjects.

7.4.
Finally, in the study published by Kolb et al. (1983), face composites were displayed upside-down and shown to brain-damaged subjects. As with the normal presentation, a bias towards the part seen in the left portion of the field was observed, except with the right-damaged subjects.

8. CONCLUSIONS
Some general comments by way of conclusion. First, we have to note that the use of unusual face-like stimuli in neuropsychological paradigms has significantly improved the understanding of the cognitive and cerebral mechanisms underlying the processing of faces. Second, we now have to design experiments with more natural faces while taking these results into account. Finally, I believe that the unusualness of the material in the studies reviewed should not be exaggerated: ecologically, experiments even with more natural faces still remains very artificial.

7. PROSOPAGNOSIAS

CURRENT ISSUES ON PROSOPAGNOSIA

E. DE RENZI

1. INTRODUCTION

There is a tendency in the literature to treat prosopagnosia as if it were a single disorder, dependent on the disruption of a unique mechanism and associated with a stereotyped lesional picture. The search for a common interpretation has from time to time privileged different aspects of the disorder, but the failure to reach a general consensus insinuates that an analytical approach, aiming at distinguishing, rather than unifying the manifestations of prosopagnosia, may be more fruitful. After all, nobody would conceive of aphasia as a single deficit and even for visual agnosia at least two forms have been envisaged.

In this paper I will draw from my experience with patients impaired in familiar face recognition to address three issues that are controversial: the functional level at which prosopagnosia occurs; its specificity for faces; and its anatomical correlates. For each of these questions I will try to show that the variety of clinical findings does not fit for a univocal interpretation, unless one is ready to force reality into a Procrustean bed.

2. TWO FORMS OF PROSOPAGNOSIA, PERCEPTUAL AND MNESTIC

There are diverging views on the functional locus of damage producing prosopagnosia, with some authors stressing a deficit in perceptual processing and others the loss or unavailability of visual memories of previously learned faces. Very few proponents of the former theory would today share Bay's (1950) opinion that subtle alterations of primary visual function are responsible for prosopagnosia and they would rather emphasise a higher level deficit in the discrimination and integration of the salient features characterising a face. A defect at this stage would prevent the patient from attaining a representation of the face suited to activate the memory units. Evidence in support of this interpretation has been sought in the failure by the patient to discriminate in daily life objects that are physically similar and in his poor performance on tasks that are perceptually demanding, but do not call for memory, such as identifying interrupted, or overlapping figures or recognising the identity of figures taken from different perspectives. Particular popularity is enjoyed by tests requiring patients to match non-identical photographs of the same unfamiliar face, taken in different conditions of illumination or from different views, or variously disguised. The ability tapped seems germane to that involved in the detection of the invariant features characterising a face and permitting its identification, despite the continuous changes through which it appears to the observer. Yet a word of caution is appropriate in evaluating the performance on these tests, since right brain damaged (RBD) patients without prosopagnosia have been repeatedly found to score poorly on perceptually demanding tasks (De Renzi, Scotti & Spinnler, 1969), in particular those involving unknown faces (Benton & Van Allen,

1968; De Renzi, Faglioni & Spinnler, 1968; Warrington & James, 1967). Benton (1980) has stressed that the ability to recognise familiar faces must be kept separate from that required to match unfamiliar faces. For instance, Whiteley and Warrington (1977) have interpreted prosopagnosia as being due to a specific deficit in perceptual classification of faces, based on the poor performance of their patients on a profile-front-view matching test. Although their scores were in fact worse than those found in any control patient, it remains to be shown that they were poorer than those of RBD patients without prosopagnosia.

3. CASE STUDIES

Thus, while a performance in the normal range on this kind of task is a strong argument for the integrity of the visuo-perceptual system, the impairment must be heavy, span on a wide range of tests, and possibly be confirmed by examples from daily life to support the claim that it is related to the disability responsible for prosopagnosia.

These requirements have been met by a few cases reported by the literature, where prosopagnosia appeared in the context of a more widespread disorder of perceptual recognition (Macrae & Trolle, 1956; Beyn & Kniazeva, 1962; Rubens & Benson, 1971; Levin, 1978; Shuttleworth, Syring & Allen, 1982; Gomori & Hawryluk, 1984). To them I will now add the following three cases.

3.1. Patient 1

Patient 1 has already been reported (De Renzi et al., 1968) and will be briefly summarised. A 54-year-old, right-handed man had suffered two years earlier from a stroke which had left a left superior quadrantopia. Inability to recognise familiar faces was his major complaint and extended to the discrimination of age and emotional expressions, but, when closely questioned, he admitted to also making errors in identifying stimuli belonging to other categories, e.g. in distinguishing an orange from a lemon, an apple from a peach, a beef steak from a veal steak, a bottle of wine from a bottle of water, the faces of playing cards, banknotes, well-known buildings. The performance on a series of tests confirmed that the patient's perceptual abilities were severely impaired well beyond the problem of face recognition. Table 1 reports his scores and the available means of RBD patients on the same tests. He performed in the normal range in naming 40 common objects, but made 11 errors with 30 coloured, realistic pictures, did not recognise any of the 11 fragmented figures of the Street

TABLE 1. Scores of patient 1 and means of RBD patients

	Patient 1	RBD patients
Wechsler VIQ	127	
Object recognition	38/40	–
Figure recognition	19/30	–
Street's completion test	0/11	5/11
Ghent's overlapping figures	15/36	22/36
Face-matching test	1.83/9	4.93/8
Recurring face test	– 3.24	14/24

completion test, missed 21 out of the 36 overlapping figures of the Ghent's test and scored remarkably worse than RBD patients in matching profile-front-views of unfamiliar faces and in recognising previously seen unfamiliar faces from new faces.

3.2. Patient 2

Patient 2 was a 68-year-old man who was admitted to the wards for the sudden onset of a severe headache and a right hemianopia. A CT scan showed the presence of a haematoma located in the subcalcarine portion of the left occipital lobe and of an area of density in the lateral part of the right occipito-temporal region encroaching upon the periventricular white matter, which was attributed to an old infarct. He was alexic without agraphia, moderately anomic and constructional apraxic. Visual acuity was 10/10 in the left eye and 7/10 in the right eye. Goldman perimetry showed a right superior quadrantopia. He could recognise familiar persons only by voice and was unable to learn to identify doctors and nurses, unless they spoke. His performance on a series of visuo-perceptual tests is shown in Table 2. He made some errors with objects and was severely impaired in recognising coloured photographs. On the test of figure-ground discrimination described by Warrington and Taylor (1973), where the subject has to identify a fragmented letter (an X or an 0) superimposed upon a fragmented background, on Street's test and Ghent's test his performance was strikingly poor. Unfamiliar face recognition was assessed with the short form of Benton's test (Levin, Hamsher & Benton, 1975): his score was severely defective according to Levin et al.'s standards. The age identification test (De Renzi, Bonacini & Faglioni, in preparation) is a test requiring the subject to rank by age 12 quadruplets of faces of the same sex. The score is in terms of errors and the maximum error score is 96. The patient made 44 errors (the worst score found in a normal subject is 24). The face memory test was given immediately after the age identification test and consisted in the presentation of 48 pairs of faces, one of which was an item shown in the age identification test and the other was new. The patient had to identify the old member of the pair. His performance was at chance level.

TABLE 2. Scores of patient 2 and 3, and means of RBD patients and normal controls

	Max Score	Pt. 2	Pt. 3	RBD Pts.	C Pts.
Wechsler VIQ		—	110	—	—
Object recognition	30	24	25	—	29
Figure recognition	30	8	10	—	27
Figure-ground discrimination	33	12	25	27	31
Street's completion test	11	0	0	5	7
Ghent's overlapping figures	36	5	0	22	32
Benton's face matching test	27	12	12	18	21
Age identification test	96 E	44 E	28 E	16 E	6 E
Face memory test	48	29	26	33	37
Recurring face test	24	—	- 1	14	—

3.3. Patient 3

Patient 3 was a 70-year-old lady with a four-year long history of progressive failure of visuo-perceptual abilities, which had resulted in an increasing difficulty in reading, sewing, embroidering, etc. Oral language was unimpaired, verbal memory was in the normal range and VIQ was 110. She was acalculic. The patient spontaneously complained that she failed to recognise well-known people by sight and that she followed TV movies only by relying on the audio information. She could slowly and laboriously read a printed text, but not one written by hand, even if written by herself, and was unable to distinguish banknotes and coins. Her scores are reported by Table 2. She had mild difficulty in recognising objects, but was severely impaired on object photographs and on all the perceptually complex tests, including those requiring discrimination and identification of faces. CT scan showed bilateral ventricular atrophy, particularly marked in the temporal-occipital lobe.

These three patients have severe problems in recognising two-dimensional, realistic representations of objects, fail perceptually demanding tests and make a striking number of errors on face tests requiring either their identification or the appreciation of the features characterising the subject's age. As only visuo-perceptual skills are involved by these performances, it seems legitimate to infer that these patients suffer from a diffuse perceptual deficit, which prevents the attainment of a face representation sufficiently clear to activate the corresponding memory unit.

The contribution to prosopagnosia of a memory component cannot be excluded, but its assessment is hindered by the disruption of the recognition process at an earlier stage.

This is not always the case with prosopagnosia. There are at least six cases in the literature (Assal, 1969; Tzavaras, Hécaen & Le Bras, 1970 Benton & Van Allen, 1972; Lhermitte & Pillon, 1975; Ross, 1980; Malone et al., 1982; Bruyer et al., 1983) who scored in the normal range on face matching tests and at least one of them (Bruyer et al., 1983) also passed a number of non-facial perceptual tests. Their inability to recognise familiar faces cannot therefore be ascribed to the defective processing of visual information and suggests that either access to facial memory or the visual storage itself was disrupted. The two following patients are an example of this pattern of impairment, their performance showing a striking dissociation between perceptual and memory tests for faces.

3.4. Patient 4

A 72-year-old public notary was still prosopagnosic 16 months following a stroke, which had also caused a persistent left hemianopia and a transient topographical amnesia. He had resumed his work with the usual proficiency, but needed to be assisted by his secretaries in the identification of old clients, although he perfectly remembered the details of their business. Also the identification of relatives and close friends constituted an insurmountable problem if he could not rely upon their voices. The extensive neuropsychological investigation of this patient disclosed a pattern of impairment quite different from that found in the three previous patients (Table 3). Not only objects and realistic figures but also fragmented and overlapping figures were well recognised. On Benton's face matching test he scored rather poorly, but not worse than the average RBD patient without prosopagnosia and he made substantially fewer errors than RBD patients on the age identification test (see Table 2 for the means of the RBD and control group). On the contrary, his performance was definitely impaired on two face tests involving memory. They were the face memory test previously described and a recurring face test, similar to the recurring meaningless figure test devised by Kimura (1963). On the latter test, where the score corresponds to the sum of correct recognitions minus the sum of false recognitions, the mean of RBD patients is 14.

3.5. Patient 5

Patient 5, a 42-year-old woman, stands apart and cannot be considered, strictly speaking, a true example of prosopagnosia, because her difficulty in recognising many persons familiar to her before the disease was framed in a picture of more widespread amnesia. Six months before examination, she had suffered from an encephalitis of probable herpetic etiology, from which she recovered in one month. She subsequently showed a peculiar clinical picture, different in many respects from the classic amnesic syndrome found

TABLE 3. Scores of patients 4 and 5

	Patient 4	Patient 5
Wechsler VIQ	124	101
Wechsler PIQ	–	116
Object recognition	30	30
Figure recognition	30	30
Figure-ground discrimination	26	31
Street's completion test	8	–
Ghent's overlapping figures	36	36
Benton's face matching test	18	23
Age identification test	10 E	6 E
Face memory test	26	32
Recurring face test	1	0

after herpes simplex encephalitis, and which will be the subject of a separate report and is here only briefly summarised. She had a profound disorder of semantic memory, which resulted in severe anomia on visual and verbal confrontation and in impaired name comprehension, but only marginally interfered with expression analysis and comprehension of running speech. Her command of phonology, grammar and syntax was perfect. As to memory, there was a striking discrepancy between a complete failure to recall general events, and a substantially preserved ability to report biographical data, namely events in which she was directly involved, whether they belonged to the remote or the recent (post-disease) past. Thus, for instance, she could tell nothing of the second World War, the Red Brigade's and Moro's affair, the earthquake that a few years ago destroyed many cities in Southern Italy, etc., while she referred in detail the circumstances of her engagement and wedding, her children's birth, how she had passed the last summer holidays, what was said and done in the course of the previous testing session, etc. Faces provide an exception to this rule. Relatives and a few close friends were recognised, but other acquaintances were not. When she returned to the high school where she had been working for many years as a secretary, most of the teachers, whom she was well familiar with, looked to her completely unknown and the same occurred with many other people. She was frequently addressed by somebody, who asked questions revealing a long, reciprocal acquaintance and whom, much to her dismay, she was totally unable to identify, having not even the slightest feeling of familiarity. If somebody reminded her of the circumstances in which she had become acquainted with that person, however, she recalled a great number of details of her/him. A typical example of the dissociation between face recognition and personal event recall was the following: on a Sunday the psychologist who had repeatedly tested her came to the wards with her child and waved to the patient when she met her. The patient did not recognise her and anxiously asked who she was. The next day the patient remembered the event perfectly, but again failed to recognise the psychologist.

It is questionable whether this case can be classified as an example of prosopagnosia, not only because the deficit was framed in a more general, albeit peculiar, memory disorder, but also because in many instances neither the voice, nor the dress helped the patient to identify a familiar person. It is, however, a striking example of the inability to recognise people, consequent to a predominantly visual mnestic deficit, as attested by her excellent performance on a wide range of perceptual tests (Table 3) in contrast to the failure on face memory tests.

The distinction between two forms of prosopagnosia, one affecting the perceptual processing of visual data and the other the memory units permitting retrieval of semantic information concerning a person, is an oversimplification, as more than one component is likely to be active at either stage of the face recognition process (Hay & Young, 1982; Ellis, 1983). Further, both levels may be impaired in the same patient. Despite these limitations, it seems useful to adopt a dichotomous classification, which is to a large extent remindful of that currently accepted for visual agnosia, where an apperceptive form is kept separate from an associative form.

4. THE SPECIFICITY OF PROSOPAGNOSIA

An issue that has been repeatedly debated in connection with prosopagnosia is whether the deficit is really confined to faces, or whether its apparent specificity is contingent on the way it is examined. A positive answer would have important implications for understanding how the face processing system is organised in the brain (Hay & Young, 1982). As the evidence from present cases suggests, in patients with apperceptive prosopagnosia the disruption of the visuo-perceptual processors is not confined to faces, but extends to other categories of stimuli, when their perceptual saliency is decreased. Even the recognition of coloured, realistic drawings was impaired in our patients in comparison to normals when assessed with a standardised test. The only case in which a face specific perceptual classification deficit has been implicated as responsible for prosopagnosia has been reported by Whiteley and Warrington (1977), but I have alredy argued why I do not think that the evidence is compelling.

When objects and figures are correctly recognised, unknown face tests are passed and the patient's complaints appear to be confined to faces, is it conceivable that a mechanism specialised in processing and/or storing facial data is selectively disrupted? Many authorities have warned against too easily accepting this view and stressed that since no prosopagnosic patient fails to recognise that a face is a face, but rather that it is a particular familiar face, also other classes of stimuli should be tested for the ability to identify a particular item of the category. Anecdotal evidence that the identification of subordinate categories differing for minor perceptual features was defective can be found in a few case reports of prosopagnosia: a patient failed to discriminate chairs from armchairs (Faust, 1955); a birdwatcher had lost the ability to identify birds

(Bornstein, 1963); other patients misidentified animal figures, especially if of similar shapes; and car makes (Gloning et al., 1966; Lhermitte & Pillon, 1975); or national coins from foreign coins (Blanc-Garin et al., 1984). Even more compelling are the cases where the deficit involved the recognition of a particular item, the patient was well familiar with, e.g. his own cows by a farmer (Bornstein, Sroka & Munitz, 1969; Assal, Favre & Anderes, 1984); and their own cars and articles of clothing by Damasio, Damasio and Van Hoesen's patients (1982). Based on these data, Damasio et al. (1982) postulated that the true dissociation of prosopagnosia is not between faces and other objects, but between the recognition of the general class to which the stimulus belongs and that of "the historical context of a given object vis-a-vis the subject" and predicted that the patient "will be just as incapable of evoking the history of a familiar object as he will be of evoking the history of a familiar face". The pre-eminence of the impairment for faces would be more apparent than real and due to the fact that for a face it is crucial to identify its individuality, while objects of the same class are more easily interchangeable in daily life.

Our fourth patient was an ideal subject to verify the hypothesis of a specific impairment in the experience of familiarity, as perceptual deficits apparently played no role in his prosopagnosia. His ability to recognise single objects or stimuli that were familiar to him from among other members of the same class was, therefore, investigated. He was requested to identify his own electric razor, wallet, glasses and neckties, when each of them was presented together with 6 to 10 objects of the same category, chosen as to have physical resemblance with the target. He was also asked to write a sentence on a cardboard and then to identify his own handwriting from nine samples of the same sentence written by other persons. Finally he was required to identify the photograph of a Siamese cat from photographs of other cats and to sort out 20 Italian coins from 20 foreign coins. On all of these tasks he performed unhesitatingly and correctly. It must be added that on inquiry both the patient and his wife denied that he had ever shown any problem in the identification of personal objects. He easily recognised his car in parking lots.

The evidence provided by this patient is, therefore, not supportive of the thesis that prosopagnosia is but a particular aspect of a more general disorder in evoking the previously learned context of a visual stimulus. The loss of the feeling of familiarity appeared to be confined to faces and this selective impairment suggests that the corresponding memory units have a specific organisation in the nervous system. No definite conclusion can be drawn based on a single case and it is highly desirable that, in the future, patients with prosopagnosia and free from perceptual impairment be carefully investigated for their ability to recognise personal objects.

5. UNILATERAL OR BILATERAL DAMAGE?

There is a substantial body of evidence pointing to the damage of the mesial occipito-temporal region as the anatomical correlate of prosopagnosia, but whether the lesion may be confined to the right hemishere or has to be bilateral remains a matter of debate.

The former thesis (Hécaen & Angelergues, 1962) was mainly advanced on the grounds of the more frequent association of prosopagnosia with left than with right visual field defect (19 versus 4 cases in the review made by Meadows, 1974), but the value of this finding was challenged by a scrutiny of the literature (Lhermitte et al., 1972; Meadows, 1974; Cohn, Neumann & Wood, 1977), which showed that in the few patients who came to autopsy there was invariably bilateral damage. Since the left hemisphere lesion was not consistently localised in the occipito-temporal region, Meadows (1974) left open the possibility that right brain damage alone can produce prosopagnosia, while Damasio et al. (1982) took a stronger stance, claiming that CT scan evidence converge with pathology in showing that bilateral lesions are necessary.

The issue needs further consideration, because there are in the literature six case reports with surgical evidence (Hecaen & Angelergues, 1962; Assal, 1969; Meadows, 1974; Lhermitte & Pillon, 1975; Whitely & Warrington, 1972) and one with CT scan evidence (Whiteley & Warrington, 1972) showing the involvement of the right hemisphere alone. To them I now add two cases. One was the fourth patient of the present series and the other a 72-year-old retired clerk (patient 6), who was admitted to the wards for a stroke dating back to a month earlier which had caused left hemianopia and route finding troubles. He was unable to recognise his relatives and to learn the faces of doctors and nurses. Two months after the stroke, his VIQ was 115, and he scored 0/11 on Street's completion test, 12/36 on Ghent's overlapping figures, 24/33 on figure-ground discrimination and completely failed on the face matching test. Six months after the stroke he no longer had trouble in taking his bearings in the town in which he lived, but still met with difficulty in recognising old friends, when he met them in the street.

The CT scan of these two patients (Figure 1 and 2) showed a softening of the right posterior cerebral artery, without any sign of abnormality in the left hemisphere. The extent of lesion was remarkably similar in both cases

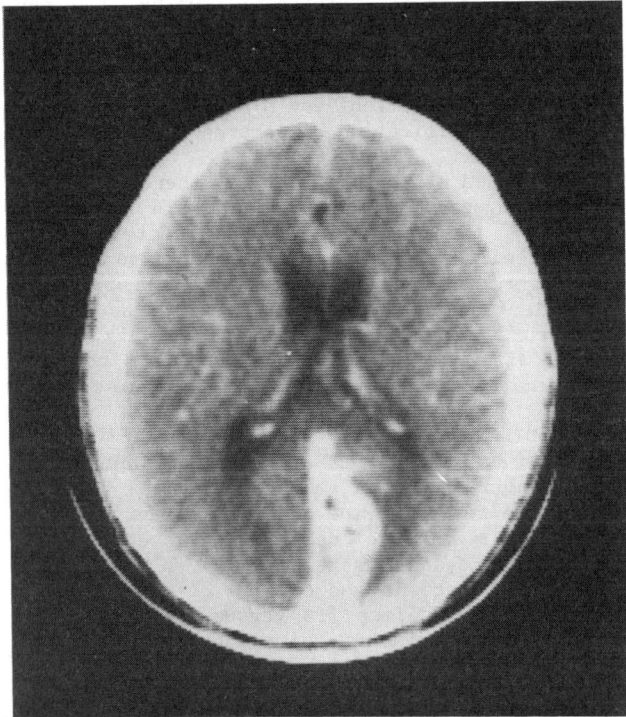

FIGURE 1. CT scan of patient 4.

and encompassed the lingual and fusiform gyri, both lips of the calcarine fissure, the cuneus, the right outflow of the splenium and the parahippocampal gyrus.

Six patients with prosopagnosia and CT scan evidence of damage confined to the right occipito-temporal region have been reported by Landis et al. (in press), three by Torii and Tamai (1985) and a patient with a right posterior haematoma is presented at this symposium by Tiberghien (1985). Thus there are altogether 19 patients, 6 surgically verified and 13 with CT scan documentation who have shown prosopagnosia after a lesion apparently restricted to the right hemisphere and in some of them the symptom has lasted for months. I believe that these data cannot be neglected, although obviously the evidence provided by CT scan is not definitive and the last word must be left to autopsy studies.

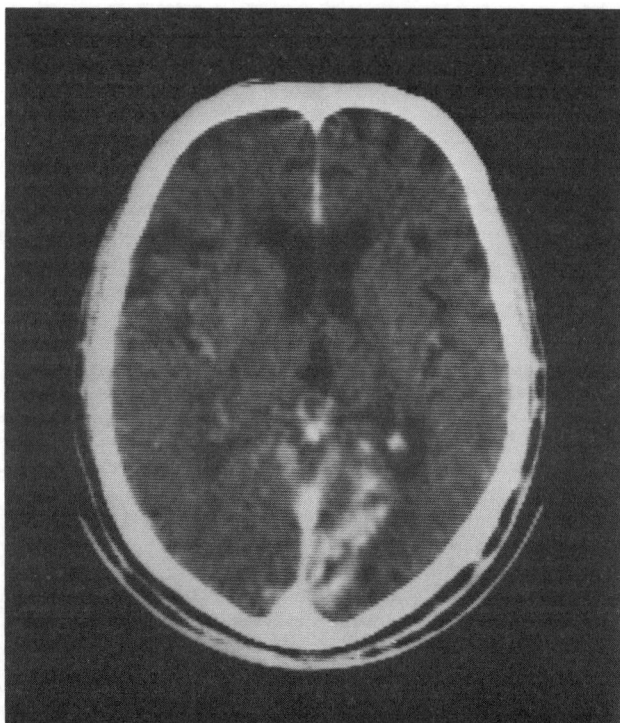

FIGURE 2. CT scan of patient 6

One may ask why prosopagnosia is such a rare symptom, if it can be produced by right temporo-occipital damge. A possibility is suggested by the extension of the lesion which was much larger in our two patients, as compared to that shown by the RBD patients without prosopagnosia reported by

Damasio et al. (1982). The involvement of the entire area of vascularisa-
tion of the right posterior cerebral artery and not simply of its inferior
sector, as it obtains in the majority of softenings, may be the critical
factor in determining prosopagnosia. Alternatively, it may be submitted
that human brains have different degree of hemispheric specialisation and
that only in a few of them the right side has gained a definite ascendancy
in processing faces. CT scan - clinical correlations carried out in a
series of unselected patients with infarcts in the territory of the right
posterior cerebral artery can help settle the issue.

THE COGNITIVE PSYCHOPHYSIOLOGY OF PROSOPAGNOSIA

RUSSELL M. BAUER

1. INTRODUCTION

Prosopagnosia is a rare neurobehavioral syndrome in which a patient with brain damage becomes unable to recognize previously familiar persons by visual reference to their facial features (Bodamer, 1947; Bauer & Rubens, 1985). It is distinct from disorders in the perceptual processing of previously unfamiliar faces (Benton, 1980) and is dissociable from specific impairments in learning new faces seen as part of a more general visual recent memory deficit (Ross, 1980). In many cases, the disorder extends to famous faces and may even prevent identification of the patient's own face in a mirror. Prosopagnosics invariably recognize faces as faces, and are able to achieve immediate and certain recognition when they hear the person's voice or when some informative extrafacial visual cue (clothing, gait, etc.) is available. Prosopagnosia cannot be solely attributed to aphasic misnaming or to perceptual impairment, since tests of language and visual perception are usually performed at normal or near-normal levels (cf. Bauer & Rubens, 1985 for review).

Neuropsychological investigations of prosopagnosia have always been guided by two basic ideas about the nature of visual recognition. First is Lissauer's (1889) classic notion that recognition occurs in two distinct stages, which he labelled "apperception" and "association". By apperception, Lissauer meant the piecing together of sensory impressions into a perceptual whole. By association, he meant the imparting of meaning to the content of perception by matching and linking it to previous experience. Lissauer's view implies that "recognition" occurs only to stimuli that have been consciously perceived and perceptually analyzed. Second is the apparent assumption that overt verbal identification is the single 'best' measure of recognition performance. Clinicians formally test recognition by requiring patients to name the stimulus, point to it when it is named, or to otherwise indicate conscious knowledge of stimulus identity.

The first part of this chapter questions the validity and utility of these assumptions by briefly reviewing evidence that stimulus identification and stimulus recognition are dissociable. Our psychophysiological studies of recognition abilities in prosopagnosia are then described. Our studies readily demonstrate that (1) prosopagnosics who are totally incapable of identifying any faces can reliably discriminate familiar and unfamiliar facial identity at the psychophysiological level; and (2) despite an ability to display differential electrodermal recognition, prosopagnosics consistently show phasic sympathetic hypoarousal to visual stimuli. The degree of hypoarousal is sufficiently profound to suggest pervasive deficits in the systems which support orienting responses and effortful exploration of relevant visual stimuli. After these findings are reviewed, their possible anatomic bases are discussed. These findings, taken together with the results of neuropsychological tests, suggest that prosopagnosia takes place in the context of (1) subtly impaired perception, (2) a failure to access stored memories, and (3) a breakdown in the cognitive system which assigns familiarity to an apprehended face.

2. THE NATURE OF RECOGNITION

Lissauer's distinction between "apperceptive" and "associative" defects of recognition is by far the most widely accepted scheme for classifying the clinical manifestations of visual agnosia. These two entities are defined by the extent to respond to stimuli they claim not to be able to see. Weiskrantz, Warrington, Sanders, & Marshall (1974) reported a patient with hemianopia resulting from the excision of an arteriovenous malformation in striate cortex who could discriminate between "X" and "O", could reach fairly accurately for stimuli, and could differentiate between horizontal, diagonal and vertical lines in the hemianopic field. The term "blindsight" has been applied to this phenomenon.

These data and many more like them cast significant doubt on the validity of the two-stage recognition model. First, there is ample evidence that certain recognition phenomena can take place before (or without) reaching the level of conscious awareness. Since positive evidence of recognition is seen in responses other than the verbal report, questions regarding the exclusive reliance on verbal report are raised. Indeed, I would argue that the classic criteria of recognition in common usage in the clinical evaluation of agnosia are specific measures of identification, not recognition in the sense implied by the above review.

A broader view is to postulate three general sets of performance criteria by which to judge "recognition performances". First is the patient's ability to overtly identify the stimulus. This category subsumes the convential criteria of naming, directed object use, and pointing mentioned above. Second is the presence or absence of responses adequate to the stimulus (e.g., nonverbal or psychophysiological discrimination, spontaneous object use). Exclusive focus on spared and impaired identification abilties in agnosics has left us with little systematic information about abilities in this category. Third is the patient's report of subjective familiarity with the stimulus. Agnosic patients who fail to identify a stimulus may nonetheless feel that they know (or should know) what it is, or more commonly may be unable to generate any familiarity response at all.

The attempt to understand dissociations among these performance criteria has guided our research on prosopagnosia and is the primary reason why we collect psychophysiological indices of recognition performance in addition to the verbal report. In the next section, I describe these studies and their basic results.

3. AUTONOMIC RECOGNITION OF NAMES AND FACES IN PROSOPAGNOSIA

3.1. The Guilty Knowledge Test

Our studies of autonomic recognition in prosopagnosia are based on an applied psychophysiological technique called the "Guilty Knowledge Test" (Lykken, 1959; 1974; 1979) that was originally introduced as a way of detecting in criminal suspects the presence of unreported information about crime details. Such procedures are necessary in situations where, because of the suspect's unwillingness to cooperate, there is reason to doubt the truthfulness or accuracy of the verbal report. The GKT begins with the basic assumption that "a guilty person will show some involuntary psychophysiological response to stimuli related to remembered details of [the] crime" (Lykken, 1959; p. 258). The differential response is based on the presumption that the correct alternative represents a singular piece of 'significant' information among the irrelevant alternatives, and is thus capable of eliciting an orienting response (Barry, 1977; Berlyne, 1960; Bernstein, Taylor, and Weinstein, 1975).

During the procedure, the subject is presented with a series of multiple-choice items, each containing one correct alternative. For example, a suspect in the theft of a camera from a private residence may be questioned regarding the type of camera stolen ("Was it a [a] Nikon, [b] a Minolta, [c] a Kodak, [d] a Pentax, or [e] a Fujica?"), the place from which it was taken ("Was it from [a] a desk drawer, [b] a knapsack, [c] a filing cabinet, [d] a walk-in closet, or [e] a safe"), and other relevant details.

During the administration of the GKT, psychophysiological measures are continuously recorded. Sufficient time is allowed between the presentation of each alternative so that autonomic reactions can independently peak and recover to each. The subject may listen passively to each item, or may be asked to select one of the alternatives after the item has been fully presented. Verbal responses are not required for the successful application of the technique. For each item, the alternative resulting in the largest phasic autonomic response is located. The number of such peak responses to relevant (correct) alternatives is then computed and compared to a binomial distribution which assumes that all alternatives have an equal a priori probability of eliciting a maximal response.

Although the clinical evaluation of patients with prosopagnosia is different in many ways from the criminologic investigation, the clinical analogy to "guilty knowledge detection" is obvious. In both criminologic investigation and agnosia assessment, the examiner's task is to determine what, if any, information the subject has about the relevant stimuli. In the criminologic investigation, the suspect does not cooperate; in agnosia assessment, the patient cannot cooperate in identifying relevant stimuli because of the recognition impairment. In the next section, the specific application of the GKT to the evaluation of two cases of prosopagnosia is described.

3.2. Initial Demonstration of Autonomic Recognition: Patient L.F.

3.2.1. Case Report. This 39-year-old right-handed college graduate has been extensively described in two previous papers (Bauer, 1982; Bauer, 1984). The patient was in good health until he suffered severe head trauma in an motorcycle accident. As a result, he suffered bilateral traumatic hematomas of the occipitotemporal regions and posterior temporal lobes, and was rendered profoundly prosopagnosic. His CT scan, taken five days post-trauma, is presented in Figure 1.

FIGURE 1. CT Scan of Patient L.F.

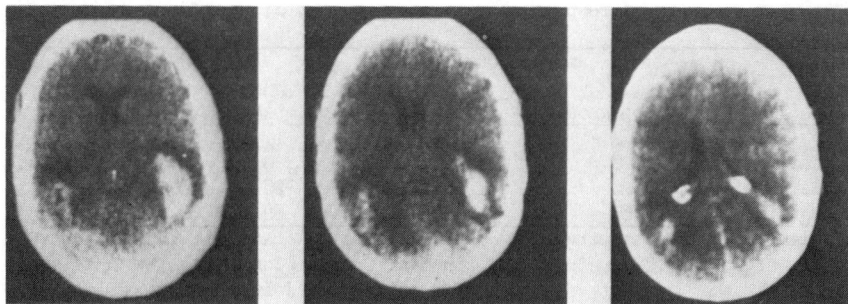

L.F. was completely unable to recognize familiar people, including his own mirror image and pictures of famous personalities. In the five years we have known him, he has never identified a face correctly, except in two rare instances where correct identification was based on the verbal retrieval of a distinctive facial feature. Even then, his identification was made without any degree of rated familiarity. His face agnosia existed despite normal performance on tests of facial matching (Benton Facial Recognition Test; Benton, et al., 1983), and took place in the context of extremely poor recent memory for faces and other visually-presented stimuli. Auditory-verbal memory was relatively intact. Visuoperceptual and visuoconstructive tests revealed mild impairments which worsened with increasing visual or visuomotor complexity. Bilateral dyschromatopsia was observed, affecting visual-visual color tasks (Munsell-Farnsworth 100 Hue Test) but not color naming.

3.2.2. Method and Results. Two sets of pictorial stimuli were used in the modified GKT. The first set contained ten photographs of famous actors, athletes, and world leaders well known to the patient. The second set consisted of eight members of the patient's family. All pictures were face-front photos masked with an oval template to include only the head area. During the GKT, each face was presented in central vision accompanied by five multiple choices of the correct name. The position of the correct name was varied randomly within and across items except that it never appeared as the first alternative in any item. The first alternative was presented solely to control for initial startle (Graham, 1973) and was not included in statistical analysis. Names were read at 15-second intervals in a neutral voice. Skin conductance (SC) and respiration rate/depth were continuously recorded, the latter serving as an artifact control (Stern & Anschel, 1968). SC was sampled for the 7 seconds preceding name onset (tonic period) and the 7 seconds following name offset (phasic period), and was measured using Ag/AgCl electrodes attached to the thenar and hypothenar eminences of the nondominant palm. A skin conductance response (SCR) was defined as any phasic change in SC greater than .02 micromho occurring in the first 1-5 seconds of the phasic period. SCR magnitude was calculated as the change in peak-to-peak conductance from the tonic to the phasic period.

On each trial, three dependent measures were recorded: (1) naming of the facial identity prior to the presentation of multiple choice alternatives (spontaneous naming); (2) selection of the correct name after all alternatives had been presented (name selection); and (3) the number of trials on which the maximal SCR occurred to the correct name (SCR recognition). Results were summed across trials and are expressed as percentage correct responses in Table 1.

TABLE 1. Percent correct responses by L.F. and controls

	Famous Faces		Family Faces	
	Prosopagnosic	Controls	Prosopagnosic	Controls
Spont. Naming	0	90	0	0
Name Selection	20	100[a]	25[b]	12.5[b,c]
SCR Recognition	60[d]	80[a,d]	62.5[e]	37.5[c,e]

Pairs with the same superscript (a,b,c,d, or e) are not significantly different at p < .05 using the binomial test. Controls are two males matched with the patient for age, education, and intellectual ability. Neither had any history of neurologic disease.

L.F. could not spontaneously name any of the famous faces, and could select only 2 of 10 correct names by multiple choice. However, he displayed SCR recognition of 60% of the correct names. On 4 trials, the patient showed correct SCR recognition in the absence of name selection. Normal controls showed the expected higher rates of spontaneous naming, name selection, and SCR recognition.

Since the family pictures were unknown to controls, we expected that they would show no spontaneous naming accuracy and chance levels of name selection and SCR recognition. Results supported these predictions. In contrast, the prosopagnosic again showed substantially higher SCR recognition than spontaneous naming (p < .01) or name selection (p < .01). L.F.'s SCR recognition accuracy can best be seen by summing across famous and family faces. He was only 22% (4/18) correct in verbally selecting the correct name, but correct SCR recognition occurred 61% (11/18) of the time. SCR recognition is three times as accurate as name selection in determining the correct identity of famous faces, and 2.5 times as accurate as name selection in detecting the correct identity of family faces.

3.3. Case P.K.

3.3.1. Case Report. This 59-year-old divorced supply technician was in good health until two weeks prior to her clinic visit when she suffered sudden severe headache, diplopia, and acute loss of vision on the left. She was admitted to a local hospital where CT scan (Figure 2) revealed bilateral occipitotemporal infarcts and an angiogram showed 50% stenosis of the left vertebral artery.

FIGURE 2. CT Scan of Patient P.K.

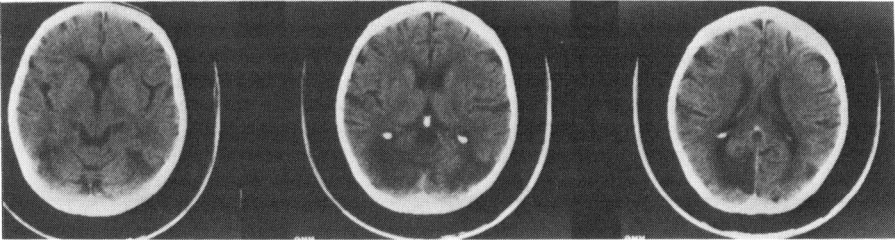

Admitting neurological examination revealed normal motor, sensory, and cranial nerve functions with no cerebellar signs or pathological reflexes. Mental status exam was normal except that she remembered only 1 of 3 items at five minutes, and was unable to distinguish colors, particularly in the upper quadrants. She could not recognize the consulting physicians upon their return for follow-up evaluation, nor was she able to learn the faces of the attending physicians and nurses who attended her daily throughout her hospital stay. Ophthalmological exam revealed corrected visual acuities of 20/40 OS and 20/70 OD. Pupils were 3.5 mm bilaterally with a 3+ reaction to light. Confrontation visual fields revealed left homonymous hemianopia, and formal perimetry revealed additional partial right upper quadrantanopsia.

Neuropsychological exam revealed a dextral, high-school-educated female with a Verbal IQ of 103 on the Wechsler Adult Intelligence Scale and a Wechsler Memory Quotient of 118. Memory testing revealed visual recent memory loss with relatively spared auditory-verbal memory. For example, she recalled 5, 9, 7, 10, and 10 words on five trials of the California Verbal Learning Test (Delis, Kramer, Kaplan, & Ober, 1983), and could to recall 12/16 words with cues both immediately and after a 20-minute delay. Delayed recognition was 15/16. On the Wechsler Memory Scale Logical Memory stories, she was able to recall an average of 10/24 items, which is a normal score for her age. In contrast, visually-presented stimuli (Rey Osterrieth Complex Figure, Wechsler Memory Scale Visual Reproductions, Milner Facial Recognition Test) were poorly recalled immediately and after delays of even a few minutes. She named real objects with hesitation, but was nearly totally incapable of naming line drawings or photographs. Mild spelling alexia was seen. She could not discern action in complex pictures, describing only a portion at a time. She had no gaze paralysis or misreaching for visual targets. She could not name colors, appropriately color line drawings, or sort colors across or within hues (Munsell-Farnsworth 100 Hue Test). She was, however, fully capable of performing "verbal-verbal" tasks of color perception.

She was profoundly prosopagnosic, failing to spontaneously recognize any of 48 famous faces shown to her. Family was unavailable. Despite failure to visually learn any of the faces of her doctors, nurses, or neuropsychology staff, if spoken to she could immediately recognize even those she had only briefly met. She could not reliably make man vs. woman or black vs. white discriminations, but could always recognize a face as a face.

Her descriptions of objects or pictures indicated extremely fragmented vision with serial scanning of details. She performed all visual tasks, not just those including faces, extremely slowly. On the Benton Facial Recognitoin Test (Benton, et al, 1983), she was 80% accurate on trials in which the comparison face was an exact replica of the target (isomorphic trials), but only 20% accurate when the comparison face was presented under different lighting conditions or at different angles than the target (nonisomorphic). Findings suggested an apperceptive defect with some of the behavioral characteristics of "simultaneous agnosia" (Kinsbourne & Warrington, 1962; Luria, 1959; Wolpert, 1924).

3.3.2. Method and Results. P.K.'s electrodermal recognition was tested using 16 facial stimuli from the Albert, Butters, & Levin (1979) Remote Memory Battery. The GKT procedure was identical to that previously described except that, by the time P.K. was tested, the presentation of facial stimuli, multiple choice alternatives, and the collection of psychophysiological data was automated and controlled by an IBM PC/XT microcomputer with an on-board A-D converter. Skin conductance data was sampled at 20Hz during the seven-second tonic and stress periods. Results of the GKT are presented in Table 2.

TABLE 2. Percent correct responses by P.K. and controls

	Famous Faces	
Response Measure	Prosopagnosic	Controls
Spont. Naming	0[a]	98[b]
Name Selection	31[a]	98[b]
SCR Recognition	63[c]	40[c]

Pairs with same superscript are not significantly different at p < .05. Controls were two women matched to the patient on the basis of age and education, neither of whom had a history of neurologic disease.

With famous faces, the patient was unable to verbally identify any of the sixteen faces (controls = 98%, p < .001), and was only 31% accurate on selection from multiple choice (controls 98%, p < .001). However, she showed maximum EDR to the correct name on 63% (10/16) of the trials (controls = 40%). On 6 of these trials, the patient showed maximum EDR to the correct name in spite of the fact that she was unable to select the correct name from multiple choice.

The patient is able to display discriminative electrodermal responses in the absence of verbal identification and multiple choice recognition. This implies that she has premorbidly stored representations of famous faces and is able to activate such representations when the correct name is given. However, such activation is somehow insufficient to result in conscious identification. The internal representation of the face which is covertly activated by this process must be an extremely flexible one, since the particular facial stimuli used in our famous faces test almost surely do not correspond in any formal way with what is stored in memory. This raises a question regarding the patient's poor performance on the Benton Facial Recognition Test. In this task, the patient must match a target face with a comparison face which is presented under different lighting conditions or at different angular orientation. To succeed at this task, the patient must form, and act upon, flexible representations of apprehended faces and must be able to imagine how each target face would appear under nonisomorphic viewing conditions. The patient performed poorly under these conditions, and the question arises whether she could display differential electrodermal recognition of correct target-test matches in the absence of the ability to overtly match such stimuli. We modified the Benton Facial Recognition Task to fit the basic multiple choice paradigm in an effort to answer this question.

Fifteen of the target stimuli from the Benton FRT were selected and individually mounted on 12.7 cm x 7.6 cm cards. For each target, five comparison faces, one of which depicted the target person, were selected (this differs from the standard FRT in which, after Item 5, 3 of 6 comparison faces depict the target person on each trial). On five trials the selected comparison face was an isomorphic representation of the target, and on 10 trials the comparison face depicted the target person under different lighting conditions or angle of view. On each trial, the target face was presented to central vision and remained in view throughout the serial presentation of the five comparison faces, which were presented with an interstimulus interval of 18 + 3" as in the famous faces test. The serial position of the correct comparison face was randomly counterbalanced across trials and never occurred in the first position. Skin conductance was sampled as described above. Once the five faces had all been shown, they were arranged in front of the patient who then pointed to the one which depicted the same person as the target. Results are shown in Table 3.

TABLE 3. Percent correct responses (nonisomorphic trials) on Modified Benton FRT

| Response Measure | Modified FRT | |
	Prosopagnosic	Controls
Spont. Naming	--	--
Correct Match	30[a]	73[b]
EDR Max to Correct Match	30[a]	54[c]

Pairs with same superscript are not significantly different at p < .05.

The patient pointed to the correct comparison face on 80% (4/5) of the isomorphic trials, but on only 30% (3/10) of the nonisomorphic trials (overall = 47% [7/15]), consistent with previous administration of the standard Benton FRT. On this task, no evidence of electrodermal discrimination was found on either isomorphic (20% [1/5]) or nonisomorphic (30% [3/10]) trials. Neither of these values is significantly different from the chance probability (.25) of obtaining a maximum EDR on any given trial.

Despite the fact that the patient showed electrodermal recognition of the correct identity of famous faces, thus implying the existence of flexible internal representations of such faces, she was unable to electrodermally discriminate correct from incorrect target-comparison matches in a task using unfamiliar faces. The modified Benton FRT, like the famous faces task, requires the patient to operate with a flexible representation of an apprehended face in performing a matching task. What distinguishes the two tasks is the fact that the representation involved in the famous faces task is one which was ostensibly formed prior to illness onset, whereas the representation involved in successful completion of the matching-to-sample task requires the patient to form a new representation of a previously unfamiliar face and to match it to a comparison face. We believe that the failure of EDR discrimination on the Modified Benton FRT is a direct result of the fact that the patient has no internal stored representation of the unfamilar faces used in this task. These results suggest that patients with prosopagnosia are able to display evidence of premorbidly stored facial representations, but are unable to form new, stable representations of faces. These data provide initial psychophysiological support in prosopagnosics for the widely-accepted distinction between familiar and unfamiliar facial processing (Benton, 1980).

3.4 Summary of Electrodermal Recognition Studies
    We have also administered the GKT to a prosopagnosic with a severe apperceptive
defect (Case 2 of Ross, 1980).   In addition, Tranel & Damasio (1985) have
demonstrated similar effects using a somewhat different procedure.   Results of all
these patients are summarized in Table 4.
    Patient G.Y. failed to demonstrate electrodermal discriminination of correct
facial identity.   We have attributed this failure to the fact that his ability to
form adequate perceptual images of faces was so disordered that they could not
effectively activate the stored representations on which electrodermal
discriminations are based.   Tranel & Damasio (1985) presented slides of familiar

TABLE 4.   Summary of Patients Tested for Electrodermal Recognition

Patient	Reference	Disorder	EDR Discrimination
L.F.	Bauer, 1984	Prosopagnosia (assoc)	+
P.K.	Bauer & Verfae- llie, in press	Prosopagnosia (mild appcp)	+ (remote) - (recently learned)
G.Y.	Ross, 1980	Visual recent memory loss Prosopagnosia (severe appcp)	-
Case 1	Tranel & Damasio 1985	Prosopagnosia (assoc)	+
Case 2	"	Visual recent memory loss	+ (recently learned)

and unfamiliar faces to a prosopagnosic patient. They found that skin conductance
responses were greater and more frequent to the familiar faces than to the
unfamiliar faces. A second patient became unable to learn new faces after a herpes
simplex encephalitis produced bilateral temporal lobe lesions.   This patient
responded more strongly and frequently to familiar faces first encountered after
the illness. This patient was not tested with faces which were familiar before her
illness since she had no difficulty recognizing previously familiar faces.   Thus
this patient showed electrodermal discrimination of newly learned and novel faces.
Although Tranel & Damasio describe this case as an "anterograde prosopagnosic", she
is more properly understood as having a visual recent memory disorder.
    Based on these five patients, several summary statements can be made.   First,
prosopagnosics with associative defects display electrodermal discrimination of
familiarity despite a total inability to identify any visually presented face.
Second, electrodermal recognition can be prevented by severe apperceptive defects
(Case G.Y.) which impair the processes of perceptual analysis and synthesis of
incoming facial information. We believe that autonomic recognition does not occur
in such patients because of an inability to collect visual information sufficient
to activate the stored internal representation of the face. Third, patient P.K.
illustrates our view that autonomic recognition in prosopagnosia is based on
activation of a premorbidly stored representation; when the patient deals with
unfamiliar or newly-learned faces, no autonomic discrimination takes place, even in
a simple matching-tosample paradigm. On the surface, this appears to conflict with
Tranel & Damasio's Case 2, who showed autonomic discrimination between faces
learned since illness onset and faces never learned. However, the conflicting
findings are more apparent than real, since their Case 2 was not classically
prosopagnosic (i.e., did not have a recognition impairment for previously familiar
faces). The "anterograde" type of autonomic recognition seen in their patient
suggests that electrodermal discrimination of unrecognized material can occur in
amnesia as well as in agnosia, which agrees with data from our own laboratory
(Bauer, et al, in preparation).

3.5 The Anatomy of Spared Recognition

It is now generally agreed that prosopagnosia results from bilateral lesions in the ventromedial aspects of the occipitotemporal gyri (Damasio, Damasio, & Van Hoesen, 1982; Meadows, 1974). These lesions not only the cortex of Areas 18, 19, and 20, but also the white matter connections of this region to temporal lobe (Benson, Segarra, & Albert, 1974). Disconnection models of prosopagnosia propose that the visual system becomes functionally incapable of accessing the memory store, resulting in disruption of the mechanism whereby current facial percepts are associated to facial memories built up from past experience.

FIGURE 3. Proposed anatomy of spared recognition ability (Vis = visual association cortex; A = amygdala; Hy = hypothalamus; STS = superior temporal sulcus; IPL = inferior parietal lobule; CG = cingulate gyrus; Aud = auditory cortex). Stippled area represents typical location of prosopagnosia-inducing lesion.

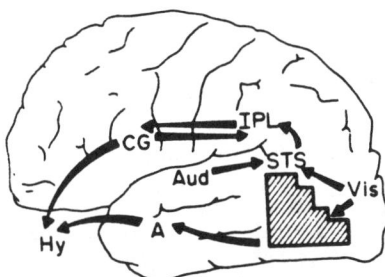

The lesions in prosopagnosia affect a system of visual-limbic connections that has been called the ventral visual-limbic pathway (Bear, 1983). The inferior longitudinal fasciculus, via the temporal lobe, has input into both the basolateral limbic circuit (amygdala, mediodorsal thalamus, orbitofrontal cortex, uncinate fasciculus; Yakovlev, 1948) and the medial limbic circuit of Papez ([1937]; hippocampus, fornix, mammilary bodies, anterior thalamus, cingulate). Data from behavioral, clinical, and psychophysiological studies suggests that the ventral pathway subserves emotional as well as memory and learning functions that are modality-specific to vision (cf. Bauer, 1984).

There is now good evidence for a second visual-limbic connection, referred to as the dorsal visual-limbic pathway (Bear, 1983). This pathway involves projections to the superior temporal sulcus (Jones & Powell, 1970; Mesulam, Van Hoesen, Pandya, & Geschwind, 1977), and thence to the inferior parietal lobule (Mesulam, et al, 1977; Pandya & Kuypers, 1969). The superior temporal sulcus also has strong "sensory" input from superior parietal lobule (somesthesis) and from the supratemporal plane (audition). The first step in this pathway thus involves multimodal convergence. From IPL, there are extensive reciprocal (limbic) connections with the cingulate gyrus and, subsequently, the hypothalamus (Kievit & Kuypers, 1975; Mesulam, et al, 1977). A large body of behavioral and electrophysiological evidence implicates the dorsal pathway and its adjacent regions in complex attentional functions, emotional arousal, and rapid selective orientation to stimuli that have motivational significance (cf. Lynch, 1980 for review; Heilman, Schwartz, & Watson, 1978; Rolls, Perrett, & Thorpe, 1980; Rolls, Perrett, Thorpe, Puerto, Roper-Hall, & Maddison, 1979).

The significance of these two visual-limbic pathways is that the lesions in prosopagnosia selectively impair the ventral visuolimbic route while sparing the dorsal connections (Figure 3). Since the ventral pathway has been implicated in object and face recognition (Mishkin, 1966; Gross, Bender, & Gerstein, 1979; Ungerleider & Mishkin, 1982; Meadows, 1974), lesions of this system are probably responsible for the defect in overt face identification. However, the patient can access limbic system by the dorsal pathway, allowing for differential autonomic reponding to the significant alternative. The anatomic data thus implies that the dorsal system contains a mechanism capable of covertly detecting significance by integrating sensory and limbic input. The important aspect of activity in this region is that such a capability does not appear to be dependent upon conscious identification.

4. AUTONOMIC HYPORESPONSIVITY IN PROSOPAGNOSIA

Up to this point, I have focused on the ability of prosopagnosics to differentially respond to the correct identity of faces within multiple choice paradigms. In this section, I emphasize the fact that, although some prosopagnosics display normal or near normal differential sensitivity to correct facial identity, they do so with extremely reduced absolute response levels. This was originally discovered when L.F. spontaneously reported that he was no longer able to become emotionally aroused by visual stimuli. He stated that natural scenery appeared dull, that he was no longer interested in looking at pretty girls, and that he had become unable to effectively judge aesthetic aspects of buildings which was previously important to him in his work as a city planner. The reduction in felt arousal appeared to be limited to vision, since he reported normal subjective reactions to music and tactile stimulation.

Prosopagnosia has been associated with bilateral damage involving the inferior longitudinal fasciculus (ILF), and may disconnect peristriate cortex from the temporal lobe. Because the ILF terminates on those areas of the temporal lobe (primarily area TE, comprising middle and inferior temporal gyri) that subsequently project to limbic system, defects in visually evoked autonomic arousal, and associated defects in emotional responsivity, are not entirely unexpected as 'neighborhood signs' of prosopagnosia. Furthermore, hyporeactivity to visual stimuli has been seen in monkeys with either bilateral ablations of basolateral temporal lobe (Kluver & Bucy, 1937) or complete visual-temporal disconnection syndromes (Horel & Keating, 1972). This latter procedure leaves the intact temporal lobe without visual input. Horel & Keating have noted that, after such ablations, the monkey displays profound hyporeactivity to visual stimuli (e.g., toy snakes, gloved hands) that had previously elicited fear and avoidance reactions.

Based on these considerations, we decided to explore L.F.'s psychophysiological reactions to emotional and nonemotional stimuli presented in either the auditory or the visual modality (Bauer, 1982). In the visual modality, the patient was presented color pictures of nudes and landscape scenes. In the auditory modality, he was asked to listen to familiar sounds (e.g., telephone ringing, typewriter), brief news stories, musical passages, and sexual narratives. Skin conductance and respiration rate/depth were recorded during the 10 seconds before stimulus presentation (tonic) and the 10 seconds after stimulus presentation (stress).

The patient shows significantly greater response to auditory than to visual stimuli, an effect which is not shown by normal controls. Within the visual modality, he showed negligible differences in responsivity between landscapes and nudes, while the controls respond significantly more strongly to nudes.

The patient's responses to nudes are significantly smaller than those of normal controls. Although not particularly germane to this discussion, it should also be noted that the patient's responses to auditory stimuli are in fact greater than those of normals. It is if he compensates for hyporeactivity in the visual modality by hyperresponsivity in the auditory domain. In describing their monkeys with visual-temporal disconnections, Horel & Keating (1972) describe the tendency which perceptual disorder is responsible for the failure to recognize. The patient with apperceptive agnosia has defects in the perceptual analysis and synthesis of information which are sufficiently severe to account for the failure to recognize. Patients with associative agnosia have no such defects, and allegedly form relatively normal percepts which have been "somehow stripped of their meaning" (Teuber, 1968). This dichotomy can descriptively accomodate nearly all reported cases of prosopagnosia. For example, several cases (Gloning, et al., 1970; Macrae & Trolle, 1956; Nardelli, Buonanno, & Coccia, 1982 [Case 2]) had severe apperceptive impairments while others (Bauer & Trobe, 1984; Benton & Van Allen, 1972; Pallis, 1955) had clear associative defects. While useful descriptively, however, the simple two-stage model (with its assumption that identification follows conscious perception) is inconsistent with an extensive amount of recent cognitive and neuropsychological data.

The literature on "unconscious" recognition processes stimulated by the "perceptual defense" movement (Erdelyi, 1974) has shown that covert discrimination can occur in the absence of overt identification of the stimulus. The phenomenon has been variously named "subception" (Lazarus & McCleary, 1951), "subliminal perception" (Adams, 1957), or "preconscious recognition". In their study of subception, Lazarus & McCleary trained subjects to discriminate shock-associated from non-shock stimuli in an autonomic conditioning paradigm. In a subsequent recognition test in which stimuli were presented at exposure durations below absolute threshold, subjects displayed discriminative autonomic responses even though the stimuli on which such responses were based could not be identified.

The work of Zajonc and colleagues (Kunst-Wilson & Zajonc, 1980; Moreland & Zajonc, 1979; Zajonc, 1980) on the "exposure effect" provide more contemporary support for this phenomenon. These researchers have demonstrated that subjects prefer previously presented stimuli to novel ones, and that this effect does not depend upon conscious identification of the stimulus. For example, Kunst-Wilson & Zajonc repeatedly presented geometric shapes at an exposure duration of 1 msec, too brief to allow for conscious identification. Each stimulus was then paired with a novel (foil) stimulus and presented for forced choice recognition. Subjects were asked (1) to choose which had been previously presented and (2) to indicate which of the two they preferred. Results showed that only 48% of the target stimuli were correctly identified. Only 21% of the subjects correctly classified targets and foils at a better than chance level. Despite this, 67% of subjects preferred targets over the foils.

Similar effects have been found in lexical priming experiments. When word stimuli are preceded ('primed') by semantically related words that are masked and presented too briefly to reach conscious awareness, the undetected primes still facilitate the processing of succeeding stimuli (Fowler, Wolford, Slade, & Tassinary, 1981). Similarly, in several dichotic listening studies (Allport, Antonis, & Reynolds, 1972; Kellogg, 1980; Rollins & Thibadeau, 1973), subjects who are asked to shadow one channel while stimuli are presented to the unattended ear can reliably discriminate unattended information despite their inability to verbally identify it. Corteen & Wood (1972) found that the occurrence of an emotional word in an unattended channel produced significant electrodermal reactions in some subjects even though they failed to identify the critical word as such.

These findings derive from diverse experiments, and involve reactions to a broad range of stimuli and tasks. One common thread, however, is that dissociations can exist between processes which lead to overt stimulus identification and those which lead to "unconscious" discrimination of targets from distractors or other performance effects (Jacoby & Dallas, 1981). Similar dissociations can be observed in the clinical symptoms of agnosia. For example, it is not uncommon for an agnosic who is unable to identify a common stimulus (coffee cup, cigarettes) when asked to name it, to be able to use the stimulus normally when formal testing is over. It is even possible for patients to appropriately

FIGURE 4. Electrodermal Hyporesponsivity to Visual Stimuli -- Patient L.F.

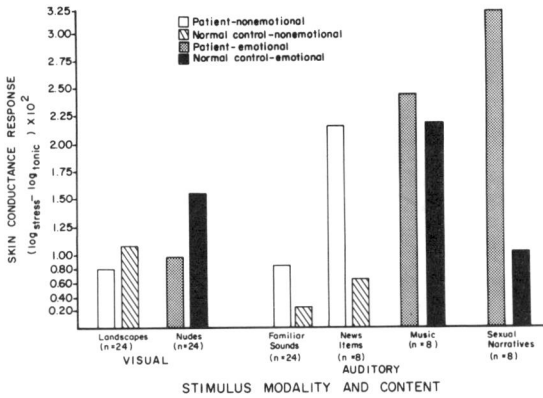

for these animals to utilize other sensory modalities in a compensatory way to achieve recognition: "It was as though all emotional reactions were available to the animal, but visual cues could not elicit them until they had been identified by another modality. Once they had been identified, usually be smelling, the animal would react appropriately to that visual cue" (p.110). Without exception, the prosopagnosics we have tested have all been autonomically hyporesponsive during the GKT as well. As an example, P.K.'s absolute responses to correct and foil alternatives are presented in Table 5 along with the responses of controls.

TABLE 5. Absolute skin conductance responses during GKT

	Prosopagnosic (P.K.)	Control
Correct Alternatives	.101 mmho[a]	.206 mmho[b]
Distractors	.043 mmho[c]	.160 mmho[b]

Entries superscripted by the same symbol are not significantly different at p < .05

Inspection of Table 5 reveals that P.K.'s responses are significantly smaller than are the responses of the controls regardless of whether targets or distractors are being viewed. Autonomic recognition as described in the previous section is based on within-subject comparisons, while the hypoarousal that is the subject of this discussion is based on between subject comparisons. On every such comparison, P.K.'s responses were significantly smaller than those of controls. The same pattern of responses was observed in the GKT data of L.F.; patient G.Y. showed the effect so strongly that he was unresponsive (SCR < .02 micromho) on the vast majority of trials.

5. THE COGNITIVE PSYCHOPHYSIOLOGY OF PROSOPAGNOSIA

The psychophysiological data, along with the wealth of behavioral data available from case reports of prosopagnosia, raise important issues that bear on our understanding of the cognitive state of prosopagnosic patients. In this section I want to discuss three of these issues and to speculate on related matters. First, I will describe an information-processing approach to the autonomic recognition data which can account not only for the spared orienting behavior of prosopagnosics, but also for the occasional finding (in normals) that identification can take place without differential autonomic responding. Second, I will suggest that the reduced overall magnitude of autonomic responding in prosopagnosia not only reflects the outcome of perceptual and cognitive analyses of stimuli, but also may actually support the recognition defect. Third I want to briefly discuss how two other aspects of prosopagnosic behavior (the extremely slow perceptual processing and the total lack of subjective familiarity with viewed faces) might relate to the psychophysiological findings discussed earlier.

5.1. An Information Processing Approach to Orienting in Prosopagnosia

Our anatomic model of spared autonomic recognition (Section 3.5) posits a "significance detector" involving the dorsal visual-limbic pathway which is capable of activating a stored representation of previous experience with a face. The notion that orienting occurs to "significance" and not just "novelty" (as implied in Sokolov's [1963] model) is consistent with recent models of the OR (Bernstein, 1973, 1979; Maltzman, 1977). The GKT is based on the assumption that differential autonomic response results from the increased "signal value" (Berlyne, 1960) of the correct (significant) alternative relative to the others. This amounts to a simple "memory" interpretation as far as prosopagnosia is concerned, since the signal value of the correct name derives from the specific presence in memory of a stored representation. This view also predicts that every time the correct name occurs during the GKT, an orienting response will occur.

We encountered a problem with this last prediction very early in our work with L.F. when it became apparent that normals could verbally choose the correct name without displaying differential autonomic responses to it. The tendency for this to occur was strongly related to the certainty with which the subject chose the correct name. That is, strong orienting took place only under joint conditions of "significance" and "uncertainty". In order to understand this, we sought guidance from models of the OR which explicitly contain information-processing concepts.

Ohman's (1979) model of the orienting response suggests that the autonomic concomitants of the OR initiate cognitive processing (and active memory search) in a central, limited capacity information processing channel. This channel, the activation of which requires cognitive effort (Kahneman, 1973), is identified with focal attention. It carries out flexible and subject-controlled processing of incoming sensory stimuli. According to Ohman's model, there are two conditions under which calls to this channel will be made. First, if a perceived stimulus arrives for which no matching representation exists in short-term memory, it will be encoded and admitted to the central channel for further processing. Second, when a "significant" stimulus arrives, it is admitted to the central channel for full analysis. According to Ohman, different autonomic responses may reflect different aspects of this process. Electrodermal responses in particular may be associated with the call for central processing, but because the EDR is also highly sensitive to cognitive effort, it may additionally be affected by processing in the central channel itself. That is, EDR may reflect "not only the call, but also part of the answer to the call" (Ohman, 1979, p. 454).

These notions may help explain not only the differential autonomic responses of prosopagnosics, but also the ability of normals to identify faces without evoking the visceroautonomic components of orienting. We believe that normals may frequently achieve overt recognition of famous faces in an effortless, automatic fashion (see Hay & Young, this volume). They seem to easily retrieve the name of the famous face they are viewing, and in most cases need not even actively attend to the multiple choice names in the GKT to achieve positive and certain identification. That is, they do not need to activate the central channel to succeed in face recognition.

Prosopagnosics, on the other hand are never successful in overtly finding a matching representation of the face because the anatomic location of their lesions prevents memory access. However, their spared differential orienting suggests that they retain certain rudimentary elements of information processing which normally lead to memory retrieval and stimulus identification. Put another way, the spared autonomic recognition may reflect the beginning aspects of the "call" for central processing, while the grossly reduced response magnitudes may mean that the call is not answered completely and that the stimulus is not extensively processed.

One important aspect of this discussion is that the rudimentary orienting responses of prosopagnosics in the GKT are not seen as simple reactions to stimuli; instead they represent the beginning activity of early perceptual and cognitive processes. The role such attenuated responses may play in supporting the overt recognition defect is discussed in the next section.

5.2. Hypoarousal and its Relationship to the Recognition Defect

A major question raised by our data is why, in the face of adequate autonomic discrimination, prosopagnosics cannot achieve correct recognition. Their defect of recognition is not just relative (as is the memory loss in amnesia, for example); it is absolute. Is it possible that the defect of function in prosopagnosia is somehow not only indexed by reduced autonomic responsiveness, but also supported by it? Several recent lines of evidence suggest that autonomic arousal can serve as a secondary signal supporting cognitive appraisal of sensory stimuli (Mandler, 1975). A simple study illustrates this point. Olivos (1967) presented voice stimuli to subjects and asked them to judge whether each voice was their own or another person's while simultaneously recording psychophysiological reactions. He demonstrated significant improvement in recognition accuracy simply by waiting for psychophysiological reactions to peak before asking for recognition judgements. He suggests that these findings indicate that two kinds of reactions are involved in such recognition experiments -- one a reaction to the stimulus, the other a reaction to the subject's awareness of stimulus identity. He states that "the perceptual experience is probably the result of a complicated interaction of these two responses involving reciprocal feedback of autonomic and cognitive information". The reduced magnitude of responding in prosopagnosia makes it virtually impossible for these patients to generate appropriate internal responses needed to assist their faulty perceptual systems in achieving positive recognition. That is, part of the prosopagnosic defect is that the amount of autonomic feedback is greatly reduced, and thus the awareness and appreciation of stimulus identity suffers. This problem may contribute to the underspecification of stimulus detail that some (e.g., Shuttleworth, et al, 1982) consider an important part of the prosopagnosic defect.

5.3. The Metacognitive State of Prosopagnosia

Up to this point, I have focused on the electrodermal recognition phenomenon and have offered suggestions regarding its anatomy and its potential importance for understanding the functional defect(s) underlying prosopagnosia. In this section, I want to suggest that the disabilities prosopagnosics encounter in the perceptual, memory, and emotional domains may contribute to a "metacognitive" state which itself is not conducive to effortful processing of faces.

Although prosopagnosia frequently exists in the context of normal achievement on perceptual tasks, it is obvious to most clinicians who deal with these patients that, in a qualitative sense, they do not perform perceptual tasks in a normal fashion. Without significant exception, prosopagnosics process faces and other visual stimuli in an extremely slow, piecemeal fashion. For example, while normals perform facial matching-to-sample tasks extremely rapidly, prosopagnosics compare faces feature-by-feature, and appear not to appreciate faces as integrated stimuli. Tasks that take normals seconds to perform may be completed, sometimes correctly, by prosopagnosics in several minutes. They may succeed in perceptually analyzing a face, but only after several minutes of tedious, step-by-step analysis of constituent features.

Associated with this 'piecemeal perception', and perhaps a result of it, is a total inability to achieve any familiarity with viewed faces. In our experience with prosopagnosic patients, we have never seen a face identified with even a hint of familiarity. Even in situations in which the patient is able to select the correct name from a multiple choice array (usually assisted by a process of elimination), such choices are made with no confidence. This feature of prosopagnosia stands in stark contrast to what occurs, for example, when a profoundly amnestic patient is asked to pick out a target word or face in a recognition paradigm. Sometimes they will do so with reduced confidence, but at other times, they will be fully confident of their (erroneous) choices. Thus, prosopagnosia involves a dissociation between processes whereby faces are perceptually apprehended and the process by which familiarity is assigned to the visual percept.

These two factors: tedious, piecemeal perception and a total absence of familiarity attribution, may eventually wear on the prosopagnosic, who may learn that regardless of how long and hard faces are studied, they do not become any more familiar. Thus, prosopagnosics may, in fact, learn to withhold concentrated effort on perceptual tasks because of its low yield. We need to better understand these "subject-based" processes and their potential relationship to hypoarousal in these patients. We do know, for example, that elicited arousal is reduced under situations of low effort or cognitive demand. The question remains, however, just how much of the hypoarousal seen in prosopagnosia results from the defect in visual-limbic 'hardware', and how much is related to a secondary reduction in effort that takes place as the prosopagnosic continues to experience chronic failure in the process of face identification.

6. SUMMARY

Prosopagnosics can electrodermally discriminate correct facial identity despite a complete inability to verbally identify any face in laboratory or everyday tasks of face recognition. This provides evidence that agnosia is not an all or none defect, and shows that prosopagnosia conforms to the now widely accepted distinction between knowledge and awareness of knowledge. Anatomically, autonomic recognition may be mediated by the dorsal visual-limbic pathway, while disruption of the ventral visual-limbic pathway precludes overt identification of the face. The spared electrodermal discrimination capacity is best viewed as orienting toward a significant piece of information in an otherwise insignificant context. Even though the ability to differentially respond is spared, the absolute magnitude of their electrodermal responses is significantly reduced relative to normal controls. The extremely small magnitudes of elicited electrodermal response need to be better understood anatomically, though psychological notions of reduced cognitive effort, and failure to fully process the facial gestalt (perceptual underspecification) may be useful in understanding the metacognitive state of prosopagnosia and its relationship to the psychophysiology of the disorder.

7. ACKNOWLEDGEMENTS

Preparation of this chapter was supported in part by funds from the Division of Sponsored Research, University of Florida, and by NIAAA Grant AA-06203 to the University of Florida. I want to especially thank Sharilyn Rediess, Mieke Verfaellie, and Philip Hanger for their contributions.

PROSOPAGNOSIA : ANATOMIC AND PHYSIOLOGIC ASPECTS

R. DAMASIO, H. DAMASIO, D. TRANEL

1. ANATOMICAL BASIS

The early descriptions of prosopagnosia indicated that the condition was associated with bilateral damage to the occipital lobes. In the 1960's when fresh neuropsychological investigations revealed the major role of right hemisphere in visual processing, it appeared reasonable to assume that the right hemisphere might possess the key to facial recognition (Meadows, 1974). Hecaen and Angelergues (1962) added strength to this hypothesis by noting that most prosopagnosic patients had left visual field defects, and suggesting that this was due to exclusive right hemisphere damage. The current view, however, is that bilateral lesions are generally necessary, although it would be unwise to rule out exceptions. This notion is based on: (1) critical review of the meaning of visual field data; (2) reassessment of post-mortem studies of prosopagnosic patients; (3) Computed Tomography (CT), Nuclear Magnetic Resonance (NMR) and Emission Tomography (ET) studies of patients with and without prosopagnosia; (4) study of patients with cerebral hemispherectomy, callosal surgery and amnesic syndromes. The fundamental evidence is as follows:

1.1.

The one patient of Hecaen and Angelergues to come to post-mortem, turned out to have a bilateral lesion. The lesion in the left hemisphere was "silent" as far as visual field findings were concerned. Similar "silent" lesions were uncovered at autopsy in patients described by Benson and by Lhermitte (Benson et al., 1974; Lhermitte et al., 1972). It is now apparent that when lesions of the central visual system fail to involve optic radiations or primary visual cortex they do not produce an overt defect or form vision even when they can cause major disturbances of complex visual processing such as a defect in recognition or color processing. While the presence of a field defect correctly indicates the presence of a lesion, its absence does not exclude focal damage. Thus while the detailed study of field defects is mandatory for the appropriate study of visual agnosia, its details can not be used for the prediction of lesion localization.

1.2.

Analysis of the post-mortem records of all patients that have come to autopsy indicate that all have bilateral lesions (see Damasio et al., 1982 and additional work of Nardelli et al., 1982). Considering the rarity of prosopagnosia it is indeed astonishing that there are 12 post-mortem cases available, spanning almost one century, and that one hundred per cent of those showed bilateral damage. The likelihood of this being a chance effect is negligible and it surely indicates that although prosopagnosia may be possible with unilateral lesions, the incidence of such cases must be small.

Those bilateral lesions preferably involve the inferior visual association cortices, i.e., the occipito-temporal region. Patients with bilateral lesions involving the superior visual association cortices, i.e., the occipito-parietal region, never develop prosopagnosia, presenting instead either a full Balint syndrome or some of its components, i.e., visual disorientation, optic ataxia or ocular apraxia. Patients with Balint syndrome can recognize faces provided their attention is properly directed to the stimuli.

1.3.

Computed Tomography (CT) has permitted the study of many cases of prosopagnosia and of numerous controls with unilateral lesions of the left or right occipito-temporal region, or with bilateral lesions of the occipito-parietal region. All cases studied in our laboratory have shown bilateral lesions (Damasio, 1985). Furthermore, numerous instances of unilateral lesion in the right and left hemispheres have been described and there has been no report of prosopagnosia appearing in those circumstances. We have heard of reports of prosopagnosia cases with unilateral lesions. We are ready to believe that they are possible. But it is important (1) to ascertain that such patients are indeed prosopagnosic (and not just partially impaired in facial recognition, or visually disoriented), (2) to verify the permanence of their prosopagnosia over time, with objective testing, and (3) to judge the appropriateness of clinical observation and CT or NMR technique. We have had the opportunity to study cases of alleged prosopagnosia in which one or all of the above criteria were violated.

Patients with bilateral occipito-parietal lesions consistently show Balint syndrome or its components but not prosopagnosia (Damasio, 1985). In the only two cases studied with nuclear magnetic resonance (NMR) the lesions were bilateral. In the only two cases studied with Single Photon Emission Tomography there were bilateral regions (our lab in both instances).

1.4.

Evidence from hemispherectomy and from cases of surgical callosal section has also been helpful. Patients with right hemispherectomy maintain their ability to recognize faces with their single left hemisphere (Damasio et al., 1975). The split-brain subjects continue to recognize faces with each isolated hemisphere although, as expected, the mechanisms of recognition appear to be different on the left and on the right (Levy et al., 1972; Gazzaniga & Smylie, 1983; Sergent & Bindra, 1981).

Other evidence for the bilaterality of damage in prosopagnosia comes from the analysis of patients with amnesic syndromes. Patients with global amnesic syndromes associated with temporal lobe damage have prosopagnosia as a symptom component (see Damasio et al., 1985). All have bilateral lesions. The finding simply underscores the fact that memory processing of the type involved in facial recognition is of crucial importance for the individual and is clearly operated by both hemispheres. This is not to say that the left and right hemispheres perform the task with the same mechanism or equally well. On the contrary, we believe each hemisphere learns, recognizes and recalls faces with different strategies and that the right hemisphere's approach is bound to be more efficient than that of the left.

Finally, we would like to point out that the report of exceptional cases with unilateral lesions of either hemisphere does not deny the fundamental bilaterality of facial recognition. To do so would be equivalent to denying the pervasive left hemisphere dominance for language just because there are some patients who develop crossed aphasia with lesions of the right.

2. THE NATURE OF THE DEFECT

There is substantial evidence against the notion that prosopagnosia is due to a primary perceptual disturbance (see Benton, 1980; Damasia et al., 1982; Damasia, 1985, cited above). Firstly, prosopagnosic patients can discriminate unfamiliar faces well. Some of these patients perform normally in Benton and Van Allen's test of facial discrimination, a difficult task in which they are called to match unfamiliar and differently lit photographs of faces but obviously not asked to recognize any of them; they can perform complex visual tasks such as the anomalous contours test and they have normal stereopsis; they can draw accurately complex figures shown in photographs, drawings or in real models; more importantly, they can recognize, at a generic level, any visual stimulus provided that no contextual memory cues are required. Secondly, severe disorders of visual perception such as seen in patients with Balint syndrome or comparable disorders, do not cause prosopagnosia. Patients with prosopagnosia can perceive and recognize accurately, many stimuli that are visually more complex than human faces, i.e., that have a greater number of individual components arranged in just as complicated a manner but crowded in smaller areas or volumes. On the other hand, there is evidence that the particular class of visual stimuli, as well as the ability to integrate facial percepts with pertinent past experience, are important factors in the physiopathology of prosopagnosia. The evidence is as follows.

Prosopagnosia does not occur in relation to human faces alone. All of the patients with prosopagnosia have defects of recognition for other stimuli. The types of stimuli for which they have agnosia, however, is rather special. They include: (a) automobiles (prosopagnosics can not recognize their own car and do not recognize different makes of cars; these patients can recognize different _types_ of car, such as a passenger car, a fire engine, an ambulance, or a funeral car); (b) clothes of the same type and general shape, i.e., dresses, suits, shirts etc.; (c) specific animals within a group (a farmer suddenly became unable to recognize, within a herd, specific animals that he could easily recognize before; birdwatchers have become unable to recognize different birds, etc.). In all of these instances, the process of recognition operates normally up to the point in which specific recognition of a given member within the group is required. In other words, all of these patients can recognize an automobile as an automobile, a cow as a cow, or a dress as a dress. They can also recognize all of the subcomponents of these stimuli correctly, i.e., eyes, noses, windshields, wheels, sleeves, etc. But when, as is the case with human faces, the patient is requested to identify precisely the specific possessor of that visual appearance, the process breaks down and the within-class-membership of the stimulus cannot be ascertained. The only exceptions to this rule appear to be for small objects that have been learned by tactile manipulation as well as sight, and even so the exception is not complete, e.g. prosopagnosics have difficulty with the recognition of some foodstuffs.

An analysis of the shared characteristics of the stimuli which can cause prosopagnosia reveals that: (a) these are stimuli for which a specific recognition is mandatory and for which a generic recognition is either socially unacceptable (human faces), or incompatible with normal activity (cars, clothing); (b) the specific recognition of all of the stimuli depends on contextual (episodic) memory, i.e, it depends on the evocation of multiple traces of memory previously associated with the currently perceived stimulus; those traces depend on a personal, temporally and spatially bound, memory process; (c) that all of the stimuli belong to groups, classes in which numerous members are physically _similar_ (in visual terms), and yet individually _different_; we have designated these stimuli as visually "ambiguous" (an operational definition of visual ambiguity is the presence in a group of numerous different members with similar visual characteristics). Prosopagnosic patients have no difficulty with the correct, individual recognition of "non-ambiguous" stimuli, i.e., visual stimuli that belong to groups with numerous members but in which different individual members have a different (distinctive) visual structure.

According to the analysis above, the basic perceptual mechanisms in prosopagnosic patients are normal. That is the only way of explaining the largely normal way in which patients recognize most stimuli in their environment. When patients are called on to recognize stimuli that belong to visually ambiguous classes, they fail to evoke the pertinent, associated traces of contextual memory on the basis of which familiarity and recognition of the stimulus would be based. Seen in this light, the defect must be described, physiopathologically, as a disorder of visually-triggered contextual memory. It is important to distinguish this from a disorder of memory in general (memory traces can be normally activated through other sensory channels) and even from a disorder of visual memory (auditory stimulation can bring forward numerous traces of visual memory testifying to the intactness of many visual memory stores). The malfunction is in the triggering system for the associated evocations. We believe this defect can be explained by one of three possible mechanisms: (1) a defect in the highest level of visual analysis, that which permits the distinction of finest structural details, (for instance, texture), necessary for the separation of visually "ambiguous" stimuli but not necessary for visually unambiguous ones; (2) a defect of the plotting of the ongoing percept into the preexisting, templated information, acquired for each specific stimulus (this mechanism would assume the normalcy of the perceptual step referred to above); (3) a defect in the activation of pertinent associated memories occurring after both steps above operate normally. Current research in our laboratory is aimed at investigating the validity of these possible mechanisms.

3. AUTONOMIC EVIDENCE FOR NONCONSCIOUS RECOGNITION

One of the intriguing problems posed by visual agnosia and, more generally, by amnesia has to do with the level at which the failure of recognition occurs. Some investigators have hypothesized that the failure to evoke both non-verbal and verbal memories capable of generating recognition, does not preclude some process of recognition at a lower, non-conscious level of processing. In other words, it is possible that some part of the brain does recognize stimulus even if the subject is not aware of that process taking place. Patients with prosopagnosia are ideal subjects to test this hypothesis and that is what has recently been accomplished using paradigms aimed at detecting autonomic responses to stimuli that patients clearly are not aware of recognizing. In both available studies, by Bauer and by ourselves, there is persuading evidence that at a nonconscious level, faces of relatives, friends, and self, generated strong psychophysiological responses clearly different from the weak or nonexistent resposes to faces unfamiliar to the subject (Bauer, 1984; Tranel & Damasio, 1985). Of course it might be argued, on the basis of the Bauer study, that the role of pure visual information was not established, because the patient also received verbal stimulation. But in our study we used a different paradigm from Bauer's. Our two patients viewed both unfamiliar faces and randomly interspersed faces of relatives but no verbal information was given, i.e. the electrodermal responses were related to visual information alone, while in Bauer's study the subject was given both faces and possible names of the depicted persons. This means that the cognitive processing of our subjects matched more closely the natural process of facial recognition. The magnitude of the responses was even higher than that reported by Bauer; the result obtained both for faces learned prior to illness and for faces that the patients came into contact with after the illness. The implications of this discovery are far-reaching. The findings support the notion that perception and recognition processes evolve by steps and that failure at the top of the cascade does not necessarily imply failure at more elementary levels. On the issue of facial recognition itself, they argue for the existence of a template system for each individual familiar face, and suggests that, at least in some of the patients, such a template system is intact.

We have attempted an interpretation of this "covert recognition" phenomenon in terms of a model of facial learning and recognition. The model includes (1) a perceptual step; (2) a template system step, in which templates are dynamic intramodal records of the elaboration of past visual perceptions of a given face; such dynamic records can be aroused by the perception of the appropriate face; (3) an activation step, in which multiple multimodal memories pertinent to a particular face are evoked; and (4) a conscious read-out of concomitant evocations which permits an experience of familiarity and a verbal account of that experience or the performance of non-verbal matching tasks. Please note that our templates are not rigid, ever-present "photographs", but rather, plastic computational records that can be activated by given perceptual processes. Note also that our model separates a "physical structure" compartment from a compartment where contextual "associated records" are kept.

The anatomical substrate of step (1) comprises bilateral visual system structures up to and including primary visual cortex; the anatomical basis of step (2) is focused on bilateral mesial and inferior visual association cortices; the anatomical basis of step (3) includes bilateral anterior temporal structures both mesial and lateral, as well as bilateral association cortices of different sensory modalities. Step (4) depends on the same association cortices.

Prosopagnosia can not be explained by an impairment of the basic perceptual step in spite of the fact that some patients have partial defects of spatial frequency analysis and texture analysis. Prosopagnosia can also not be explained by an impairment of associated memories because they can be easily evoked through other channels. The defect may be explained, however, by an impairment of the activation step, which would either not take place or take place inefficiently. That, in turn, might be due to a dysfunction of the template system, which could be (a) intact but inaccessible to ongoing percepts, (b) destroyed, or (c) intact but prevented from activating multimodal memory stores. It appears that in some cases facial templates are intact: the electrodermal "recognition" can be interpreted as an index of successful matches between percepts, i.e., correctly perceived target faces, and templates of those faces. The prosopagnosia of the two subjects we studied with electrodermal responses can be conceptualized as a complete or partial blocking of the activation that normally would be triggered by template matching. Considering the anatomical specifications of the model, the blocking occurs either in (1) white matter connections of the occipito-temporal region (linking both visual cortices to anterior temporal cortices, and the latter to multimodal sensory cortices), or (2) in anterior temporal cortices. We expect that in cases of prosopagnosia caused by slightly differently positioned lesions - a likely possibility - different mechanisms might apply.

Be that as it may, the understanding of the most frequent anatomical basis and possible physiopathologic mechanism of prosopagnosia, is progressing at good pace.

FACES AND NON-FACES IN PROSOPAGNOSIC PATIENTS

J. BLANC-GARIN

1. INTRODUCTION

The manifestations of the prosopagnosia syndrome are often used as arguments in favour of the existence of a face-specific processing system in the brain. This syndrome is indeed sometimes considered as visual agnosia restricted to faces, or the inability to process human faces. This view, which isolates faces from other objects of the visual environment was very attractive; nevertheless, no argument appeared very convincing; above all, no clear definition was given and, as stressed by Hay and Young (1982), several meanings are in fact used. Recent data and some speculations invite us to examine the findings more carefully, in order to clarify the concepts (see in particular, Benton, 1980 and Damasio, 1985).

When reviewing papers describing prosopagnosic patients, we are confronted with a wide range of approaches, various underlying models (be they implicit or explicit) and different terminology. A given expression, recognition, for instance, is used to describe very different tasks (either matching or remembering) and thus covers various processes. So, the restrictive definition given by Mandler (1980) as "a judgement of previous occurrence" appears necessary. Here in this paper, the term will be used in an even more conservative way, and means: experiencing a previous occurrence (not just deducing it), with evocation of a déja-vu or a familiarity feeling about the current visual display. This moment in the information processing may precede access to the person's identity, and we must note the differences, as stressed by Hay and Young (1982, p.191), between stimulus recognition, face recognition and person recognition, between identifying a person and naming him. Likewise, we think it would be useful to distinguish the notion of "face" (the stimulus) from "physiognomy" (a mental representation). Another necessary distinction should be made between a true feeling of familiarity (experienced by subjects when physiognomes of real, well-known persons are evoked from long-term memory) and a brief familiarisation imposed by an experimenter in laboratory conditions (photos of unknown individuals are used and no information is available about actual persons).

A part of the confusion that exists with respect to terminology is probably due to the fact that the notion of "specificity" has been applied to the stimulus (the face). It is the dissociation at the stimulus level that has been stressed (faces vs non-faces) rather than that of the processes involved. However, no coherent specificity model has been proposed, although some arguments have been put forth. The opposing hypothesis leads us to look for processes which can be relevant to the analysis of more general, perceptuo-cognitive mechanisms. Indeed, a few long-known facts are now taking on importance in light of new data. They have suggested that the relevant dissociation does not occur at the stimulus level, but at the process level, i.e. evocation of familiarity and individuality by visual image versus discrimination of features and inference of identity (see Blanc-Garin, 1984; Grusser, 1984).

2. VISUAL PROCESSING IN PROSOPAGNOSIA

From the analysis of various case reports of prosopagnosic patients (cf. Damasio et al., 1982; Blanc-Garin, 1984), some generalisations can be made and consistent disturbances can be summarised (very schematically) by 3 points:

    a. Prosopagnosic patients are able to process faces.
    b. Prosopagnosic patients are unable to recognise the individuality of a face.
    c. A similar dissociation is observed with various other objects of the visual environment, but great individual differences are found.

a. Prosopagnosic patients can, indeed, extract various kinds of information from a face:

- A face is always identified as a face and differentiated from other visual objects (in the actual environment as well as in photographs).
- The parts of faces are easily discriminated, identified, pointed to, named, drawn and memorized.
- Face gestalts can be extracted and differentiated from non-faces (scrambled drawings).
- Prosopagnosics can match face stimuli in a multiple choice display;
- Despite their failure to visually recognise the persons portrayed, prosopagnosics can sometimes develop strategies which lead them to the identity of the person they are seeing. They can deduce it from a detail they have memorised.

b. The basic impairment in face processing is concerned with recognition of well-known persons. Prosopagnosics do not experience déja-vu, or any feeling of familiarity from the sight of the face. Nevertheless, information about the person is available and accessible from other cues (voice, for instance). Moreover, when a characteristic visual detail helps them to access information about the person, his identity or name, they do so slowly; usually they add that they are not certain, and require confirmation. Thus, this is not true recognition, automatically evoked, but is the result of an inference generally based on a characteristic feature, a local and verbalisable detail.

A response (the identity of a person) can thus be accessed by two different visual routes (either recognition or inference), one of them being destroyed in prosopagnosics. The first one, by activating the visual template of an individual physiognomy, a "face recognition unit" (Hay & Young, 1982), brings on a feeling of familiarity and certainty of déja-vu; this stage is quick and automatic. Then, context elements lead to the person's identity and to his name. This route, which is the usual one, is not available to prosopagnosics who must rely on a second route, an indirect path, which is less efficient, slow and requires effort. It starts from salient features, local and verbalisable cues and does not give rise to a familiarity feeling, relying on inferences.

c. The essential dissociation thus opposes prospagnosic utilisation of available details to the evocation of a visual gestalt stored in LTM. This dissociation is not only observed for human face stimuli but is also found for certain other objects (see Table 1). Disturbances most often reported are in connection with remembering well-known particular places. The contrast between knowledge and the feeling of familiarity is explicitly brought out by the patients. "The road seemed completely strange to me though I knew it well... The surroundings (....) appeared unfamiliar (....). Though I knew it was my home, it seemed strange to me", as Bornstein and Kidron's patient reported (1959, p.125). Poncet's patient (1980) expressed a similar impression: "When I walk in Marseilles, where I have been living for 30 years, it's always like the first time I went to Alicante".

For both places and faces, the ability to describe visual features, to infer identity is not disrupted. The disorder is in the ability to recognise the "individual" image, to evoke the particular place. Again, we find prosopagnosic failure to feel familiarity and to link the current perception to an individualised representational image.

Prosopagnosic difficulties involving other visual objects also fit these characteristics. These may be less serious or less detrimental to personal adaptation (and thus, less often expressed voluntarily), but they show the same kind of cognitive disturbance: inability to recognise an individual, yet ability to extract perceptual features. One patient (Blanc-Garin, Poncet & Abonnel-Orlando, 1984) complained of difficulties when using coins and banknotes in daily life situations. In the first three tasks, in an experiment designed to analyse this difficulty, this patient was able to sort out forty coins rapidly and correctly, using various criteria (size, colour, engraving) – criteria which can be said to be perceptual or present in the visual display. In the fourth task, each coin's familiarity, only available in representational memory, was to be used as a criterion for sorting French vs foreign coins. She sorted at random and when asked to repeat the task a second time, she turned the coins over to read the inscription of the country.

Following Faust's interpretation (1955) it is sometimes said that prosopagnosics cannot perceive individuality within a wide class of objects (either faces or cars, for instance). Several formal tests show that they are able to perceive individuality; they do extract some details, using them to access semantic memory. The trouble lies in recognising an individual object as they used to. Complaints bear mainly (in recognition situations) on certain categories, where individuals are "ambiguous", to quote Damasio who stated (1985, p.134): "numerous members are physically similar (in visual terms), and yet individually different".

For a better understanding of the prosopagnosic disturbance, these difficulties should be documented in further investigations:

- by exploring spontaneous complaints and their relationships to the personal history of the patient;
- by invesigating special abilities the patient had developed, due to his high motivation in a hobby or his competence in a profession, for instance;
- by analysing types of errors (rather than setting a performance level), in discrimination and in recognition tests designed for this purpose;
- by studying the compensation strategies (cf. Christen et al., 1985) and the temporal course of recovery (cf. Malone et al., 1982).

Although disturbances in object recognition are irregularly reported in prosopagnosic cases, when they are, the dissociation is clearly of the same type as that observed with faces. As stressed by Damasio et al. (1982, p.337), "the generic class to which the stimulus belongs presents no difficulty, but recognition of an individual member of that class, whose identity has previously been learned is impaired". However, we must add that this only applies to some objects, and a greater or lesser number of categories of objects is affected, depending on the subject.

3. INDIVIDUAL DIFFERENCES

One might object to the fact that individual differences are so great that no generalisation can be made. Are these individual differences randomly distributed? Can they be regarded as noise in the system, which clouds the general process? Or can they take on a true meaning?

Individual variability, that is, degrees of freedom within a system, can be viewed as an indicator of the complexity of this system (Lautrey, 1984). We must therefore expect such variability in cognitive functioning and then analyse it. Different types of strategies can thus be regarded as "vicarious processes" (Reuchlin, 1978), which are implemented according to various factors related to the subject (cognitive style, previous learning) and to the situation (type of task, instructions).

In prosopagnosic difficulties, inter-individual differences are observed in the types and the ranges of objects for which recognition is disturbed. These difficulties often do not show up in formal tests, which generally involve discrimination tasks, but they are sometimes spoken of by the patients during examination. Since they do not involve discrimination but rather the evocation of a feeling of familiarity, they are linked to the subject's past experience and to his personal interest.

Most prosopagnosics complain about being unable to recognise cars "like they used to". Since their stroke, they must read the insignia in order to identify the make of a car, or read the licence plate to find their own car in a parking lot. Michel's patient, like Damasio's patient 1, had some difficulties in selecting "articles from the shelves of the supermarket", but she does not complain of great difficulties about cars. However she had never been interested in cars and had always used various strategies to identify automobiles whose makes were always poorly defined in her mind. The classification as "car", the colour, and the licence plate number provided sufficient cues for her limited acquaintance with cars. Many of us function similarly with respect to most animals (except our own dog or cat). To take another example, two farmers (patients of Bornstein et al., 1969 and of Assal & Favre, 1984), stressed their previous "special ability" to recognise their cows and "to call each of them by his own name". Both patients unknowingly relied on processes which were disturbed at the same time as the face-recognition process. The second farmer stated that, following his stroke, like for human faces, his cows "had lost their personality". On the other hand, another farmer did not complain of such a difficulty (Bruyer's patient). Was his capacity maintained, not destroyed by brain damage, or had "this special ability" not been constructed before his stroke? Perhaps he had a "herd" (without individualities), whereas the other farmers had individual animals, each with a personality and a name.

The range of categories of objects for which individualisation is defective is thus of variable size. This range is often narrow. It can be reduced to faces, as in the study done by De Renzi (1985). Nevertheless, in most cases, spontaneous complaints are made about a few types of objects in the visual environment (cars and playing cards, for example). This leads us to believe that, before their stroke, these patients used special processes or had built particular images for only certain categories of objects.

Therefore, it appears that the prosopagnosic disorder isolates different categories of images for each patient. In some areas, where motivation required the differentiation of a large number of similar individuals, efficient strategies had been set up that functioned both automatically and rapidly and which, since the stroke, are no longer available.

4. PHYSIOGNOMIES

Is prosopagnosia an "attenuated object agnosia", as proposed by some investigators (Gloning et al., 1970)? Currently, this opinion is not set forth. However, we should reconsider visual agnosia data by analysing both kinds of disturbances according to a model of visual environment processing (cf. Warrington, 1978; Ratcliff & Newcombe, 1982). The similarities and the differences between the two (in lesion location as well as in type of cognitive defect), will shed some light on visuo-cognitive mechanisms, and enrich the models used to account for them. Some facts observed in visual agnosic patients can illustrate the complex relationships between these two types of disturbances. Lhermitte et al.'s patient (1973) had severe object agnosia and limited prosopagnosia (she recognised a few old friends and relatives): she did not know what paintings were supposed to represent, although she was sure "they were Van Gogh's". On the other hand, Poncet's patient (1980) had severe prosopagnosia, great disturbances with recognition of places and mild difficulties with some common and personal objects (tools, belongings, handwriting). She could describe paintings, but did not recognise "Renoir's way", although she previously had been very fond of this painter.

As stressed by Damasio (1985), the question of what are the possible mechanisms of the prosopagnosic disturbance is not answered. In the processing course, what is the "locus" of the defect: the perceptual analysis, the access to the representational templates or the representational store itself? However, the analysis of facts concerning prosopagnosia show us the importance, in cognitive functioning, of a route which, rather than maintaining a list of features, allows us to store a configurational image, a physiognomy.

The physiognomies of familiar faces that we store can be thought of as slowly constructed images, kept in a visual format. These gestalts maintained in LTM rely more on relations between inner features than on external details (cf. Ellis, 1981; Ellis et al., 1979). These prototypes must undergo various alterations; they are "somehow equipped with transformational rules that permit unique configurations to be correctly classified" (Ellis, 1981, p.197). They must integrate modifications of emotional expressions, transformations across time (age, for instance). These facial images are thus flexible prototypes.

Given the emotional and social importance of person differentiation, the human face class is obviously the object category that most often requires such efficient processing strategies. Various authors agree with the idea that "faces may represent the non verbal extreme in a continuum of more or less verbally codeable stimuli" (Christen and Landis, 1984). The analysis of the prosopagnosic defect suggests that similar processes must be hypothesized for different kinds of stimuli in the visual environment (either familiar places, well-known animals, often-used objects, personal belongings...). Probably, during our experience with our visual environment, according to the expression of Grusser, some "visual patterns have gained a kind of physiognomic property" (1984, p.188).

5. CONCLUSIONS

The notion of face-specificity (a special cerebral mechanism for faces) appeared as an appealing asasumption, but it was often accepted as a postulate, rather than an hypothesis to be tested. Currently, it turns out as not supported by findings obtained from prosopagnosic patients: we must accept that this "splendid isolation" of face stimuli is not the way the system actually works. Nevertheless, if we absolutely wish to maintain the "specific view", we could say that we use a special mechanism to treat many things in our visual environment, as faces, but only things which, for us, possess a face, or to which we have given a physiognomy, as a result of personal interest or motivation.

OBSERVATIONS ON A CASE OF PROSOPAGNOSIA

JULES DAVIDOFF, W. BRYAN MATTHEWS AND FREDA NEWCOMBE

1.INTRODUCTION

A single case-study of prosopagnosia with extensive behavioural data and detailed examination of sensory studies is presented. Such published cases are still rare. Accordingly, it has been difficult to reach an agreed taxonomy of the disorder and to specify the underlying mechanisms. It is nevertheless certain that there are varieties of prosopagnosia (see Meadows, 1974). However, the classification is based mainly on clinical description; it requires amplification, taking into account relevant theoretical advances in the understanding of how face recognition is accomplished by normal subjects.

Most current models of face recognition concentrate on an information processing analysis centred around the store of face representations called face recognition units. The best proof of the existence of these units in normal subjects comes from priming studies (Bruce and Valentine, 1985). However, there is evidence that, at least in some cases of prosopagnosia the face representations in long-term memory are not lost: autonomic recordings show that prosopagnosics respond differentially to familiar and unfamiliar faces without conscious recognition of familiar items (Bauer, 1984; Tranel and Damasio, 1985). It therefore seems unlikely that representations of faces known over a life-time are lost in prosopagnosia: rather, it is difficult to access them or to make use of them. For this reason, we believe that it is necessary to determine what aspects of the stimulus are used in face recognition and by what skills recognition is achieved.

Contemporary theoretical accounts of face recognition do not make sufficiently clear the distinction between perceptual and memory processes. In contrast, Marr's (1982) proposal for object recognition makes it plain that the structural description (corresponding to the object-centred view) is not part of a semantic system since it is not necessary to know what an object is in order to recognize it. A defect at the level of a structural description – as Marr suggests for some of Warrington's (1982) agnosic patients – should properly be described as a perceptual loss. In the present study, we will use the term 'perceptual' in Marr's sense and thus are a long way in processing terms from the sensory factors considered by those authors who claim that their prosopagnosic patients are perceptually intact. Moreover, as far as we can ascertain, a detailed analysis of a prosopagnosic's perceptual abilities has not been reported. Thus, our aim is to 'locate' the functional deficit in a case of prosopagnosia, in terms of the pattern of impaired and intact perceptual skills. Only then can a presumptive loss of mnestic skills be properly interpreted.

2.CLINICAL HISTORY

In May, 1975, Mr. R.B., a successful heating and lighting engineer, aged 47, awoke one morning feeling 'light-headed', as if suffering from a hangover. He tried to 'work it off' but noted that his vision was altered:

he failed to recognise familiar faces and could not work effectively, being unable to match embossed wallpaper patterns or judge when pipes were correctly soldered. The condition persisted and during the next three months he became increasingly withdrawn, depressed, weepy, and unable to understand his symptoms.

In August of that year, he was admitted to hospital elsewhere. Gamma and CT scans were interpreted as normal. He was, therefore, treated with monoamine oxidase inhibitors and a course of eight unilateral ECT. There was some improvement in mood but his visual difficulties persisted. A second CT scan, carried out in October, 1976, revealed a small, low density area in the posterior region of the right hemisphere.

In August, 1975, testing by a clinical psychologist suggested a right temporo-parietal lesion. But, five months later, the possibility of an early dementia was invoked on the basis of 'mild word-finding difficulties' and 'concrete thinking'. In November, 1976, the psychologist reported an average IQ 'with no evidence of any organic intellectual impairment'. He performed at chance level, however, on facial and verbal recognition tasks, and the deficit was described as 'pseudoamnesic'.

In April 1977 he was referred to the University Department of Clinical Neurology, Oxford for a second opinion, at the instigation of his wife who suspected an organic basis, for the disorder. The problem of differential diagnosis was resolved by the typical clinical history, supplemented by visual field studies showing the left upper quadrantanopia (Figure 1) commonly found in patients with prosopagnosia (Meadows, 1974).

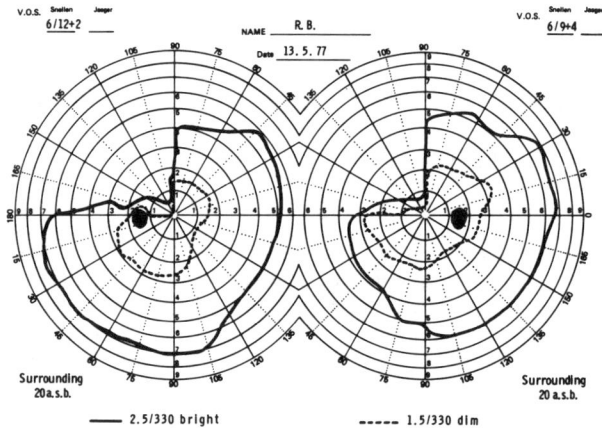

FIGURE 1. RB's visual fields plotted on a Tubingen perimeter. The numerator in the key is the size in millimetres of the target, the denominator is the distance in millimetres of the subject from the perimeter.

The CT scan reports had varied according to the technical facilities available. Repeat scans in 1976 and 1977 confirmed the right posterior lesion but one of the five scans indicated an area of diminished uptake in the left parietal region. The last scan in 1980 left no doubt about the bilaterality of the lesions. It showed a low density area in the right hemisphere at the low occipito-temporal junction, close to the ventricle and the trigone, underneath the occipital horn. A symmetrically placed but smaller lesion was seen in the left hemisphere. In addition, there were two, ill-defined, low density areas around the posterior aspect of the body of the lateral ventricle, beneath the temporo-parieto-occipital junction, more extensive in the left than the right hemisphere. The lesion, involving the white matter and the fusiform and lingual gyri at the temporo-parietal junction, was consistent with cerebrovascular pathology.

Clinical interview in 1977 revealed a history of a disproportionately severe difficulty with familiar face recognition. He could usually identify his family in a familiar context, but failed to recognise his wife and daughter on one occasion in the hospital corridor when he had not expected their visit. Since the sudden onset of his illness, he had consistently failed to recognise old friends and customers; and by the time he was admitted to our department, he was using characteristic cues for identifying staff - voices, distinctive clothing, paraphernalia (spectacle-frames, beards, hairstyles) and context.

He spontaneously reported that he had other visual symptoms. Thus, he could easily recognise object categories (e.g. cars, flowers and racehorses) but not specific exemplars. Moreover, the emotional content of visual images had disappeared: landscapes and photographs of pin-up girls no longer evoked sensations of pleasure or interest - the 'visual hypoemotionality' described by Bauer (1982).

He found his visual disabilities inexplicable and disquieting. He would have preferred the handicap of a paralysed limb that would have been comprehensible to himself and others. In addition, he could no longer work at his trade. Depression and unemployment led to a rift in the family; the patient lived on his own for several months before an eventual reconciliation. The opportunity then arose to work at a less skillful level in the small building firm of a friend. He was able to paint and decorate slowly but adequately until a more appropriate job as a porter was secured.

We had the opportunity to follow his progress for eight years. During that time, his symptoms have remained constant, but he has refined and added to his repertoire of strategies to facilitate face recognition. These include a meticulous study of facial features with particular emphasis on hair-line and the shape of individual facial features, especially the size and contours of mouth and lips.

3.SENSORY STATUS

When examined on 12 May, 1977, visual acuity was as follows: left eye, Snellen 6/12 + 2 (uncorrected) and with PH; right eye, Snellen 6/9 + 2 (uncorrected), 6/9 + 4 with PH. The patient had colour deficiences which were initially suggested by large error scores on the Farnsworth-Munsell 100 Hue test on two examinations (separated by 2 weeks): left eye (corrected) error scores 396 and 231; right eye (corrected) 504 and 311. The patient was subsequently examined by Dr. John Mollon. The patient wore spectacles and worked under CIE illuminant C. He could correctly order stimuli that varied along two dimensions of colour space - lightness and saturation: Munsell gray chips were correctly placed in order; and he could make gross discriminations of hue: he correctly ordered Munsell chips varying in chroma but of constant hue and value (using series 5 BG/6, 10 G/6, 5 R/5). The Ishihara-Ohkuma test revealed a deficiency on the most difficult plates - a moderate red-green deficiency of indeterminate type, not clearly resembling either of the common congenital anomalies.

On the Farnsworth Tritan plate, he was able to describe the light-green square (which is missed by tritans) but was unable to identify the light blue square (which is missed in red-green deficiences). He could nevertheless identify individual blue dots but remained unable to report the square when the card was presented at a distance. Dr. Mollon commented: "he appears to have difficulty in integrating elements in the visual field that are differentiated from the ground only by slight differences in hue".

Visual sensory status was examined by Professor Donald MacKay and Dr. David Foster. In summary, of all the systems examined, RB was most efficient at motion perception. He also performed normally on tasks of acuity (grating processing), long-term signalling, contrast acuity, and figure-ground perception. Movement illusions were seen both binocularly and monocularly. He had no difficulty in matching random dot patterns, whether identical or rotated in 45, 90, 135 or 180 degrees. With Julesz patterns, there was a clear stereoscopic effect with a 70% correlation of two images, slight differences with 60% and no effect with 50%. Complementary after-images, however, were weak and he had a marked difficulty in detecting contrasts in texture density, that is a difficulty in detecting static changes or fine discontinuities in grain. This was demonstrated by his failure to detect simple shapes cut out of photographed sandpaper and superimposed on photographed sandpaper of a slightly different texture.

Pattern reversal visual evoked potentials were recorded in July, 1980 and September, 1982 by Marian Small who used the method described by Matthews et al. (1977). Visual acuity was corrected to 6/6 right and 6/9 left.

On the first occasion, monocular recordings showed a double peaked positive response from each eye, with latencies of 89 and 140 ms from the right eye and 91 and 145 ms from the left (mean of two recordings from a central electrode referred to FZ). The amplitude of the major positive wave was low, 2.7μv on the right and 2μv on the left.

On the second occasion, there was a single positive wave of delayed latency, 122 ms from the right eye and 125 ms from the left (normal mean 98.9 ms, s.d. 5.1 ms). Binocular stimulation of the right half field confirmed the delayed P100 but was otherwise normal. Left half field stimulation produced a very low amplitude double peaked positive response from central and lateral occipital electrodes without the normal asymmetry.

The recordings suggested some disorder of central vision in addition to that of the left visual field.

4. INITIAL NEUROPSYCHOLOGICAL ASSESSMENT
4.1. Verbal ability

The main outline of cognitive performance was initially mapped more than two years after the onset of his disorder. His difficulty in processing faces and some other patterned visual stimuli was disproportionately severe, emerging against the background of average verbal skills (WAIS verbal IQ, 104; Mill Hill vocabulary IQs, 98 and 104) intact language comprehension (quick and accurate responses on the Token test), and normal spontaneous speech; he made only two errors – a normal score – on a formal test of confrontation-naming (Newcombe et al., 1971). He read with understanding and was able to detect the incongruous word in short paragraphs, as witnessed by a normal performance on Chapman's speed-of-reading test.

4.2. Performance ability

His WAIS performance IQ of 86 was reduced by one very low subtest score (Object Assembly, 4). Otherwise, his performance was at least average on a wide range of visuospatial tasks, including Gollin figures, the Ghent-Poppelreuter overlapping figures, Benton et al.'s line orientation, Money's road map, and Ratcliff's cube counting test (on which he was the only neurological patient we have thus far tested to get a maximum score).

4.3. Picture description

He was able to interpret pictures succinctly and appropriately. His response to the classical Bobertag picture was given without hesitation: "It's about a kiddy who's smashed a window and the person is coming out of the house to tell him off, but ... she's got the wrong one ... he's hiding". The misidentification of gender however, was, interesting: the irate householder is usually taken to be male.

4.4. Memory

Short-term digit span was normal for his age (7 digits forward) but long-term story recall was variable. Immediate recall of narrative was normal (W.M.I. story scores 13 and 9) but delayed recall, an hour later without forewarning, was poor (scores $7\frac{1}{2}$ and 0 - 5 [the latter score with an initial cue]). Short-term non-verbal span was normal (Corsi blocks - a sequence of 5) as was his performance on a short-term visual pattern recognition task (Warrington & James, 1967a). He was able to match to sample chequerboard patterns, with a stimulus-presentation time of 5 sec and a delay of fifteen seconds (score 18/20). Long term non-verbal memory, however, was significantly impaired (Rey Osterrieth geometrical design (A) copy score 27/36 delayed recall from memory 45 minutes later, without forewarning, $9\frac{1}{2}$/36). Similarly, scores on Benton's visual retention task were low (Form C 6/10, D 3/9, E 7/10: one item was inadvertently missed on Form D).

5. EXPERIMENTAL STUDIES

These studies will be considered in three sections: early sensory processing, pattern matching, and face processing.

5.1. Early sensory processing

The relationship between 'higher-order' cognitive deficits - specifically, the agnosias - and subtle sensory loss is still controversial. A classical early paper of Ettlinger (1956) demonstrated that sensory loss (carefully measured according to the then existing techniques) was not a sufficient cause of agnosic disorder. But impairments at relatively early stages of sensory processing have not always been comprehensively studied in such patients. Accordingly, we examined the ability of RB to detect (non-facial) stimuli when these were either briefly exposed or degraded by masking.

5.1.1. Tachistoscopic recognition thresholds.

A highly significant increase in tachistoscopic recognition thresholds for object silhouettes (Kinsbourne and Warrington, 1962) was found, using a central stimulus within less than 4 degrees of fixation point. Only one of eight silhouettes was perceived at 50 milliseconds of exposure, two at 100 ms, five at 120 ms, and six at 140 ms. Silhouettes of a yacht and a cat were not seen until 0.5 and 2 seconds, mainly because of persistent paranopsias: the cat was seen as a teapot or a jug from 120 millisecs, and the yacht as a bell. When all eight achromatic silhouettes had been identified, eight pairs of objects, in vertical alignment, were successively presented to the right of fixation. One object-pair was seen at 50 ms. three object-pairs at 100 ms. seven at 120 ms, eight at 150 ms, ten at 170 ms, twelve at 600 ms, fourteen at 1 second and sixteen at 2.5 seconds. RB was, always aware however, that two stimuli were simultaneously presented.

5.1.2. Detection of structure.

The patient also proved to have difficulties in detecting structure in visual displays (Frith, 1976). Frith's experimental stimuli consist of 80 x 80 black or white squares, divided experimental stimuli consist of 80 x 80 black or white squares, divided into four quadrants: only one of the quadrants has structure (symmetry). Normal subjects take less than two seconds to decide which of the four quadrants is symmetrical whereas the patient's latencies were measured in minutes.

5.1.3.Stimulus degradation. The patient had marked difficulty in interpreting visual stimuli with reduced cues. Specifically, when photographs of objects, and lower case letters were masked by filters of different opacity, he was markedly different from normal control subjects who had little difficulty in recognising the masked stimuli (Table 1).

mask opacity	objects		letters	
	RB	controls	RB	controls
4	12	2.8 (0-4)	26	0.5 (0-2)
3	8	0.4 (0-2)	15	0
2	7	0.2 (0-1)	8	-
1	1	-	0	-
0	0	-	-	-

TABLE 1. Errors made by patient RB and control subjects on two identification tasks, comprising 20 objects and 26 lower case letters, presented for inspection under masks of different opacity (uniformly spaced block dots of the following approximate diameters and distribution: condition 4, 2.5 mm at 3 dots per cm; condition 3, 1.75 mm at 4 dots per cm; condition 2, 1 mm at 6 dots per cm; condition 1, 0.75 mm at 9 dots per cm.).

5.2.Pattern matching

These experiments addressed the issue as to whether the patient had perceptual problems when matching non-facial stimuli and whether the difficulty in processing face-stimuli was disproportionately severe.

Latencies on matching to sample tasks were relatively long for non-verbal stimuli and disproportionately long for faces. The achromatic stimuli (Figure 2) included words, nonsense syllables, birds, Caucasian faces, African faces and nonsense figures (Attneave and Arnoult, 1956). His performance was compared with that of men of similar age with chronic unilateral missile-injury brain wounds and of age-matched male control subjects. Difficulty level alone cannot explain the patient's long latencies in matching faces. Moreover, the stimulus-related nature of his problem was shown by using different types of patterned stimuli (Figure 3): RB showed disproportionately long latencies for matching more densely patterned stimuli as compared with linear geometrical patterns (Figure 4).

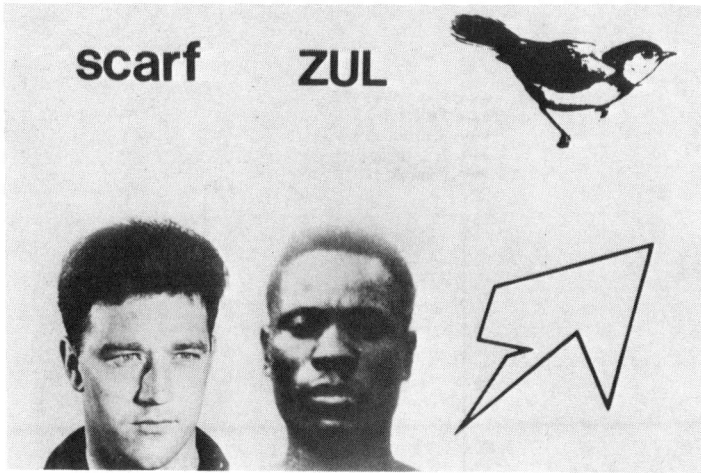

FIGURE 2. Examples of stimuli used in a matching-to-sample task: words, nonsense syllables, birds, Caucasian faces, African faces, and nonsense figures.

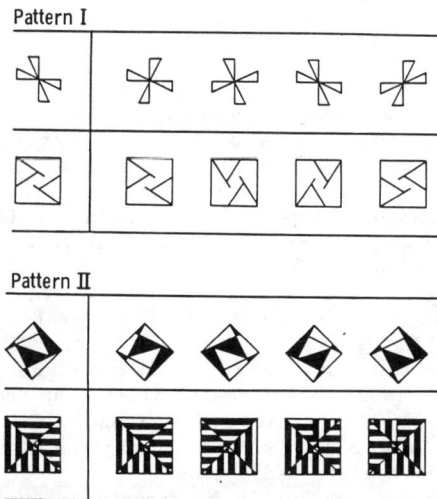

FIGURE 3. Examples of two types of patterned stimuli used in a matching-to-sample task.

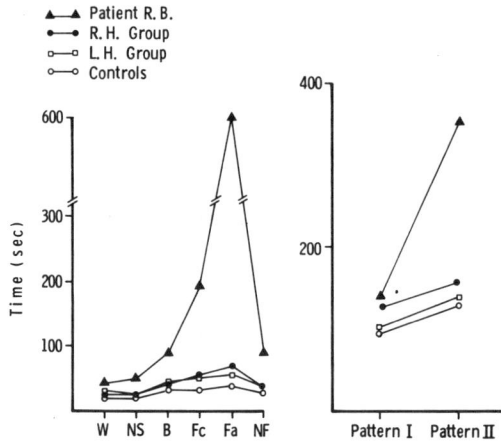

FIGURE 4. RB's latencies on matching tasks, compared with those of normal male control subjects and exservicemen with unilateral chronic missile injuries of the left hemisphere (LH) or the right hemisphere (RH) of the brain. The figure on the left shows latencies for matching the stimuli illustrated in Figure 1: words (W), nonsense syllables (NS) birds (B), Caucasian faces (Fc), African faces (Fa), and nonsense figures (NF). The figure on the right shows latencies for matching the patterns illustrated in Figure 3.

The patient spontaneously commented on a difficulty in identifying cars although he himself had been an owner-driver of several different makes of car. On a task designed for the purpose, he failed to identify the make of 27 of 34 achromatic photographs of cars, a performance well outside the range of male control subjects who make an average of 12 errors. Similarly, he made 17 errors when asked to identify 26 colour photographs of common garden flowers, a performance again outside the range of normal male controls whose mean error on this task is 9.5.

5.3.Face-processing
5.3.1.Famous faces. He recognised 13 of 20 photographs of famous faces widely known to his generation, a performance more than one standard deviation below the mean of men with chronic right posterior lesions. Of 26 photographs of more recent celebrities, he recognised only 10, a performance again well outside the range of normal controls (1-8 errors). He recognized only four of 28 cartoon drawings of contemporary celebrities (of political or media fame).
5.3.2.Unfamiliar face-matching. At a perceptual level, he showed clear-cut difficulties in matching photographs of unfamiliar faces, whatever the experimental paradigm. For example, presented with three photographs of faces of young men (two identical and one of a different person) and asked to point to the odd man out as quickly as possible, he made no errors but

took notably longer (mean 5.9 secs per item) than any control subject.
5.3.3.<u>Schematic faces - sorting</u>. The patient was examined by Dr. Chris
Frith who asked him to sort schematic faces that varied on nine features
(Frith and Frith, 1978). Dr. Chris Frith commented that his performance was
very unusual compared with that of control subjects in that he took a long
time, produced few groups using a small number of features, and furthermore
selected unusual features as criteria for sorting (e.g. upper hairline,
lower hairline, and chin). He did not show the 'multiplicative
classification' (attending to 'several dimensions of similarity at once')
that emerges after the age of eight (Frith and Frith, ibid).
5.3.4.<u>Unfamiliar faces - recognition</u>. His performance was at chance level
on a face-memory task in which he was shown eight photographs of faces of
young servicemen (presented individually for two seconds each) and then
asked to recognise them among a collection of 36 decoys, each target
appearing thrice in pseudo-random positions. His performance was outside
the range of older veterans with chronic unilateral missile injuries of the
brain and young uninjured servicemen (Table 2).

	age		recognition score	
	$\bar{x}$	(sd)	$\bar{x}$	(sd)
LH group (n = 18)	58.7	(3.1)	49.4	(4.1)
RH group (n = 17)	60.9	(4.6)	48.1	(5.3)
servicemen (uninjured) (n = 52)	21.0	(0.7)	53.5	(4.1)
patient RB	47	-	39	-

TABLE 2. Performance (mean and standard deviation of correct responses)
on a 60-item recognition task (unfamiliar faces) of older exservicemen with
long-standing unilateral cerebral missile injuries of the left hemisphere
(LH) or the right hemisphere (RH) and younger, uninjured conscript
soldiers.

6.DISCUSSION
This patient clearly does not belong to those groups of prosopagnosic
patients in which the symptom can be associated with a global amnesic
disorder or a gross perturbation of visual spatial functions. On the
contrary, many aspects of spatial orientation were well-preserved or even
better than average (e.g. judgement of visual and tactual line orientation;
cube counting); and he had no problems with map-reading tasks (Money map
and locomotor mazes). He did show, however, an impairment of long-term
visual memory and he had difficulty in learning a visually-guided stylus

maze, comparable to that of men with chronic, right posterior missile injuries. But, unlike them, the maze-learning deficit was not supramodal: he was quick to learn a tactually-guided maze and in general performed well on tactual tasks. The suggestion, therefore, is that in RB's case the disorder is specific to the visual modality but is not restricted to face-processing. It is clearly stimulus-specific and seems to be linked to the complexity and texture of surface pattern, rather than contour and orientation. He seems unable to integrate the features of a complex patterned display (see also Newcombe, 1979) in order to arrive at a global perception of a face- or indeed any complex pattern - in what Mooney (1960) called an 'initial single brief glance'. Whether he is looking at a face or a tritan colour plate, he appears to be detecting and evaluating features rather than a Gestalt. We therefore concur with Dr. Frith's comment that the patient seemed unable to group the details of high density patterns (whether faces or abstract designs) into higher order units which make search and detection easier and quicker. It is his inability to do so which, we claim, is central to his face-processing disorder. It is responsible for his difficulty with familiar faces by making it hard for him to create a proper structural description of a face.

It is clear that the structural description (and indeed most other descriptions) for faces must be visuospatial in nature. Common sense suggests that the small differences between faces could only be resolved in pictorial terms; experimental research has confirmed the obvious. Verbal descriptions are not helpful in memorizing faces (Malpass et al. 1973; Chance and Goldstein, 1976; Goldstein et al. 1979); it is other visual not verbal tasks which interfere with face memories (Cohen and Nodine, 1978). It will therefore help us define prosopagnosia if we ask what is being computed from the visual stimulus to distinguish familiar from unfamiliar faces.

There is some preliminary support for a processing difference between familiar and unfamiliar faces from a study of two aspects of face-processing in patients with unilateral cerebral lesions (Warrington and James, 1967b): there was a trend for patients with right parietal lesions to perform less well on a task involving the recognition of unfamiliar faces whereas the right temporal group were poorer at recognising photographs of famous faces. Furthermore, experimental studies (Ellis, Shepherd and Davies, 1979) suggest that different mechanisms are involved in processing familiar and unfamiliar faces: familiar faces are better recognised from the internal face features (eyes, nose and mouth) whereas unfamiliar faces can be equally well recognised from internal or external features (hair outline). The prosopagnosic patient RB reports that from choice he uses the hairline in face processing tasks. It should therefore be asked whether there is any perceptual processing ability which he has lost that makes it difficult to carry out face recognition tasks using the internal face features. We suggest that there is. The patient has difficulty in dealing with rapidly-presented pattern stimuli and we posit that this makes for considerable difficulty in dealing with internal face features. This difficulty obliges him to use compensatory strategies which may sometimes result in an error-free performance but, as reported above, with excessively long latencies.

In our view, the processing skills that are needed for the recognition of familiar faces can be seen to parallel those used to explain word superiority effects in Seymour's (1979) model of visual cognition. A familiar letter string such as a word is recognized more quickly than a non-word (word superiority effect); Seymour explains this effect by assuming that the after-effect of the word is held longer at a register by

top-down action from the representation of the word in a mental lexicon
The analogous face superiority effect (better recognition of a face than a
non-face) would have a similar explanation. The mental representation of
faces, which we presume to be held in Seymour's pictorial data-store, would
keep the after-effect of a face active longer in the pictorial register.
However, there are differences between words and faces. Besides the ability
to generate an image (face) from the data-store, the face superiority
effect also requires the ability to integrate over more than one internal
face feature and the need to do it quickly. Davidoff (1986a) has shown that
after a face has been exposed for 500 msecs the face superiority effect
disappears i.e. a feature from a face is recognized no better than from a
jumbled version of the same internal face features. We therefore should be
enquiring whether prosopagnosic patients exhibit the normal face
superiority effects. RB for one does not and therefore he is unlikely to
use the internal face features for recognition and should experience
difficulty with familiar faces. Whether or not there will be a comparable
difficulty with unfamiliar faces will depend on the strategies available
for RB to deal with the task.

A prosopagnosic disorder can therefore arise not because the mental
representations of familiar people have been erased but rather from the
loss of a requisite skill to make use of them. Put this way, we might look
for impairments in the recognition of other classes of objects,especially
if faces are not a unique stimulus type (see Davidoff, 1986b for arguments
on this issue). While faces are an unusual stimulus-category in terms of
their processing demands - requiring both recognition of an outline, as for
all shapes, and an integration of internal features - they are not unique.
The ability of our prosopagnosic patient to deal with other classes of
stimuli for which both these aspects are essential was therefore examined.
It was found that RB does indeed have problems with other such stimuli.
Whereas he was exceptionally good at a visual spatial task (cube counting)
and a task involving mental rearrangement of outline shapes (Hebb's
blocks), he had difficulty matching patterns composed of black and white
segments and could not recognise photographs of common flowers and
vegetables or distinguish between different makes of car.

On theoretical grounds, a prosopagnosia attributable to a loss of
perceptual skills rather than to a loss of stored face-representations is
unlikely to produce a specific face recognition disorder. Presumably,
perceptual impairments would affect a wide range of complex visual patterns
besides faces. A prosopagnosia attributable to a loss of face
representations would more readily permit a category-specific disorder for
which there is evidence in the verbal domain (Goodglass et al. 1966;
Yamadori and Albert, 1973; Hart et al. 1985). However, a similar argument
for visual stimuli is less plausible. Comparability of familiarity between
categories of visual (as compared with verbal) stimuli is much harder to
achieve; and we can never be sure that absolute differences in latencies or
errors are not artefacts of similar differences in familiarity. Moreover,
no unique processing procedure used for faces but not used for objects has
been demonstrated, despite some honourable failures (see discussion in
Davidoff, 1986b). Indeed, we believe that the best candidate is rapid
visual integration and even this process, we have argued above, need not be
face-specific.

Our analysis of RB's inability to recognize faces and difficulty in
matching complex visual patterns suggests that the important loss is of a
perceptual skill. In which case, is it proper to call his disorder
prosopagnosia? Certainly not,if a memory loss is necessary for this term to
be used. Moreover, it is our belief that there is no reported case in which

memory loss in a face recognition disorder is proven. All reports in which perceptual loss is excluded fail to take account of the perceptual processes necessary for face recognition. Even in cases of error-free performance, latency measures, which could point to defective perceptual mechanisms, have seldom, if ever, been reported. We prefer to consider RB as providing an example of one of the ways in which a processing disorder could affect the recognition of both familiar and unfamiliar faces. In his case, a perceptual disorder makes the rapid integration of patterned information difficult. In other cases, the difficulty in recognising familiar faces could have a different source. It could, for example, result from an inability to generate an image (Farah, 1984) to match the integrated pattern. In yet others, and we do not completely rule it out despite the present lack of substantial evidence, prosopagnosia could result from the loss or disconnection of the stored face representations. In RB's case, however, a perceptual disorder appears to be sufficient to explain his face-recognition disorder.

8. BRAIN PATHOLOGY

FACIAL PROCESSING IN THE DEMENTIAS

JR CRAWFORD, JAO BESSON, HD ELLIS, DM PARKER, EA SALZEN, HG GEMMELL, PF SHARP, DJ BEAVAN and FW SMITH.

1. INTRODUCTION

A number of studies have investigated facial processing ability in different dementing conditions (e.g. Kurucz et al., 1979; Biber et al., 1981; Wilson et al., 1982). However, there has been no attempt to directly compare the performance of different diagnostic groups on the same facial processing tasks. This makes the delineation of communalities and differences in performance between different groups hard to assess. Such comparisons, were they to provide evidence of clear differences in facial processing ability between these groups, would also have the practical value of allowing facial processing tasks to be used as tools in differential diagnosis. This would be of particular value in differentiating between Dementia Alzheimer Type and Multi-Infarct Dementia as existing clinical and psychometric methods have their inadequacies (Liston and La Rue, 1983).

In addition to a lack of comparative studies on facial processing in different dementing conditions there has also been no systematic attempt to examine a broad range of facial processing abilities in the same cases. The few studies that do exist in the literature have typically concentrated on only one aspect of facial processing such as facial memory (Wilson et al., 1982) or facial discrimination (Eslinger and Benton, 1983). Studying a range of tasks would help to determine which aspects of face processing are most compromised in dementia and which show relative preservation. An interesting question in this regard is whether, as has been demonstrated in cases with focal lesions, (e.g. Benton, 1980; Ellis, in press), patients with dementia show dissociation in performance for different aspects of face processing. Eslinger & Benton (1983) administered the Benton Facial Recognition Test (Benton et al., 1983) and the Judgement of Line Orientation Test (Benton et al., 1978), a test of visuospatial ability, to a group of patients suffering from dementia. They reported a substantial dissociation in performance on these two tests in a large number of cases. The demonstration of dissociation in performance on a facial task and another visuoperceptual task raises the possibility that dissociation may occur between measures of different aspects of face processing. The only study to have directly tackled this issue suggests that this is indeed the case (Kurucz and Feldmar, 1979). In this study a group of patients classified using DSM II as suffering from "chronic organic brain syndrome" was administered a test requiring identification of photographs of familiar faces (i.e. ward personnel, relatives, public figures) and a test requiring the correct identification of photographs and line drawings representing the facial expression of affective states. The correlation between performance on these two tasks was low and non-significant suggesting that the two abilities could be dissociated. It should be noted however that the familiar faces test by its nature contained a memory component (requiring recognition of the face and recall of the name of the person depicted). Had some other test of facial processing ability which makes no memory demand been administered then this confounding factor would have been removed.

Both the studies cited above made no attempt to differentiate between different dementing conditions. In the Kurucz & Feldmar (1979) study the sample included patients with a history of alcohol abuse, patients with evidence of vascular disease and an unknown proportion of patients presumably suffering from primary degenerative dementia (Dementia Alzheimer Type); while in the Eslinger & Benton (1983) study the sample contained patients with dementia related to primary degenerative disease, vascular disease, alcoholism, anoxia, drugs and hormonal or metabolic defects. Thus it is not known whether particular etiologies/pathologies are likely to give rise to dissociation. It might be expected for example that dementia associated with vascular disease (Multi-Infarct Dementia) would be more likely than other conditions to give rise to dissociation because of the relatively more focal effect on brain tissue.

The aim of the present study was to fill in some of the gaps in our knowledge of this area by examining the performance of dementing groups over a range of facial processing abilities.

2. METHOD

2.1. Subjects

Four clinical groups were studied – Dementia Alzheimer Type, Multi-Infarct Dementia, Alcoholic Dementia and Korsakoff Psychosis. In addition a control group of comparable age and educational level was recruited. The demographic characteristics of these groups are presented in Table 1 below.

TABLE 1   Demographic characteristics of clinical groups and controls.

	MEAN AGE	AGE RANGE	MEAN YRS. EDUCATION	Numbers tested on each facial task			
				FACIAL MEMORY	FAMOUS FACES	BENTON	AFFECT RECOGNITION
DEMENTIA ALZHEIMER TYPE	66.9	57-77	10.3	16	17	8	8
MULTI-INFARCT DEMENTIA	66.5	46-85	9.4	9	9	6	6
ALCOHOLIC DEMENTIA	52.2	42-63	8.4	17	17	10	10
KORSAKOFF PSYCHOSIS	62.6	48-81	9.8	12	12	10	11
CONTROLS	59.1	43-80	9.5	18	18	13	10

Dementia Alzheimer Type (DAT) is a progressive dementia associated with degenerative nerve cell changes in hippocampus and association areas of cortex. At the neurochemical level acetylcholine deficiency has been strongly implicated as a causal factor in the striking cognitive impairments shown by such cases (Coyle et al., 1983; Perry et al., 1978).

Multi-Infarct Dementia (MID), as the term suggests, results from multiple strokes. In the early stages it has a stepwise course and, to a degree, behavioural deficits reflect focal lesions as they occur. However, as more tissue suffers infarcts a picture of severe general deterioration emerges (Lezak, 1983).

Alcoholic Dementia is a broad term used to refer to cases with a history of alcohol abuse who do not exhibit the full-blown amnesic syndrome, but in whom there is evidence of cognitive impairment persisting three weeks after cessation of drinking.

Korsakoff Psychosis is characterised by a severe amnesic syndrome, generally considered to be the result of damage to mesial diencephalic structures particularly the dorsomedial thalamus and mammillary bodies. However, a recent neuropathological study (Arendt et al., 1983), which provided evidence of degeneration in the Nucleus Basalis de Meynert, has led Butters (1985) to suggest that this maybe the crucial lesion.

Following neurological and psychiatric examination, and laboratory investigations (see Glen and Christie, 1975) to exclude metabolic or endocrine causes, cases were assigned to diagnostic groups according to DSM III. Differentiation between Dementia Alzheimer Type and Multi-Infarct Dementia was carried out on the basis of Hachinski (1975) ischemic scores. This scoring system, which is based on clinical features of atherosclerotic disease, has received neuropathological verification (Rosen et al., 1980) and its predictive utility has been further demonstrated using NMR imaging and regional cerebral blood flow imaging (Ebmeier et al., 1985).

Regional cerebral blood flow imaging using 123 Iodo-n-isopropyl-amphetamine (IMP) was carried out with all cases in the present series. The distribution of this substance in the brain following intravenous injections reflects the distribution of cerebral blood flow and uptake by the cells of the brain . Areas of low activity in the cerebral cortex can therefore be indicative of local pathological change.

2.2 Materials

Four facial processing tasks were administered as part of a larger research battery which included tests of verbal and non-verbal memory.

Benton Facial Recognition Test, Short Form (Benton et al., 1983). In this test of facial discrimination subjects are simultaneously presented with a photograph of an unfamiliar face and a multiple choice display which contains one or more examples of the same face. Subjects are required to identify those examples. The multiple choice display includes identical front-view photographs, three-quarter view photographs and front-view photographs taken under different lighting conditions.

Affect Recognition Test. This test uses sixteen cards each bearing photographs of the faces of two people with the same emotional expression. The cards belong to a series prepared by A. Young and D. Hay of Lancaster University from the Fairburn System of Visual References Set No. 2. There are four cards for each of the expressions, Happy, Unhappy, Surprised and Angry. Subjects are first required to read these four emotion terms from a printed card. They are then asked to use these terms to identify the expressions on the sixteen test cards.

Facial Memory Test (Munn, 1961. In this test subjects are presented with an array of twelve unfamiliar faces for a period of two minutes. After a four minute delay they are required to identify these from a larger array of 25. False identifications are subtracted from correct identifications to yield a final score.

Famous Faces Test. This test consists of a series of twenty photographs of public figures which subjects are required to name or, failing this, to provide information unique to the individual portrayed.

3. RESULTS AND DISCUSSION

In Table 2 the mean scores of the clinical groups and control group on the four facial processing tasks are presented.

TABLE 2   Mean Scores (and S.Ds) for clinical groups and controls on four tests of facial processing.

Mean (S.D.)	FACIAL MEMORY (Max score=12)	FAMOUS FACES (Max score=20)	BENTON (Max score=54)	AFFECT RECOGNITION (Max score=16)
DEMENTIA ALZHEIMER TYPE	2.00 (1.33)	5.76 (4.98)	41.50 (5.09)	13.00 (2.27)
MULTI-INFARCT DEMENTIA	1.33 (1.94)	7.89 (5.3)	39.5 (5.75)	9.00 (3.29)
ALCOHOLIC DEMENTIA	5.82 (2.96)	15.18 (7.89)	45.50 (4.33)	13.80 (1.75)
KORSAKOFF PSYCHOSIS	1.25 (1.91)	5.92 (4.32)	41.73 (3.74)	11.09 (1.64)
CONTROLS	8.67 (1.25)	19.11 (1.18)	51.08 (2.9)	14.10 (0.88)

3.1. Performance of the DAT group. In Figure 1 the mean scores for the DAT group are presented as a ratio of the control group mean. Analysis by t-tests revealed that the DAT group performance was significantly poorer than the control group on the Facial Memory Test ($t = 10.02$, $p < 0.0001$), the Famous Faces Test ($t = 10.76$, $p < 0.0001$) and the Benton Facial Recognition Test ($t = 5.52$, $p < 0.0001$). The highly significant difference between the DAT group and controls on the Benton is partly due to the above average performance of the control group (the standardisation sample mean was 45.4).   In addition, the mean score for the DAT group obscures the fact that there was a great deal of variability in performance within this group.   Fifty percent of the DAT group obtained scores in the normal range.   The striking impairments on the facial memory and famous faces tests shown by DAT cases, given the relatively milder impairments shown on the Benton and Affect Recognition Test, is probably largely attributable to the mnestic component in such tasks rather than being a facial processing deficit per se.   This conclusion is supported by an examination of the correlations between these tests and other memory items in the full battery.   The facial memory test shared a markedly greater amount of variance with these tests (Logical Memory, Visual Reproduction, and Digit Span from the Wechsler Memory Scale) than with the Benton or Affect Recognition Test.

The DAT group did not differ significantly from controls on the Affect Recognition Test (t = 1.3, p = 0.227).   The preservation of the ability to process faces for affective meaning is in marked contrast to the results for the other aspects of facial processing investigated. However it becomes all the more striking when set in the context of the severe general impairment of cognitive function demonstrated by this group's performance on the full research battery.   Of the 21 tests which make up the full battery, the Affect Recognition test was the only test in which the DAT group did not differ significantly from controls.

Fig. 1

PERFORMANCE OF DAT AND MID GROUPS EXPRESSED AS

A RATIO OF CONTROL GROUP MEAN

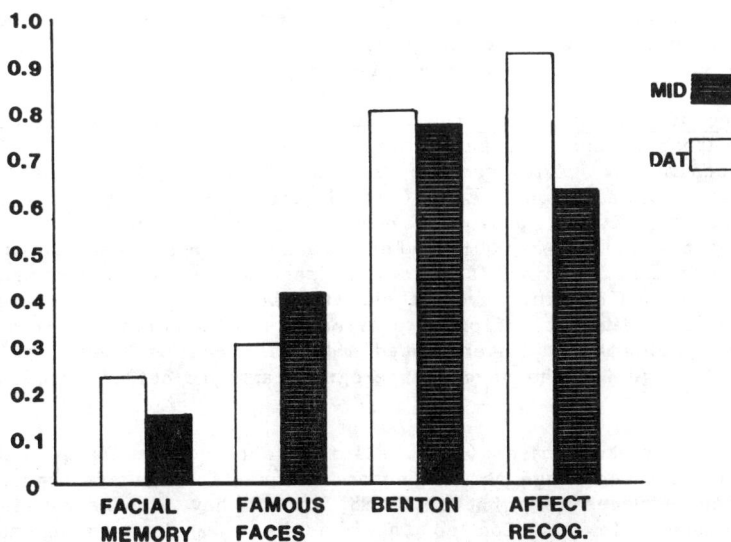

3.2. Performance of the MID group.   The MID groups performance on all four facial tasks was significantly poorer than the control group (Facial Memory, t = 10.04, p<0.0001;   Famous Faces, t = 6.27, p<0.0001;   Benton, t = 4.66, p = 0.003; Affect Recognition, t = 3.72, p = 0.014). Again the performance of the control group exaggerates the impairments shown by this group on the Benton and the mean score obscures considerable variability. Thirty three percent of the MID group obtained scores in the normal range. Performance was most impaired on the Facial Memory Test.

3.3. Comparison of DAT and MID groups. The DAT and MID groups performance is compared in Figure 1. Analysis by t-tests revealed no significant differences between the two groups' performances on the Facial Memory Test (t = 0.77, p = 0.451), Famous Faces Test (t = 1.01, p = 0.322) or the Benton (t = 0.69, p = 0.504). It would appear then that these tests have no utility in the attempt to differentiate between Dementia Alzheimer Type and Multi-Infarct Dementia using psychometric instruments. The difficulty in achieving this objective is attested to by the large number of unsuccessful attempts reported in the literature and the failure, in this regard, of the other tests in the present battery. A significant difference, in favour of the DAT group, was obtained in a comparison of the two groups' performances on the Affect Recognition Test (t = 2.7, p = 0.019) which suggests that this test may have discriminatory ability. However, it can be seen that the difference between the group performance was significant only at the 0.05 level suggesting that it would be of only limited value in differential diagnosis in the individual case. This was confirmed by the degree of overlap in scores between these two groups. This overlap, however, arises because of the greater variability in the MID group (which might be expected given the variability in the distribution of lesions in this condition). None of the DAT group scored less than 60% correct on the test whereas four of the six MID cases fell below this point. Thus, although a high score on this test would be of little significance, in cases where MID & DAT are competing diagnoses, a low score (less than 60% correct) may prove to be uncommon in Dementia Alzheimer Type and thus of some diagnostic usefulness. However, as numbers in both the MID and DAT cohorts are small it would clearly be unwise, at the present time, to attach too much significance to these findings.

Performance of the Korsakoff group. In Figure 2 the performance of the Korsakoff group on the four facial tasks is presented as a ratio of the control group means. This group's performance was significantly poorer than controls on all four tests (Facial Memory t = 11.08, p<0.0001; Famous Faces t = 10.33, p<0.0001; Benton t = 6.89, p<0.0001; Affect Recognition t = 5.16, p<0.0001). Performance was most impaired on the Facial Memory Test. This test was the best discriminator between the Korsakoff group and controls amongst the full battery. The task demands, requiring correct identification of previously seen material after a four minute delay filled with interpolated material, can be viewed as well suited to highlighting the severe anterograde amnesic deficit present in such cases.

Three of the Korsakoff cases (27%) fell in the borderline range and two (18%) in the impaired range on the Benton. These findings are consistent with previous studies (see Butters, 1985) which have demonstrated that Korsakoff cases, in addition to their obvious impairments on memory tasks, also commonly show impairments on measures of other cognitive abilities.

Fig. 2

PERFORMANCE OF KORSAKOFF AND ALCOHOLIC DEMENTIA

GROUPS EXPRESSED AS A RATIO OF CONTROL GROUP MEAN

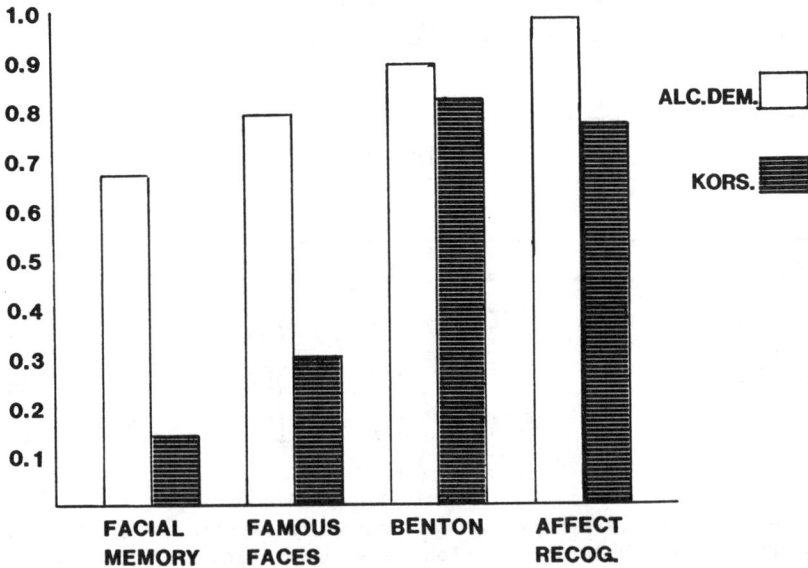

To our knowledge no previous attempt has been made to study facial affect recognition ability in Korsakoff Psychosis. The performance of the Korsakoff group in the present study suggests that they do show impairments of this ability. The Korsakoff group performed significantly more poorly on this test than did the Alcoholic Dementia group (t = 3.66, p = 0.002) and the DAT group (t = 2.14, p = 0.048).

Performance of the Alcoholic Dementia Group. The Alcoholic Dementia group performed significantly more poorly than controls on the Facial Memory Test (t = 3.45, p = 0.002), the Famous Faces Test (t = 2.77, p = 0.013) and the Benton (t = 3.7, p = 0.001). This group however was the least impaired of the four clinical groups studied. The significant difference in performance on the Benton test is due to the above average performance of the control group. Only one case (10%) fell in the impaired range on this test. There was no significant difference between the Alcoholic Dementia group and controls on the Affect Recognition Test. The impairments shown by this group then are, almost exclusively, limited to facial tasks which involve a memory component. On these tasks their impairments are considerably milder then those found in the other clinical groups.

Evidence of dissociation of performance. Raw scores on the Benton and Affect Recognition Test were converted into standard equivalent scores yielding a record of an individual's performance on these two tests expressed as the number of standard deviations below the mean of the

TABLE 3

FREQUENCY OF DISSOCIATION IN PERFORMANCE ON BENTON FACIAL RECOGNITION TEST AND AFFECT RECOGNITION TEST

	STANDARD DEVIATION UNITS				
GROUP	1	2	3	4	5
KORSAKOFF	40%	20%	10%	0%	0%
ALCOHOLIC DEMENTIA	78%	44%	22%	11%	0%
ALZHEIMERS	50%	50%	50%	38%	25%
MID	83%	67%	17%	0%	0%

control group.   Dissociation was operationally defined as a difference of more then one standard deviation between performance on these two tasks.   The results of this procedure are presented in Table 3.
   It can be seen from Table 3 that the majority of cases showed some degree of dissociation in performance on these two tests and that in many cases this dissociation was marked.   In the DAT group the dissociation was without exception a result of superior performance on the Affect Recognition Test.   In the other groups however, although most dissociation was obviously in line with the trends for the group as a whole, a substantial number of cases showed dissociation which went against the group trend.   Thus, although as a group the Alcoholic Dementia cases showed greater impairment on the Benton and 55% of this group showed dissociation in this direction, 22% showed dissociation of over two standard deviations in favour of the Benton.   As one might expect,because of the variability in the distribution of infarcts and the relatively more focal effect on brain tissue, the MID group showed the greatest amount of dissociation and this dissociation was as likely to occur in favour of one test as another.   The data presented above, we believe, have two main implications. Firstly, Dementia Alzheimer Type, and to a lesser extent Alcoholic Dementia, have commonly been viewed as giving rise to a general, uniform decline in cognitive abilities.   The degree of dissociation observed in the present study between the Benton and Affect Recognition Tests (despite their communalities) suggests such a view is untenable.   Secondly the degree of dissociation observed also suggests that different functional systems (Luria, 1973) and neurological substrates underlie the facial processing involved in discriminating between individuals (Benton) and discriminating between facial expressions (Affect Recognition).

Fig. 3

Performance on the Affect Recognition Test expressed as
a ratio of control group mean.

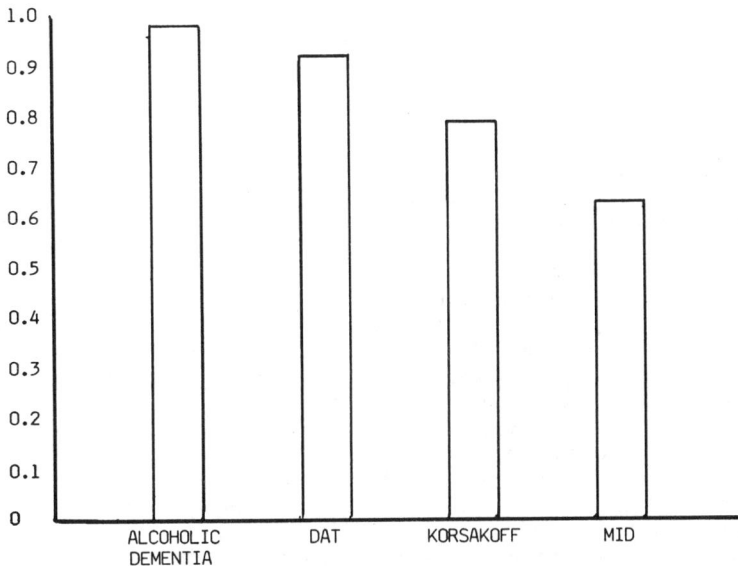

Affect Recognition Test. In fig. 3 the performance of all four clinical
groups on the Affect Recognition Test are presented as a ratio of the
control group mean.   On the basis of what is known of the neuropathology
of these conditions, the performance of the clinical groups on this test
suggests that structures other than neocortex (with the limbic system and
diencephalon being particularly strong candidates) play the major role in
processing faces for affective meaning.   Dementia Alzheimer Type, and to
a lesser extent Alcoholic Dementia are associated with degenerative
changes in the neocortex (Perry & Perry 1982; Adams & Victor, 1981).
With the clear exception of the hippocampus, Dementia Alzheimer Type is
not characterised by severe degeneration in limbic and diencephalic
structures (although a recent study (McDuff and Sumi, 1985) suggests that
degeneration in the thalamus and hypothalamus may be more common and
extensive than was previously thought).   In contrast, Korsakoff cases
typically show little neo-cortical pathology with damage limited largely
to limbic and diencephalic structures (Victor, et al., 1971; Mair, et
al., 1979).   The results of regional cerebral blood flow imaging carried
out with cases in the present series are consistent with the above
findings.   The DAT group showed striking reductions of perfusion in
neocortex particularly in occipito-parietal watershed areas (Gemmell, et
al., 1984).   The Alcoholic Dementia group also showed reduction of
perfusion although this was more variable.   In contrast the Korsakoff
group showed little or no reduction in these areas (Sharp et al., 1985).
As both the DAT and Alcoholic Dementia groups did not differ
significantly from the control group on the Affect Recognition Test,
whereas the Korsakoff group performed significantly more poorly than all
of these groups, it can be argued that the relative integrity of limbic/
diencephalic structures is of considerable importance in the processing
of faces for affective meaning.

THE MATCHING OF FAMOUS AND UNKNOWN FACES, GIVEN EITHER THE INTERNAL OR THE EXTERNAL FEATURES : A STUDY ON PATIENTS WITH UNILATERAL BRAIN LESIONS

E.H.F. DE HAAN and D.C. HAY

1.INTRODUCTION

On the view that prosopagnosia represents a specific pathophysiologically based inability to recognize familiar faces (Bodamer, 1947), two basic questions arise. First, there is no unequivocal agreement as to whether a unilateral lesion is sufficient to cause the syndrome (c.f. De Renzi, this volume; Meadows, 1974; Damasio and Damasio, this volume). The second question is concerned with functional mechanisms: if faces are processed differently with respect to other visual stimuli, where do these differences occur and what effect will disruption at different stages of processing have? Relevant information on both topics, lateralization and process analysis, can be expected from studies of patients with relatively circumscribed and stable brain lesions. The underlying premiss is that if this severe and comparatively rare inability to recognize faces has a specific neuroanatomical substrate, then less flagrant forms of face recognition impairment may be found in larger numbers of patients with cerebral damage (Benton and van Allen, 1968).

Evidence for this assumption can be found in the clinical literature. De Renzi and Spinnler (1966) reported that a group of patients with right hemisphere (RH) lesions was impaired, in relation to a group with left hemisphere (LH) lesions, on tasks involving immediate memory for faces and abstract designs. Benton and van Allen (1968) also obtained a significant RH effect using a simultaneous matching paradigm with face stimuli but, unlike De Renzi and Spinnler, they found no correlation with visual field defects, nor any clear cut association with type of lesion or intra-hemispheric locus of lesion. Other results consistent with RH involvement come from the studies of Milner (1968), Yin (1970) and Warrington and James (1967).

The research of cognitive psychologists with respect to face-processing has focussed on experiments with normal subjects using tachistoscopic presentation in the two visual half-fields. Overall, the results strengthen the key role of the RH (Ellis, 1983; Rhodes, 1985), although some studies have reported a LH advantage (Marzi and Berlucchi, 1977; Sergent and Bindra, 1981). This should make us aware of possible face recognition problems after LH damage (see also Benton, 1980).

Another important contribution is the development of face processing models (Hay and Young, 1982; Bruce, 1983; Ellis 1983) that allow predictions concerning the nature of the impairments that may and may not occur in patients. A cardinal feature of all models is that known and unknown faces are (partly) processed in a different manner. Support for such a dissociation (see also Warrington and James, 1967) was obtained by Ellis, Shepherd, and Davies (1979) with normal subjects, using a task in which either the internal features (eyes-nose-mouth) or external features (hair-ears-chin) were the stimuli for the recognition of previously shown familiar and unfamiliar faces. For familiar faces, subjects were more accurate with the internal than with the external features; for unknown faces, there was no difference in performance using either cue. Ellis et al. argue that the internal features are important because they are more crucial in social interaction, hence receive more attention which in turn could lead to a better memory representation. When an unknown face is presented for later recognition, the hairline is just as good a cue as the eyes. Endo, Takahashi and Maruyama (1984) replicated the Ellis et al. study and also showed that the advantage of the inner features became apparent when subjects had to give attributional judgements (e.g. likability and intelligence) when the faces were being learnt, but not when they were instructed to try to memorize them for later recognition. This result is consistent with the explanation proposed by Ellis et al. At this point, it is also possible to argue that the enhanced performance on the internal features of familiar faces results from the fact that the subjects have stored semantic information in connection with the face, which could facilitate recognition (i.e. "There is the ugly one again"). In our view, it is more likely to be the result of a better memory representation. An experiment of Klatzky and Forrest (1984) where subjects performed better on remembering famous faces even when the subjects could not tell anything more than that the face was familiar to them, strengthens this idea.

Using only famous faces, Young (1984) found a left visual field - RH advantage for the recognition of whole faces, internal features and external features (in increasing order of difficulty), but not for inverted faces. Thus the RH advantage holds for both the internal and external features. This result cannot be attributed to a RH advantage for complex visual stimuli per se, since the effect does not show up with the inverted faces.

In our study we investigated the ability of patients with unilateral lesions to match either famous or unknown faces using either internal or external features, in a reaction time paradigm. Two questions are addressed in this experiment. First, the results should show whether one hemisphere is better than the other in matching faces. More interesting is the question whether the two hemispheres use a qualitatively different mode of processing faces (see Benton, 1980; Sergent and Bindra, 1981). If so, a different pattern should emerge with respect to the two factors (Famous/Unknown; Internal/External features) depending on which hemisphere is damaged. However, if a similar pattern appears, it could be argued that there is no difference in the way the two hemispheres deal with faces.

With reference to problems raised by Hay and Young (1982) when identical photographs are used (i.e. the possibility that subjects will make use of stimulus-matching strategies), two different pictures of each individual were used in the "Same" condition, forcing subjects to rely on person matching.

2.METHOD
2.1. Subjects

This experiment is part of a larger research programme still in progress in the MRC Neuropsychology Unit at Oxford. The experimental group is drawn from the UK sample of ex-servicemen who sustained a penetrating head injury during the Second World War and who are participating in this follow-up. Twelve patients who sustained a LH missile injury and twelve patients with a comparable lesion confined to the RH, were selected. No finer categorization of lesion site will be attempted here because of the relatively small numbers. There was no difference in the frequency of visual field defects between the two groups. The control group consist of 12 paid volunteers, all male, recruited locally and selected on the basis of age and educational level. Means and standard deviations for age were respectively; Control subjects 67.2 (3.5); LH patients: 65.3 (5.5), and RH patients 62.6 (3.5). All subjects were right-handed.

2.2.Stimuli

Two black and white photographs were presented simultaneously and in a vertical alignment. Half of the faces were famous, i.e. people well-known in Great-Britain (politics, TV, cinema, royalty and sports), the other half were unknown: (local celebrities in a provincial town, foreign politicians and unknown actors and actresses). None of the people whose faces were used wore spectacles, hats, beards or moustaches. The top picture was always a full view and the bottom one was restricted to either the internal or the external features of the face. This resulted in four sets of stimuli: Internal features – Famous faces; Internal features – Unknown faces; External features – Famous faces; External features – Unknown faces, presented in this order. Each set contained eight practice and twenty experimental trials. In half of the trials, the two pictures were different photographs of the same person (Same condition); the other half consisted of pictures of two different people (Different condition), arranged in a pseudo random order.

For the choice of stimuli in the Same condition, matched sets of pairs of photographs had been constructed in order to control for familiarity of the famous faces and the differences between the two photographs (of both famous and unknown faces) in orientation and expression. The Same pairs were selected from a large pool of photographs of the same person's face. Five independent judges rated the extent to which the two pictures differed in expression and orientation of the face; they also rated the familiarity of the famous faces. The sets of faces for each condition were also equated for the number of male and female faces, and were matched by eye to achieve comparable ages and comparable ranges of hairstyles and picture quality. Figure 1 shows some examples of the stimuli used.

2.3.Apparatus

Stimuli were presented with two Kodak S-AV 2050 carousel slide projectors, operated by an Electronic Developments three-field tachistoscope. The stimuli were simultaneously projected in the middle of a white screen of 115 cm. by 125 cm., behind which the subject was seated at a distance of 145 cm. The visual angle was approximately 10 degrees. A remote control button operated by the experimenter activated the exposure sequence. An electronic Developments digital timer was triggered by stimulus onset. The clock was stopped by the subject closing a switch, operated by a lever, situated in front of his body. The lever was approximately 15 cm. high and placed on top of a wooden base (15 x 28 x 24 cm.), which housed the lever mechanism. Closure of the switch required a 2 cm. movement of the lever. However, in order to monitor the response, two additional switches were placed at the points of maximum lever displacement (approx. 10 cm.). These were linked to two lights on a display monitored by the experimenter. On top of the leverbox were two paper signs (Same; Different) indicating the direction to move for a specific response.

2.4.Procedure

All subjects completed the four conditions in a fixed order (see 2.2. above). After the subject was seated comfortably in the chair behind the screen, he was instructed to decide as quickly but also as accurately as possible whether the two photographs of faces, of which one showed only part of the face, were taken from the same person or two different people. Then the leverbox was put in front of him and its operation explained. He

FIGURE 1. Examples of stimuli used in the experiment (reproduced by kind permission of the Press Association).

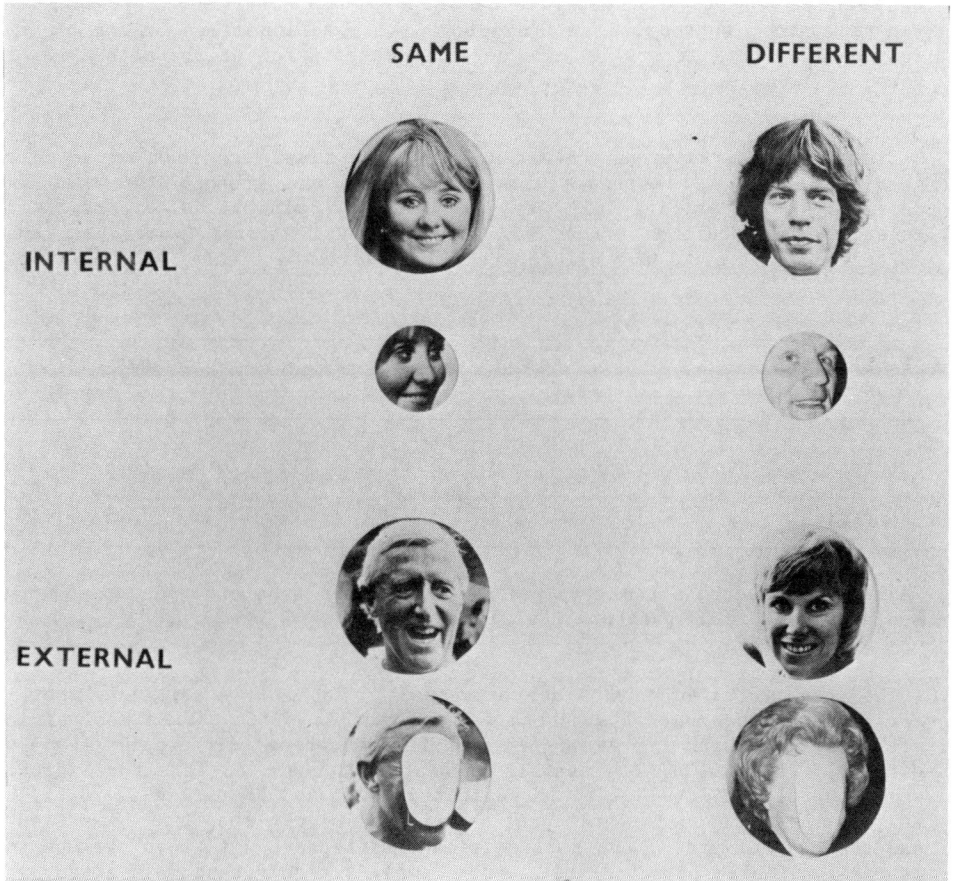

was told to respond by moving the lever forward for Same and backward for Different. All four conditions commenced with a practice series of which the data were not analyzed, followed by the test series. The exposure time was set at 4 sec. The experimenter started each trial by pressing the remote control button and recorded both the reaction times of the correct responses and the errors. A more detailed description of the method can be found in Young et al. (in press).

3.RESULTS

Since the objective was to measure reaction times and thus to keep the number of correct responses comparable over the groups, the task was designed to be sufficiently easy to ensure a minimum of errors. As a consequence, a ceiling effect was expected on the error scores, at least for the control group and all interactions had to be treated with caution.

| Familiarity | Famous | | Unknown | |
Features given	Internal	External	Internal	External
Control Subjects	0.33 (0.78)	0.83 (1.11)	1.17 (1.03)	0.83 (0.72)
LH patients	0.42 (0.79)	1.08 (1.00)	1.92 (1.08)	1.25 (0.87)
RH patients	2.08 (0.67)	2.25 (1.29)	2.08 (1.38)	2.17 (1.19)

TABLE 1. Mean errors and standard deviations (in brackets) for the control subjects (N=12), LH patients (N=12) and RH patients (N=12).

The mean number of errors are presented in Table 1. A ceiling effect is apparent for the control subjects and for the LH patients. An analysis of variance, however, revealed a significant group difference ($F=14.4$; d.f.=2,33; $p < 0.001$). The overall percentage correct for the three groups was: control subjects, 92.1; LH patients, 88.3; and RH patients, 78.6. The RH patients performed significantly less accurately than the LH patients and the control group, but no significant difference was shown between the latter two (Tukey post hoc test, $\alpha = 0.05$). A significant main effect was also found for the factor Famous/Unknown faces ($F=10.8$; d.f.=1,33; $p < 0.001$): more errors were made when the faces were unknown. In addition, two interactions reached statistical significance. First, Group and Famous/Unknown faces ($F=4.3$; d.f.=2,33; $p < 0.025$): the accuracy advantage for famous faces was largest in the LH group and somewhat smaller in the control group (ceiling effect), but completely absent in the RH group. Second, Region of the face given for matching and Famous/Unknown faces ($F=4.9$; d.f.=1,33; $p < 0.025$): with internal features all subjects made significantly more errors (Tukey post hoc test, $\alpha = 0.05$) on the unknown (mean error = 1.72) than on the famous faces (mean error = 0.94). Matching on external features was comparably accurate on both famous (mean error = 1.39) and unknown faces (mean error = 1.42).

Response latencies of the correct responses are shown in fig. 2. Despite a significant three-way interaction between Familiarity of the face, Region of the face, and Same/Different condition, the data presented here have been collapsed over the correct Same and Different responses. This interaction is due to the fact that Same responses for matching unfamiliar faces with the external features took a curiously long time. Our view is that this reflects a tendency for subjects to be cautious in deciding that external features of unfamiliar faces belong to the same person. Alternatively, it could be argued that different processes are involved in Same and Different responses, but then it is difficult to explain why this happens in only one out of four conditions. The key point, however, is that this holds equally across all subject groups (i.e. for controls, LH patients and RH patients).

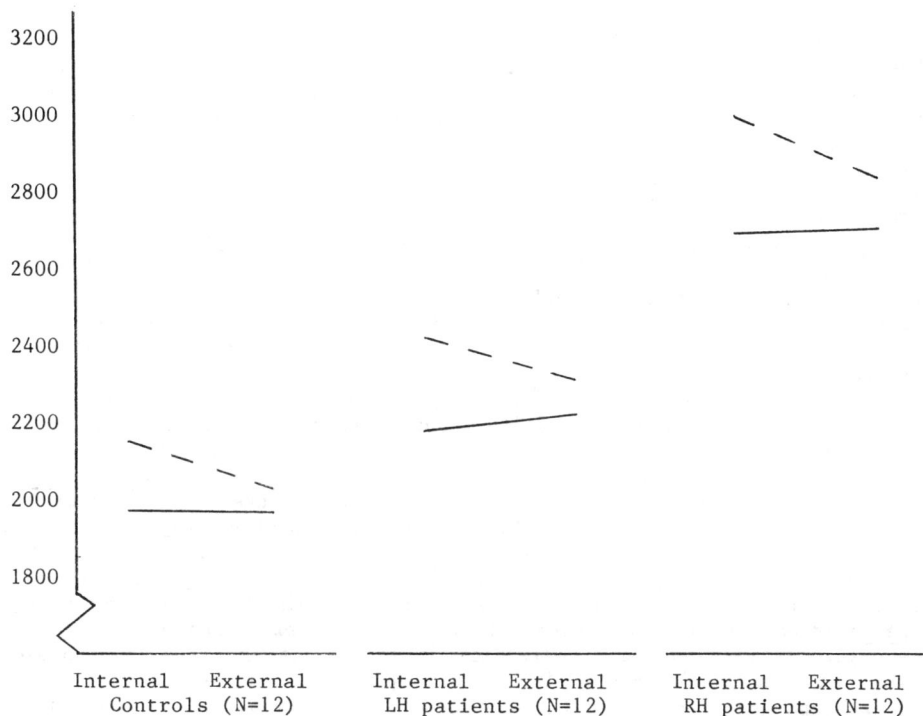

FIGURE 2. Mean latencies of correct responses in milliseconds for matching famous (———) and unknown faces (— — —) on internal or external features.

A three-way analysis of variance again revealed a strong group effect (F=10.1; d.f.=2,33; p 0.0005) with the RH patients being the slowest (mean RT = 2810.67), followed respectively by the LH patients (mean RT = 2294.63) and the control subjects (mean RT = 2149.82). The RH group was significantly slower than both the LH group and the control subjects (Tukey post hoc test, ∝ = 0.05), but there was no significant difference between the latter two. Famous faces were recognized faster than unknown faces (F=19.4; d.f.=1,33; p 0.001) and the interaction between Familiarity and Internal/External features was also significant (F=8.2; d.f.=1,33; p < 0.025), showing a similar pattern to the error scores. With internal features, matching of the unknown faces is slower (and less accurate) compared with famous faces. No difference in RT was apparent when either the famous or the unknown faces were matched on the external features. All three groups showed this interaction. None of the other F-ratios exceeded the value of 0.87.

4.DISCUSSION

The overall inferior performance of the RH group compared with the LH group and the control subjects, on both the error scores and RTs, is in accordance with the clinical literature. On both indices, the RH group differed significantly from the other two groups, while there was no significant difference between the patients with a LH lesion and the control subjects. This result gives further evidence for the hypothesis that the RH is more involved in face processing than the LH.

Apart from the presence of slower reaction times in the patients with RH lesions, the pattern of the RT results is identical for all three groups. Thus the interaction between face familiarity and use of internal or external features must be considered to be very robust. With respect to the factors Familiarity and Internal/External features, there is no qualitative difference in the processing of faces between patients with a right or a left hemisphere lesion. This points to a efficiency problem in matching faces for the RH patients.

The interaction between Familiarity and Region of the face is comparable with previous findings (Ellis et al., 1979; Endo et al., 1984). There is, however, a difference in the absolute performance pattern. In their experiments, the subjects performed equally well with unknown faces, whether internal or external features were given. In the present study, matching was slower and less accurate with the internal than with the external features, if the faces were unknown. When famous faces were used, the pattern was reversed. In the previous studies, famous faces were recognized better on the internal features whereas in our data there was no difference between matching on either cue. It is possible that this discrepancy is caused by a difference in relative task difficulty between the internal and the external feature conditions in the three studies. If in the present study, for example, the conditions requiring subjects to match internal features with famous and unknown faces had been easier, then the same pattern might have emerged as in the other two studies. A more plausible explanation of the discrepancy is that both previous studies used a recognition paradigm. Compared with recognition, simultaneous matching on the external features might be relatively easier. It is therefore proposed that it is relatively more difficult to memorize (for later recognition) the external than the internal features both with famous and unknown faces.

The contribution of the present data in this respect is to suggest that with external features, there is no significant difference between matching famous and unknown faces, whereas famous faces are matched better than unknown faces on internal features. The fact that this effect shows up on both indices (errors and RTs) rules out the possibility of a trade-off between speed and accuracy. Theoretically, this has three implications. First, famous and unknown faces show different properties, which supports the position that they are (partly) processed in a separate manner. Second, when there is a difference in performance, famous faces are processed more effectively than unknown faces. Finally, the advantage in matching famous compared with unknown faces is restricted to the internal feature cue. Thus famous faces are probably better encoded in terms of these internal features.

With respect to the lateralisation of function issue, our findings clearly indicate that patients with posterior lesions of the right cerebral hemisphere perform less well than patients with left hemisphere lesions and control subjects. Thus there may be grounds for the hypothesis that milder forms of face-recognition disorders in association with unilateral right hemisphere lesions may be found more frequently than the rare and florid prosopagnosias usually attributed to bilateral cerebral damage.

In terms of process analysis, all three subject groups show the same qualitative pattern of performance. These results emphasize the importance of the right hemisphere in face-processing, but suggest that – at least in the experimental conditions described above – both hemispheres use the same mode of processing.

FACE RECOGNITION DYSFUNCTION AND DELUSIONAL MISIDENTIFICATION SYNDROMES (DMS)

A. TZAVARAS, J.P. LUAUTE, E. BIDAULT

1. INTRODUCTION

It is well known, from the neuropsychological literature, that dysfunction of face recognition is common following brain damage. On the other hand, in several psychopathological conditions, handling of the face as a stimulus could be a central problem; i.e. the recognition or identification of one's own face, or of another person's face could be part of the mental dysfunction. Capgras' syndrome is a typical such case. As defined by Critchley (1979), the Capgras' syndrome is "the non-recognition of familiar persons, with the postulation of imaginery differences and the further expressed belief that the real person has been replaced by a double".

This type of phenomenon is also observed in several other syndromes, which are grouped under the label "Delusional Misidentification Syndromes" (DMS), which are frequently associated with each other. It should be recalled that the Capgras' syndrome was initially described as an identification agnosia (Capgras & Reboul Lachaux, 1923) and thus it would be tempting to reconcile it with agnosia for faces as Bodamer isolated and described it in 1947.

However, at a clinical descriptive level, it is known that the two types of disorders were distinguished from each other and could even present opposite characteristics (Luaute et al., 1978, 1982; Bidault et al., in press).

Prosopagnosia, a rather rare clinical phenomenon, has been studied thoroughly only in the last twenty years and several experimental studies have explored the disorders of visual recognition of the human face following brain damage. In almost all cases, the stimulus material (faces) is unknown to the subject. In brain damaged patients, who did not exhibit clinical signs of prosopagnosia, poor performance in various face recognition tests has been viewed as an infra-clinical prosopagnosic disorder (Bruyer, 1983).

According to these findings and hypotheses, poor performance at a face recognition test, a "prosopagnosic symptom", has been proposed as a possible support for the existence of DMS by several authors.

However, the small number of clinical cases that have been studied and the controversial findings of the different studies leave open the possibility of a link between a prosopagnosia-like disorder and DMS. So, from published relevant data, two papers reporting cases with DMS describe normal performance at a face perception test (Bogousslavsky & Salvador, 1981; Synodinou et al., 1977) and two papers report pathological performance at a face perception test (Luaute et al., 1978; Shraberg & Weitzel, 1979).

There is another phenomenon described in neuropsychology, namely reduplication behaviours (Weinstein & Kahn, 1955; Alexander et al., 1979; Dennis, Staton et al., 1982) which may relate to space, time, persons and body, that may be present in the behaviour of DMS patients. Although this analogy is tempting, it should be reminded that patients suffering reduplication phenomena are (a) brain-damaged, and (b) those phenomena are usually not isolated to persons, but also relate to space, time and body. "It is thus likely that the various forms of reduplication are not discrete mechanisms but represent different elements of the basic reduplicative pattern" (Weinstein & Kahn, 1955, p.59).

Finally, we have to take into account, previous observations with DMS patients, who suffered from pathological perception of details, a kind of piecemeal perception of the human face (Luaute et al., 1982).

The present work was designed to verify the following hypothesis: a possible link exists between DMS, prosopagnosia and poor performance in a standard neuropsychological test for face perception.

2. SUBJECTS

The sample consisted of a) The critical pathological population (P1), which involved ten patients who have expressed during an acute psychiatric episode an isolated or an associated DMS. Only two patients (cases No.6 and 8), suffered from a patent organic brain lesion. b) The control groups, one pathological (P2) and one normal (P3), were formed in such a way that for every P1 subject two P2 and two P3 subjects were studied. Care was taken to ensure matching for sex, age and IQ between the three populations. P1 and P2 populations were also matched for clinical syndrome context. All groups were divided into two subgroups according to their IQ level in the following way: first subgroup = IQ $\geq$ 100 and second subgroup = IQ < 100. The total number of subjects and their general characteristics are shown on Table 1.

TABLE 1. Description of the three groups

	Subjects (N)	Male	Female	Mean Age
Pathological group with DMS (P1)	10	5	5	45
Pathological control group without DMS (P2)	20	10	10	45.7
Normal control group (P3)	20	10	10	43.8

Two different studies were carried out, at two different clinical moments for P1; a) an experimental study of face perception during the acute phase with active DMS, and b) performance on the Rorschach Test once the acute phase was over. Some of the results of this study are soon to be published (Bidault et al., in press) so here a new analysis is presented, focussed in neuropsychological data.

3. FACE RECOGNITION
3.1. The Test

An abridged version of the face recognition test presented by Tzavaras et al. (1970) was used. The test consists of six photographs in black and white of front-view male faces, without extra-facial visual cues (7.5 x 9 cm). Apart from the demonstration series consisting of the six photographs, the test is composed by the following four series: a normal series similar to the demonstration set (T1), the original series modified by accessories (T2), or by lighting effects (T3), or by mimics (T4).

3.2. The procedure

All subjects were shown the Face test in a set order (T1, T2, T3, T4); stimuli were presented in a standard randomised order, under two experimental conditions, with a 20 sec delayed short memory with occupied-interstimulus-interval (M1) and immediate perception by matching (M2).

4. RESULTS

Table 2 presents means and standard deviations of performance for all three groups (or six subgroups), to the four subtests (T1 to T4) and to the two experimental conditions (M1 and M2). Performances are presented as correct responses with a maximum score of 6 for all conditions.

Inspection of the results for the normal control group (P3) shows almost perfect scores for all subtests and conditions with the exception of scores for the short memory (M1) conditions and the T2 and T3 subtests for the IQ < 100 (G6) subgroup.

4.1. Statistical Analysis

The analysis of variance was presented in Bidault et al. (in press) which showed that the three experimental groups had different results: subjects of group P3 give the highest performances, subjects of group P1 the lowest, with subjects of P2 being in the intermediate position. The short-term memory experimental condition (M1) is more difficult than the matching perceptual (M2) for all subjects. The performances to the four faces subtests are different with increasing difficulties from the unchanged faces (T1), to mimics (T4), to lighting effects (T3) and to accessories (T2). Two interactions reach significance: T x M (Faces subtests x experimental condition) thus pointing to the fact that performance at the difficult face subtests is more affected by the difficult experimental condition of short memory; and N x M (intellectual level x experimental condition), meaning that subjects with IQ < 100 present poorer performance in the short-term memory task. An analysis of means, between groups and conditions, by student t-test for paired groups, was then performed.

Comparisons shown on Table 3 lead to the following observations. DMS patients with an IQ greater than 100 (G1) differentiate from normal subjects with a similar IQ (G5), only in the relatively easier parts of the Face Perception Test, light and mimics. This may indicate that complication of the task is not sufficient to explain their difficulties.

DMS patients with an IQ less than 100 present by far the poorest performance when compared with subjects in all other four groups.

It is interesting to note that psychiatric patients without DMS and with an IQ lower than 100 (G4), are the only ones that perform poorly in the short-term memory test for normal face, when compared with normal subjects and psychiatric patients without DMS having an IQ greater than 100 (G3). A possible explanation could be that these patients are better motivated when the task is more complicated.

Finally, among normals, the only statistically significant difference between the two subgroups is noted at the rather easier task (light), but only at the most difficult condition (short memory).

5. DISCUSSION

The study of face perception by a standard neuropsychological test, in patients suffering from an acute psychiatric episode and presenting DMS in view of the results of the analyses of variance and the comparisons by t-tests points to the following:

a) The group of normal controls (P3) as expected, presented the better performances at all subtests and at both experimental conditions. The

TABLE 2. Means and SD of performances to the face tests, presented according to two experimental conditions; short memory and matching perceptual and to the four subtests (11, 12, 13, 14). Maximum score of correct responses per subtest = 6

EXPERIMENTAL CONDITION		SHORT MEMORY (M1)				MATCHING PERCEPTUAL (M2)			
EXPERIMENTAL GROUPS (G) FACE SUBTESTS		T1	T2	T3	T4	T1	T2	T3	T4
P1	IQ > 100 (G1)	5,6 (0,55)	4,0 (0,00)	4,6 (1,68)	4,4 (1,82)	6,00 (0,00)	4,8 (1,30)	5,4 (0,89)	5,2 (1,30)
	IQ < 100 (G2)	4,6 (2,19)	2,00 (1,22)	3,2 (0,84)	3,6 (1,95)	5,8 (0,45)	3,8 (1,48)	4,6 (0,89)	4,8 (0,84)
P2	IQ > 100 (G3)	5,8 (0,42)	4,2 (1,40)	4,9 (1,60)	5,6 (0,52)	5,9 (0,32)	5,0 (0,94)	5,6 (0,70)	5,7 (0,67)
	IQ < 100 (G4)	4,6 (1,26)	4,1 (1,37)	3,6 (2,07)	4,5 (1,27)	5,6 (0,97)	5,0 (1,89)	5,4 (0,97)	5,1 (1,91)
P3	IQ > 100 (G5)	5,7 (0,67)	4,9 (1,91)	5,9 (0,32)	5,9 (0,32)	5,9 (0,32)	5,7 (0,48)	6,0 (0,00)	6,00 (0,00)
	IQ < 100 (G6)	5,8 (0,42)	3,7 (1,70)	4,5 (2,01)	5,2 (1,32)	6,00 (0,00)	5,2 (1,32)	5,7 (0,48)	5,9 (0,32)

TABLE 3. Summary of comparisons that reached statistical significance between groups at all experimental conditions. Performances of the second group in each pair of comparisons are always better. Values of Student t-test for paired group. * indicates p <.05, ** p < .02, *** p < .01

			\multicolumn{8}{c}{Task}
			\multicolumn{2}{c}{Normal}	\multicolumn{2}{c}{Accessories}	\multicolumn{2}{c}{Light}	\multicolumn{2}{c}{Mimics}
			M1	M2	M1	M2	M1	M2	M1	M2
G1	vs	G5					**	**	**	
G2	vs	G1			***					
G2	vs	G3			***		*	**	***	**
G2	vs	G4			**					
G2	vs	G5			***	***	***	***	**	***
G2	vs	G6						***		***
G2	vs	G3	***							
G4	vs	G5	**				***		***	***
G4	vs	G6	***							***
G6	vs	G5					*			

subjects of the present study gave comparable performances with the subjects of the control groups used in the initial studies with this face perception test (Tzavaras et al., 1970).

b) The general trend of performances of all three groups present a progressive increase in difficulty among subtests and experimental conditions. So, the short-term memory condition is more demanding than the immediate perception of faces for all subjects, and subtests are ranged according to increased difficulty in the following order: T1 (unchanged face), T4 (mimics), T3 (light effects) and T2 (accessories).

c) In spite of the general trend showing that normal subjects perform better than subjects belonging to the pathological groups, there is a further differentiation among the performances of subjects of the pathological groups, i.e. the DMS subjects are more vulnerable to the different transformations of the target faces with a maximum effect at the accessories subtest (T2).

d) An unexpected finding of our study is the negative influence of IQ < 100 to the performance of subjects belonging to all groups, especially in the short-term memory experimental condition as shown by the analysis of variance (Bidault et al., in press). It is interesting to note that G1 patients when compared to G5 subjects differed, only in the easy parts of the test. There can be no unique explanatory hypothesis about these results for the effect of the IQ on performance that can be found in any published material. If, in addition, we take into account that the splitting of the initial pathological group led to the arbitrary limit value of IQ = 100, the explanation might be even more difficult. There is another factor which, in our view, should be taken into account, namely the attention span of the subjects during the test procedure. Low attention span might interfere with the piecemeal strategy used by DMS patients for the recognition of faces. In any case, new data are neded taking into account current and previous treatments of our subjects (neuroleptics, ECT, etc) especially as they were psychiatric patients.

e) Finally, it is interesting to note that the comments of subjects of the critical pathological group during the performance to the tests are characterised by a speedy, fragmentary judgement which is reminiscent of the confabulated response to the Rorschach test, i.e. responses determined by small details of the pictures rather than responses determined by the configuration which results from the immediate apprehension of the whole picture.

6. CONCLUDING REMARKS

This experiment was designed to study the visual-perceptual status and style of a special group of psychiatric patients who suffer from DMS. As it has already been mentioned, the same question has been put forward by a few authors (including, Christodoulou, 1977; Luaute et al., 1978, 1982 and Shrabert & Weitzel, 1979) in case studies, where there has been a systematic exploration of face recognition. Findings of these studies have been controversial, as in a few of them experimental investigation of face perception has shown normal recognition by DMS patients, whereas in others the performance of such patients was abnormal.

The main advantage of the present study is that the performance of a group of ten DMS patients was compared to that of two control groups, one consisting of normal subjects, and one of non-DMS psychiatric patients.

a. DMS patients show lower performance at the face test when compared to the performances of subjects of both control groups. Their difficulties increase when the task gets complicated by the changes of the target faces, or when memory mechanisms are solicited by the task. So, although it is not possible by clinical observation to state that DMS patients suffer from prosopagnosia per se, their performances at the face test may be considered as an infra-clinical prosopagnosic symptom. This finding can be related to the general observation about "organic", i.e. brain damaged patients; among these patients, the prosopagnosic ones may have a normal performance at a face perception test, whereas the ones that do not present clinical prosopagnosia may show poor performance at a face perception test (Benton, 1980). So, by analogy, we could argue that in DMS patients there might be an "organic" component, the nature of which is difficult to determine at least for the present. However, a systematic investigation into the possibility of existence of organicity in patients suffering from DMS should be undertaken.

b. We should, however, take into account interpretations put forward in related studies, namely the two neuropsychological mechanisms underlying the perceptual behaviour of DMS patients. One is memory disorder, thus assimilating the Capgras' syndrome to paramnesia of reduplication (Alexander et al., 1979). The other is the mechanism of depersonalisation-derealisa-tion, that would place the Capgras' syndrome among phenomena of the "deja vu" and "deja vecu" type, related to temporal lobes pathology (Christodoulou, 1977).

c. Nevertheless, as the main characteristic behaviour of DMS patients is the piecemeal-style perception, the two above mentioned mechanisms are not sufficient to account for it. The piecemeal-style perceptual style reminds us of three phenomena of different order; (i) The analytic way of perceptual functioning of the left hemisphere of right-handed people, thus pointing to a possible dysfunction of the right hemisphere in DMS patients (Bruyer, 1983). (ii) The way children perceive faces up to adolescence, thus pointing to a possible mechanism of regression operating in DMS patients (Bruyer, 1983). (iii) Both clinically and experimentally, the behaviour of DMS patients reminds us of the behaviour of patients suffering from frontal lobe agnosia, as described by Luria (1978).

d. Lastly, the DMS phenomena may relate to another psychopathological phenomenon, namely the "grafted delusions" observed after somatognosic disorders, also labelled "somatoparaphrenia" (Gertsmann, 1942). If this is the case, DMS might be associated with prosopagnosic disorders or connected with a prosopagnosic background. Thus DMS might be called "prosopara-phrenia" by analogy with "somatoparaphrenia". This speculative hypothesis cannot be retained, for at least two reasons: (i). a review of the relevant literature reveals that no prosopagnosic patient was ever deluded over his disorder; and (ii) the postulated clinical characteristics of such "prosoparaphrenia" do not correspond to the DMS as they are described to date.

In order to put in evidence and comprehend the neuropsychological mechanisms operating in DMS patients, the above mentioned interpretative hypotheses should be taken into account and specific studies should be conducted with a greater number of patients.

Acknowledgements: The authors are grateful to Professor Olga Maratos for revising the English version of this manuscript.

9. FACIAL EXPRESSIONS

FACIAL EXPRESSION PROCESSING

N.H. FRIJDA

1. INTRODUCTION

This paper presents a theoretical analysis of the process of recognising facial expressions. That process is interesting in its own right, since it touches upon the general problems of knowing other minds and of social communication. In addition, analysis of facial expression processing may contribute to understanding face recognition generally.

"Recognition of expression" refers to a type of semantic recognition. It involves, not the assessment of familiarity or identity as does face recognition, but recognition of meaning. Recognition of expression implies reference to something else than the expressive pattern as such. To understand the process of recognition, a distinct conception of that "something else" is indispensable. What does the meaning of facial expression consist of?

The question can be phrased in several alternative, equivalent ways. What does the information processed in expression processing consist of? Or: what is it that is recognised when recognising expressions? Or: what is the nature of the coding system onto which expressions are assimilated when they are recognised? Or again: what types of responses are made which give evidence of recognition; because "recognition" may be said to have occurred when the expression stimuli are responded to in differential and systematic fashion.

Answers to these questions can be sought by analysing those recognition-evidencing responses. The first kind of response to consider is labelling: labelling the other person's expression or state. Expressions, or people, are labelled "angry" or "happy" etc. Labelling, however, cannot be considered the most elementary response mode to expression; nor is it a very enlightening one, for the present purpose. For one thing, labelling would not seem to be what people generally do in daily interactions, when they respond to other people's expressions; labelling is a conspicuous response mode only in expression recognition experiments (or similar situations), because there it is what subjects are requested to do, and because they can do little else under those circumstances. For another thing, expressions are also responded to meaningfully by certain preverbal and nonverbal organisms. Most importantly; labelling just begs the question of the nature of expressive meaning, since the words used hide the meanings sought.

There are other modes of response to expression, and which provide more insight in those meanings. Three modes of response can be distinguished. They can be distinguished behaviourally; and also in the verbal statements people give when interpreting expressions. The present distinctions are derived from the protocols of an old experiment in which subjects were presented with a series of brief film fragments, each fragment showing an expressive response; fragments contained the person's head and shoulders only, and thus her facial expression and head position. Subjects were asked to provide free descriptions of that person's "inner state", for each fragment (Frijda, 1953, 1956).

We call the three response modes the contextual mode, the interactional mode and the observational mode, respectively. The three modes, we will argue, correspond to three different types of observational setting, or of relationship between perceiver and perceived; and they correspond to three different "coding systems", or kinds of internal representation, for expressive meaning. All three can readily be manifested at non-verbal levels, and by non-verbal organisms. They may be held to represent more elmentary and more natural ways of responding to expressions than attaching labels, or even the explicit attribution of inner states.

2. THE THREE MODES OF EXPRESSION RECOGNITION
2.1 Contextual mode

In most situations of daily life, a person seen to respond emotionally is seen behaving within an environmental context and as responding to that context: as acting upon it, reacting to it, and modifying his or her relations with it. Expressions are, or are part of, activities of accepting or rejecting an event, pausing to watch it or absorb it, opposing it, etc.

Under these conditions, recognising or "understanding" expression means that the behaviour is seen as fitting the nature of the environmental context; or else that that context is scanned with the expectation of finding a fitting event: a potentially fearful or aggravating or amusing etc. one. Seeing someone get startled makes one look around for the startling event; seeing someone's grief leads to a compassionate "what happened?" One is puzzled and "does not understand" when a fitting event cannot be located. In recognising expression, expression points to a particular feature of the environment.

Alternatively, or complementarily, expression points to behaviour likely to follow. Understanding behaviour as "joy" implies the expectation of continued vivid interaction with the eliciting event; signs of anger elicit the expectation of aggressive outbursts if the event persists, comes closer or presses harder.

Recognising other people's emotions is equivalent to the emergence of the above kinds of expectation; and of course in emergence of those expectations lies the social value of that recognition. "Recognition of expression" consists of accessing the internal representations corresponding with these expectations.

In the expression-recognition experiment referred to the contextual mode of coding and responding is expressed in comments like "she looks the way you look at a small kitten", or "she looks as if on the point of exploding" or "he looks as if has just been told some terrible news". Comments like these appear to come more naturally than categorical labels such as "she feels endearment" or "he looks stunned", they also catch more of the expressions' content.

2.2. Interaction mode

Often, expressions are perceived while the perceiver participates in an interaction with the person observed. Expressions then appear to be coded primarily in terms of their significance for that perceiving subject, as the target of the other person's actions. The other is seen as threatening, or frightening, or intimidating; or as inaccessible, immovable; or as open, reassuring, or appeasing, etc. These terms do not denote feelings in the other; rather, they denote his or her readiness or unreadiness for action towards the subject, or for responding to actions by the subject. Recognition of expression thus is evidenced by that subject's own emotions: his or her feeling of being threatened, frustrated or reassured.

Recognition consists of accessing internal representations corresponding to these emotions, and to the expectations upon which they are based. Verbal statements manifesting this mode of recognition parallel the epithets just given: "she looks in an intimidating way"; or even: "his way of looking makes me feel ill at ease".

One may assume this mode of seeing and coding to be the most primitive one – that of a human infant smiling at a mother's smile, or of an infant monkey frightened by an aggressive monkey face (Sackett, 1966).

2.3. Observational mode

Expressions are sometimes truly observed: watched in detached fashion, and cut loose from an environmental context which they might be responses to; they are seen without the perceiver orienting towards that environment and without his being engaged in interaction with the person observed.

Watching a face or facial photograph is of that nature; so is observing expressions in an expression interpretation experiment; and so is watching a theatrical performance such as ballet; or waiting for things to happen, as when feeding your restive infant; or watching a tightrope walker.

Under these conditions, expressions are coded in terms of one's own experiential and behavioural potentialities. They are recognised as familiar: that is, here, that they are felt as similar to one of the things one oneself could feel or do. Recognition consists of accessing the internal representations corresponding to one's own matching potential. The statements in interpretation experiments manifesting this mode of recognition do refer to feelings, and use the subjective terminology of tendencies and intentions: "She feels tension rising within her"; "he feels inhibited, blocked, cluttered up", "she is abandoning herself to what she hears or sees". On occasion, the mode of coding which underlies such statements translates itself into actual feeling or actually manifesting activation of one's own potential: that is, it translates in emotional contagion, sympathetic experience (suffering with the suffering actor on the screen), or motor mimicry.

Sympathetic experience and motor mimicry are to be considered as manifestations of a particular mode of coding and recognising. They are not sources of recognition, as they were held to be in classical theories of expression perception (e.g. Lipps, 1907). There are several arguments. First, sympathetic experience and motor mimicry do not always occur when expressions are recognised, that is, responded to differentially and systematically. Their occurrence appears very much restricted to the conditions outlined: that is, to conditions which preclude coding in other fashions. Second, motor mimicry is itself an interpretative response. Interpretation of expression, at least to some extent, precedes and does not merely follow it. It cannot be the intermediary for understanding which Lipps and others have seen in it. Several observations support this position. In the experiment on interpreting filmed expressions (Frijda, 1953), involuntary imitations of the expressions shown occurred, and occurred not infrequently. Some of these "imitations" were similar in intent but not in shape to the expressions which triggered them. For instance, seeing a film episode in which the subject clenched and tensed her mouth made an observer involuntarily clench his fists; seeing a sigh of relief made an observer make a smile. In another experiment, subjects were asked to put on the same face as one shown on a slide; the imitations were photographed. The subjects were subsequently asked to verbally intepret the expression seen; the interpretations often differed considerably from the true state of affairs. New subjects then had to judge which of the two descriptions, the true one or the imitator's, best fitted the expression.

Matches were made significantly more often with the imitator's interpretations than with the description of the true state of affairs; this finding supports the point that imitations (voluntary ones, this time) followed interpretation rather than preceded it. Which is not to deny that, on occasion, imitation or empathy is called upon to help in interpretation and understanding.

3. THE NATURE OF EXPRESSIVE MEANING

The above description of the three modes of expression recognition demonstrates that such recognition does not necessarily involve labelling another person's state, nor even attribution of feelings, as classical theories (Lipps's, 1907, or Bain's, 1859) would have it. Recognition can remain at a level of "perception of meaning" and of the emergence of expectations regarding what the other might do or what the environment will contain. The analysis thus accounts for the immediate, intuitive, perceptual character of expression recognition.

The analysis also provides clues as to the nature of the information which the three recognition modes employ; it thus clarifies the meaning of expression and the nature of the information that expression processing processes. That information consists of what the three modes of recognising and coding have in common.

What they have in common is their reference to the individual's relational activity and state of activation — two aspects of momentary state which together be called "state of action readiness" (cf. Frijda, in press). The meaning recognised, first place, and which gives rise to the expectations etc. discussed, is the perceived individual's readiness to act or to react, or not to act or to react; and his or her readiness to relate or not to relate to the environment in some particular fashion. It can be argued (Frijda, in press) that every expressive pattern is the manifestation of a particular kind of action readiness.

This analysis of the meaning seen in expressions implies that expressions are not perceived as mere movements, but as acts or attitudes. They are perceived as stances taken with respect to some event, as modes of behaviour or as parts of such modes. As data for perception, expressions have an "intentional" character ("intentional" in the wider, philosophical sense; cf. Dennett, 1969), implying relationships between a subject and an object towards which that subject orients.

This intentional, relational aspect of expression will be referred to as the "sense" of expression. That "sense" may or may not correspond to some inner feeling or intention (in the strict sense); by itself, it is a category of perceived behaviour.

It merits emphasis that the various forms of "sense" correspond closely to the structural features of the expressive movements. "Sense" and expressive pattern correspond in about one-to-one fashion. "Approach" is forward movement towards an object, "alertness" is manifest activity of eyes or ears; "reserve" is active restraint of forward movement and of sensory receptivity, etc. Further, "sense" is quite close to what is meant by "emotion". "Emotion" can be considered to refer primarily to action readiness (to various modes of action readiness) and "action readiness" to readiness for behaviours with the sense as indicated. "Emotion", in fact, can be considered to denote changes in action readiness as elicited by particular kinds of (to the subject) meaningful events; a given emotion as a given mode of action readiness elicited by a given kind of event. When recognising "emotion", on the basis of expression, cognitions regarding the nature of the eliciting event are added to the perceived change in action readiness.

4. EXPRESSION PROCESSING

"Sense" and facial expression features, as said, closely correspond; they are, however, not identical. "Sense" is a translation of the expression features into behavioural, that is, intentional, terms. Widened eyes and raised brows become passive acceptance of stimuli; forward movement becomes approach, etc. That is to say: in recognising expression the feature of intentionality, the asymmetrical relationship between subject and object, and the recourse to something outside the perceived subject, are added to the perceived facial features as such.

The addition meant is illustrated most clearly by the way eyes are perceived - someone else's eyes. Eyes are not just glossy globes. They appear to look, and they look at something; or they look at you. They show direction. They manifestly link the individual to his environment (in the contextual mode), to you (in the interactional mode) or to the completion of his intentions (in the observational mode).

Modes of looking and not looking are obvious constituents of facial expression. Other expression aspects fit the translation-through-addition scheme ("sense" is features provided with intentional content) equally well. The frightened face - frown, narrowed eyes, hunched shoulders, contracted mouth - is one which shrinks from the environment; the desirous face - eyes opened, head forward - advances; the laughing face shrinks nor advances but still responds to, and remains in contact with the event; sadness's downward glance and drooping features manifests giving up striving and interest in what is.

Now, if this is so - if indeed expression is perceived as facial and other features clad with intentional reference - there are several interesting implications. First, it explains the intuitive process of expression recognition. Sense is grasped whenever the translation is made - whenever links between movement and environment, or movement and its completion, can be made and are made. Second, the translation involves the application of quite general principles. Extrapolations as indicated - from forward movement to approach, from glossy globes to looking - are not tied to previous experience with particular expressions, but to acquisition of grasp of sensory and motor functioning generally. Relevant knowledge can even have been acquired outside the domain of expression, because what is relevant are notions like "forward movement leads to proximity and continued interaction", "glossy globe shift means response to events in that direction", "looking in a certain direction precedes locomotion in that direction", and the like. The meanings involved probably are not all acquired. Being-looked-at, in particular, may well be innately meaningful. Whatever their origin, such meanings serve as principles in the sense that other meanings - subdued looking implies reticence, moderated advance implies softness, etc - are derived from it. Grasping the sense of expressions involves grasping "intelligible" variations of the general principles.

A third implication of the preceding: if expression is perceived as facial features given intentional, relational reference, the process of expression recognition derives from a perceptual process of a quite particular kind. We called it addition, or extrapolation: linking a perceptual given to some other perceptual given as its reference point, or linking a movement to its potential completion. There are few other perceptual processes which appear to involve similar cognitive activity. The only one which comes to mind is the perception of causality (Michotte, 1946), which also links two givens in dynamic and asymmetrical fashion (and which, in fact, readily blends over into intention perception; cf. Michotte, 1950; or else perceptual anticipation of movement completion, as in catching a ball or a fleeing prey.

This kind of perceptual extrapolation, then, might be the particular of expression recognition, and, thus, of the perceptual process underlying it. It may not be involved in all expression recognition. Some expressions probably function as simple signs, and their meaning have been acquired by simple sign-learning; the social smile could well be an example. But most expression recognition would seem to require the process. As to the process's further nature, I have no suggestions to make. Ideomotor theories (like Lipps's) invoke actual or potential evocation of one's own motor schema's; eye-movements may be supposed to be involved; earlier discussions with regard to the nature of perception of causality probably all are relevant here.

5. CONCLUSIONS

Recognition of expression, we have argued, has as its core recognition of the "sense" of expression: of the individual's readiness to relate with and respond to the environment, and the kind of, accepting, rejecting etc., relationship he or she is ready to engage in. Recognition of "sense" and thus of intentionality, derives from extrapolating from the facial and other features to their relations with the environment which they intend or imply. That extrapolation, in turn, derives from general principles of what perceived movements and actions of the senses are for or lead up to; and, in addition, it presumably is based upon the organism's ability to perform such extrapolations. We suggested that extrapolation towards relations between a subject and an object, or the perception of intentionality, set the process of expression processing off from other perceptual processes.

One may venture the hypothesis that this process is not particular merely to expression processing, but participates in face processing generally.

Faces are "expressive", in the sense in which this notion has been used above; their expressiveness is what makes them a separate class of stimuli. Faces look; they are not just inert patterns. Also, faces represent different modes of habitual or current relational readiness or unreadiness, in precisely the same way, and by the same sort of features, as emotional expressions do: drooping eyelids imply weakness of attention, full lips readiness for sensory acceptance at that level, etc. Note that we are not concerned here with whether these features "truly" represent the corresponding relational modes; we are concerned merely with how they strike the eye of the beholder; that is, we are concerned with their "sense".

It is plausible that these expressive features contribute to face recognition, as much as does the more objective coding of these features, or as do the truly objective characteristics. There is some evidence that this is actually the case. In a recent study (Frijda & Kroon, in preparation), subjects were asked to describe the face of some person they were familiar with - a parent, partner or friend - by freely listing characteristics. Items listed were classified as referring to objective characteristics ("dark hair", affective judgements ("handsome") or expressive qualities ("friendly face", "searching eyes"). Expressive qualities comprised 21% of the items listed. They appeared to serve particularly to get at the more individual features of the face. That is, they occurred more frequently in later serial positions in the listing; their average serial position was 7.5 while that of the objective features was 5.2. Of course, the hypothesis that "expressive features" contribute to face recognition is in line with other evidence to the effect that face recognition involves conceptual, and not merely "pictoliteral" representations (Klatzky, this volume). If this is true, and if face recognition does indeed involve some particular faculty which is different from visual pattern recognition generally, the particular faculty may well reside in "intentionality extrapolation" as outlined above. The hypothesis leads to two predictions. First: individual differences in quality of face recognition should correlate with individual differences in quality of expression recognition. Second: both should correlate with performance in perception of causality and/or perceptual anticipation. These correlations should hold particularly when face recognition is seriously disturbed, as in prosopagnosia. But perhaps there is already information available which refutes these predictions.

THE PERCEPTION OF ACTION VERSUS FEELING IN FACIAL EXPRESSION

E.A. SALZEN, E.A. KOSTEK and D.J. BEAVAN

1. INTRODUCTION

After an exhaustive and critical review of studies of facial expression Ekman, Friesen and Ellsworth (1972) concluded that there were seven emotions that could be reliably identified. The seven emotions were Happiness, Surprise, Fear, Sadness, Anger, Disgust/Contempt and Interest. In their own strictly empirical studies Ekman and co-workers have substantiated and minutely delineated the specific expressions for these emotional categories. What they have not done is explain why these particular facial movements and postures are associated with their corresponding emotional states and feelings. In a review and analysis of the perception of emotion in faces Salzen (1981) used ethological evidence and theory to provide an explanation of affective expressions in terms of incipient or thwarted actions and action states. In essence Salzen identified eight classes of behavioural actions representing functional states that may occur in all possible types of motivational state or arousal. These actions, which include facial actions to varying extents, can be equated in an heuristic oversimplification with eight emotions for which these actions are the basic but not the exclusive action tendencies. Table 1 is a revised version of the original tabulations by Salzen (1981) of the hypothetical corresponding Action states, Facial actions, and Emotional states. In this Table Surprise is treated as a special Attention response and is equated with Interest. It is, however, a rather special form of interest being equivalent to "Alarm" responses in animals. Sadness is postulated as a combination of Fatigue with Appetence or Protective actions and may occur in prolonged Desire or Distress respectively. The emotion of Distress corresponds with Protective effort and pain reactions. Many studies of facial expression make no distinctions between Sadness and Distress. Similarly Desire corresponds with Appetitive approach tendencies and is an affective condition which surprisingly is not often included in studies of facial expression. In some studies Interest is recognised as a category of emotion. In the sense that Interest is a prominent element of Desire it may be that these are effectively equivalent categories of emotion. But not all states of Interest can be said to be affective and it might be better to use the term Desire. It should also be noted that in Table 1 the Actions of Weeping and Crying have been placed in the Rejection category. This reflects the similarity of incipient crying and incipient disgust expressions, particularly evident in children. The salivation and lacrimation actions of crying may originally have been part of the disgust reaction in which they serve to counteract and wash away any irritating and offensive substances in mouth, nose and eyes.

This analysis of Action systems in emotional expression was applied by Salzen to a series of Frois-Wittman photographs (Hulin & Katz, 1935) that he had selected as representing various forms of the eight basic emotional expressions. These photos were used to illustrate the association of observable facial Actions with inferred Feeling states or emotions. The present study began as an attempt to see if adults and children, who were not familiar with ethological or psychological theories of facial expression, would perceive and identify these same Action patterns in the same Frois-Wittmann photographs. This test of the recognition of Action

TABLE 1. Eight functional states and facial actions which predominate in
eight classes of emotion according to Salzen (1981).

ACTION STATE	DESCRIPTION OF FACIAL ACTIONS	EMOTIONAL STATES
ATTENTION	Focal stare, frown, tense mouth, head forward, (Interest). Phasic, open eyes, raised brows, open mouth, head back, (Surprise).	Interest, Curiosity, Wonder, Awe, Surprise, Astonishment.
APPETANCE	Lips and tongue protrude, mouth open and attention for oral intake.	Want, Longing, Desire, Cordiality, Caring, Tenderness, Love, Devotion, Greed, Lust.
AVERSION	Gaze aversion, head turning and abduction, eyes close (cut-off or hide).	Fear, Dread, Horror, Panic, Terror.
REJECTION	Raised upper lip, nostril dilation, depression of mouth corners and ejection action of tongue with lower lip eversion. Eyes close or gaze aversion with head turning lateralization of rejection. Salivation, Lacrimation.	Disdain, Contempt, Disgust, Loathing, Dislike, Weeping, Crying.
AGGRESSION	Attention, tense or open mouth of intention bite with expiration (shout).	Grumble, Annoyance, Anger, Rage, Hate, Fury.
PROTECTION/ EFFORT	Eyes close, lips retract, close glottis with expiration (scream) or hold breath and clench teeth (grimace).	Tension, Effort, Pain, Anguish, Suffering, Distress, Screaming.
FATIGUE	Open mouth and glottis for in-halation, flaccid eyelid droop and jaw drop. Residual effort may give frown/oblique brow and clenched teeth with retracted lips.	Tiredness, Listlessness, Despondency, Dejection, Despair, Impotence, Exhaustion, Sadness, Grief.
ACCEPTANCE/ RELIEF	Relaxation of other facial actions especially from Protection (smile) and Scared-Threat (laugh or play face). Relaxation oscillations of muscular, autonomic, and respiratory systems.	Comfort, Security, Satisfaction, Enjoyment, Pleasure, Happiness, Bliss, Joy, Delight, Elation, Rapture, Ecstacy.

systems in facial expression was extended by adding a series of photographs of\ emotional expressions published by Ekman & Friesen (1975) and based on a considerable body of evidence on the validity and reliability of the judged affective character of the facial patterns. The actions in these expressions were determined empirically and have not in any way been considered in terms of potential functional systems. Both adults and children were tested with these two series of photographs for the following reasons. Adults have firmly established cognitive concepts of the conventional categories of emotion and their corresponding facial expressions. They may have difficulty, therefore, in consciously identifying the functional actions underlying or contained in these expressions. Children have to acquire the adult cognitive concepts involved in perceiving emotional categories of expression and in using the appropriate verbal labels. Honkavaara (1961) has provided evidence that the perception of action may precede the perception of feeling in facial expression in children and that the latter is not well developed before 6 years of age. Young children, therefore, may have less difficulty identifying action systems in the photographs of facial expression and more in perceiving and labelling them in terms of affective constructs. Therefore both types of subject were used.

2. PROCEDURE

Two series of photographs of facial expressions were used; one set of ten Frois-Wittman (F-W) photos taken from Hulin & Katz (1935), and one set (E&F) of ten male and ten female photos taken from Ekman & Friesen (1975). The precise identifications of the photographs and the emotional states they are supposed to present are given with the results in Tables 4 & 5. The F-W photos (See Fig. 1) were selected independently by D.J.B. from the set used by Salzen (1981) to illustrate his action analysis. They represent eight emotions with Surprise as an extra form of Interest and with two forms of Happiness (smiling and laughing). The E&F photos included an expressionless "Neutral" photo, and "full expressions" of Surprise, Fear, Sadness and Disgust for both male and female faces, and two each for Happiness (smile and laugh) and Anger (tense- and shout-mouth) for the female. The nearest equivalent pairs of male faces for Happiness were a "smile" and a "grin", and for Anger were "angry eyes" and an "anger-surprise" expression. Desire and Distress were not represented in the book by Ekman & Friesen (1975) from which the descriptions in quotations are taken.

Twenty adults (20 - 30 years) naive to studies of emotional expression and twenty schoolchildren (4.5 - 5.5 years) were successfully tested by E.A.K. Each subject was asked to say "what the man/lady in the picture is doing" for each photograph first of the F-W, and then of the E&F series, with randomised order of presentation within each of the two series. Having completed this test the process was repeated but the subject was asked "what the man/lady is feeling". Responses were free and were tape recorded. For the children the test was split into two sessions a week apart. The recorded labelling responses were transcribed by E.A.K. and D.J.B. into quotations of 1 - 5 words which contained an action or feeling term according to whichever was present. These quotations were the data which were then classified into as many categories as appeared necessary by E.A.S. and E.A.K. on an agreed basis, with the judgements of E.A.K. taking precedence in case of disagreement, because E.A.K. was not party to the hypothesis being tested.

FIGURE 1. Frois-Wittman photographs representing nine categories of emotional expression as follows:- 1. Interest, 30. Desire, 29. Surprise, 46. Fear, 36. Anger, 33. Disgust, 54. Sadness, 9. Distress, 69. and 72. Happiness.

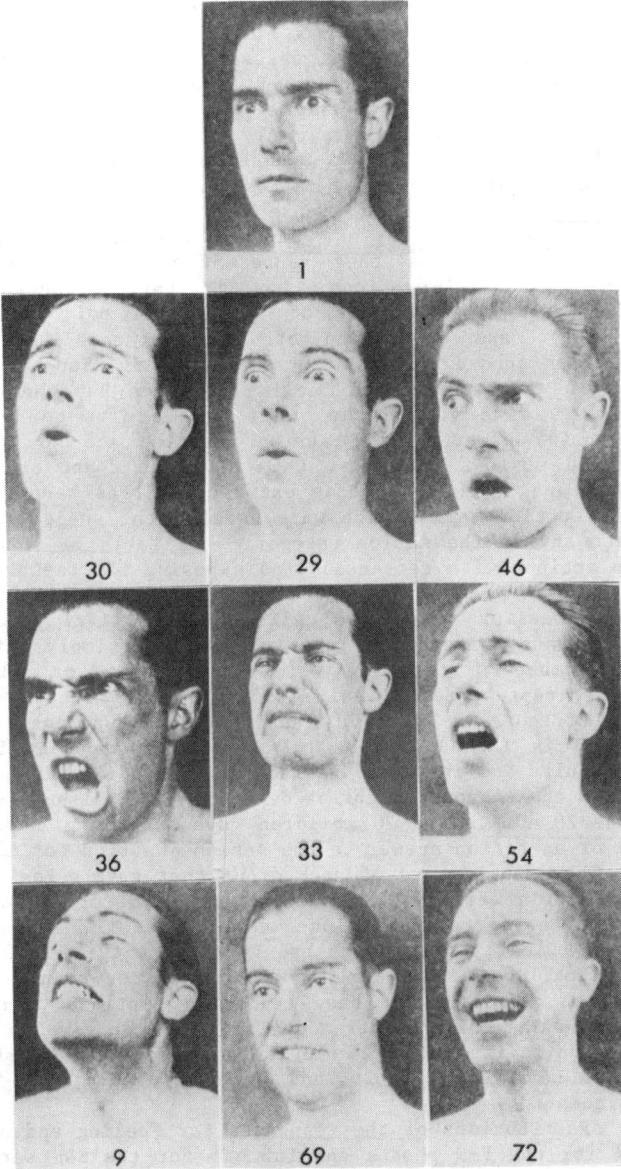

3. RESULTS

Tables 2 & 3 show the Feeling and Action categories that were used in the analysis of the data and the actual terms that made up each category. The numbers in the Tables are the frequencies of occurrence of the terms (or their grammatical variants) over the whole study for F-W and E&F photos combined. Every term whose frequency was at least 5% of the total responses for its category is included in the Tables. The Action categories correspond with those described in Table 1. No subject used any terms corresponding with Desire or Appetence and so these categories are absent from Tables 2 & 3. The Terms Surprise and Pain were always categorised as Feelings when given in response to a Feeling question or when the response phrase clearly indicated that the person was <u>feeling</u> surprise or pain. However both Surprise and Pain were categorised as Actions when given in response to an Action question without being qualified by a feeling phrase. This was done on the assumption that these two terms can refer to specific motor patterns derived from behaviours of "attentive alarm" (Surprise) and of "tense clenched-teeth protective pain reflexes" (Pain). The terms Crying, Smiling and Laughing were always categorised as Actions because they represent specific motor patterns probably derived from "reactions to irritating substances in mouth-nose-eyes" (Crying), relaxation of "protective pain reflexes with screaming" (Smiling), and relaxation of "scared-threat vocalizations" (Laughing). Children tended to volunteer "smiling" or "laughing" for the Happiness photos in response to the Feeling question but these were not classed as Feeling answers. On the other hand adults tended to give "happy" responses in answer to the Action question and so they scored poorly, despite the obvious fact that they could no doubt recognise the actions of smiling and laughing. Three extra categories were required to contain meaningful action terms which were used by the subjects but which did not fall into any of the Action categories of Table 1. One category represents mouth actions with retracted lips exposing the teeth. A second represents descriptions of an open mouth and inferred vocalizations. The third refers to expressions that were called "funny" (i.e. peculiar), or were seen as deliberate grimaces, or that the subject simply imitated. A relatively small number of responses were idiosyncratic or ambiguous in meaning yet clearly represented a Feeling or Action of some character not assignable to any of those in Table 1. These form the "Unclassified" categories included in Tables 2 & 3. It should be apparent from these Tables that both adults and children did indeed volunteer Action terms that are consistent with the Action categories delineated by Salzen (1981).

Not all of the 20 adults and 20 children gave a Feeling answer to the Feeling question or an Action answer to the Action question for each of the 30 photographs. The mean numbers of each group that gave a Feeling answer to the Feeling question were 19.0 for adults and 10.8 for children. The means for an Action answer to the Action question were 11.7 for adults and 12.6 for children. Clearly the adults had no difficulty with the Feeling question, but the children did. Adults were no better than children in answering the Action question, but they tended to continue to reply with Feeling answers while the children were equally likely to give no answer or a Feeling answer when failing to supply an Action term. The children found the Action question no more difficult, and for some photos less difficult, than the Feeling question.

The frequency distributions of the responses for Feeling and Action are given in Table 4 for the F-W photos and Table 5 for the E&F series using the classifications of Tables 2 & 3 and including the Unclassified

TABLE 2. Feeling categories used in Tables 4 & 5. The Feeling terms used by Adults (A) and Children (C) are listed according to their assigned Feeling category. The numbers are the frequencies of the terms and their grammatical variants. All frequencies ≥5% of each category total are included.

EMOTION	A/C	FEELING TERMS used by ADULTS/CHILDREN (A/C)
Neutral	A	Content(15),Nothing(7),Relaxed(4),Vacant(3),Normal(3).
	C	All right(4),Quiet(1).
Interest	A	Puzzled(16),Uncertain(4),Confused(3),Receptive(3),Serious(2), concerned(2),Thoughtful(2),Interest(2).
	C	Serious(4),Interest(1).
Surprise	A	Surprise(57),Shock(16),Disbelief(8),Amazed(4),Astonished(4).
	C	Surprise(17),Amazed(3),Shock(1).
Fear	A	Fear(10),Fright(9),Horror(7),Worried(6),Alarm(3),Suspicion(2).
	C	Frightened(10),Scared(7),Nervous(2),Worried(1).
Anger	A	Angry(57),Annoyed(19),Aggressive(4),Frustrated(3).
	C	Angry(45),Cross(32),Mad(13),Grumpy(11),Annoyed(9).
Disgust	A	Disgust(13),Not impressed/caring/satisfied(11),Distaste(7),Dislike(7).
	C	Dirty(1),Nasty(1),Rotten(1),Stinks(1),Doesn't like(1).
Distress	A	Pain(29),Anguish(3),Distress(2).
	C	Pain(1),Broken bone(1).
Sadness	A	Sad/Sorrow(25),Disappointed(6),Unhappy(5),Depressed(3),Upset(3).
	C	Sad(42),Unhappy(3).
Happiness	A	Happy(73),Pleased(12),Amused(4),Smug(4).
	C	Happy(76),Joy(3),Nice(2).

TABLE 3. Action categories used in Tables 4 & 5. The Action terms used by Adults (A) and Children (C) are listed according to their assigned Functional Action categories. The numbers are the frequencies of the terms and their grammatical variants. All frequencies ≥5% of each category total are included.

ACTION	A/C	ACTION TERMS used by ADULTS / CHILDREN (A/C)
Passive	A	Pose-photo(11),Nothing(6),No reaction(4),No expression(3),Natural(3),Impassive(3),Blank(2).
	C	straight,Straight-mouth/lips/face(16),Close mouth(4),Pose-photo(2).
Attention	A	Concentrate(13),Listen(10),Think(9),Watch(7),Stare(7),Question(6),Look(5),Frown(3).
	C	Look(25),Stare(13),Think(5),Frown(5),Watch(4),Sees something(2).
Surprise	A	Surprise(54),Shock(10),Startle(2).
	C	Surprise(15),Open eyes(3),Show eyes(1).
Aversion	C	Run/move away(3).
Aggression	A	Shout(14),Fight(6),Threat(5),Argue(3),Go to hit(3),Tell off(3).
	C	Shout(35).
Rejection	A	Bad taste/smell(10),Cry(9),Disagree(3).
	C	Cry(9),Sniff/blow/screw nose(4).
Protection/Effort	A	Pain(12),Lift weight(9),Doing sport/running/exercise(6),Strain(3).
	C	Dig hole(1),Exercise(1),Stretch(1).
Fatigue	A	Ending race(3),Exhausted(2),Sleepy(1).
	C	Tired(4),Sleepy(1).
Acceptance/Relief	A	Smile(17),Laugh(11),Greeting(3),Agree(2).
	C	Smile(84),Laugh(27).
Show/Close teeth	C	Show / Close /Brush teeth(13).
Open/Vocal mouth	A	Talk(8),Sing(3),Whistle(2).
	C	Open mouth(13),Talk(7),Whistle(7),Sing(6),Growl(5),Saying Oh(4),Blow(4),Yawn(4),Round mouth(2).
Make/Funny face	A	Making face(12),Funny face(1).
	C	Funny face(10),Imitate face(8),Making face(5),Yuk(2).

categories. The underlined entries are frequencies that are at least 2 SD's greater than would be expected if the responses bore no relation to the categories and so would be distributed equally among the categories. If attention is directed to these more significant entries, then a general pattern emerges for both series of photographs. In general the expected Feeling identifications were made by adults for all the F-W photos except Interest, Desire and Sadness, and for all the E&F photos without exception. The alternative labels given for the F-W Fear photo suggest that this is a compound expression of Fear, Anger and Surprise. Similarly the E&F Anger photos appeared to include Fear and Surprise elements. The children's Feeling labelling was less frequent than that of the adults but was appropriate for Surprise, Anger, Sadness and Happiness in the F-W photos and for all the E&F photos except Disgust and Neutral. In general the expected specific and appropriate Action terms were given by Adults for all the F-W photos except Desire, and for all the E&F photos except Fear, Anger and Sadness. In fact the labels that were actually used for the last three expressions are not inappropriate because the Fear expression has elements of Surprise, the Anger expression is the tense mouth with a frowning stare of Attention, and the Sad expression was labelled as "crying" which we have classified as Rejection. The expected element of Fatigue in Sadness was perceived in the F-W photo but not in the E&F photos. In addition the Adults used Open/Vocal mouth descriptions for the F-W photo of Desire, and Make/Funny face descriptions for the E&F Disgust photos. The childrens' Action labelling largely paralleled the adult responses in the E&F series although the children failed to give any predominant Action for the Fear photos and the Sad photos were labelled as Attention or Passive. They used the Open/Vocal mouth descriptions for Anger and the Make/Funny face responses for the Disgust photos. In the F-W series the children gave appropriate Action labels to Interest, Anger, Disgust and Happiness photos. They used Show/Close teeth responses along with the terms "smile" for the Distress photo and Open/Vocal mouth responses for the rest of the expressions - Surprise, Desire and Fear.

Specific correspondences between the perception of each Feeling and Action category can only be said to have occurred when the same person attaches the corresponding labels to the same photograph. All the occasions where this occurred have been collected from both series of photographs and are presented in Table 6 which shows the direct relationships between Action and Feeling categories independent of the hypothetical nature of the expressions of the individual F-W and E&F photographs. The underlined numbers in Table 6 are at least two SD's greater than the numbers that might be expected if all the Action categories were equally likely to be the associated with each Feeling category. Table 6 shows that for Adults there is a reasonable correspondence between the Action and Feeling categories for Passive with Neutral, Attention with Interest, Surprise with Surprise, Aggression (primarily 'shouting') with Anger, Rejection (primarily 'bad taste/smell') with Disgust, Protect/Effort (primarily 'pain' and 'effort') with Distress, and Accept/Relief (primarily 'smile' and 'laugh') with Happiness. These are all consistent with the hypothesis of Salzen (1981). Sadness is coupled with Rejection and not Fatigue as the original hypothesis would suggest. It would seem that the E&F Sad expression was seen as incipient crying and it is suggested that this should be classed as a Rejection action. If the element of Fatigue is present it is clearly not the predominant feature in the E&F photos, but some Fatigue responses were made to the F-W photo for Sadness. The Table also shows that Fear was coupled

TABLE 4. Feeling and Action responses of 20 adults and 20 children to 10 Frois-Wittmann photographs (Hulin & Katz, 1935). The column headings are the photograph number and its assigned emotional character. Table entries are the numbers of subjects giving responses classified according to Tables 2 & 3. Underlined entries are at least 2 SD's greater than expected for an equal distribution across all Feeling or all Action categories for each photograph.

F-W PHOTOGRAPH	1 Int A	1 Int C	29 Sur A	29 Sur C	30 Des A	30 Des C	46 Fear A	46 Fear C	36 Ang A	36 Ang C	33 Disg A	33 Disg C	9 Dist A	9 Dist C	54 Sad A	54 Sad C	69 Happ A	69 Happ C	72 Happ A	72 Happ C
FEELING																				
Neutral	6	3																		
Interest	3	3	1					1												
Surprise	1		18	4	4	3	1		1		2									
Fear	4	4	1		2	1	6	3	2			5								
Anger	1						2		20	10	9									
Disgust							5	5		1	5	7	1							
Distress						3	1						15		1					
Sadness						2					3				11	3				
Happiness		2		3	2												15	7	20	13
Unclassified	2	2			2	1								3			2	1		
ACTION																				
Passive	3	1			1															
Attention	8	12	1		1	2	2	3									2	2		
Surprise	4			11	1	2	1													
Aversion							3	3				1		1						
Aggression	1		1		1		2		9	8	2	6	2		4	2				
Rejection																				
Protection/Effort				1						3	3		16		7	5				
Fatigue																				
Acceptance/Relief														1			3			
Show/Close teeth			2										5	6	5	6	10	4	7	17
Open/Vocal mouth				8	5	9		5					1	1	1					
Make/Funny face	2	1	3		1	2	1				1				1	2	1	2	2	1
Unclassified		1											2		2				1	1

TABLE 5. Feeling and Action responses of 20 Adults and 20 Children to 10 male and 10 female facial expression photographs taken from Ekman & Friesen 1975. The column headings are the Figure number and intended emotional character of the expressions. Table entries and underlinings are the same as in Table 4.

E&F PHOTOGRAPH	32B/45C		32A/33A		11B/11A		22A/22B		33A/42A		40/42B		29B/30		60B/60A		44A/50A		44B/50B	
FEELING	Neut A	C	Int/Ang A	C	Sur A	C	Fear A	C	AngA A	C	AngB A	C	Disg A	C	Sad A	C	HapA A	C	HapB A	C
Neutral	**21**	3	1	2												1	5			
Interest	5	2	**14**				1													
Surprise					**38**		8	2												
Fear					5	8	**25**	2	1											
Anger		4	10	14			4	6	**24**	**24**	**26**	**18**	2	13						
Disgust			1	4			2			2		1	**30**	7	1	4				
Sadness				1			5							2	**30**	**22**				
Happiness																2	**34**	**23**	**39**	**13**
Unclassified	2	3	2	3	1	2	3	2	3		2		4	2	4	1				
ACTION	A	C	A	C	A	C	A	C	A	C	A	C	A	C	A	C	A	C	A	C
Passive	**20**	10	5	3		1		1	1	3		2	1			4	2	3		3
Attention	**15**	5	5	**21**	4	5	4	3	5	5	2		1	3	4	6	2	4		3
Surprise			1	2	**31**	9	2	3	1	2	1							1		
Aggression						2		3			**13**	**14**		5		5				
Rejection																				
Fatigue																				
Acceptance/Relief		**8**		1		2		4		1				1	1	2	12	**27**	12	**32**
Show /Close teeth						4		3		3				2				1		1
Open/Vocal mouth	1	1		1	1	4	2	2	2	4	1	2	2	5	1		1		1	
Make/Funny face						3		3		1		2		1		1				
Unclassified	1	3			1	3		3		3		1		1		1				1

with the Action of Surprise rather than with Aversion which the hypothesis requires. However, the E&F photos of Fear have eyes that could be seen as Surprise and also lack any clues to a withdrawal action. The equivalent F-W photo has a lateral withdrawal action but it too has wide-open eyes as in Surprise. Attention labels were used not only in association with the Interest labels but also with Neutral and Anger. The latter association may reflect the frown and stare element in the tense-mouth Anger photos of the E&F series since terms such as 'frown', 'stare' and 'glare' were classed as Attention actions in order to maintain consistency and objectivity rather than make inferences as to the Aggressive nature of these attention responses. Clearly, intense focal attention is part of incipient attack states and the conjunction of Attention and Anger might be expected. The correspondences in Table 6 for the childrens' responses are less evident, largely because there are so few instances. In fact few children were able to give both a Feeling and an Action label to the same picture. The children varied in their ability to offer Feeling labels, from being able to label very few to almost all of the expressions. The significant Action category entries in Table 6 for the emotions of Surprise, Anger, and Happiness correspond well with those used by adults. In addition the children used Open/Vocal mouth and Make/Funny Face responses with the Anger judgements.

4. DISCUSSION

As expected adults had no difficulty in supplying unequivocal and appropriate Feeling emotional labels for the photographed expressions with the exception of Desire. Many of the children had great difficulty in supplying Feeling or emotional labels but Happiness, Anger and Sadness were the more frequently identified emotional expressions while Disgust, Neutral and Desire were not named. Yet the children were slightly better at giving Action terms than Feeling terms and as good or better than were the Adults. Honkavaara (1961) found that 3 - 4 year old children gave more correct action answers to photographed expressions when asked "Happy or Sad?" and then "Laughing or Crying?", and she concluded that perception of action precedes comprehension of expression in development. Izard (1971) has shown that children discriminate emotions earlier than they can label them. He found that recognition of Anger, Enjoyment, Surprise, and Fear developed fastest, with Disgust and Contempt the slowest, and Interest and Distress falling between them. The present results for children match this finding closely. Much earlier Gates (1923) found that children had increasing difficulty in recognising Laughter, Pain, Anger, Fear, Surprise and Scorn. But what is important is that the recognition of expression that occurs before emotional labelling develops must involve perception of action as Honkavaara proposed and the present results confirm. Furthermore the actions perceived are the types of action outlined by Salzen (1981). Both adults and children gave Action terms that could be assigned to seven of the eight categories proposed by Salzen. Furthermore, these categories were used in a manner consistent with the hypothesized relationships between Action categories and the Emotional character of the different expressions. In those instances where adults were able to give both Action and Feeling labels to the same photos there was a good correspondence with the hypothesized pairings, i.e. that Action and Feeling categories appear to be related in the manner of Table 1 with the exception of Fatigue and Sadness, and of course the absence of Appetence and Desire. These two exceptions have been considered in detail in the Results where possible explanations were outlined. In summary it was suggested that

TABLE 6. Correspondence of Action and Feeling categories. The categories refer to Tables 1, 2, & 3. The Table entries are the numbers of occasions that the corresponding Action and Feeling terms were given by the same subject to the same photograph. Underlined values are at least 2 SD's greater than an equal distribution of frequencies across all the Action categories for each Feeling category or Emotion.

ACTION / FEELING	Neut		Int		Sur		Fear		Ang		Disg		Dist		Sad		Happ	
	A	C	A	C	A	C	A	C	A	C	A	C	A	C	A	C	A	C
Passive	_18_	2	3						1	3					2	2	6	4
Attention	_6_	1	_13_	1	5	3	2		_9_	_8_					4	3	5	3
Surprise	2	1	1		_42_	6	_6_		1	1	3				1	2	1	
Aversion					1				5	1	3		4	1	1		1	
Aggression			2		1	1	1	1	_19_	_10_			1	1				
Rejection											1				_10_	1		
Protection/Effort						1		1	3		_12_		_15_	2				
Fatigue																		
Acceptance/Relief				1	1					1	1			2		1	_29_	_31_
Show/Close teeth			1		2	3		1	1		1					1		2
Open/Vocal mouth	2				4	2	2	1	1	_8_	3				1	2	1	2
Make/Funny face															1		1	2
Unclassified	1				5		2	1	4	4	2	4	1	1	1	1	3	3

recognition of Appetence and Desire may be dependent on knowledge of a goal or appeted stimulus. In the absence of this information this expression may be interpreted simply as Interest because of the Attention element. The Sadness expression has been given the Action category of Rejection because it was labelled as incipient crying which we regard as a Rejection action. There is a confusion in the use of the term Sadness. In the cry expression of the E&F photograph the term Sadness is applicable in the sense of Unhappiness. The F-W photograph for Sadness did produce some Fatigue responses and here Sadness is applicable in the sense of Despair. It is this latter connotation of Sadness that we would consider is related to Fatigue.

Of course Action terms were not confined to their corresponding Feeling identifications and this should be expected since composite and conflicting action states were invoked by Salzen to explain the full range of naturally occurring emotional expressions and states. It is not surprising, therefore, that Attention and Surprise actions were frequently used for Anger and Fear expressions since such actions may well be present in these expressions in addition to the incipient Attacking and Retreating actions respectively. Furthermore, in the critical Action x Feeling pairings in Table 6 Attention appears as a significant action for Neutral and Anger feelings as well as for Interest. The Action responses that were not assignable to the eight functional categories were Open/Vocal mouth action and Make/Funny face. These occurred significantly in relation with a specific Feeling label only for children in the case of Anger (c.f. Table 6). A few children were able to give both Action and Feeling labels significantly but only for Anger, Happiness and to a lesser extent Surprise. This matches the early development of recognition of these emotions claimed by Izard (1971).

In conclusion, Tables 4 & 5 show that the adult Action labels were not simply inferences made after identifying an emotional expression, because they are similar to the Action labels used by children who were often unable to make the emotional identification. The data also show that the Action terms volunteered by these unsophisticated subjects correspond with seven of the eight categories of Action identified by Salzen as the constituent elements in the perception and identification of emotional expressions. Table 6 shows that five of these seven Action categories were each associated with particular inferred Feeling categories of emotion as hypothesised. It must be admitted that most of the Action patterns responsible for the significant entries in Table 6 are the rather obvious specialised patterns of Surprise, Crying, Smiling/Laughing, Shouting, Pain and Nasty taste/smell. Some of these patterns are generally believed to be ritualised emotional displays evolved from other original functional patterns (c.f. Salzen 1981). Therefore the demonstration of their correspondence with specific feeling states may be regarded as trite or as truism. But as Honkavaara (1961) has shown, even Laughing and Crying may not be synonymous with Happiness and Sadness for young children. And such specialised Action displays shade into the less obvious i.e. less ritualized Action/Feeling combinations shown in Tables 4 & 5 so that it could be said that the present study has produced results that were not all totally predictable without recourse to the analysis of Action in Emotion outlined by Salzen (1981). In fact the analysis cannot be tested properly by using still photographs of "en face" expressions with no clues as to the movements of the whole head, let alone of the whole body, in relation to the stimulus sources. Indeed Ekman & Friesen (1975) in constructing the series of photographs which we have used note (p. 17) "We decided to leave out the primitive forms of some of the emotional expressions - that is the most extreme, least controlled versions of some of the emotions. These primitive expressions, which some scholars have said are the innate forms of emotions, are rarely shown except by an infant or young child, or by an adult under unusual and extreme distress. When they are seen they are readily understood. Their message is obvious and their message is almost always repeated in a simultaneous voice sound" We suggest that using E&F photos lacking some of these primitive expressions and their voice sounds provides a severe test of Salzen's analysis and that the outcome is not unfavourable to it, supporting the view that the socialised expressions described by Ekman & Friesen are indeed based on primitive expressions which are understandable as specific action patterns belonging to one or more of the categories defined in Table 1 and explained in more detail in Salzen (1981).

TOWARDS THE QUANTIFICATION OF FACIAL EXPRESSIONS WITH THE USE OF A MATHEMATIC MODEL OF THE FACE

I. PILOWSKY, M. THORNTON, B.B. STOKES

1. INTRODUCTION

This paper reports on an approach to the quantification of facial expressions based on a microcomputer. It is predicated on the assumption that it should be possible to relate any individual facial expression to a number of 'pancultural expressions'.

We have developed a mathematical model of the face so that digitised information from a photograph allows a line drawing of 'essential' information to be generated. As well, measures are derived based on distances between facial landmarks. These are normalised by dividing them by a distance between fixed facial points. The size of these measures indicate the distance between landmarks, and thus the degree of action of facial muscles.

With this method, facial expressions can be presented as a series of measures, and offer a basis for studying the onset and offset of individual expressions over time, as well as a method for delineating more quantitatively the differences between expressions. The line drawings can also be used to obtain judgements of facial expressions, based on facial data from which information concerning sex, age, etc. has been removed.

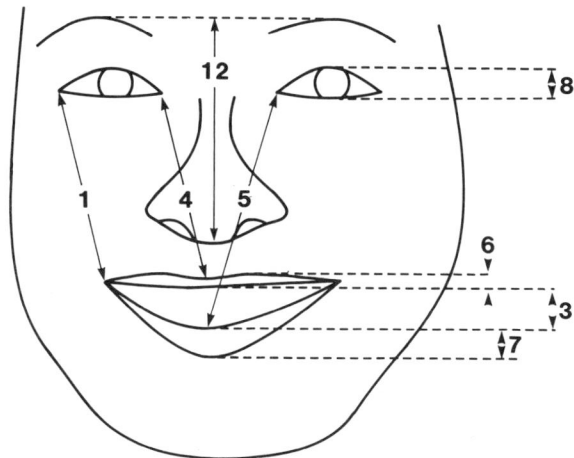

VERTICAL MEASURES

1, **4**, **5**, **8** and **12** are measured on each side of the face, and averaged.

2. MEASUREMENT OF EXPRESSIONS

To date, the most systematic approach to measuring facial emotions has been that of Ekman and Friesen (1976) who have developed a method for scoring the activity of the facial muscles which subserve these emotions. While this technique represents a considerable advance, it has the disadvantage of requiring trained raters to carry it out, and of not providing a direct quantification of the emotion being displayed, but rather of the muscle activities involved.

In an attempt to facilitate the study of facial expressions, we have been developing a computerised method based on a mathematical model of the face (Thornton, 1979; Thornton & Pilowsky, 1982; Pilowsky, Thornton & Stokes, 1985).

Our approach is influenced by the observation that certain facial expressions (fear, anger, sadness, happiness, surprise, disgust) are pancultural phenomena (Ekman & Friesen, 1971). In the light of this finding, the possibility arises of using such expressions as templates against which to match any facial configuration. In other words, it becomes theoretically possible to quantify the extent to which any given facial expression matches any one of these fundamental expressions.

3. METHOD

Against this background, a mathematical model of the face has been developed which allows the quantification of facial expressions (Thornton & Pilowsky, 1982). Using the model involves the digitising of up to 100 specified facial points from a photograph, on to a graphics terminal. Curves are then drawn through the points by the computer using a B-spline technique, thus generating "anonymous" line drawings of the face which can be manipulated by mathematical "muscloids". These "muscloids" are simply lines joining specific points, and represent the actions of muscles. By

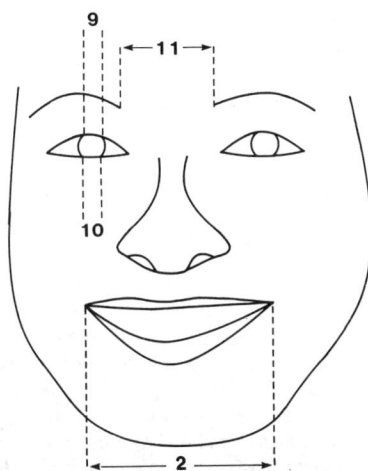

HORIZONTAL MEASURES

9 and **10** are measured on each side, and averaged.

FIGURE 2. Horizontal face measures

"contracting" or "relaxing" these "muscloids" we are able to produce graded series of facial expressions (Thornton & Pilowsky, 1982). The line drawings, whether unchanged or modified by muscloid action, make it possible to obtain observer judgements of facial expressions, when only the essential features are available, i.e. without information concerning identity, sex, age, social class, etc.

In addition, we are seeking to establish the relationships between certain facial measures and specific expressions, beginning with the smile. The measures are distances between key facial "landmarks" and are shown in Figures 1 and 2, classified as "vertical" or "horizontal". Each measure is normalised by dividing by a constant "vertical" or "horizontal" measure, shown in Figure 3. Thus the raw distances between landmarks are divided by the appropriate reference distance to compensate for head movements and to facilitate comparisons between different subjects.

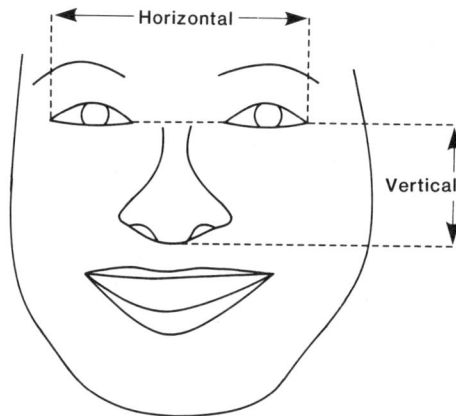

FIGURE 3. Reference measures

4. QUANTIFICATION

In order to establish which measures have the closest relationship to a particular expression, we can correlate specified distances with the degree of an expression by digitising a series of faces taken from one expression sequence. This is illustrated in Figure 4 which shows the changes in three measures during the course of a smile lasting approximately three seconds. The measures (with their identifying numbers in parentheses) are Mouth Width (2), End-Lip-Raise (1) and Eye-Opening (8). As can be seen, Mouth Width increases, and the distance between the outer corner of the eye and the corner of the mouth (End-Lip-Raise) decreases, as the smile emerges. Eye opening is maximal at first, but then decreases, with two blinks evident. As might be expected, the correlations between the first two measures and degree of smile are very high (r = 0.9). (See Table 1).

TABLE 1. Correlations between degree of smiling and face measures (N = 10)

Face measures	r	p
1	− 0.85	0.002
2	0.82	0.004
3	0.30	ns
4	− 0.79	0.006
5	− 0.30	ns
6	0.24	ns
7	− 0.90	0.000
8	− 0.73	0.016
9	− 0.18	ns
10	0.71	0.022
11	0.58	ns
12	− 0.77	0.009

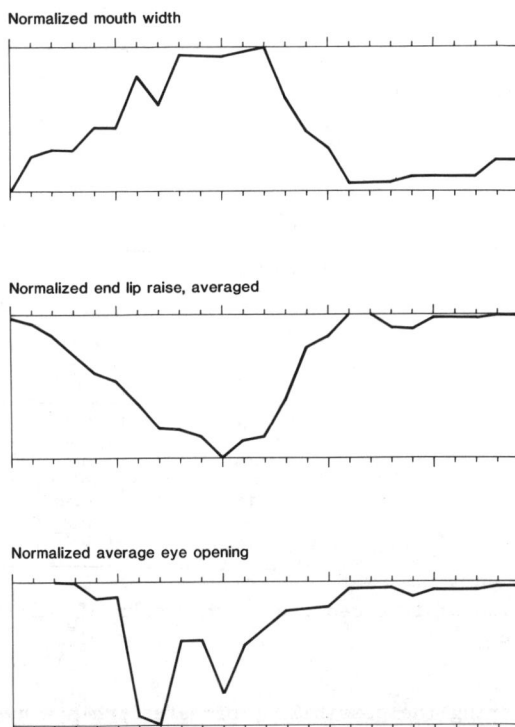

Normalized mouth width

Normalized end lip raise, averaged

Normalized average eye opening

FIGURE 4. Changes in 3 face measures sampled on 25 occasions during smile sequence (3 seconds)

Figure 5 includes the facial measures (for ease of reference) and the correlation value of each measure with the degree of "intensity" of smiling. As can be seen, the measures with highest correlations with the degree of smiling, are lower lip thickness (– 0.9), mouth width (.82), and end–lip–raise (– 0.85).

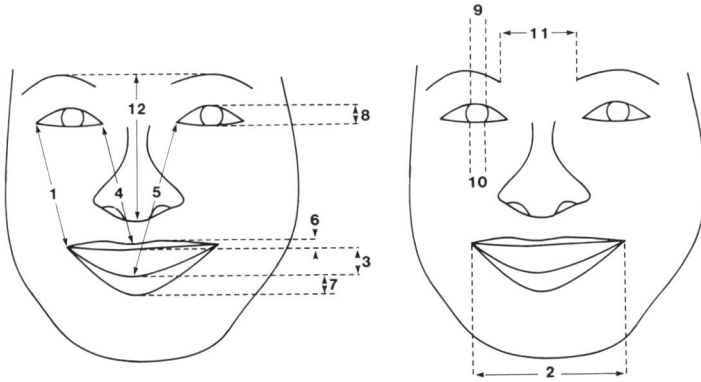

Spearman correlation coefficients of degree of smiling and face measures. (N = 10)	Face measures	r	sig r
	1	-0.85	0.002
	2	0.82	0.004
	3	0.30	n.s.
	4	-0.79	0.006
	5	-0.30	n.s.
	6	0.24	n.s.
	7	-0.90	0.000
	8	-0.73	0.016
	9	-0.18	n.s.
	10	0.71	0.022
	11	0.58	n.s.
	12	-0.77	0.009

FIGURE 5. Correlation of face measures with degree of smiling

We are also exploring the possibility of establishing threshold values for the presence of a smile, i.e. a facial expression which will be perceived as a smile. Figures 6 to 8 show face measure values in 10 smiling faces as compared to 10 neutral faces. It is clear that the measures which distinguish rest are the "lower eyelid iris intersect", "mouth width",

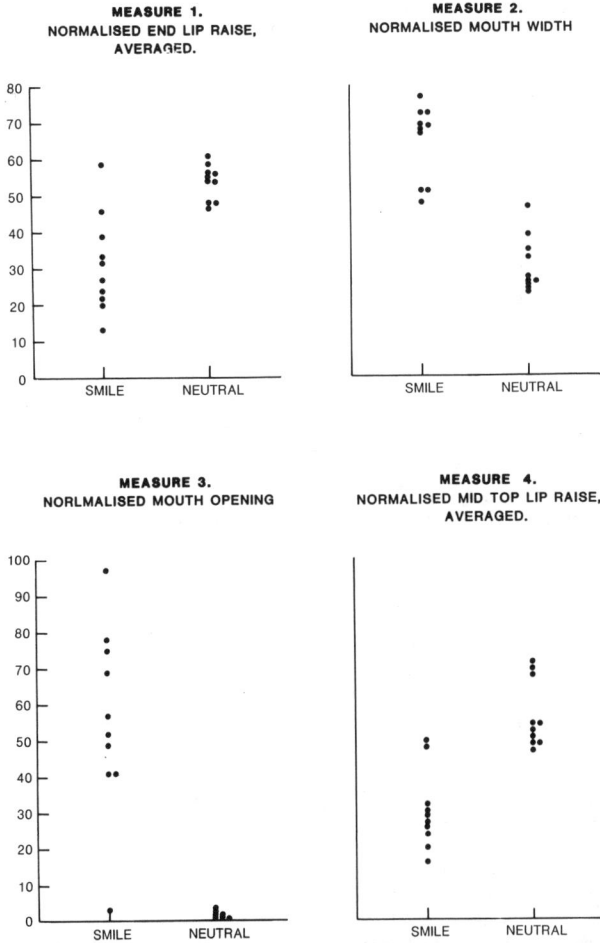

FIGURE 6. Scattergrams comparing face measure values in smiling and neutral faces (measures 1-4)

end-lip-raise" and "mouth opening". This does not, of course, mean that any one of these values will be specific for a smile. It will be necessary to establish which are more specific and which combination of measures will maximise the probability of the value referring to a smiling face.

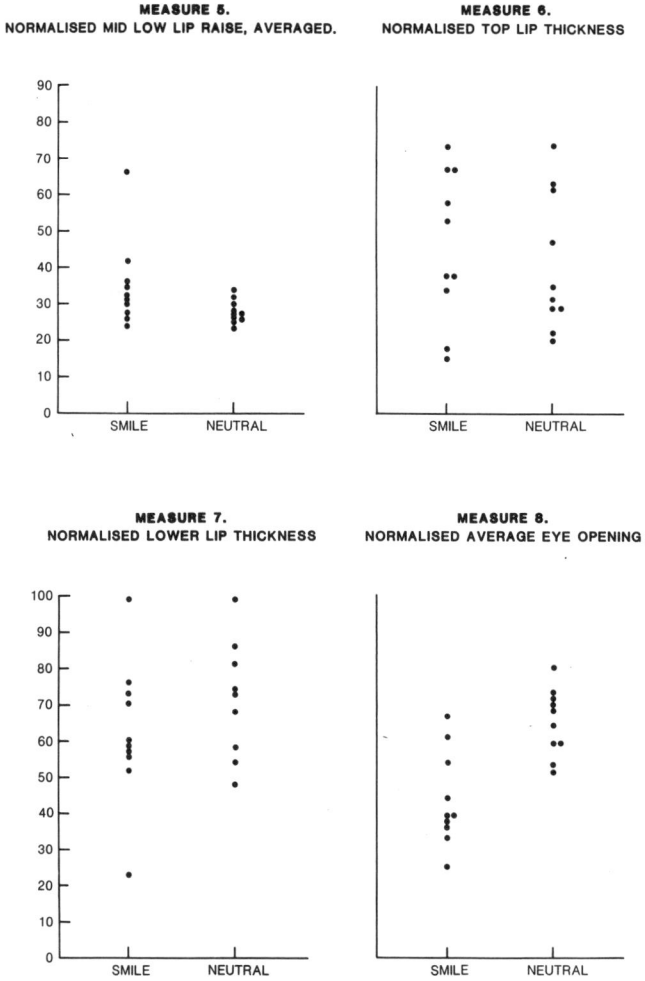

FIGURE 7. Scattergrams comparing face measure values in smiling and neutral faces (measures 5-8)

5. CONCLUSIONS

In this paper we have described an approach to the quantification of facial expressions with the use of a microcomputer. This method obviously has considerable potential for use in a number of contexts. The following constitute a few of the possibilities:

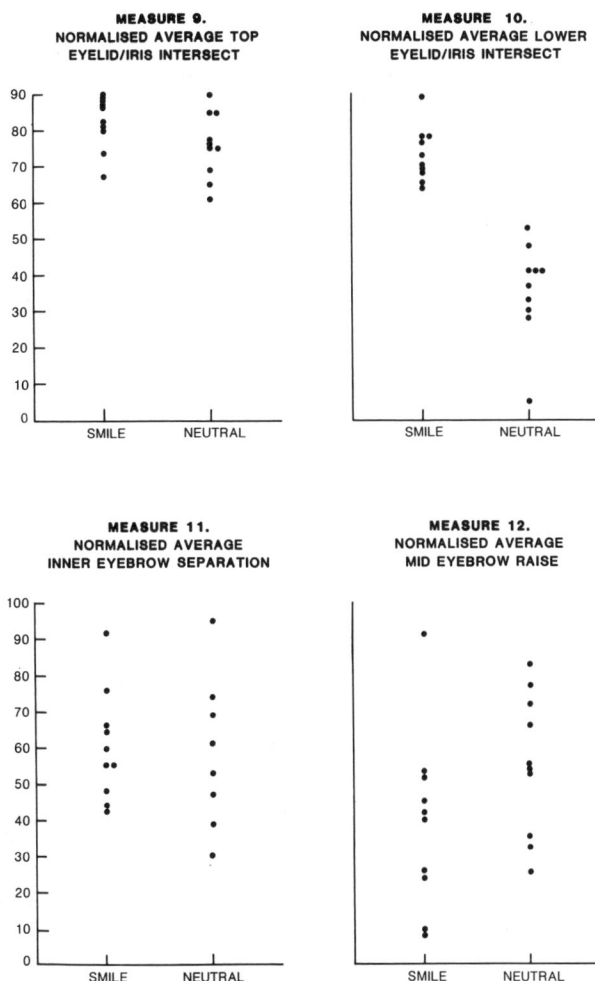

FIGURE 8. Scattergrams comparing face measure values in smiling and neutral faces (measures 9-12)

1. Establishing the minimal information required to detect a facial expressions.
2. Estimating the extent to which a particular facial configuration represents a specified expression.
3. Establishing "norms" for particular expressions in terms of facial measures.
4. Developing a taxonomy of facial expressions based on facial measures.
5. Studying the range and mobility of facial expression in medical conditions known to impair emotional display (e.g. Parkinson's disease, depression).

6. Monitoring changes in facial expression and mobility during the course of treatment.
7. Studying the emergence of facial expression in infancy.
8. Investigating asymmetries in mouth movements which may be related to hemispheric linguistic dominance.

IS THE FASTER PROCESSING OF EXPRESSIONS OF HAPPINESS MODALITY-SPECIFIC ?

P. FEYEREISEN   , C. MALET & Y. MARTIN

1.INTRODUCTION

Like the comprehension of verbal, written, or pictorial material, the processing of facial expressions of emotions involves several cognitive operations (Frijda, 1969). This behavior may be disrupted by brain lesions in association with various disorders and, accordingly, diverse interpretations have been given to the impairments of facial expression comprehension (Feyereisen, in press): for example, the deficit could be related to other perceptual disorders in the visual modality or to amodal disorders of emotional processing.

In fact, cognitive mechanisms involved in the recognition of emotion are still inadequately described (Feyereisen & de Lannoy, 1985). For instance, little attention has been given to the consistent emotion category effect in recognition studies: higher percentages of correct responses are observed for happy faces, both in children (Reichenbach & Masters, 1983; Felleman et al., 1983; Bullock & Russell, 1984) and in adult subjects (Bassili, 1979; Carlson et al., 1983; Kirouac & Doré, 1984; see Table 4.4 of Ekman, 1982, for review of previous studies). This advantage is also observed with the response time as the dependent variable (Ducci, 1981; Kirouac & Doré, 1983). A similar emotion category effect showing a consistent advantage of happy expressions in percentage of correct responses and in response time is regularly noted in neuropsychological studies with lateral presentation of facial stimuli to normal subjects for different tasks: semantic decision on target emotions (Ladavas et al., 1980; Pizzamiglio et al., 1983; Stalans & Wedding, 1985), same/different judgments (Strauss & Moscovitch, 1981, Exp. 1, ANOVA on "type of affect"; Thomson, 1983), selecting the side of the emotional face (Reuter-Lorenz & Davidson, 1981; Reuter-Lorenz et al., 1983; Duda & Brown, 1984), and naming or intensity rating (Hirschman & Safer, 1982).

Several hypotheses could account for such an advantage of happy faces: 1) The size of the emotional set: A two-stage categorization process would first distinguish positive and negative expressions, then apply finer distinctions to the primary emotions. As there are fewer positive emotions than negative ones, the chance of error is reduced. 2) The visual properties of the happy faces: Happy expressions would either be simpler, in terms of the number of action units involved, or more salient than other expressions. The advantage of happy expressions would be then restricted to the facial modality. 3) The conceptual organization of the emotional field: The pleasant-unpleasant dimension would be the major structuring axis of the emotional field, whatever the modality of the emotional expression: facial, postural, vocal, or verbal. Happiness would then be the unmarked pole of that axis and thus the simplest to process.

The aim of the present study is to compare happy and sad expressions in two modalities, verbal and facial. Two tasks were devised: emotion categorization and same/different judgments.

2. CATEGORIZATION TASK
2.0. Introduction
In a pilot study, 24 subjects (12 female and 12 male students) first classified as "pleasant" or "unpleasant" words expressing positive or negative emotions and faces with happy or sad expressions presented in a mixed list of words and faces. The response times (RTs) were recorded. In the second condition, the subjects rated the same stimuli on a seven-point pleasant/unpleasant scale. Main effects of modality (words vs faces) and emotion (happiness vs sadness) were observed with the correct RTs and the ratings as dependent variables. The interaction between these two effects was significant in the judgment condition only, the two sets of words receiving equal rating scores on the intensity scale, whereas the happy faces were judged as more expressive than the sad ones. Thus, words referring to happiness were classified faster although no difference appeared in the judgment condition. In the present study, a new sample of subjects classified another series of words and faces. A methodological modification was made by presenting blocks of words and faces.
2.1. Method
Subjects were 16 female student volunteers, 20 to 25 years old, native French speakers.

The stimuli were 16 words of six to eight letters long expressing happy states (heureux(-se), content(e), amusée, radieux(-se), épanoui(e), réjoui(e), jovial(e), allègre) or sad states (sombre, abattu(e), maussade, morose, affligé(e), peinée, éploré(e), chagriné) and 16 facial expressions from the Ekman & Friesen (1975) series (4 women and 4 men, with happy and sad expressions). The stimuli were presented until the subject responded.

These words and faces were presented twice in blocks of 32 slides, each block preceded by eight practice trials. The order of the blocks was balanced across the subjects.

The instructions were as follows: "You will see slides of happy and sad expressions, facial or verbal. Press the plus key if happy, the minus key if sad with the index finger of the left and right hands". The position of the two keys was balanced across subjects.

2.2. Results
2.2.1. Global analysis. Four-way ANOVAs (mixed models) were used to determine the influence of order of blocks, modality, emotion, and presentation (first vs second). The subjects' means of correct RTs were first computed. Main effects of emotion and modality were qualified by an order of blocks-by-modality-by-emotion interaction ($F_{1,14} = 9.32$, $p < .01$): see Figure 1. RTs were also faster in the second presentation than in the first, but this effect did not interact with any others. The same results were obtained with an analysis of the median RTs of the subjects.

Stimuli mean RTs were then computed across subjects. A new ANOVA showed a main effect of modality qualified by a modality-by-emotion-by-group of subjects interaction ($F_{1,28} = 10.73$, $p < .005$). Thus, the results of the first analysis were replicated.

Unexpected was the absence of difference between faces with happy and sad expressions. In order to check this result, and to verify the intuition of a differential processing of male and female faces, an analysis was conducted on facial stimuli only.

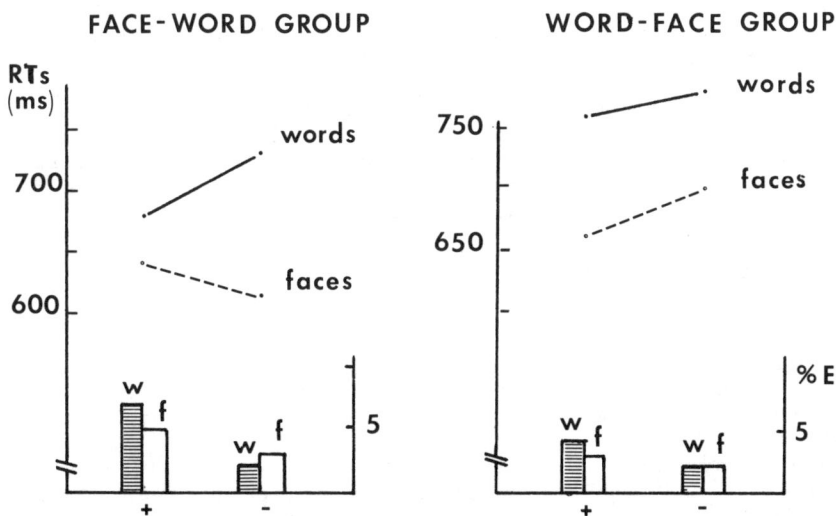

FIGURE 1. Mean categorization times and error percentages for words and faces expressing happiness (+) or sadness (-): the group-by-modality-by-emotion interaction.

2.2.2. Categorization times for faces. A four-way ANOVA (mixed model) was used to analyze the influence of order of blocks, sex of the model, emotion, and presentation (first vs second) on the median RTs of subjects. A main effect of the sex of the model ($F_{1,14} = 17.99$, $p < .001$) was qualified by a trend toward a sex-by-emotion interaction ($F_{1,14} = 3.27$, $p < .10$): RTs for facial expressions of happiness were faster than expressions of sadness with female faces but not male faces. The male faces expressing happiness were more slowly processed than the corresponding female faces, whereas no difference appeared with facial expressions of sadness. A second ANOVA was used for the same variables for mean stimuli RTs. This time, only the main effects of the within-variables, order of blocks, and order of presentation were significant (F1,12 = 45.85 and 37.18, p < .001). Thus, the sex-by-emotion effect was not replicated when treated as a "between" factor.

2.3. Discussion

We found evidence for some advantage in processing time of happy expressions in the happy-sad categorization of words referring to emotional states. Thus, bias in sampling the emotion set or visual characteristics of the happy faces are not the only explanations for the faster or more accurate recognition of facial expressions of happiness.

However, conclusions supporting the hypothesis of conceptual differences between emotions have to be qualified by possible interactions between modality and emotion, which partially depend on procedural variables (order of blocks). Similarly, the difference in the processing of male and female faces suggests that the advantage of happy faces could also partially depend on the visual properties of faces.

The comparison of words and faces in Posner's paradigm could provide stronger evidence for or against the competing hypotheses. In same/different judgments where same responses correspond either to physically identical stimuli or to conceptually identical stimuli, the visual characteristics of the face are assumed to influence the physical judgment as well as the conceptual one, whereas pure conceptual difference between happy and sad expressions will affect the conceptual judgment only.

3. SAME/DIFFERENT JUDGMENT

3.1. Pilot study

3.1.1. Method . Subjects were 16 female students (new sample) receiving either the physical or the conceptual condition first.

3.1.1.1. Physical identity condition. The stimuli were two blocks of 32 pairs of words and 32 pairs of faces. 16 pairs were physically identical expressions of happiness or sadness (8 pairs each). The different pairs bore either visual resemblance (words of the same length with the same initial letter, faces of the same person posing for different emotions) or conceptual resemblance (words or faces expressing the same emotion).The stimuli were taken from the same set as in the categorization task. The instructions were to press the plus key if the two slides were strictly identical, the minus key otherwise.

3.1.1.2. Conceptual identity condition. The stimuli were three blocks of 20 pairs of stimuli (words, faces, or word-face). The mixed pairs were always the last presented. Five pairs of happy expressions and five pairs of sad expressions required the response of "same", ten other pairs the response of "different". The instructions were to press the plus key if the two slides represented the same emotion, and the minus key if they did not. In both the conditions, the stimuli were presented until the subject responded.

3.1.2. Results

3.1.2.1. Physical identity matching: "same" responses. A three-way mixed model ANOVA (order of blocks-by-modality-by-emotion) was conducted on the means and medians of subjects' correct RTs. Both the analyses revealed only one significant effect, a main effect of emotion (slower RT for negative expressions): F 1,14 = 11.15 and 22.12, $p < 0.005$ and 0.001 respectively. There was also a trend toward slower processing of words (F 1,14 = 4.20 and 4.57, $p < 0.10$), but no interaction between these two effects.

3.1.2.2. Physical identity matching: "different" responses. A three-way mixed model ANOVA was used to determine the effects of order of blocks, modality, and nature of distractors (visual versus conceptual) on the mean and median subjects' correct RTs. In both the analyses, significant main effects of the modality and of the distractors were revealed. Facial expressions were processed faster (F 1,14 = 8.32 and 7.19, $p < 0.025$) and the responses were slower to visual distractors (F 1, 14 = 22.13 and 31.91, $p < 0.001$). These two effects did not interact.

3.1.2.3. Conceptual identity matching: "same" responses. A three-way mixed model ANOVA was applied to the mean and median subjects' correct RTs (order of blocks-by-modality-by-emotion). Significant main effects of modality were observed: words pairs were processed more slowly, mixed pairs had intermediate RT and face pairs were the fastest (F 2,28 = 38.75 and 37.88, $p < 0.001$). Emotion also significantly influenced processing time, and the RTs to happy expressions were faster (F 1,14 = 38.24 and 17.74, $p < 0.001$). These two effects did not interact, but the modality did interact with the order of blocks (F 2, 28 = 4.16 and 4.09, $p < .05$): There was less difference between words and faces in the word-face order than in the inverse.

3.2. Replication

3.2.1. Method . Subjects were the 16 female students who were the subjects in the categorization task. Same/different judgments always followed.

Stimuli were four blocks of 48 pairs of stimuli, presented in the ABBA or the BAAB orders (two presentation of word and face blocks). Twenty-four pairs required the response of "same": 12 were physically identical, and 12 were conceptually identical. In each case, six pairs represented happy expressions, and six pairs sad expressions. The 24 different pairs were words or faces of different persons expressing different emotions. The stimuli were taken from the same set as previously used (words of the categorization task and faces of the Ekman and Friesen series).

Instructions were the same as in the conceptual condition of the pilot study.

3.2.2. Results

3.2.2.1. Global analysis. A four-way ANOVA (mixed model) was used to determine the influence of order of blocks, same/different responses, words or faces, and presentation (first and second) on the subjects' means of correct RTs. Three main effects were observed, showing faster RTs for the same responses, the faces, and the second presentation. The only significant interaction was between stimulus modality and presentation, which was probably a floor effect for the faces in the second presentation.

3.2.2.2. Analysis of the "same" responses. A four-way ANOVA (fixed model) was conducted, comparing mean subjects' correct RTs to physically and conceptually similar stimuli, to happy and sad expressions, and to words and faces in the first and the second presentation. The four main effects were significant. Physical versus conceptual identity interacted with emotion (F 1,15 = 6.69, p < .025) and with modality (F 1,15 = 7.93, p < .025), as well as modality and emotion (F 1,15 = 14.73, p < .005): see Figure 2. Special attention was paid to the emotion-by-presentation interaction, since some of the subjects reported interference with the categorization task because the pairs of sad stimuli, which previously elicited the minus response were now to be responded to as "same". Such an interference would equally affect words and faces, but would be reduced in the second presentation. This interaction was not significant (F < 1), nor were the triple interactions involving emotion and presentation. The four-way interaction tended to be significant, due to the reduced difference between physically similar happy and sad words in the first presentation (F 1,15 = 3.97, p < .10).

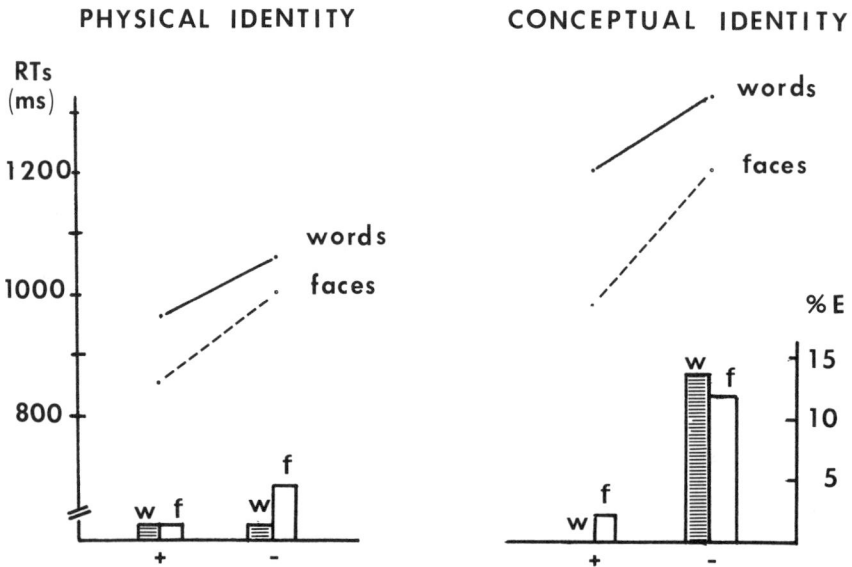

FIGURE 2. Mean RTs and error percentages for "same" responses for words and faces, happy (+) and sad (-) expressions in the physical identity and the conceptual identity conditions.

3.3. Discussion

The pilot experiment provides contradictory results. On the one hand, the advantage of happy over sad faces in the physical identity condition suggests differences in the visual characteristics of facial expressions of emotions. But, on the other hand, a similar effect with words raises a serious interpretation problem. The second study shows an identity- by- emotion interaction, that does not differ for faces and words: here, the greater advantage of happy expressions in the conceptual rather than in the physical matching supports the hypothesis of a conceptual difference between happiness and sadness. However, emotion also interacts with modality, showing greater advantage of happiness for faces than for words. Thus, faster recognition of happiness cannot be explained only by the structure of the emotional field.

4. CONCLUSION

The present study suggests non-additive influences of modality-specific and non-modality-specific factors in the processing of emotional expressions.

Further research would have to control variables such as word frequency and face quality and to assess the role of specific (e.g. open versus closed smile) and unspecific (e.g. intensity) factors that may influence the processing of emotion in the different modalities.

PRIMARY STAGES IN SINGLE-GLANCE FACE RECOGNITION:
EXPRESSION AND IDENTITY.

Gé CALIS and LUCAS MENS

1. INTRODUCTION

All faces share the same global spatial structure (eyes above nose, above mouth, etc.). Thus more specific classifications, for instance of identity and expression, should be compared to the classifications of a single letter written in a specific way, rather than to just letter recognition. Yet, in no more than a fraction of a second, we do not only see a face as a face, we also notice its individual uniqueness. We see its age, gender, race, beauty and emotional expression. Moreover, under conditions of adequately stored information, we even identify it within the same split second. Thus face perception is perception par excellence.

From age to identity, all these types of information are veridical, visible and ultimately based on (high-speed) abstractions of different spatial invariances. However, as shown in perceptual learning, the perceptual potential to 'select new features into existence' seems to be inexhaustible. There may even be completely different features or procedures which are sufficient to identify the face. In proposing theoretical constraints it is therefore not enough to give a more exact geometrical specification of whatever features (though this already proves to be paradoxically difficult). We must somehow also unravel the perplexingly ambiguous nature of the perceptual selection mechanism (Calis, 1984).

Face recognition, like any other act of visual perception, may be based on a general visual input system or module (cf. Marr, 1982), which optically infers the shape of the distal object from its retinal projection. This shape, however, is nothing more than the information about the spatial structure and orientation of a real (but still unknown) visual object in the world, put into an appropriate format for a more central identification system. Now it seems both unlikely and inefficient that the central system would just blindly try all possible object classifications by some sort of direct template matching. Introspectively it is more likely that the identification starts with an abstract categorization of the global object-structure in terms of a limited set of common and simple geometrical shapes (including for example 'oval' and perhaps even 'face'). Such evidence for a "global precedence" (cf. Navon, 1977) comes especially from those single-glance situations in which we are confronted with a familiar face but only perceive this as a sort of general face that certainly has a specific orientation but no identity or expression. Thus, in an early stage of processing, the infinite number of possible object classifications seems to be reduced to one basic category 'face'. The most efficient subsequent reductions would now consist in going down the implicational hierarchy of the basic category, while the given spatial structure may serve as a basis for reality testing at each level. Evidence for such a hierarchical-sequential or microgenetical identification of faces (each level may evoke extensive parallel processing) was proposed by Calis et al (1984).

Fodor (1983) presents good arguments for his view that it is in fact the input system which autonomously infers basic categories (like 'face') and thus presents a ready-made hypothesis to the central system. Similar bottom up processes may apply to certain expressions, gender, etc. Only higher face-recognition would be a central process because now all kinds of knowledge may have selective top down effects. (note: It may be clear that neither a general input system, nor central identification can account for a specific agnosia for faces resulting from localized brain damage. Prosopagnosia must be either a symptom of a more general disturbance - in which case the name is not adequate - or there must be a specific module for faces.) Because of the encapsulation of input systems Fodor proposes a "principled distinction" between input and central systems. And again he has good arguments. However, we do not like the conclusion that in fact only the modular processes are perceptual. We think that a principled distinction between perception and cognition should be looked for in a difference between codes which preserve geometrical information, and codes which do not.

However, what sometimes looks like perception (i.e. seems to involve geometrical information) may, even in case of a single glance, actually result from more abstract thinking. Bruce and Young (1985) distinguish "visually derived semantics" (i.e. geometrical surface information) from "identity specific semantics" which are secondary, resulting from a subsequent classification. In our opinion, the best example of such identity specific semantics is a name. You cannot visually derive the name when you see a face. A name is derived from the seen identity. Things get complicated, however, when we realize that some visual information (age, gender, etc.) may also be derived from the identification. Once we identify somebody we have access to all the associated knowledge in the semantic machinery of our minds. There may even be restorations of spatial information which was either defective or not actually derived visually. The fact that we can see something does not automatically imply that we do see it. And the fact that we can visualize (point at, cut out, draw, describe, etc.) almost any feature, does not tell us whether it constituted recognition or emerged from it. Such a feature may even be an 'ad hoc invention'. The same could be true for the features related to the recognition of an expression. Most likely, however, both identity and expression ultimately depend on a basic categorization of a spatial structure as a face.

The relation between identity and expression is not so obvious as the one between each of them and a basic face category. In principle we cannot derive expression from identity as we can do with age or gender, nor can we derive identity from expression. Of course some faces may laugh very specifically, very frequently, or both; some faces may even show an habitual expression of happiness. In other cases, for example when we must differentiate between identical twins, recognition of an expression may even be a necessary and sufficient condition for identification. In general, however, detection of an expression cannot be very efficient in reducing the number of possible faces as any face can show any expression.

Still, the relation between expression and identity has considerable theoretical importance, because there may be other reasons (apart from identification per se) which require that the expression is taken into account first. If identification is based on the abstraction of a simple feature like the breadth of the mouth, then it would be affected by a laugh which precisely changes these types of measures. So we would first require information about the non-rigid transformations of the face that we call expressions, before adequate measurements are possible. We would need a normalization (cf. Valentine and Bruce, 1985) for plastic deformations of the face comparable to the ones which are sometimes suggested for spatial transformations of the retinal image produced by translations and rotations of rigid bodies. Perhaps expressions are detected by an "affective" system that operates earlier and easier than the one which "infers" higher-order cognitive aspects (cf. Zajonc, 1980), especially those expressions which also produce specific emotional arousal in the perceiver (cf. Mueller et al, 1983; Burt Thompson and Mueller, 1984). Physiological evidence for such a system is that expression detection is handicapped selectively in case of right posterior brain damage (Christen et al, 1985). On the other hand, if identification is based on the abstraction or "extraction" of higher order invariants (cf. Gibson, 1979) then expressive variation of the face might be irrelevant for the process of identification. Because we only discus single-glance or snap-shot face recognition, we do not consider the possibility here that shape may be inferred from translations and rotations of the face during the perceptual process (Ullman, 1979), or even from the temporal structure of movement patterns of the expressional event.

Galper and Hochberg (1971: 354) were probably the first who noted that "manipulations of expressive variation thus appears to be a promising means of determining the nature of the information on which face recognition is based". In the same paper they actually defend a moderate dependency between expression and identity because they found that a change of expression influenced recognition memory. Sorce and Campos (1974: 71) go one step further; "Facial expression is apparently a parameter of facial recognition".

Independence, however, is claimed by many other investigators. Kurucz and Feldmar (1979) describe two "unrelated" types of prosopagnosia, one for identity and one for expression. Zajonc (1981: 151) asserts that affective and cognitive discriminations "are under control of separate and partly independent systems that can influence each other in a variety of ways, and that both constitute independent sources of effects in information processing" (but see Lazarus, 1984). Winograd (1981: 189) presents the interesting suggestion that manipulations of facial distinctiveness may in fact only influence "the probability of encoding distinctive features", facilitating recognition memory, while Parkin and Goodwin (1983) seem to add that even this does not occur in case of remembering facial expressions. Also Hay and Young's (1982) and Ellis' (1983) models of face recognition suggest an essentially independent processing of identity- and expression information. Experimental evidence that identity and emotional expression can be treated as independent sources of information by adults with intact right hemispheres was presented by Etcoff (1984: 292).

Investigating the relation between expression and identity within the time course of single-glance face recognition may contribute to these lines of research. Our experimental technique is both inspired by research into the microgenesis of visual perception (cf. Froelich et al, 1984) and by the motion picture (see also Calis et al, 1981, 1984 and Leeuwenberg et al, 1985). Its essence is that two pictures are presented like a very short movie. These two pictures share the coarse layout of a frontally viewed face as in a movie sequence of the same portrait, though in fact portraits of different persons are used. The perceptual processes, started by the first portrait, 'asking' for information in order to refine the identification may or may not be disturbed by the features and completely different identity in the second picture. The subject's identification-response reveals such disturbances.

2. METHOD

2.1. Subjects

Seventeen volunteers were run individually. All were very familiar with the models whose portraits we used as stimuli.

2.2. Stimuli

Using positive colour film, the faces of 8 male staff-members of our department were photographed en face against a white background while looking neutrally and while showing the biggest smile possible. They were about 40 years old and had no exceptional characteristics, like beards. Clothing was not visible. The sizes of the portraits only varied with the natural sizes of the faces. The upright and frontal position of the faces and the localisation of the eyes on the slides was approximately standardized by the photographers vision. The 16 portrait stimuli were grouped in 2 subsets: 4 models wearing glasses (the same horn-rimmed spectacles during the photosessions) and 4 models without glasses.

2.3. Apparatus and Procedure

Two computer controlled Random Access slide projectors, A and B, provided with a central-type shutter in front of the projection lens, each contained copies of the 16 original slides. The aperture of A was set at f/5.6 and that of B at f/8 so that A produced brighter portraits in case of simultaneous projection (cf. Calis et al, 1984). The setting of B was such that a correctly exposed new picture from the screen on a film of ISO 100 would require 1/125 sec and f/2.8. The projected portraits almost fully covered the same small projection screen (25 x 25 cm) which was placed at a distance of 2 m in front of the subject in a moderately tube-lighted room. Thus the sizes of the portraits were about the same as those of natural faces at that distance (visual angle about $7°$).

Trials were self-initiated. After the starting key was pressed, immediate presentation of the two portraits (10 msec each) followed with one of 3 different onset asynchronies (SOA): 0, 10 or 50 msec. Projector A always contained the 'first' slide (in case of SOA = 0 there is of course not really a first and a second slide !). A trial was completed when the subject selected one out of 16 response keys which were grouped in two rows of 8 buttons along with the names of the 8 models printed in alphabetic order: the upper row for neutral expressions, the lower for laughs. Thus each response indicated perceived identity and expression at the same time. The instruction was to identify the most clearly perceived face and whether this was laughing or looking neutrally. There was a training session of 20 trials. The experiment took about 45 minutes per subject.

2.4. Design

According to the constituent portraits (laughing-neutral) we distinguished 4 types of 'portrait-films': LL, NN, LN, NL. Each of these types contained all combinations of different faces with glasses: 12 combinations, and without glasses: also 12. The total series (4 conditions x 3 SOAs x 24 combinations = 288 trials) was presented in a random order.

2.5. Hypotheses

- 1 Normalization should manifest itself as a difference between the conditions with similar expressions (LL + NN) and those with different expressions (LN + NL).
- 2 If typical expressions also make the identity more distinctive we may expect differences between LL and NN.

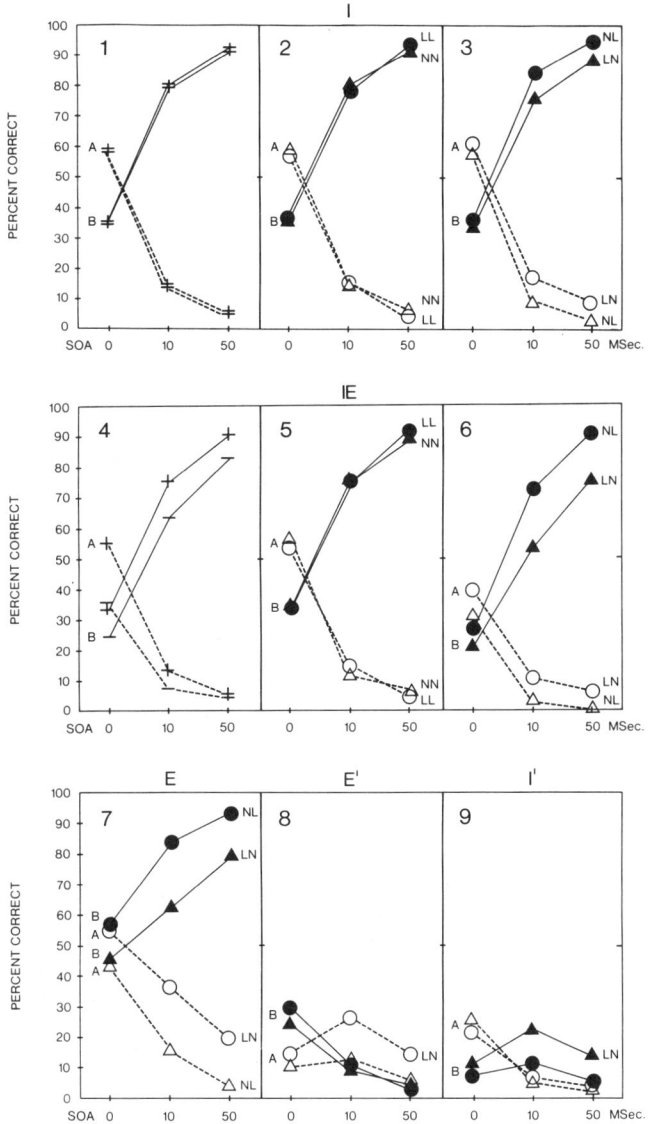

Figure 1–9
Percent correct recognitions of the Identity and Expression of the superposed slide projections of two different familiar faces, A (double intensity) and B, as a function of Stimulus Onset Asynchrony and the similarity/dissimilarity of their expressions

I   (Id   cor; Exp cor or incor)
IE (Id   cor; Exp correct   )
E   (Exp cor; Id   cor or incor)
E' (Exp cor; Id   incorrect   )
I' (Id   cor; Exp incorrect   )

A   △ – – – Neutral   ▲ ——   B
    ○ – – – Laughing   ●——

+ (Expression of A and B similar ; NN+LL)
– (Expression of A and B different; NL+LN)

- 3 If expression and identity are completely independent there is no reason to expect any differences between LL, NN, LN and NL.

3. RESULTS AND DISCUSSION
3.1. Identity
Both LL+NN and LN+NL form completely counterbalanced conditions of all 16 portraits. Let us call the one with similar expressions '+' and the one with dissimilar expressions '-'. The averaged proportions correct A- and B-names irrespective of the expression chosen, called 'I', are compared in Fig. 1. We can see the effect of the brighter A-faces in case of SOA=0. We can also see that the preferences for A decrease and for B increase as a function of SOA. The latter may be explained in terms of visual masking or in terms of a transfer of information from A to B (cf. Calis, 1984; Leeuwenberg, Mens and Calis, 1985). Of interest here is that there is no difference whatsoever between the I-curves in '+' and in '-'. Consequently, we conclude that there is no normalization for emotional expression (plastic deformation) as hypothesized before. In Fig. 2. the I-scores of LL and NN are compared. Again there are no differences. Thus we also reject our second hypothesis. However, we cannot simply accept the third hypothesis.

Fig. 3 shows that there is at least one effective expression factor associated with the order LN vs. NL. Both within the A- and the B-identifications there is a significant, but opposite, main effect of Order ($F(1,16)= 12.74$ and 7.27, $p<0.001$ and $p<0.01$, respectively). Apparently, this effect is due to a dominance of the laughing face (and thus completely cancelled out in Fig. 1). There is also a (not significant) tendency toward an interaction Order x SOA. So the question is how to explain this relation without reintroducing the rejected notions of normalization and distinctive help. For this purpose let us suppose: 1. That detection of an expression is indeed neither necessary nor helpful for the identification of a face (i.e. that the expression only conveys additional information about an emotional state of the perceived model while recognition of identity is based on higher-order invariants). 2. That expression is indeed detected earlier than identity. 3. That in our experiment the laugh is a more informative (or 'real') expression than neutrality.

Now consider condition LN. Once we detect that the (first) face is laughing, we have selected an informational framework which is more suitable for the first face than for the subsequent non-laughing face. Consequently the chance of identifying the first face is greater than in condition NL. In condition LL this is of course not the case. In condition NL the second face creates the framework so that also the identity of the second face stands out most clearly. This is not happening in NN. Thus the relation of expression and identity is not one of normalization or help, but one of a framing confinement. In case of SOA=0 there are no first and second but only simultaneous portraits. Accordingly, confinement cannot have forward or backward but only instantaneous and thus less selective effects. Therefore, an eventual interaction of confinement with SOA would be understandable. Despite the statistical significance of the main effect of confinement, it may be clear from a closer inspection of Fig. 3 that it influences identity only marginally. Let us therefore now also consider expression itself.

3.2. Expression
First we shall have a look at the scores which are correct both with respect to identity and expression. These are called 'IE' and are and presented in Figures 4, 5 and 6. The difference between '+' and '-' (Fig. 4) is clearly due to the LN vs. NL effect (Fig. 6); LL vs. NN (Fig. 5) again shows no

differences. We shall therefore only analyse LN vs. NL. Comparison of the data of Fig. 3 and Fig. 6 reveals that the main effect of Order (LN vs. NL) has been increased, both within the A- and the B-scores (F(1,16)= 31.34 and 22.83, p<0.001 in both cases). Again the interaction with SOA is not significant. Moreover, now NL has a better total result (A + B): (F(1,16)= 4.69, p<0.05) and both the totals of NL and LN are better with large SOAs: (F(2,16)= 26.09, p<0.001). These findings are in line with the proposed confinement effect.

Further analysis, however, reveals that the confinement effect is only part of the story. The fact that the B-level of LN is much higher in Fig. 3 than it is in Fig. 6, implies that there are many identifications of the second portrait which are 'erroneously' completed with the expression (laugh) of the first portrait. These 'slipped-through' B-name identifications are presented separately in Fig. 9, and the corresponding 'freefloating' A-expressions in Fig. 8. LN is better than NL for both A (Fig. 8) and B (Fig. 9): (F(1,16)= 19.68 and 21.31, p<0.001, respectively). Thus the inhibition of the second portrait's identity (Fig. 3) is only a minor effect: identity and expression are largely independent.

Final support for this thesis can be found in an analysis of 'E', the recognitions of expression irrespective of correct name-identifications. Here, of course, only a comparison of LN vs. NL makes sense because in LL vs. NN we do not know whether a correctly recognized expression should be assigned to A or B. The corresponding data are presented in Fig. 7. Again there is a large main effect of Order (LN vs. NL) which is now completely identical for the A- and the B-recognitions because these are of course inversely proportional (F(1,16)= 77.38, p<0.01). Interestingly, in case of SOA=0 no effect of the brighter A projection is present in contrast to Fig. 3 where the brighter A dominates in the identity response. Again we see that the processing of identity and of expression do not coincide. Discrimination of expressions is more swift and less liable to subtle stimulus aspects than recognition of identity. Perhaps we are indeed talking about an early and rapid warning system which 'simply' recognizes expressions as such, not especially for the sake of successive identification, but for its own sake.

3.3 Final remarks

The LN vs. NL order-effect is of course an artifact of our non "ecologically valid" way of experimenting. Nevertheless we strongly feel that it reveals the logic of the perceptual system.

We suggested that it is more likely that face recognition is based on higher-order invariances than on simple features. However, more specific statements about these invariances must of course await future research.

It is possible that it was in fact not (perceived) expression which accounts for the effective differences between our experimental conditions. We can think of an associated brightness factor, not unlike the one we introduced deliberately and which was effective with respect to the identities in our simultaneous projection of the two portraits. A big smile, for example, often correlates with a brighter area of bare teeth. For this very reason, however, control conditions with white lips or a white area instead of a mouth, may also provide the single-glance abstraction: 'laugh'. At this moment we can only say that it was our (and our subjects') impression that we primarily perceived laughing faces rather than bright areas. Nevertheless, this point may also need further deliberation and research.

AFFECTIVE AND COGNITIVE DECISIONS ON FACES IN NORMALS

M. REGARD, T. LANDIS

A face not only carries different meanings, but also carries meaning differently than for example a word. A face is stimulus and response in one, a stimulus which changes over age, changes with the affective state of beholder and perceiver and which exists in its strict spatial arrangement of eyes, nose, mouth and ears in an indefinite number of exemplars. Considering the great amount of different information which can be extracted from a face and considering the biological importance of this stimulus we expect different processing systems, and thus different parts of the brain to be involved when it comes to deal with faces. Aspects of faces such as emotional expression, gender, age, identity etc. are all known from clinical observation and experimentation (for review see Davies et al. 1981) to interfere with or to facilitate face recognition. Confronted with faces it may not be random which aspect triggers our prime interest and thus influences our perceptual decisions. We conducted a simple concept sorting test with photographed faces and observed that kind and order of concept identification was not at random. When 35 men were presented with 8 faces which could be sorted correctly according to 5 different concepts (sex, age, emotion, headgear, fame), we found that the emotional concept (friendly-unfriendly) was chosen first (mean rank 2.1) and by most subjects (n=33), followed immediately by sex (2.2, n=30), then headgear (2.9, n=29). Age ranked next (3.5) and was only identified by 22 subjects and fame (identity) ranked least (4.0) and was correctly sorted by 16 subjects only.

This finding let us to reexamine data of tachistoscopic hemi-field experiments with faces, all conducted over the last few years in our laboratory for different reasons. Since decisions on facial aspects are not arbitrary but triggered first by the emotional concept and last by the identity of a person, we analyzed our data with respect to these two extremes, i.e. affective and cognitive decisions. Affective decisions were measures of preference, i.e. subjects had to decide which face they liked or disliked most; and cognitive decisions were measures of accuracy, i.e. subjects had to match, detect or recognize faces. Expecting that affective and cognitive decisions be differentially processed by the two hemispheres, we specifically looked for dissociated effects of visual-field of stimulation (laterality) and type of perceptual decision (affective vs. cognitive).

The Szondi-Test is an established projective test in personality assessment (1947) using photographed faces of mentally ill representing, according to Szondi´s analytical theory, a wide range of drives in their pathological state (sex disorders: hermaphrodism-sadism, paroxysmal disorders: genuine epilepsy-hysteria, schizophrenic disorders: catatonia-paranoia, and cyclic disorders: depression-mania). The original task requires their affective judgment in two conditions, one a sympathy and one an antipathy choice. We adapted this test for tachistoscopic stimulation (note 1). We presented pairs of photos, simultaneously one in each visual field for 120 ms. 32 men were once required to indicate which one of the two faces they preferred and once which one they disliked most. There were two runs in each condition. If "feelings preceed thinking" (Zajonc 1980), we would expect a preference effect only to first but not second presentation. Since in brain damaged patients characteristic affective changes were observed according to the side of lesion (see Heilman and Satz 1983), we expected different preferences depending upon the psychopathological category of the photographs and the visual field of presentation.

As illustrated in Fig. 1 we found an overall difference in affective decision: the photos presented to the RVF (right visual field = left hemisphere) were more often liked and those presented to the LVF (left visual field = right hemisphere) more often disliked. However, this interaction of visual field of presentation and affective choice disappeared in a second run, indicating that a second stimulus presentation weakens its affective attractiveness. No differences were found among the psychopathological categories but, similar to data obtained with the normal (non-tachistoscopic) Szondi-Test, we found some items to be collective favourites (Fischer 1985). Our results suggest that the right hemisphere more readily reacts with antipathy, i.e. behaves socially less attractive than the left hemisphere with its preponderance of sympathy judgments, which may represent already censured affective decisions. Our result is well in line with a the performance of a split-brain patient observed by LeDoux et al.(1977) who consistently rated affectively high loaded words as "bad" when presented to the LVF "...as if the right hemisphere was in a bad mood" (p.420). Therefore, it may well be that each hemisphere has its inherent affective bias which is largely stimulus independent. Thus, hemispheric differences in cognitive decisions of prerated bipolar stimuli such as happy and sad faces in numerous studies may well represent an artifact of this demonstrated hemispheric dichotomy in affective decisions.

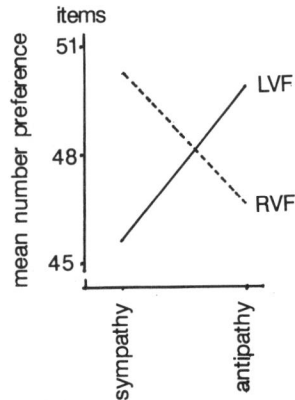

FIGURE 1. Significant interaction of choice condition and visual field of presentation of the Szondi faces with more sympathy choices to RVF and more antipathy choices to LVF presentation.

We approached the role of affect in face processing also in another manner, using a lateralized and modified version of the experimental paradigm of Kunst-Wilson and Zajonc (1980) (note 2). Pairs of stimuli consisting of an oval target face and a distractor, were tachistoscopically projected, one to each visual field. The target face appeared randomly in the LVF or RVF. Each experiment was conducted at a different exposure duration (exp. I subliminal: 1ms, exp. II liminal:

5-7ms, exp. III supraliminal: 20ms). After this exposure phase subjects were centrally shown for 1 sec. pairs of vertically arranged faces, to one of which they had previously been exposed. They were asked to choose the face they liked better (affective decision) and to indicate the face they previously had been shown (cognitive decision). The influence of exposure duration and field of presentation upon subsequent affective and cognitive decision was studied. As Fig. 2 (left hand side) shows, supraliminal (and liminal) presentation had no significant effect on the subsequent affective choices, but subliminal presentation elicited dissociated visual field effects: faces subliminally presented to the LVF were significantly not liked (or avoided) and those presented to the RVF tended to be preferred. Both hemispheres, therefore, react affectively to a face, but only when presented below the level of conscious perception. The left hemisphere tends to prefer a face previously exposed to, while the right hemisphere "dislikes" such a face, i.e. maybe prefers the novel (Goldberg & Costa 1981). We conjecture that the inherent opposite hemispheric bias for affective decisions as shown in the previous experiment is enhanced by the absence of conscious perceptual control, an idea as old as psycho-analytical theories. Conscious perceptual control, however, was certainly present at supraliminal exposure (20 ms) where, as shown in Fig. 2 (right hand side), affective decisions were random but accuracy of cognitive decision displayed the well known pattern of LVF advantage for the recognition of faces. This study suggests that affective decisions take place at an early stage of processing (see Dixon 1980, Moscovitch 1979) and are dissociated with respect to overall affective tone (like vs. dislike) and hemisphere involved, but not in terms of overall affective hemisphere dominance, a finding very similar to that obtained with the Szondi faces. At later stages of processing, however, affective decisions maybe overridden by cognitive decisions for which the two hemispheres compete for relative dominance.

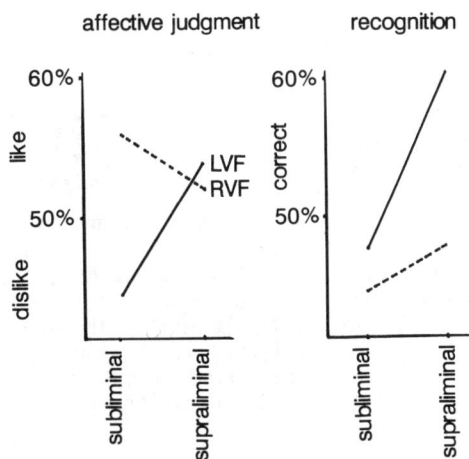

FIGURE 2. Effect of visual of presentation and exposure duration on affective decision (left hand side) and cognitive decision (right hand side).

This theory predicts hemispheric differences in affective decisions to be primarily dependent upon the inherent affective bias of each hemisphere, (i.e.the preference for liking of the left hemisphere and the preference for disliking of the right hemisphere), but not upon stimulus type (e.g. faces vs. words). Whereas for cognitive decisions the reverse is predicted: hemisphere differences are expected to be primarily dependent upon stimulus type and relatively resistant to changes in physical characteristics such as changes in exposure duration etc. We therefore expect a consistent relative dominance for all experiments using the same biologically meaningful stimulus category (e.g.faces) when measuring cognitive decisions, irrespective of the design used. Accordingly, we reanalyzed our data from studies measuring response accuracy.

Patients suffering from prosopagnosia are known to rely heavily upon paraphernalias for the recognition of familiar faces (Tzavaras et al. 1970). In order to investigate right hemisphere function, we therefore designed a pure facial matching task, using faces stripped of all external features as illustrated in Fig. 3 and also tested the effect of manipulations of stimulus exposure duration on laterality (note 3). We thus presented these faces at short (20ms) and long (150ms) exposure duration. According to the finding of Rizzolatti & Buchtel (1977) we expected an impaired RVF performance, but a stable LVF performance at reduced exposure duration, thus resulting in an enhanced LVF advantage at 20 ms. 20 right-handed men participated in the experiment. They had to indicate if two vertically arranged faces to the left or right of the central fixation point were identical.

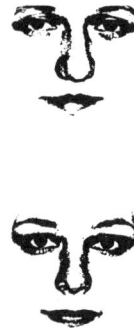

FIGURE 3. Stimulus example of
a pair of different faces in
the pure facial matching task

The analysis of the hits revealed a significant LVF advantage at both exposure durations and a significantly better performance for both visual fields at the shorter exposure duration of 20 ms (Fig. 4). This strong effect of exposure duration violates a basic rule in psychophysics which predicts better recognition with longer stimulus exposure due to enhancement of stimulus energy. This result is also not in agreement with Hellige et al. (1984, exp.1) who found improved recognition for both visual fields with increasing exposure duration from 10 to 55 to 100 ms.

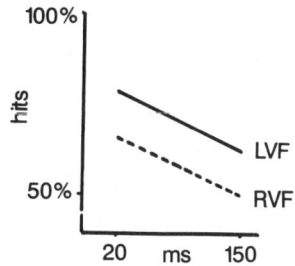

FIGURE 4. Results of the pure facial matching task: LVF advantage at both exposure durations with a significantly higher hit rate at 20 ms than at 150 ms.

This effect is similar to findings by Christen et al.(note 4) who also found no impairment of performance in a <u>face detection task</u> with a decrease in exposure duration. They used a double simultaneous go no-go facial decision paradigm and asked 28 subjects to respond only when they detected a correct face which appeared randomly at the left or right of central fixation. The target stimuli were faces always having the same frame of hair and ears, but with different features, and the non-targets were faces having a identical frame, but with displaced features, i.e. the position of the nose and the eyes was exchanged (Fig. 5). There were two runs, one at 20 ms and one at 100 ms.

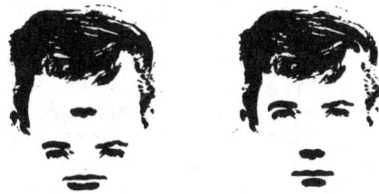

FIGURE 5. Stimulus example of the face detection task with the target on the right side and the non-target on the left side.

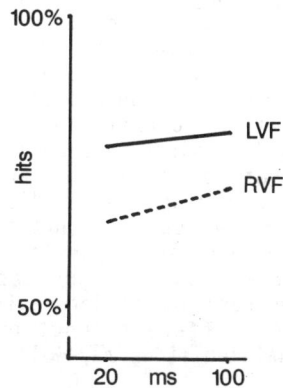

FIGURE 6. Result of face detection task: LVF advantage with no effect of exposure duration.

Fig. 6 illustrates the significant LVF advantage found at both exposure durations. This result, together with the finding of the above reported study using pure faces, suggests the existence of a processing system specific to face discrimination with a relative right hemisphere dominance, one that cannot profit from longer exposure duration and one that is not disturbed by perceptual degradation evoked by short exposure duration (Hellige et al. 1984, Sergent 1982).

A right hemisphere advantage even remains when the faces display a strong emotional expression, provided however that the decision is a cognitive and not an affective one. We conducted an experiment in which 24 subjects had to match faces for three emotions (angry, happy, astonished). At an exposure duration of 150 ms we found that most subjects reacted significantly faster to LVF presentation, whereas the same subjects showed an opposite visual-field advantage in performing a similar concept match with objects. (Landis et al. 1979).

Two main conclusions can be drawn from the reanalysis of our data: 1) processes involved in perceptual decisions on faces depend on the kind of decision required, and 2) the kind of decision required activates different hemispheric processes and presumably involves different anatomic structures. We found that affective decisions on faces lead to dissociated visual field effects depending on the choice that has to be made, whereas cognitive decisions, be it comparision, detection or recognition, revealed a consistent right hemisphere advantage. Affective decisions, perhaps on any stimulus, as for example suggested by the observation of hemisphere dependent word ratings by LeDoux et al. (1977), elicit a right hemisphere advantage for more positive values and a left hemisphere advantage for more negative values. It is also tempting to conjecture that these findings support early ideas regarding the left hemisphere as a censure of spontaneous emotions and the right hemisphere as the place for primary emotional activation (Tucker 1981). Affective decisions may activate an earlier stage of processing while the clearly lateralized cognitive decisions may follow in a second stage of processing. The right hemisphere advantage found for cognitive decisions was present if faces were presented with or without paraphernalia and even when faces displayed strong emotional expressions. The alteration of physical characteristica such as the time to perceive a stimulus, which have repetitively been shown to interfere with dominance (Sergent 1982) have not played a crucial role in our experiments. This may suggest a hierarchy among factors influencing the relative dominance in cognitive decisions. According to our data the stimulus type and its biological relevance (e.g.meaningful faces) is the strongest predictor for cerebral laterality provided the experiment measures accuracy.

In summary knowledge about faces is at least twofold, affective and cognitive. We conjecture that hemisphere differences obtained from affective decisions dependent little on stimulus characteristics, but rather reflect a general tendency of the left hemisphere to like and of the right hemisphere to dislike. On the other hand, for cognitive decisions, we suggest that it is the stimulus "face" and its biological relevance which is responsible for the relative dominance of the right hemisphere. However, our approach of a separate view of affective vs. cognitive decision in laterality research should not be confused with a notion of different functional systems for affect and cognition since perceptual decisions may well be contingent upon affective arousal.

ACKNOWLEDGEMENTS

Thanks are due to Jules Davidoff for letting us use his stimulus material, to Maya Cajöri, Lisanne Christen and Andreas Müller who collected and analyzed some of the data. This work was supported by Grant Nr. 3.884.0.83 from the Swiss National Science Foundation and by a twinning grant of the European Science Foundation.

REFERENCE NOTES

1. Cajöri, M.(1985).(Affective hemisphere differences: the tachistoscopic Szondi-Test). Diploma thesis, Institute of Applied Psychology, Zürich.
2. Landis, T., Christen, L., Graves, R. From subliminal to conscious processing: dissociated hemispheric and stimulus effects upon affective choice and recognition. Submitted for publication.
3. Regard, M., Landis, T., Müller, A. Fast exposure duration enhances right hemisphere advantage in pure facial matching. Unpublished manuscript.
4. Christen, L., Davidoff, J., Landis, T., Regard, M. (1985). Opposite hemifield advantage for "face" and "nonsense face" decisions. Journal of Clinical and Experimental Neuropsychology,7,141.

10. APPLICATIONS AND COMPUTER TECHNOLOGY

DYNAMICS OF FACIAL RECALL

K.R. LAUGHERY, C.DUVAL, M.S.WOGALTER

1. INTRODUCTION

The purpose of this chapter is to examine some of the dynamic properties of facial memory, particularly facial recall. Most research to date on face memory has employed recognition as opposed to recall procedures. One reason for this emphasis is that while facial recognition is a frequent, everday activity, facial recall or description of someone is much less common. Hence, the study of facial recognition processes has ecological validity. A second reason is essentially methodological. How does one adequately assess facial memory through recall? Having witnesses provide drawings presents the problem of artistic skills. Having witnesses provide verbal descriptions presents the problem of describing a complex spatial configuration. In both cases, the difficulties at the response level precludes knowing whether the witness possesses more facial information than shown in the resulting external representation.

In one applied context, witnesses recalling faces of criminals, research has been carried out on various techniques for constructing hard-copy representations from the witness's memory. Primarily, this research has focussed on the sketch-artist, identikit and Photofit. These techniques involved the witness subject: (1) recalling information about the face from memory, (2) describing the face to the artist or operator, (3) responding to questions posed by the artist or operator about the face, and (4) reacting to the constructed image to suggest changes. This work has been discussed elsewhere (Laughery & Fowler, 1980; Ellis, Shepherd & Davies, 1975).

In this chapter we will examine some of the dynamic properties of facial memory in two of these construction tasks – the sketch artist and the identikit. We are concerned with the memorial acts/processes occurring over time. Putting it differently: What is going on inside the witness's head while performing facial recall tasks? Towards this end, several behavioural indices will be presented and inferences drawn about the recall process. More specifically, we ask questions such as: "What strategies do witness subjects use when they try to remember and when they try to recall a face? Are there individual differences in strategy usage?"

Most of the data to be reported came from a large study carried out on sketch artist and identikit techniques (see Laughery & Fowler, 1980). The task procedure involved pairs of witness subjects meeting with an experimenter and a white-male target for a small group discussion lasting approximately eight minutes. The recall task immediately followed. One witness subject met with a sketch artist and the other with an identikit technician to construct images of the target. None of the subjects had ever done this task before. Generally, one target was used per pair of witnesses, but because of subject no-shows some sessions were held with only one witness subject. Witness subjects were told of the subsequent memory task before seeing the target; however, expectancy/intentionality has not been found to affect recall measures (Ellis, Davies & Shepherd, 1978).

A variety of data were recorded: (1) Construction sessions were tape recorded, transcribed, and timed, (2) Adjectives describing 23 facial parts/features were sorted to comprise an adjective dictionary, (3) Post-session questionnaires were completed by witness subjects following the construction, and (4) Judged similarity scores were obtained as a measure of performance.

Five analyses were carried out and concerned: strategies witness subjects reported using to remember faces; time-line data describing some of the frequency and time properties of feature production; time-line data describing feature sequencing during production; post-session responses describing features that were easy/difficult to remember/describe and vocabulary used in describing faces.

2. STRATEGIES USED TO REMEMBER THE FACE

This section deals with the strategies used by witness subjects to remember the target face. On the post-session questionnaire, witness subjects wrote down the methods and strategies that they used during initial exposure to remember the target face. The specific question asked: When you viewed the target, what did you do to help you remember the face? Since witness subjects knew in advance they would be attempting to recall the face, it seemed reasonable to assume they would employ some strategy to remember the target. Responses to the question yielded verbal statements from 121 witness subjects. In an effort to find a way to make some sense of these statements the following analysis was carried out. Twenty-seven additional subjects performed an unconstrained sorting task (Bookman & Arabie, 1972) on the statements. Prior to the sorting task, these subjects looked at a face and then wrote down how they would try to remember it. This first step was to acquaint them with the task. In the unconstrained method of sorting, each sorter can place responses into any number of similarity piles. Using the sortings, a nominal cluster analysis (Bhat & Hampt, 1976, p.61) was employed. This analysis identified an organisation consisting of three strategy clusters: (1) comparison or association with a known person (n = 18), (2) feature analytic (n = 75), and (3) forming a mental picture, wholistic processing (n = 28). These clusters are illustrated by the statements shown in Table 1.

The issue of cluster reliability is important. To what extent are the witness's responses characterised by the clusters? An estimate of the overall reliability of the cluster structure would be helpful. A commonality score was developed that measured how much a given witness's response had in common with responses in each of the three clusters. Conceptually, commonality was based upon the extent to which a response was assigned to the same or other groupings in the sorting task. An analysis of these cluster commonality scores indicated that the above cluster structure accounted for 56% of the variance.

The issue of performance characteristics for persons using these strategy groupings was addressed by examining the quality of facial images produced. Another group of subjects provided ratings of goodness-of-fit (or similarity scores) between the images and photographs of the target from 102 of the 121 witnesses. The mean standardised similarity ratings as a function of strategy grouping is shown in Table 2.

An analysis of variance of the similarity scores for the three different clusters yielded a marginally significant result, $F(2,99) = 2.26$, $p < .07$. The fact that both clusters 1 and 3 involved visual imaging of the whole face prompted recalculating the analysis of variance with groups one and three combined. The result was significant though small, $F(1, 100) = 4.50$, $p < .05$. The means for this analysis are shown in Table 3. As can be seen

TABLE 1. Examples of statements describing strategies reportedly used to examine the target's face during study.

Cluster 1: Comparison or Association to Known Person

He looked very similar to a friend of mine - colouring, hair style, and general shape of face. I noted basic differences between my friend and the target - glasses, smooth skin, and no sideburns.
I tried to remember someone he reminded me of.
I compared his moustache and beard to a very close friend of mine and they were very similar. I tried not to forget my first and last impressions. I noticed how his face changed as he did different things - squint, smile, etc.
I tried to get a good fixed picture of him in my mind, and imagined certain features of his face with someone else I knew.

Cluster 2: Feature Analytic

I looked at each feature of the face and tried to remember the most noticeable thing about them.
I checked the length and width of the eyes, and their depth in the face; size of lips and position on face; and shape of the nose. Also, I checked wrinkles and identifying marks.
I tried to look at each of his features - his colouring, the shape of his face, his hair, his glasses, shape of his ears, and his upturned chin.
Looked at features of his face, how large was his nose, colour of eyes and hair, position of features.

Cluster 3: Forming Wholistic Mental Picture

I glanced at the target from the hair on his head to his chin. Then I shut my eyes and tried to visualise what he looked like. My second look at the target was another glance. By this time, I was able to close my eyes and see his face clearly.
I tried to visualise an image.
I looked at him, then got a visual picture in my mind, I kept this up for the entire time.
I looked at him, looked away, looked back; each several times to commit his face and stature to memory, and then to check the accuracy of the impression.

TABLE 2. Mean standardised similarity rating as a function of strategy grouping (lower score indicates higher similarity).

Cluster 1	Cluster 2	Cluster 3
.284	- .177	.276

TABLE 3. Mean standardised similarity rating for a two-strategy grouping (lower score means higher similarity).

Strategies 1 & 3 Wholistic/Gestalt	Strategy 2 Feature/Analytic
.280	- .177

in this table, as well as Table 2, recall performance was better for witnesses who reported using a feature analytic strategy than those reporting a wholistic or gestalt type of processing.

These two general groupings of witness subject responses, wholistic processing and feature analytic strategies, correspond to the views most commonly held to account for facial information processing (Bradshaw & Wallace, 1971; Nielsen & Smith, 1970). Indeed, Bartlett (1932) found two "natural groups" based on individual differences: (1) persons who relied mainly upon visual images, and (2) persons whose responses were predominantly determined by the use of language. We will return to this issue of wholistic versus feature processing in the discussion.

3. TIME-LINE DATA DESCRIBING FREQUENCY AND TIME PROPERTIES OF FEATURE PRODUCTION

Protocol analysis (Newell & Simon, 1972) involves a detailed accounting of the behaviour of an individual as the person works toward some specified goal. The purpose of such analysis is to provide information from which to infer the internal representations of the subject's knowledge as well as the processes employed by the person when performing the task. Both the content of the person's statements as well as the temporal properties of the process are examined.

A number of molar properties of the order and timing of feature descriptions during image generation were examined by a type or protocol analysis. The data was 64 witness subject protocols (34 sketches and 30 identikits) which consisted of tape recordings and transcripts. Twenty-five targets were described by one witness working with the identikit and a second witness working with the sketch artist. Nine of the remaining 14 targets were described only with the sketch, and the other five only with identikit. Summary statistics of this data are presented in Table 4.

The frequency and time measures in this table quantify the following: (1) how many different features were described (Number of Feature Codes - NFC), (2) how many times features were described (Number of Feature Stops - NFS), (3) a measure reflecting the amount of "moving around" or feature refinement during construction (Ratio of Feature Stops to Feature Codes - RFSFC), (4) the duration of the image generation session (Total Elapsed Time - TET), (5) the Time per Feature Code - TFC), and (6) the Time per Feature Stop - TFS). Several t-tests were carried out to determine if the technique differences were statistically significant. It should be noted from this table that witness subjects using the sketch technique reported information on more features, switched features more often, refined the features more often, and spent more time describing features than witness subjects using the identikit. On the other hand, identikit witness subjects spent more time per feature on any one occasion (a feature stop). No difference between the two techniques was found for TFC, the time spent per feature. The RFSFC measure is essentially a token to type ratio. It is an indicant of how much "moving around" between features occurred in the generation session. A witness subject with RFSFC equal to 1, the lower bound of this measure, means he or she did not refine the description of a feature once it had been given. Though the RFSFC measure for identikit appears close to one, statistically it is significantly different from 1.0 (p .001).

Correlations were computed between the frequency and time measures and the goodness-of-fit of the constructed images. None of the correlations approached statistical significance.

TABLE 4. Time-line measures for both production techniques

	Sketch	Identikit	t	p
Frequency Measures				
Number of Feature Codes (NFC)	13.32	8.10	8.08	.001
Number of Feature Stops (NFS)	30.41	12.33	8.13	.001
Ratio of Feature Stops to Feature Codes (RFSFC)	2.26	1.48	6.33	.001
Time Measures				
Total Elapsed Time in sec. (TET)	2069	1368	4.63	.001
Time Per Feature Code (TFC)	156.0	171.9	1.07	.05
Time Per Feature Stop (TFS)	72.5	118.0	4.55	.001

The amount of time witness subjects spent describing the five most frequently mentioned features (the set was the same for both techniques) are presented in Table 5. This ordering of features by elapsed time corresponds, in part, to the ordering of parts of the face that were most helpful to facial recognition as reported by Goldstein and Mackenberg (1966). They determined that the upper portions of the face (hair-hairline and eyes) were more helpful to identification than the lower portions (mouth and chin). Other research has shown that the upper face features: (1) are selected first during reconstruction using the Photofit (Ellis, Shepherd & Davies, 1975), (2) are better recognised (Goldstein & Mackenberg, 1966; Fisher & Cox, 1975), (3) lead to more description with the face present (Shepherd, Ellis & Davies, 1977) or absent (Ellis, Shepherd & Davies, 1980), (4) lead to faster judgements for same/different comparisons of facial changes (Matthews, 1978), and (5) produced fewer confusions (Davies, Ellis & Shepherd, 1977). These results indicate the greater importance or salience of the upper features for identifying a face. Of course, this ordering may in part also reflect the complexity and distinguishability of these features. We will elaborate on this point later.

Table 5. Mean elapsed time to describe the most discussed features. (Mean times between features beginning at the same margin were not significantly different.)

Features	Mean time (sec)
Eyes	338
Hair/Hairline	334
Nose	230
Chin	134
Mouth-Lips	116

It should be noted that to some extent the above measures are almost certainly task driven. The longer times for sketches are partially determined by the fact that artists usually require more time to draw a feature than identikit operators require to select it. But the difference also reflects that the witness subjects in the artist situation are thinking and describing the features in greater detail than witnesses in the more wholistic identikit situation.

4. PRODUCTION SEQUENCING USING TIME-LINE MEASURES

The time-line data was also used to try to understand the progression of the recall/production effort. The purpose was to describe some of the molar properties of production sequencing in feature description. A measure was developed to quantify order properties. Three production sequencing variables were derived to represent the relative amount of new feature activity during the First 30%, Middle 40% and Last 30% phases of the construction process. More specifically, these measures reflect the degree to which subjects describe a quantity of new features relative to a quantity of feature stops within three specific time periods for each construction. In other words, they represent the relative amounts of new feature activity during the early, middle, and late phases of the construction process. To some degree, like the RFSFC measure, they describe how much "moving around" (amount of new feature activity vs new feature refinement) that occurred in the description.

The measure is a score that represents the Ratio of the number of New Feature Codes to the total number of Feature Stops during the First 30%, Middle 40%, and Last 30% of each subject's total elapsed time (TET). These scores are calculated differently from the RFSFC measure that was described earlier. When work on a feature overlapped an interval boundary, which was most of the time, one was added to the number of new feature codes in the interval where the code description began. However, the feature stop values added to the time intervals were proportioned on the basis of the time spent on the feature in the two intervals. For example, if a new feature description took five seconds in the first 30% interval and 15 seconds in the middle 40% interval, .25 stops and .75 stops were added to the first and middle intervals respectively. The ratio of new feature code to feature stop scores produced values that ranged from near 0 to slightly above 1.

A high production sequencing score indicates more complete effort on new features (features not previously described). A low score indicates more going back to features already described - an indicant of the refinement process. Mean production sequencing scores for both techniques are shown in Table 6. The first 70% of the identikit generation time is spent on new features. On the other hand, only the first 30% of sketch generation time is spent on new features; the latter 70% is spent on refinement. An analysis of variance confirmed this Technique by Time period interaction, $F(2,124) = 4.09$, $p < .05$.

TABLE 6. Mean production sequencing scores for time intervals broken down by recall technique.

Time Interval	Sketch	Identikit
First 30%	.842	1.083
Middle 40%	.479	.998
Last 30%	.195	.577

The production sequencing scores were correlated with the goodness-of-fit ratings. Only one significant relationship was found. For the middle 40% time period and the identikit constructions, there was a significant relationship with performance (similarity ratings), $r = .66$, (43% of variance). Because a low similarity rating indicates better performance, this positive relationship shows that identikit witness subjects were more accurate if they had lower production sequencing scores (indicating more refinement) during the middle 40% interval. More broadly, this relationship suggests that those witnesses using the identikit, who make preliminary selections of features early in the process and then return to refine the selections, will do better than witnesses who try to complete work on each feature and do little refinement. It should be noted, however, that not many of the identikit witnesses followed this more effective strategy. No comparable relationships were found for users of the sketch technique.

A cluster analysis was performed on the production sequencing data in order to explore the feature production process further. The analysis identified groups of individuals who share similar production strategies as represented by time-line/order measures. Using the 64 witness protocols

that were coded for time-line, three groups of subjects were identified.
Descriptions of these cluster groups are shown in Table 7.

TABLE 7. Descriptions of production sequencing cluster groups.

Group 1 production strategy (10 SK, 4 1DK):
  There was a preliminary selection/definition of most of the facial
  features to be described, followed by both refinement of these features
  and the addition of some new features.

Group 2 production strategy (20 SK, 6 1DK):
  These witness subjects made no special attempt to make preliminary
  selections of features. They worked on a group of a few features at
  a time which would then be refined until the witness subject was satisfied
  that the best representation had been obtained. They then continued
  the same pattern with a new set of features. The feature groupings
  were generally composed of facial parts in close proximity.

Group 3 production strategy (3 SK, 21 1DK):
  These witnesses worked on one feature at a time until they were satisfied
  and then moved on to the selection of another feature.

Table 8 shows the time-line measures as a function of the three production
sequencing strategy clusters. In particular, note that subjects in cluster
2 took the greatest total time to produce the construction, produced the
greatest number of features, features stops, and tended to "move around"
most frequently. In regards to these data, note how different clusters 2
and 3 are. It is interesting that membership in cluster 2 was dominated by
sketch users and cluster 3 was dominated by identikit users. However, these
two production strategies did not appear to differentiate greatly on
goodness-of-fit scores (similarity ratings) as shown on the bottom row of
the table.

Cluster 1 consists of fewer subjects than clusters 2 or 3 and slightly
more than two-thirds worked with the sketch technique. As indicated by the
RFSFC scores, these subjects did less refinement than subjects in cluster 2
and more than those in cluster 3. Their similarity scores, however, were
high (poorer performance) compared to the other groups.

What then are some of the dynamics of facial recall? In the identikit
construction task, most subjects work on features one at a time. Getting to
and working on any given feature takes on average a longer time than with
the sketch technique. With sketch artists, the most common strategy is to
do some preliminary work on a number of features and then refine them.

To what extent are the production strategies task driven? Although the
sketch and identikit techniques were represented in all three strategy
groups, the pervasiveness of task demands seems apparent. A significant
majority of subjects in clusters 1 and 2 worked with sketch artists and with
the identikit in cluster 3.

Task influence may come about as a result of general procedures or
training and experience of the artist and operator. These factors could
lead to a systematic ordering of feature selections which in this sense may
be beyond the witness's control. While these possibilities certainly exist,

TABLE 8. Time-line measures for three production sequencing strategy clusters.

	Production Clusters		
Frequency Measures	1	2	3
Number Feature Codes (NFC)	11.7	13.5	7.6
Number Feature Stops (NFS)	22.7	33.7	11.5
Ratio of NFS to NFC* (RFSFC)	1.9	2.5	1.5
Time Measures			
Total Elapsed Time (TET)	1781	2187	1188
Time per Feature Code (TFC)	154	162	163
Time per Feature Stop (TFS)	78	70	108
Similarity	.345	- .419	- .361

* Calculated from means rather than individual scores

there were 13 subjects who worked with the technique that was not dominant in the three clusters. Hence, on the basis of these data alone there is subject control over the sequencing of work on features.

5. POST-SESSION RESPONSES TO QUESTIONS ASKING WHAT FEATURES WERE EASY DIFFICULT TO REMEMBER/DESCRIBE

As noted earlier, the post-session questionnaire was used to gain information about strategies the witness subjects used when studying the target. The post-session questionnaire was also used to gain information about which features witness subjects' thought were easy or difficult to remember or describe. The following questions were asked: (1) What parts of the face were easiest to remember?, (2) What parts of the face were difficult to remember?, (3) What parts of the face were easiest to describe?, and (4) What parts of the face were difficult to describe? Table 9 presents a summary of the results for the six most commonly mentioned features. Entries in the Table are the percent of total subjects who listed the feature in response to the particular question.

It is not our intent to make too much of these data, but they do contain some interesting observations. First, almost without exception, subjects reported that remembering faces was easier than describing them. This conclusion is based on two types of comparisons; the easy to remember vs easy to describe and the difficult to remember vs difficult to describe. The only exceptions occurred with the mouth/lips and eyebrows where more subjects listed them as more difficult to remember than difficult to describe. However, the percentages in these cells are close.

A second observation concerns the description of facial features. In the facial memory literature it has generally been concluded that people are not

TABLE 9. Percentage of witness subjects reporting features as easy or difficult to remember or describe collapsed across techniques.

	Easy to Remember	Easy to Describe	Difficult to Remember	Difficult to Describe
Eyes	43	38	35	45
Nose	36	26	37	43
Mouth/Lips	34	31	29	25
Eyebrows	26	20	14	12
Hair	49	46	8	26
Chin/Jaw	48	39	52	53

particularly good at describing faces (Shepherd, Davies & Ellis, 1978; cf. Davies, 1983). The results in Table 9 indicate that people's reports of ease or difficulty of description varies from feature to feature. More people find it difficult to describe the eyes, nose and chin/jaw features. However, more people report it easier to describe mouth/lips, eyebrows and hair. Indeed for hair the difference is almost twofold. Shepherd, Davies & Ellis (1981) in a review of the literature on cue saliency for faces point out that the most consistent finding across several methodological paradigms was that hair is the single most important feature. It is interesting to note in this regard that hair, more than the others, is probably the feature that we do describe verbally in our everyday activities. We talk about different hair styles or we describe to our barber or hair stylist how we want our hair to look. Hence, hair may be easier to describe because we are more practiced in such descriptions. This point is further addressed in the next section.

6. VOCABULARY IN DESCRIBING FACES

In our everyday memory, faces are not usually verbally described. On occasion, we may attempt to describe what someone looks like and we find we are at a loss for words. The sketch and identikit both require the recall of features, and this recall is usually accompanied by verbal description. In this section, some aspects of verbal description of faces are examined.

The interaction of the witness subject with the sketch artist produces more verbal description than with the identikit technician ($p < .01$). At the start, at least, sketch production is primarily a recall/generation task. There are no exemplars from which to choose as is the case with the identikit. Adjective words must be generated to describe the target. As the artist completes more and more of the sketch, the task increasingly becomes more recognition-like. On the other hand, the identikit produces an initial "lay-down" and becomes more of a recognition task early in the procedure. Hence, less verbal description is needed to communicate change with the identikit.

A correlation between the number of words produced by the witness subject during construction revealed no statistically significant relationship between number of words and goodness-of-fit scores ($p > .10$). This particular result may be due to the relatively large subject variance in this measure. This point can be illustrated by the following scenerio:

Some witness subjects who "seem" to have a good memory for a feature will give a description that is brief and concise, while others with good memories will attempt to elaborate at length. A similar point can be made about witness subjects who "seem" to have a poor memory: Some may not waste time (and words), and others may talk about features as if they are hoping some memory will emerge.

Though no relationship was found between the total number adjectives and quality of image, we were curious about the construction time differences for individual features shown in Table 5. Are there differences in the number of adjectives used to describe the different features? Table 10 shows the proportion of the total number of adjective descriptors during the construction phase that was used for several features. The table also presents results from a study by Ellis, Shepherd & Davies (1980) using the Photofit. Despite differences in the categorisation of features between studies (e.g. the features mouth, lips and face shape were categorised differently), note the similarity in the results. Note also that there are considerably more adjectives used to describe hair. This result may be related to the earlier point about practice in describing hair and may further indicate a richer vocabulary for this feature.

One of the findings that has shown up repeatedly in research on facial memory concerns a sort of top-down ordering of feature importance. Ellis, Shepherd and Davies (1975) found that subjects constructing the Photofit preferred to select the features in the order: hair-forehead, eyes, nose, mouth and chin. Ellis, Davies & Shepherd (1977) noted that subjects took much more time selecting hair and eyes than other features. Upper features have been shown to be better recognised than lower features (Fisher & Cox, 1975). In addition, Matthews (1978) subjects make same/different judgements on simultaneously presented pairs of identikit faces with different combinations of features. Reaction times indicated that changes to the hair, eye, and chin region were detected the fastest, while eyebrows, and nose and mouth changes were slowest. Thus, in general, the upper features of the face seem more important to memory, which is consistent with the results reported here for more processing time (Table 5) and verbal descriptors (Table 10).

We also examined those adjectives used most often (50 times or more) by witness subjects across all features. Table 11 shows the frequency of

TABLE 10. Proportion of descriptors allocated to various facial features (adapted from Ellis, 1984).

Ellis, Shepherd & Davies, 1980		Present Research	
Feature	Proportion	Feature	Proportion
Hair	.27	Hair	.23
Eyes	.14	Eye-Eyelashes	.15
Nose	.14	Nose	.13
Face structure	.13	Eyebrows	.09
Eyebrows	.08	Mouth-Lips	.09
Chin	.07	Chin	.07
Lips	.06	Face shape	.05
Mouth	.03	Facial hair	.04

TABLE 11. Frequency of adjectives used in the description of all faces along with root word count per million (A = 50-100 per million, AA = 100 per million or over) from Thorndike & Lorge (1944).

Frequency	Adjectives	Thorndike-Lorge Count
735	long, longer	AA
639	straight, straighter	AA
556	thin, thinner	AA
540	wide, wider	AA
405	round, rounded, rounder	AA
351	thick, thicker	A
272	short, shorter	AA
260	full, fuller	AA
251	small, smaller	AA
248	dark, darker	AA
245	curly	14
232	curve, curved	36
222	part, parted	AA
216	large, larger	AA
201	prominent	25
196	down	AA
191	big, bigger	AA
174	square, squared	AA
166	narrow, narrower	AA
150	smooth	A
156	turn-	A
145	light, lighter	AA
141	point, pointed	49
134	high, higher	AA
131	bushy	4
121	wave, wavy, wavier	2
117	cover-	AA
114	slant-	AA
108	move-	AA
107	oval	5
105	heavy, heavier	AA
102	flat, flatten, flatter	A
99	deep-	AA
95	angle, angular	33
78	brown	AA
76	average	A
76	broad, broader	A
75	stick-	AA
70	low, lower	AA
69	arch, arched	38
63	blocky, block-	A
63	crease, creases, creasing	3
61	normal	41
60	fat, fatter	AA
53	medium	23

adjectives used in the description of all faces along with the root word language count from Thorndike & Lorge (1944). There are two things to note about this list. Most of the adjectives were size and shape measurement terms (e.g. long, straight, thin, wide, round, and short). Also, most were very high frequency terms in the language. In general, they are feature independent; that is, these adjectives are general-use, relative-size descriptors that could be used to describe most geometric shapes, such as parts of buildings. In an imaginary word association test, it seems unlikely that a facial feature would be given to most of them. This generalisation must be qualified because there are a few terms that appear to be frequently associated with hair (e.g. curly, wavy, and bushy). A few of the adjectives might be regarded as prototypical words - average, normal, and medium. Are the features for which these words are used actually prototypical features or are subjects just "filling in the blanks" in their memory? Probably there is some of each. The important point from these data is that there does not appear to be much linguistic richness in our vocabulary to describe faces.

7. SUMMARY AND CONCLUSIONS

In this paper we have explored some of the properties of facial memory in the context of a memory recall task. The task consisted of generating from memory a hard-copy representation of a face using two techniques employed in law enforcement - the sketch artist and the identikit. In addition to the constructed facial images, the results included tape recordingsa of each session and a post session questionnaire. Time-line and vocabulary data were compiled from the tape recordings. The constructed images were assessed by having a separate group of subjects rate similarity between the images and photographs of the actual faces.

An analysis of acquisition strategies was carried out by examining subjects' responses to a question in the post-session questionnaire. The question asked what they did during exposure to the target person to remember his face. A cluster analysis revealed two general strategies which we have characterised as wholistic and feature analytic. These results are consistent with previous findings that have identified similar strategies for processing facial information. The number of subjects in these two categories, 46 in the wholistic and 75 in the feature analytic, indicated a sizeable majority who processed the facial information at the level of features. This result does raise a question about some earlier conclusions of Woodhead, Baddeley & Simmonds (1979) that most subjects process faces at a wholistic level. On the other hand, Woodhead et al. based their conclusions on the failure of a feature-oriented training procedure to improve performance on a facial recognition task which may be better served by a wholistic strategy. It should be noted that subjects in the current study were told in advance of seeing the target person that they would be constructing a facial image; a procedure that may have induced many to examine the face at a feature level. This point is supported by the fact that constructions by the feature analytic group were rated better than those of the wholistic group. Hence, it seems appropriate to conclude that people may process facial information either wholistically or at a feature level, depending on the purpose for which the information will be used. The observation that faces are normally processed wholistically may be due to the fact that facial information is typically used for recognition purposes.

Protocal analyses using time-line and feature description data revealed a number of interesting findings. In addition to sketch and identikit differences, there were significant differences in the amount of time spent on different features. Features at the top of the face, hair and eyes, received the greatest description time, with a decreasing amount of time for features lower in the face. As noted earlier, this top-down emphasis is consistent with previous findings showing greater importance or salience for the top features.

A cluster analysis of the time-line feature data revealed differences in strategies employed by subjects in the construction task. These strategies differed in terms of how much "moving around" or refinement was involved. One group of subjects was characterised by a procedure in which some preliminary work was done on each feature early in the construction, and the remaining time was used for refinement. At the opposite end of the refinement continuum was a group who completed work on each feature before moving on to the next. In between these groups was a number of subjects who worked on several features during a time period, and after completing work on them moved to another set of features. In general, the strategy of working on one feature at a time was associated with the identikit technique, while the two strategies involving refinement were associated with the sketch. These results would indicate the construction strategies may be task driven. However, there were many exceptions which indicate the strategies are at least in part task independent.

Differences in feature processing were also revealed in the answers to other questions in the post-session questionnaire. Subjects were asked to note which features were easy or difficult to remember or describe. Not surprisingly, most features are easier to remember than to describe (or more difficult to describe than to remember). This finding is consistent with other work that has indicated people having difficulty verbally describing faces. This difficulty may be due in part to lack of practice, since most facial memory activity involves recognition. An exception in the current findings was hair, which was frequently listed as easy to describe. Since hair is a feature that we probably do describe more than others, this result is consistent with the practice notion mentioned above.

The vocabulary used to describe facial features also revealed some interesting results. The number of descriptors used for different features reflected the top-down importance or salience of feature and was consistent with earlier results reported by Ellis, Shepherd & Davies (1980). Perhaps even more interesting, however, are the vocabulary items used to describe the facial features. Most of the adjectives are high frequency words that describe size and shape. Moreover, they are words that are not specifically associated with facial features; but instead might be used to describe any structure. A few words such as curly and wavy might be associated with facial features, but these terms are exceptions. This outcome also helps to explain the difficulty people have in describing faces. In addition to the lack of practice, our vocabulary is not well suited to the description.

One of the issues that cuts across the above analyses and findings is the extent to which strategies and processes employed by subjects are task driven or subject determined. Several of the findings are unbdoubtedly influenced by the memory construction task. As already noted, strategies employed by subjects to remember the target person were probably influenced by the fact that they were informed that they would subsequently be doing the construction task. Similarly, the greater time spent on the hair and eyes as well as the number of vocabulary items used in describing these features may be because the features are more complex and take longer to construct - especially in the sketch technique. A third example of task determined strategies is the greater "moving around" or refinement that occurs in the sketch technique. This result is probably influenced by the sketch artists who usually try to get some preliminary outline information about the different features before filling in details.

These task driven strategies and processes to some extent reflect adaptive characteristics of memory. However, not all of the subjects' behaviour is determined by the task. Vocabulary items used to describe the features are more a function of the language experience of the subjects. Also, there were individual differences in the strategies employed. Thirty-eight percent of the subjects used a wholistic processing strategy during initial exposure to try to remember the face. The time-line data indicated that strategies during construction varied between subjects within each of the construction techniques. Hence, the dynamics of or processes employed in facial memory are both a function of the task to be performed and the experience and capabilities of the person.

In the opening paragraph of this paper the problem of response competence was raised as a methodological problem in examining facial recall. The goodness-of-fit of the recalled face (the constructed image) cannot be regarded as an accurate reflection of the subject's memory. Other significant sources of error or variance are important. These sources include the limitation of the identikit foils to represent features, the skills of the artist or operator, and the verbal skills of the witness subject. Each of these factors limit how good the representation can be. Virtually everyone who has attempted the construction task notes that his/her memory is better than the constructed image. But these observations should not preclude the use of recall procedures to study memory for faces. Protocol analyses such as those presented here provide information from which memory processes and strategies can be inferred. In the present study, these analyses have identified task driven as well as subject determined strategies.

THE RECALL AND RECONSTRUCTION OF FACES:
IMPLICATIONS FOR THEORY AND PRACTICE

GRAHAM DAVIES

1.FACE RECALL TECHNIQUES

As these proceedings illustrate, interest in the theoretical mechanisms underlying face recognition has increased dramatically in recent years. The study of face recall, by contrast, has been somewhat neglected. Yet any comprehensive theory of face memory must take account of recall and recognition. Most work on recall has been couched in terms of the practical problems surrounding the identification of criminals.

The French policeman Vidocq (1775-1857) appears to have been the first systematically to use verbal descriptions and pictorial representations as aids to the identification of criminals (Thorwald, 1965). Since that time police forces around the world have developed their own specialised techniques. Extended reviews of recall procedures have been provided by Davies (1981; 1983a) and the aim of the review below will be to complement, rather than recapitulate this earlier material.

1.1.Verbal Descriptions

Most police forces will use some form of cued recall or check-list procedure for describing the appearance of a wanted person. Facial information is not generally regarded as critical in the immediate follow-up to a crime. The standard Field Interview Report used by the Los Angeles Police Department, for instance, refers only to hair and eye detail. Greater priority is accorded to other aspects of person information such as height, weight, age and clothing which are probably more discriminable cues for officers on mobile patrols (LAPD, 1974).

Information on the facial appearance of the suspect assumes a greater priority if a decision is taken to follow up the crime with an extended witness interview. Most forces will employ a form of check-list, though its use is not mandatory in the United Kingdom. There are national and regional differences in the make-up of these, though they share common headings. A typical list used by a Canadian Regional Force asks for information on the face shape of the suspect; hair colour and type; eye colour and type; eye defects; nose; mouth; chin; ear type and defects; eyebrows; facial hair; scarring and complexion. For each feature there is a selection of alternative descriptors to assist witness and police officer; thus, for nose:'large/small/pug/straight/pointed/flat/broken/convex/concave'. Such information can then be used to direct an album search of mugshots of selected suspects or as the initial description for production of a facial composite picture.

Such check-lists are clearly useful, though the lack of a standardised format within and across forces must hinder the rapid transmission of suspect information. Moreover, it is unclear whether witness and interviewer share a common understanding of terms such as 'concave' nose or 'cleft' chin: there is no empirical evidence that witnesses can use such terms with the precision of language that they demand. Information is available from free verbal descriptions of faces collected in Houston (Laughery, Duval and Fowler, 1977) and Aberdeen (Shepherd, Ellis and Davies, 1977) which could provide a basis not only for the selecting of appropriate descriptors, but also those attributes of the face to which witnesses most readily attend.

1.2.Pictorial Representations

The oldest form of visual representation involves the use of a police artist working with the witness and this technique is still common among the larger metropolitan forces in North America. Such artists rarely receive any formal training and each has evolved an individual style and technique (Davies 1985b).

One experienced artist has recently described the stages in sketch production which he employs (Homa, 1983). The session begins with a preliminary discussion between witness and artist which is designed both to establish rapport and to gauge the likely quality of information available to the witness in the light of the circumstances in which the suspect was observed. Next, a detailed description is taken covering all aspects of facial appearance. On the basis of the description the witness is referred to illustrative material (typically mugshots) to confirm the appearance of different features. From this information a preliminary sketch is then improvised around a framework of lines showing the usual position of the major facial features. The witness can then suggest modifications to this initial sketch from which a final sketch is developed. At the conclusion, the witness is encouraged to comment on the quality of likeness using a ten-point scale.

Even in the United States, only the major forces can afford to retain full-time artists. The great majority of composites will be composed from Kits of selected facial features of which Photofit and the Identikit are the best known. The design and operation of the Kits has been fully described elsewhere (see Davies, 1981; Shepherd and Laughery, this volume), so they will only be briefly discussed here. Both Kits contain a range of parts including eyes, noses, mouths, chins and hair sections, which have been abstracted from monochrome photographs. Photofit has a repertoire of some 560 different features while the revised Identikit contains a similar range of pieces. The features in Photofit are printed on to thin card which can be slotted together in a special frame to produce a composite 'face'. The features in the Identikit are printed on to transparent acetate sheets and the face created by superimposing relevant sheets, one on top of the other.

Compared to the police artist, such composite systems have certain inherent inflexibilities. While both systems allow some manipulation of the configuration of the face, it is impossible to alter such relational cues as the distance between the eyes and very difficult to amend the relative proportions of the face. There have been criticisms from police operators over deficiencies in the range of features available, in particular lack of specifically youthful features and contemporary hairstyles (Venner, 1969; Kitson, Darnbrough and Shields, 1978).

Both Photofit and Identikit have been the subject of extensive laboratory evaluation. Laughery and Fowler (1980) compared the performance of trained sketch artists with Identikit Operators. Faces were constructed by the operators either in the presence of the model ('from view') or indirectly from a witness description ('from memory'). Sketches produced by artists received higher ratings of likeness that did the composites. Further, sketches 'from view' received higher evaluations than those 'from memory', a result not found for the Identikit. A later study by Laughery and Smith (1978) confirmed that the superiority of the sketches extended to a mugfile search task where the actual face had to be identified in a sequence of photographs. The Identikit system employed in these studies was the original Kit which used drawings rather than the revision which employs a photographic representation. Unaccented line drawings of faces are notoriously difficult to identify (Davies, Ellis and Shepherd, 1978a; Davies, 1983b).

It is conceivable that Photofit or the new Identikit with their larger and more realistic range of features might have performed rather better against the sketch artist (c.f. Davies, 1985b). However, laboratory studies on the effectiveness of Photofit offer little support for this view. Parallelling Laughery and Fowler's results, Ellis, Davies and Shepherd (1978) also found no difference in Photofit quality between faces made in the presence or absence of the target. Christie and Ellis (1981) compared the effectiveness for recognition purposes of the original descriptions furnished by witness subjects and their subsequent Photofit pictures. Judges given the descriptions were able correctly to identify twice as many faces from an array than those who were provided with the Photofits. Clearly, in this latter study, information available to the witness was actually being lost in the transition from verbal description to pictorial representation.

1.3.New Systems for Facial Reconstruction

Not surprisingly, researchers and manufacturers are anxious to develop new techniques which will transmit more effectively the information available to the witness. Recently, researchers at Aberdeen had the opportunity to examine the prototype of Magnaface, a Kit designed to produce a realistic composite portrait in full colour. Construction begins from 'a clone', a featureless face which is attached to a magnetic board. The individual facial features incorporate a metallic backing so they can be laid smoothly and securely on to the clone allowing a complete face to be composed feature by feature. The final stage involves placing a special colour overlay over the composite which serves to harmonise the skin tones of the separate elements. Minor amendments to the face can then be made with cosmetic pencils and colouring supplied with the Kit.

Magnaface is currently only available in an Afro-Asian version, so a comparison trial was conducted between it and the Afro-Asian supplement of Photofit. Both kits were employed to make up a series of three African and one Asian face, half the faces being made 'from view' while the remainder were constructed 'from memory'. Subsequently volunteers attempted to identify which in a set of seven photographs a given composite was meant to represent. On this measure Magnaface enjoyed a 10% overall advantage over Photofit, though this was almost entirely confined to the 'from view' condition.

While differences in the size of feature repertoire between the two Kits must qualify any interpretation, it did appear that the employment of colour improved the overall quality of likeness of the composites. The fact, however, that the difference arose disproportionately from the condition in which the witness viewed the composite directly during construction cautions undue optimism. It appeared that either the witness failed to encode spontaneously the additional colour information into memory or, alternatively, the operator was unsuccessful in interviewing the witnesses in a way which enabled the information to be retrieved effectively.

Colour also plays an important part in another composite system which has received considerable publicity of late. BBC Television's 'Videofit' is used to 'improve' and colour composites which are shown to viewers in the course of the 'Crimewatch' programme. The latter reconstructs unsolved crimes and then appeals to the public to assist by furnishing information and possible identifications.

Contrary to popular belief, Videofit is not in itself a composite production system, rather it is a specialised use of the standard Quantel 7001 'paint-box' computer graphics package. The orthodox Photofit picture is electronically processed to remove the boundary lines between features and colour added to different parts of the face such as the eyes, flesh or hair. Features or accessories can be tranferred between pairs of composites to demonstrate appearance with or without disguise. No objective assessment of this system's effectiveness has yet been conducted, but undoubtedly criminals have been caught through its use. It is difficult, however, to decide whether this success reflects Videofit, the quality of the composite from which the finished picture was derived or the immense exposure enjoyed by the picture in question.

The BBC envisage that Videofit might be extended to include a range of features stored on disc and a graphics package for manipulating and fusing these features into a completed 'face'. The use of computer graphics for face production offers many advantages over cardboard or acetate. Difficulties over manipulating the position of features relative to each other can be resolved and individual features can be bent or stretched to give an infinite number of variations. One such computer-based system was created by the Computer Aided Design Centre in Cambridge, using the Photofit library of features. However, evaluation tests against the standard Photofit Kit suggested that further development work was required before a viable system could be produced (Christie, Davies, Shepherd and Ellis, 1981).

Like their predecessors, these new systems have been developed by technicians with little input from psychologists with a knowledge of face processing. Consequently, the choice of features and techniques of facial synthesis reflect a logical rather than a psychological analysis of the process of face memory. In principle psychologists should be capable of shedding light on the processes underpinning facial recall from the extensive studies of face recognition. But how is face recognition related to face recall? Does it utilise the same processes or are different mechanisms involved? If recall and recognition are not continuous processes how might the mechanisms postulated for face recognition be manipulated to achieve recall? And do such mechanisms shed any light on how recall might be achieved more effectively? These are questions which are addressed in the subsequent sections of this paper.

2.THE RELATIONSHIP OF FACE RECALL TO RECOGNITION

It cannot be assumed that face recall necessarily draws upon the same cognitive mechanisms and processes as face recognition. Whether recall and recognition are continuous or discontinuous processes is, of course a major question in cognitive research (Tiberghien and Lecocq, 1983). The continuous position argues that recall and recognition represent differentially sensitive tests of retrieval from long-term memory. While a simple differential threshold model is untenable, more sophisticated versions of the theory can be readily defended (Tulving 1982).

The alternative, discontinuous position has assumed many forms with differing degrees of overlap between the two retrieval processes (Kintsch 1970; Anderson and Bower, 1972). One of the more extreme disjunctions between recall and recognition is proposed by Johnson (1983). Recall and recognition are seen as the products of two quite separate cognitive systems: recall operates through a higher-order planning system (the reflective system) while recognition draws on a lower level perceptual system. Drawing on neuropsychological data, Johnson claims that total disassociation can occur between the two systems resulting in recall in the absence of recognition and vice versa.

Virtually all the evidence underlying such rival hypotheses are derived from studies of learning and memory for verbal stimuli, though it is equally appropriate to pose the same questions in relation to memory for faces. Do the effects of variables known to influence face recognition extend to recall? Is there a strong relationship between face recall and recognition at a within-group level? Does prior recall influence subsequent recognition and vice versa? To the extent that positive answers are found to these questions, the continuity position will receive support.

2.1.Do Memory Variables Influence Recall and Recognition Uniformly?

Davies (1983a) reviewed the extant literature on the impact of mnemonic variables on verbal recall and composite production. He noted a reasonable concordance between results from the two measures of recall but noted that verbal recall had generally proved the more sensitive of the two. Thus, Ellis, Shepherd and Davies (1980) reported a significant decline in the length and accuracy of a verbal description of a face from one hour to one week after original observation. However, the finding has not been replicated with Photofit as the measure of facial recall, a result more attributable to the vaguaries of the latter medium rather than any fundamental difference between the two measures (Davies, Ellis and Shepherd, 1978b).

Davies (1983a) considered the impact of the variables of race of face, delay and sex of observer and suspect on recall and recognition. He concluded that while race and delay had parallel effects upon recall and recognition, findings for sex were more equivocal. Since the publication of this review, two more variables have been examined for their impact upon face recall: encoding instructions at presentation and the age of the observer.

Wells and Hryciw (1984) presented subjects with a target face made from Identikit components and asked them to make a series of trait judgements (ratings on honesty, likeability etc.) or physical feature judgements (distance beetween the eyes, length of nose etc.) Subsequently, the subjects either recalled the face using the Identikit to construct a likeness or to recognise it in an array of photographs of similar composite faces. Consistent with earlier findings (Memon and Bruce, 1983), trait judgements led to superior recognition accuracy compared to physical features. However, the position was reversed when face recall was required; physical feature judgements produced more accurate Identikit likenesses than trait judgements. The Wells & Hryciw interpret this finding in terms of the differential processing demands of the two tasks: the Identikit relies upon knowledge of specific features while recognition involves configurational encoding. Their conclusions are worth quoting in full:

"Our conceptualisation suggests there is some orthoginality in the types of retrieval cues involved in these face memory tasks: Recognition memory favours interfeature retrieval cues; reconstruction of faces favours intrafeature cues; verbal recall favours neither inter-nor intrafeature cues" (Wells and Hryciw, 1984, p.343).

Unfortunately, the authors did not include any measure of verbal recall in their study, though they note that Brigham and Wolfskeil (1984) found no difference in quality or style of verbal description following either a trait or feature judgement task. If this result can be replicated using a real face as the original target, then it appears to offer an unequivocal example of a disjunction between recall and recognition and also between the two measures of recall.

A rather greater concordance between recall and recognition has emerged from a study by Markham, Flin and Davies currently being conducted into recall of faces by children. Children aged 8 and 11 years constructed two of a set of target faces, one being made from view while the second was made from memory. Comparison with adult data suggest a clear developmental improvement in the quality of likeness achieved by subjects at different ages. Such a finding seems at variance with the views of Carey (1981) who hypothesises that young children encode faces in terms of piecemeal features while adults are biased toward configurational information. In the light of the findings of Wells and Hryciw one might have expected an absence or even an reversal of the normal developmental trend. However, the findings for composite production complement those for face recognition for the age ranges tested.

In summary, existing studies of face recall show some parallels with the recognition data but also an interesting discrepancy. If the finding of Wells and Hryciw is a robust one, then it raises the possibility that processing strategies appropriate for recognition may be less effective for certain forms of a recall and vice versa. However, all the studies reviewed involve comparisons across groups. A more sensitive measure of the relationship of recall and recognition involves a within-group comparison: is a given subject's ability to recall a face correlated with their aptitude subsequently to recognise it?

2.2. Is there a Strong Relationship Between Recall and Recognition Within Groups?

Irrespective of the measure employed, there is no good evidence for a relationship between recall and recognition at the level of individual subjects. Davies et al. (1978b) and Laughery and Fowler (1980) found no relationship between an individual's ability to recognise the face of the target person and the quality of composite produced in a prior task. Similarly, Goldstein, Johnson and Chance (1979) found no correlation between subjects' fluency in describing faces and their ability to recognise them. Finally, Brigham and Wolfskiel (1984) examined directly the adequacy of a witness's verbal description of a face and their ability subsequently to recognise the person concerned in any array: correlations were uniformly close to zero.

Such results appear clearly at variance with the continuity position. It can always be argued, of course, that special factors might be responsible for these results. The two measures of recall are not significantly correlated themselves at an intra-subject level (Christie and Ellis, 1981) and perhaps a check-list procedure might yield results more consistent with the continuity position. On the existing evidence, however, the findings provide powerful support for the discontinuity position.

2.3.Does recall influence subsequent recognition?

If recall and recognition are drawing on the same trace information, then it might be expected that under some circumstances, prior recall should influence subsequent recognition of the same face. Davies (1981) reviewed three studies which had examined the impact of composite production on recognition, two of which showed a significant effect of prior recall. Only one (Davies et al., 1978b) showed no effect, a result more consistent with the discontinuity standpoint.

One of the three studies (Mauldin and Laughery 1981) demonstrated a facilitation to recognition from prior construction of the face with the Identikit, a result also reported by Thomson and Laughery (1979). The authors draw parallels between this finding and the report of Read (1979) who demonstrated that mental rehearsal of a face subsequently facilitated its recognition. However, the parallel, while attractive, is not perfect. Read reported equivalent facilitation when subjects rehearsed verbal descriptions, while Thomson and Laughery found no equivalent effect of verbal recall on recognition.

The final study (Hall, 1977) found a significant decrease in recognition accuracy for subjects who had collaborated with artists in producing a sketch of the target person. Thomson and Laughery note that the artists used in this study were inexperienced and they hypothesise that witnesses may have been pressed to fabricate detail thus biasing their subsequent recognition. There is certainly evidence that the incorporation of erronous detail into composites can marr subsequent recognition performance (Jenkins and Davies, 1985) but the interpretation of this and the other findings in terms of recall amending an existing trace is challengeable.

Morton, Hammersley and Bekerian (in press) have proposed a 'headed records' approach to memory which incorporates the assumption that each encounter with a given stimulus leads to the setting up of separate memory records rather than accessing the same original trace. Applied to the studies reviewed above it would imply that both observation of the target and constructing the composite produced separate records. A major assumption of the model is that access is always to the final record. Hence, recognition performance on the final task could be good, bad or indifferent depending on the quality of the final likeness achieved by subjects in the composite task. Support for such an interpretation comes from an unpublished study by Jenkins (1985) which demonstrated that the impact of misleading composite information on subjects' recognition behaviour could be ameliorated by instructions which enabled subjects to access their record of the initial observation of the target. It appears then that this last line of the evidence like the other two provides no compelling proof that recall and recognition necessarily draw on the same stimulus information.

It appears that these three strands of information provide support for only the broadest link between recall and recognition performance. While it is implausible, given the findings on memory for words, that the two processes are totally divorced, there is no evidence to support a complete identity between recall and recognition. Face recall, for instance, might utilise the mechanisms involved in face recognition, but in a different way, consistent with the demands of verbal description on the one hand and composite production on the other. The final section considers how the various hypothesised components of the face recognition process might contribute to recall.

3.MODELS OF FACE RECOGNITION: LESSONS FOR RECALL

The current 'modal model' of face recognition incorporates three major components. The central feature is some form of face recognition unit which fires in response to a familiar face and recruits a new unit when confronted with a novel face. This, in turn, is connected on the input side to a system for the detection and analysis of facial stimuli. Face recognition units in turn are interconnected with a third system which is concerned with knowledge about the person concerned (see, for instance, the chapters by Bruce and Young for further elaboration). It seems likely that all three components of this system play a role in face recall. What follows is largely descriptive but provides one sketch of how such a system might be adopted to cope with the vaguaries of the recall process.

Face recognition is hypothesised to procede from detection, through stimulation of recognition units to access to semantic information about the person concerned. The simplest conception of how recall might function would be simply to posit the reverse process. In Bartlettian terms, the witness 'turns about on his own schemata': a bottom-up recognition processing system is operated top-down. One theory of verbal memory which assumes recall and recognition are discontinuous processes provides a plausible model for the relationship of recall and recognition.

Anderson and Bower (1972) have proposed that a distinction be drawn between recognition, where the unit of information is present and the subject's task is to retrieve the appropriate context, and recall, where the context is defined by the experimenter and the subject's task is to use this to retrieve the information unit. Thus with recall of a face, the subject might begin by recalling the physical context in which the person had been encountered. Such information would presumably be subsumed in the 'person knowledge' component of the modal model.

If this is correct then one might predict that the more effectively contextual cues were stimulated, the more facial information might be retrieved. This seems indeed to be the case. Davies and Milne (1985) report a study in which the quality of composites produced by witness subjects was significantly improved by stimulating context. This was achieved either by physically placing the witness in the same room in which the target 'suspect' was observed or by giving instructions designed to stimulate affective and cognitive cues associated with the original incident. These effects were independent and additive, suggesting that information on facial appearance is accessed selectively rather than on an all-or-none basis, in line with recent thinking on differing codes for face recognition (Bruce and Young, 1985).

It is also worth noting in passing that the idea of priming of face recognition units by person-related semantic information has some interesting implications for the recognition of composites. It might suggest that if the appropriate information was not stimulated, even a good composite might remain unrecognised, rather in the manner of Tulving and Thomson's (1973) demonstration that words will not be recognised in an amended context.

As regard the central components, the characteristics of the face recognition units themselves, their nature is unclear. Most theories (e.g. Hay and Young, 1982) make a distinction between dedicated units concerned with an individual face and undedicated units. However, is a dedicated unit created in a single operation or can such a unit be incremented by further information through more frequent encounters with the individual concerned?

It is tempting to opt for the latter given that verbal recall of a face tends to be richer and fuller for persons whose face we know well than for strangers (Shepherd, Davies and Ellis, 1978). Likewise, the vividness of imagery associated with the recall of friends and relatives tends to be stronger than for photographs of persons seen briefly in a laboratory (Morris, 1985). It could, of course, be argued that verbal recall and imagery are not the direct output of recognition units, but rather, reflect the products of the person information store, much in the manner of Johnson's 'reflective memory'. Such a viewpoint might help to explain the generally poor relationship of recall and recognition at an inter-personal level. Clearly, however, while parsimony favours the former, further research is called for to clarify this issue.

Turning finally to the basic mechanisms underlying the detection of faces at input, it is important that forensic systems for constructing and recalling faces should be compatible with what is known about basic encoding processes. Studies of face recognition have laid an increasing emphasis upon changes in the variety and types of information which subjects utilise to recognise a face as it becomes more familiar. Ellis, Shepherd and Davies (1979), for instance, reported a greater reliance on interior parts of the face compared to exterior features for familiar faces. Likewise, Sergent (1984) reported a shift in emphasis from feature information to configurational cues as familiarity with a face increased. As has been noted, most commercial composite systems are inadequate in their ability to manipulate the relation of one facial feature to another.

On the basis of neuropsychological evidence, Hay and Young (1982) disassociate expressive cues from feature information with only the latter mediating recognition. There is an interesting discrepancy here between their views and those of some police artists (Davies, 1985b) and professional portrait painters (Gombrich, 1972) who see expression as the key to achieving a likeness. Certainly, on the basis of available evidence it would be premature to dismiss the possibility that expressive information might contribute to the representation of a face as it becomes increasingly familiar. All will know the experience of glancing at photographs of themselves or friends and exclaiming "that one looks like you-but that does not" a discrimination which seems based ultimately on the expressive content of the pictures concerned (c.f. Yarmey 1982).

4.CONCLUSION

Some years ago, Baddeley (1979) distinguished between what he termed 'cognitive applied' and 'applied cognitive' research. By 'applied cognitive' he referred to the application of cognitive models to concrete issues such as memory for faces. He perceived this endeavour as a superior and more productive exercise than cognitive applied research which he characterised as atheoretical and problem-orientated. The current review of the issues of face recall suggests that perhaps this perspective may be a little overdrawn. There is a role both for the applied cognitive, in the shape of laboratory research on face recognition and the cognitive applied in the form of research on face recall. To produce a comprehensive and general theory of face memory requires a process of assimilation and accommodation. Assimilation of the new theoretical insights generated by basic research on face recognition and accommodation of these theories to the elusive and ill-understood processes of face recall. As long as practical composite systems remain exclusively the domain of the commercial manufacturers and academic psychologists concentrate on recognition processes, it is unlikely that either endeavour will be crowned with success.

Note   Thanks are due to Dr. R. Markham for valuable discussion of the recall/recognition issue.

AN INTERACTIVE COMPUTER SYSTEM FOR RETRIEVING FACES

J.W. SHEPHERD

1.INTRODUCTION

The evidence of eyewitnesses plays an important role in the work of the police and security services. The use of identification parades and mug-shot albums is an integral part of the investigative aspect of police work, while the evidence of eyewitnesses often forms a major part of the prosecution's case. It is therefore not surprising that for many years police forces have tried to improve the efficiency of methods of obtaining identification evidence from eyewitnesses.

The use of illustrative aids has a long history (see Davies 1981 for a review) and these are still popular with the police forces in most countries. Those in use in the United Kingdom, the United States and some parts of Continental Europe usually either involve some variant of a jig-saw principle in which separate parts of the faces (hair, eyes, mouth, etc.) are selected from a number of alternatives and are assembled to make a composite of the face, or involve an artist producing an impression of the target from the description provided by the witness.

These methods share the common difficulty that they require the witness to recall all the major features of the face of the target or at least be able to recognise each of the major facial elements from among a large number of alternatives. However, people often find great difficulty in recalling the features of faces even of familiar people, and, as Klatsky and Forrest (1984) report, subjects were unable to report details about the faces of people they had just been shown. For example, they were often unable to report whether the person's mouth had been open or closed. Failure to select the appropriate feature in composite construction may lead to grossly misleading end products, even if other features are a good fit. An additional problem of many such systems is that the range of alternatives available in comparison with the population of features they are supposed to sample is so small that a good match for any feature is difficult to make. The advent of computer techniques (see Laughery, Rhodes and Batten 1981 for a review) has enabled more flexibility to be introduced into the construction process but even these do not overcome the limitations of recall in the witness. For even when subjects are asked to reproduce from memory a Photofit composite they have just seen they are seldom able to make a perfect match (Ellis, Shepherd and Davies 1975).

The alternative to asking a witness to provide a composite construction or verbal description of a suspect is to ask him to search for a photograph of the person from among a collection of mugshots. The advantage of a photograph is that instead of having to recall a face, a witness has only to recognise that suspect, a task at which people in general are highly efficient. Most police forces retain collections of photographs of previously convicted offenders, and these are frequently assembled into albums through which witnesses can search in an attempt to identify a suspect. Apart from the requirement that the suspect must have a previous conviction for this method to be used, the main problem with it is that the witness may be required to look through a very large number of photographs, possibly a thousand or more, with the attendant risks of interference, change in criterion or fatigue (Davies, Shepherd and Ellis, 1979; Laughery, Alexander & Lane, 1971). Where the police make up a special album, for particular kinds of offence or categories of person, there are considerable time demands on the police personnel.

Ideally a witness should be presented with a subset of faces selected by searching the complete set of faces available on the basis of information provided by the witness and by other means of investigation, so that only the most likely items in the collection are included in the set to be searched. Such a preliminary search is a task for which a computer is clearly ideally suited.

The application of computers to this search problem has taken two main forms. One approach has been to obtain some form of graphic input, from an artist's impression or Identikit or Photofit construction, and run this through a pattern matching algorithm. This approach does not surmount the problem of detail recall facing the witness. The alternative is to use a coded verbal description of the suspect to search through a database of coded descriptions of the faces on file (e.g. Goldstein, Harmon & Lesk, 1971), and to produce a list of the faces which fit the initial description most closely (see Laughery, Rhodes and Batten, 1981 for a review). This is the approach which has been the basis of the method adopted at Aberdeen, where FRAME, Face Retrieval And Matching Equipment, has been developed in collaboration with the Home Office.

2.THE FRAME SYSTEM

In its present form FRAME comprises a videodisc on which photographic images of 1000 faces are stored, a database of 1000 records of these faces coded on 50 attributes or parameters, and a program which compares a set of input parameters for a face with each of the records in the database, ranks records in their order of similarity to the input, and displays the corresponding facial images via a video disc player on a television monitor in this order.

Setting up the system involved three stages: assembling a collection of photographs to provide the basis of the prototype system, coding the photographs to form the database on which the search program operates, and evaluating the system.

2.1. Assembling the collection

Two considerations entered into decisions about the nature of the collection. Since this was to be a prototype for a police system the size of the collection should be such that it would give some indication of its applicability to the mug-shot system which might be held by a moderately sized police force. It was decided that 1000 faces would meet this requirement, for although many police forces would have photographic collections larger than this, the size of the collection to be searched could be reduced by preliminary screening, for example using the nature of the offence. The second guiding consideration was that the sample of faces should be representative in age distribution, and the presence of beards, moustaches and spectacles of the population of men convicted in the courts, whose photographs were likely to form the basis of police collections. Consequently, the sample had a high proportion of men in the younger age groups (16 to 25 years) with diminishing proportions of men in the older age groups. The men were recruited by being approached on the campus of the University or in the streets in the centre of the city. The nature of the project was explained and the subject was invited to accompany the investigator to a temporary studio which had been prepared nearby. A high compliance rate was ensured by offering the participant the opportunity to win a cash prize.

The temporary studio was used in an attempt to get the maximum uniformity of pose and photographic quality, and was equipped with three Olympus OM cameras each with a 135 mm lens, and each yoked to a Bowen's 200 monolight electronic flash head with an umbrella for bounced flash. The cameras were set up at a distance of 173 cm from the subject's nose. Two of the cameras were set at an angle of 90 degrees to give a full face and right profile view, while the third camera was set at 45 degrees to the others to give a semiprofile. All three cameras were fired simultaneously by an electronic firing mechanism, and were loaded with Kodak Ektachrome 64 ASA slide film.

2.1.1. <u>Procedure</u>. On arrival at the studio subjects were told the purposes of the research and were asked to sign a form of agreement for the specific uses of their photographs. Each subject put on a green surgical gown to conceal his clothing, was seated in a specially adapted dental chair, and was asked to adopt a relaxed expression. The dentist's chair was used to enable the position of the subject to be adjusted in the vertical plane to the level of the cameras, and was fitted with a specially constructed neck rest to ensure that the head was held at the correct angle in the frontal plane. This was important since these photographs were to be used to take physical measurements of the subjects' faces.

The 3000 slides comprising 3 poses for each of the 1000 subjects were transfered by Thorn-EMI to a VHD videodisc, which when used with a Thorn-EMI Videodisc player model 3D01 permits random page access and a still page display of the image on a T.V. monitor.

2.2. Development of the database

There are a number of ways in which a retrieval system may store information relating to images. FRAME, in its present version codes information about the facial images in terms of 50 parameters for each face. Some of these have been obtained by direct physical measurements from the image, some are based upon ratings from trained judges of qualitative features of the image, while three parameters were obtained from the subjects themselves namely those for height, weight and age of the subject.

As a first step to obtaining these values, a group of graduate students were trained to make ratings of 38 attributes of the faces on five-point scales, and a further 9 attributes on dichotomous scales.

These scales were based upon previous work by Shepherd, Ellis and Davies (1977) and Jones, Hirschberg and Rothman (1976), and describe attributes relating to the general shape of the face, complexion, hair, forehead, eyebrows, eyes, ears, nose, mouth, chin, facial hair, physical peculiarities such as scars or squint, and accessories such as eyeglasses or earrings. The mean value of the ratings for the ten raters for each face on each parameter was used as the data point. Ratings were carried out with all three poses of each face projected simultaneously on to a screen.

2.2.1.<u>Physical measurement</u>. The second stage was to substitute for the ratings physical measurements taken from the facial image, where this was appropriate. This was accomplished by means of a Summergraphics Bitpad. The pad is approximately 25cm by 25cm in size with a resolution of 0.1mm., providing coordinates of 2500 by 2500 within which points could be defined.

Images were projected on to the Bitpad from a Kodak Carousel projector via a mirror to give a projected image of approximately 20cm by 10cm. Digitising was accomplished by touching each of 37 defined points with a stylus in a specified order. These points were based mainly upon the work of Jones et al. (1976) and are illustrated in Figure 1. Linear and area measurements were derived from the coordinates of these points.

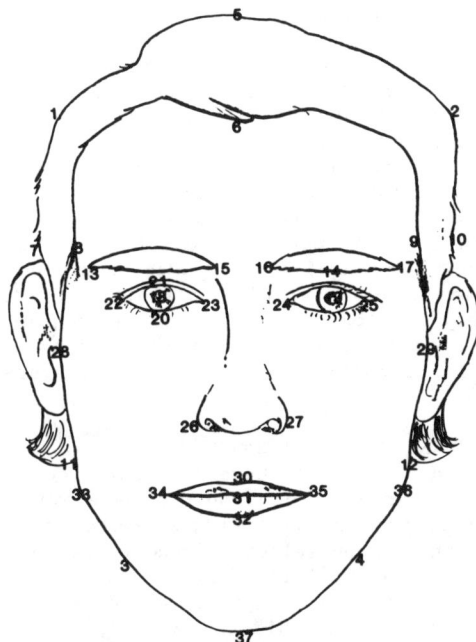

FIGURE 1 Points digitised in coding faces.

These measurements were scaled to values on a 5 point scale by using the equation for the regression of the rating scales on to the corresponding, physical measurements and these were substituted for the ratings in the database. Where no physical measurement was possible, as for example in rating hair colour or eye colour, the original rating was retained. The database thus comprises 1000 records, each with fifty parameters, of which 21 are based upon physical measurements, 26 on ratings, and 3 on data obtained from the subjects.

2.3.<u>The search program</u>

The FRAME search and retrieval program operates by comparing a set of input parameters with each of the records for the 1000 faces in the database. For each record a matching score is computed, which is the proportion of the input parameters which match the corresponding parameters in the database record. The criterion for a match is defined by specifying a range of tolerance values around the entry in the record within which the input parameter must fall. At present this tolerance range is set at +/- 0.5 of a scale point.

After comparing the entered set of parameters with all the records, the program ranks the matching scores and produces a retrieval list of record numbers in order of similarity to the input parameters.

The images for these records may be retrieved from the video disc and displayed automatically on a television monitor, or may, of course, be retrieved manually from a file of photographic prints.

2.3.1.Facilities available with FRAME. If the intial search does not result in the retrieval of a target face in, say, the top ten records of the retrieval list a number of options are available to a witness. The input parameter values may be re-entered but with specified parameters given an additional weighting so that in computing the matching score such parameters contribute proportionately to the weight given to them. The value of this option is that it enables witnesses to give an additional weighting to features which are particularly salient or about which they are very confident while correspondingly reduced the contribution of less certain judgements in the search algorithm. A second facility enables the witness to substitute for any parameter the value of the parameter in any of the retrieved images. So, for example, the witness may observe that the eyes of one retrieved image are similar to those of the target, the nose of another retrieved image matches the nose of the target, and the hair colour and hair length of a third image correspond to the target. In this way it would in principle be possible for the witness to select instances of every attribute from the set of displayed images, though in practice this never occurs. A variation of this option allows the parameter value for a particular feature to be averaged across a set of faces.

3.TESTING THE DATABASE

A number of laboratory studies have been carried out to test the utility of the system. The three to be reported here were designed with three objectives. First, to test whether the system could retrieve a target described from a photograph selected from the set of faces in the system. This would ensure that the appearance of the target had not changed between the time at which he was photographed for the system and the time of his presentation to the subject. Second, to test its effectiveness with a live target who may have changed in appearance between the time of photographing and the time of presentation of the subject. Third, to compare the performance of subjects using FRAME with subjects using the conventional album method.

3.1.Experiment 1

This experiment set out to provide a simple trial of the system by requiring a subject to produce a description of a target, and using this description to locate the target in the database.

3.1.1.Targets. Eight targets were randomly selected from the database using random number tables.

3.1.2.Subjects. Thirty two members of the public and undergraduates served as subjects of whom 26 were female and 6 males. Four subjects were randomly assigned to describe each target.

3.1.3.Procedure. A subject was presented with one of these targets on a 26 inch television monitor for 10 seconds. At the end of this period the image was removed and the subject was asked to describe the target to the experimenter. Using this free description the experimenter obtained from the subject a rating on a five point scale on those parameters which the subject had spontaneously mentioned. These values were then entered as the initial search parameters. If, after the first search, the target did not appear in the first ten of the retrieval list the subject was asked whether she wished to amend any of the search parameter values. This could be done either by substituting for the initial entry the value for that parameter in any of the faces in the retrieval list which the subject thought resembled the target, or by the subject rescaling her own values on the basis of anchor values derived from the faces in the retrieval list. In effect the subject would use the faces in the list as a means of calibrating her own scaling system. Up to four searches were permitted. The criterion of a successful retrieval (a hit) was that the target appeared in the first ten retrieval positions and was recognised by the subject.

3.1.4.Results. On the first trial, 56 per cent of subjects achieved a hit, and the experiment was terminated for these. This rose to 72 per cent after the second search, 78 per cent after the third search and 84 per cent after the fourth. All targets were retrieved at least once over the four searches, and 7 out of 8 targets were retrieved at least once on the first trial.

This experiment demonstrated that subjects could retrieve faces from the database using the coding scheme we had developed when the imges they were describing were as they appeared in the system. These conditions represent the most favourable for a subject working from memory. As some kind of approximation to the circumstances in which an operational system might be used, the second experiment involved using live targets which the subject would be required to describe from memory.

3.2.Experiment 2

The aim of the second experiment was to test the utility of the system when the subject was asked to recall a live target.

3.2.1.Subjects and targets. For this experiment the subjects were senior students from the department of psychology at Aberdeen University and the targets were four members of staff who had been photographed during the initial collection of the database.

3.2.2.Procedure. Each student was tested individually, and was asked to describe a member of the staff of the department from the list of targets whom he or she knew by appearance. The procedure for describing the target and completing the ratings was the same as that adopted in experiment 1, except that no initial presentation of the target occurred. The criterion for a hit was that the target should appear in the top ten of the retrieval list. This task was in some ways a more exacting test for the system, for while the subjects could claim a degree of familiarity with the appearance of the targets which a photographic presentation of a few seconds could not attain, they were trying to retrieve photographs of these targets which had been taken some three years earlier.

3.2.3.<u>Results</u>. The results did not indicate that the task was more difficult. On the first search there was a 70 per cent hit rate which rose to 80 per cent after three searches. Thus, apparently, the system had shown itself to be effective when subjects were describing a target whom they had encountered in the course of normal daily life, and whose appearance may have changed over the course of time. While it appears that the majority of subjects were able to retrieve a target from the database, it is not obvious that their performance was any better than could have been achieved using the traditional album method. In the final experiment to be reported here, the performance of subjects using the traditional album method was compared with that of subjects using FRAME.

3.3.Experiment 3

In this experiment, in addition to the comparison of FRAME with the album method for selecting mugshots the effect of two other variables was examined. The first of these was the distinctiveness of the target. There is evidence that the similarity of the target to the distractors in a recognition test affects the performance of the subject (Davies, Shepherd & Ellis, 1979a), and that the "typicality" of a target also reduces the readiness with which it can be recognised (Light, Kayra-Stuart & Hollander 1979). A target which had a distinctive feature might therefore be expected to be more readily recognised in an album than a target without a distinctive feature, since the distinctive feature should make the target both less similar to the distractors and less "typical" than the non-distinctive target. The distinctiveness of the target should have little effect on the probability of a retrieval using FRAME since the faces in the retrieval list might be expected to have the same distinctive feature as the target and thus, paradoxically make the task more difficult with FRAME than with an album, but no more difficult than with a target without the distinctive feature.

The second additional variable was the position of the target in the album. It has been shown by Davies et al. (1979) and by Laughery et al. (1971) that the later in a series of distractors a target appears, the less the likelihood of it being identified. In this respect FRAME should prove more effective than the album method when the target appears later in position in the album.

3.3.1.<u>Selection of targets</u>. A person unconnected with the project was asked to select from the set of 1000 faces four nondistinctive and four distinctive faces (i.e. with a beard or moustache or glasses or bald). These were the target faces and were presented in 3/4 profile pose.

3.3.2.<u>Procedure</u>. Following the presentation by one experimenter of a single target projected on a screen, a subject went through a search procedure with a different experimenter, using either the FRAME method or the album method. Subjects using FRAME went through the procedure of describing the face and coding descriptors on the list of parameters as in the previous experiments. These were entered as the initial search parameters and a search initiated. If the target did not appear in the top six retrievals, a second search was carried out making use of two of the facilities offered by FRAME for modifying the subject's input mentioned earlier, the alteration of a parameter's value, or adding a weight to any parameters about which the subject was confident. Up to four searches was allowed, and a trial was regarded as successful if the target appeared in the first six of the retrieval list on any of the four searches.

For the ALBUM condition subjects were asked to give a description of the target and were then asked to look through the albums to try to pick out the target. They were told the target's photograph might or might not be present in the albums.

For this condition full face colour prints, 13 cm by 9 cm, of all the faces were arranged four to a page in four albums, each album containing 250 faces. Each target was placed an equal number of times in one of four positions: 97, 353, 649 and 898.

3.3.3.Subjects. A total of 128 subjects, undergraduates at Aberdeen University, were run with 2 subjects being assigned to each target at each position in the album, and a parallel subject being run for each of these subjects in the FRAME condition. Thus 64 subjects were run in the album condition and 64 subjects used FRAME.

3.3.4.Results. Each subject's outcome was scored in one of four categories. A HIT was recorded when the subject correctly identified the target, a FALSE ALARM meant the subject had mistakenly selected a face which was not the target, a MISS occurred when the subject failed to identify the target when he appeared and did not make a false alarm, a NON RETRIEVAL could occur only under the FRAME condition when the subject failed to get the target into the top six positions within four trials.

For the distinctive faces the results for the two methods of search are similar. The hit rate for FRAME is 75% compared with a hit rate of 78% for the album condition. The false alarm rate and misses are low and also similar. For the nondistinctive faces, however, the results are rather different. The hit rate of 69% for FRAME is not significantly different from the 75% hit rate for the distinctive faces. For the album method the hit rate drops significantly to 44% with a corresponding increase in the false alarm rate, as indicated in Figure 2. (For Hits Chi square = 9.06, df = 1, p < .01).

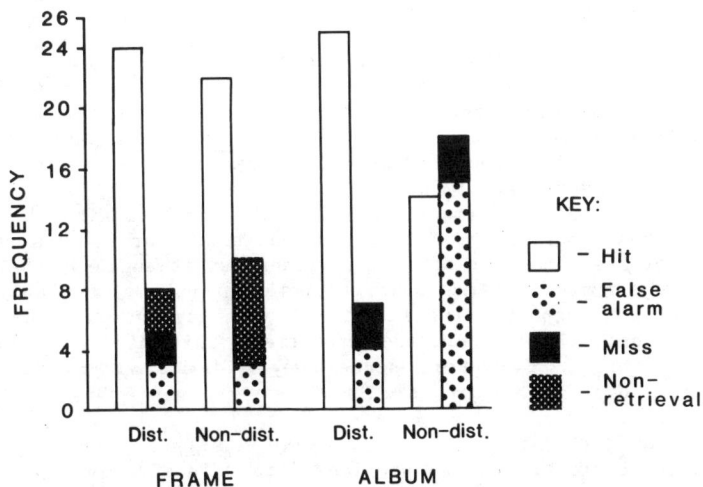

FIGURE 2. Hits, false alarms and misses for Frame and Album procedures on distinctive and non-distinctive targets.

This drop in performance for the album condition is due mainly to the effect of the target appearing in the later positions, and, as Figures 3 and 4 show there is a clear position effect for the nondistinctive

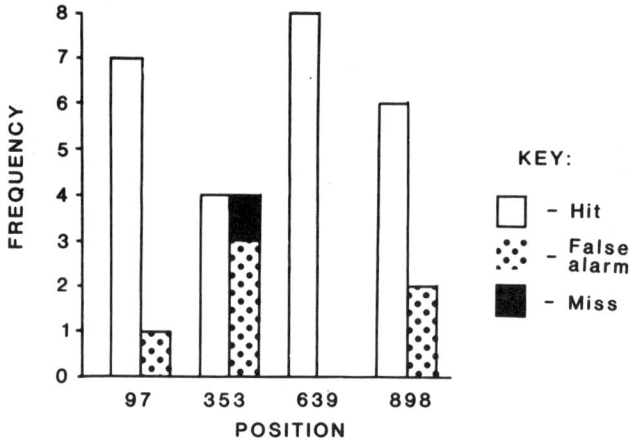

FIGURE 3.   Position effects for album search.
Distinctive targets.

faces but not for the distinctive faces, with the former showing a monotonic fall in hit rate and increase in false alarms as the position of the target in the album occurs later. This result is similar to that obtained by Lenorovitz and Laughery (1984), who also obtained a position effect using Identikit composites as their stimuli and a smaller set than was used in the present experiment.

The increase in false alarms which occurs in parallel with the fall in the hit rate has important practical implications. For if this is in any way typical of the behaviour of police witnesses, it suggests that giving witnesses large numbers of mug-shots to work through may not only reduce the chance of the suspect being identified, but may increase the risk of misidentification. In the present experiment this did not occur when subjects used the FRAME system, since they did not view more than 24 different faces over four search trials.

3.4.Parameter usage
The database currently in use provides data points for 50 parameters. While it would be possible to ask witnesses to rate a target on each of these parameters, such a practice would be unwise since we have found that subjects are unable to remember faces in the detail such a task would require. For example, in Experiment 2 above, the retrieval rate on the first search was 70 per cent. When a search was carried out on the basis

of ratings by colleagues of the targets on all 50 parameters, a hit rate of 46 per cent was achieved. What parameters a witness uses will vary

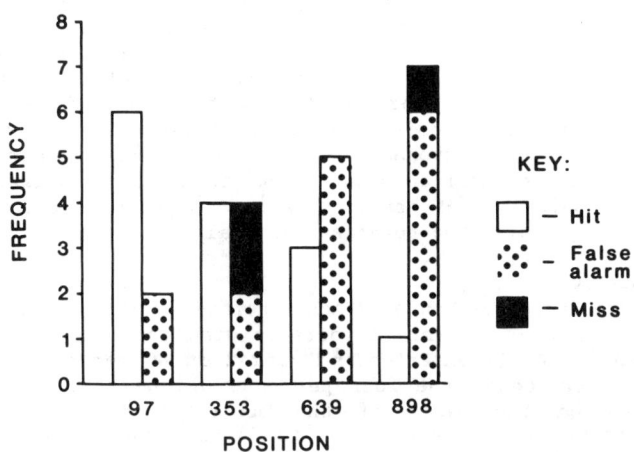

with the nature of the target. Nevertheless, across different experiments using different targets some parameters are used very frequently while others are rarely used. Table 1 lists the parameters used by one half or more of the subjects who took part in the experiments reported above. It is clear from this table that upper features of the face and particularly the hair are most salient in physical descriptions of male targets, a finding that has been reported many times before (Shepherd, Ellis & Davies, 1981).

TABLE 1. Frequency of parameter usage in experiments 1,2 and 3.
(Only those parameters are listed which were used spontaneously by 50 per cent or more of subjects in that experiment).

Experiment 1 n=32		Experiment 2 n=20		Experiment 3 n=64	
Parameter	freq.	Parameter	freq.	Parameter	freq.
hair length	32	hair length	18	hair colour	57
hair colour	32	hair colour	18	eye colour	55
hair texture	27	hair texture	18	hair length	51
eye colour	27	face fatness	15	hair texture	47
eyebrow thickness	24	baldness	11	eyebrow thickness	34
lip thickness	19	face length	11		
		complexion	11		
		hair greyness	11		
		eyebrow thickness	11		
		mouth size	11		
		nose length	10		
		lip thickness	10		

A further significant aspect of Table 1 is that the most frequently used parameters are those relating to the length and colour of the targets' hair both for photographic and for live targets. While this may not seem intuitively to be very remarkable, it does have implications for the policy of the police in photographing and coding faces for storage and retrieval by computer. With colour such an important cue for witnesses, it is clear that computer records of facial codes will have to include details of colour of hair and eyes. However, this makes more difficult the task of devising purely automatic means of coding physical characteristics of faces. At present a practical system for coding monochrome photographs of faces entirely of computer does not exist, though work by Craw and Lishman of the departments of mathematics and computing science at Aberdeen University is directed towards that goal.

4.CONCLUSION

The prototype version of FRAME reported here has produced retrieval rates which compare very favourably with those of other systems so far reported. In experiments 1 and 2 in 80 per cent of trials the target occurred in the four per cent of the faces in the database selected on the basis of the subject's description, while in experiment 3 the face occurred in 75 per cent of trials in the 2.4 per cent of faces selected from the database. These rates were achieved with a database of 1000 faces, which is of modest size compared with the number of faces which might be expected to be held in the criminal record files of a metropolitan police force. However, the size of the database to be searched could be reduced on the basis of the category of the crime, so that a set of say 10000 might be selected. If FRAME produced results in line with those of experiments 1 and 2 above, a witness would expect to retrieve a target within a set of 240 faces to inspect in 80 per cent of cases, and in 56 per cent of cases within a set of 60 faces. This clearly represents a considerable saving in time and cognitive effort for the witness.

The algorithm used with FRAME is a sequencing algorithm, which Laughery et al. (1981). contrast with a matching algorith. The essential difference between these algorithms is that the former retains all the cases in the database throughout its search and selects the most likely cases at the end of the run on the basis of some "distance" measure between each record in the database and the input. The matching algorithm, on the other hand, eliminates from the search those cases which fall outside the value of each search parameter so that the set to be searched is reduced as each feature's value is entered. On the basis of their own research compared with the results of previous work, Lenorovitz and Laughery (1984) claim to have demonstrated the superiority of the matching algorithm. However, the results obtained with FRAME raise doubts about the empirical justification for their claim. At present, it would clearly be premature to advocate either of the options as being superior.

Acknowledgements.   The work reported here was carried out under contract from the Scientific Research and Development Branch of the Home Office.   Frank Smith of the Home Office was primarily responsible for writing the FRAME program, while the work at Aberdeen was carried out in collaboration with Hadyn Ellis, Graham Davies, Rhona Flin, Steve Greentree, Alan Milne and Jean Shepherd.

INVESTIGATING FACE RECOGNITION WITH AN IMAGE PROCESSING COMPUTER

NIGEL D. HAIG

1. INTRODUCTION

All of us participating in this conference will, at some time or other, have ruminated deeply about faces and how we recognise them. The human visual recognition process is so astonishingly effortless, however, that most people take it entirely for granted, without questioning the extended complexity of neural processing that must be involved. So much so that it is sometimes difficult for people to realise just how complex is the process of visual perception, quite apart from the additional burden of recognition. Indeed, the Nobel Prizewinner Francis Crick (1979) expressed the problem well when he said "Few people realise what an astonishing achievement it is to be able to see at all". One of the aims of my group at RARDE is to attempt an understanding of visual recognition, in order that it may be modelled and, ultimately, simulated by computers and electro-optic imaging systems. Clearly, an early stage in the development of modelling must involve the collection of relevant data in several different fields of human endeavour, such as physical optics, psychology and neurophysiology. The decision to use faces as recognition targets was based on their essential ubiquity and familiarity; observers would not require special training to recognise them. Having selected a class of targets for exploration, the nature of the exploration has to be decided. As I have pointed out elsewhere (Haig, 1984), many useful and interesting experiments concerning face recognition have been reported, but they have each asked slightly different questions, and have thus received different answers that are difficult to inter-relate.

In this paper, I shall attempt to show how useful an image-processing computer can be in probing face recognition. The advantages of such a system include; the ability to insert new targets into digital storage by way of a CCTV camera, the ability to control and to change brightnesses and contrasts both locally and globally, the ability to move the targets around, change their size and orientation, to present them for a wide range of fixed time intervals, and the great blessing of running experiments automatically, collecting the data and analysing the results. Among the disadvantages are the capital cost, the need to write one's own specialised software and ensure its validity, and the limited resolution and storage capacity of a single framestore. In my case, an additional constraint is the lack of colour: My image processor is a purely monochrome system. Notwithstanding such limitations, I hope to demonstrate the versitility and usefuless of the system by briefly reviewing some experiments in face recognition that I have undertaken with it. Since the image processor was the same for all the experiments, I will begin by summarising its characteristics and the observers' viewing facility.

2. THE IMAGE PROCESSING SYSTEM

The heart of this system consists of a very early model of a Microconsultants INTELLECT Series 1 image processor. The host computer is an LSI-11, having a MOSS operating system, and the image processing is performed by means of the moderately high-level language ART. The INTELLECT 1 contains only one framestore of 512 x 512 pixels, (to an accuracy of 8 bits) which thus permits 256 grey levels from black to peak white. Additional digital picture storage was available by means of a Perex PERIFILE digital cassette recorder, although the access time in this mode was very slow. In contrast to this, the INTELLECT processing time was very rapid; an advantage that was seriously offset by the limitation of integer-only operation. Such a limitation had the practical effects of fixing a low ceiling on program length and storage space, together with a prohibition on fractional computations during data reduction.

The database of target faces, taken under reasonably standardised conditions from the direct frontal aspect, consisted of a random selection of more than 100 Ministry of Defence employees. The resultant black and white photographs were re-imaged, via a Link Electronics Model 109B CCTV camera and the image processor, into storage on digital tape cassettes. Experimentation showed that the face pictures were rendered with high quality if contained within 128 x 128 pixel squares, thereby permitting 4 x 4 = 16 such pictures to be stored within the single framestore. Care was taken to register the head positions accurately and reproducibly by fixing the positions of the eye pupils within the squares. This procedure accurately fixed the Interpupilary Distance (IPD) at 30 pixels, except for a few special cases that will be mentioned later.

The output from the INTELLECT drove a broadcast quality Pye TVT monitor, which had a 15 inch screen with a green (GH) phosphor. Mean display luminance, for all of the experiments that I shall describe, was 64 cd.m^{-2} , and there was a large cardboard screen-surround illuminated to match the screen colour and luminance as closely as possible. With a viewing range of 2.0 metres, the square raster subtended 6.5 x 6.5 degrees, giving a single pixel size of 0.45mm which corresponds to 0.76 min of arc. The retinal image size was thus equivalent to an average human face, at a range of 10 metres, containing considerable detail, but without the distraction of resolvable raster lines.

As regards software, the ART language possesses certain fundamental functions that operate on the data stream into, out of, and within the framestore. Programming the INTELLECT is thus a matter of chaining together the required functions in such a way as to act upon the specified parts of an image in a defined sequence. Programmes were written that performed such operations as grey-level shifting, contrast stretching and compression, generalised histogram modification, image shifting, image stretch and compression both vertically and horizontally, contrast matching, picture blanking, windowing and so on. All of these operations, and more, were utilised in preparing and running the experiments to be described in this paper. It should not be assumed that the mere possession of an image processing computer necessarily makes experimentation any easier, nor does it generate ideas. Rather, it allows the researcher to attempt different tasks, particularly those involving considerable data collection, and it guarantees an almost absolute reproducibility. By way of contrast, it is worth pointing out that conventional photography can unwittingly introduce considerable stimulus variability, by virtue of the considerable non-linearity inherent in the several processing steps. We have found, at RARDE, an additional benefit from ready access to an image processor, namely the ability to try out new ideas very quickly. Once appropriate software has been written and target imagery is available, via the CCTV camera or from tape, preliminary experiments may be assembled and tested very rapidly. I hope to illustrate the versatility and usefulness of the image processing approach by describing some experiments that I have undertaken, over the last two years, to probe face recognition.

3. FACE DISTORTION EXPERIMENTS

This set of experiments has already been published (Haig, 1984) and I will therefore summarise them only very briefly. Nevertheless, the stimulus material, the presentation technique and the results demonstrate the value of the thoughtful use of an image processor.

The aim of this experiment was to measure the sensitivity of adult observers to slight positional changes of prominent facial features. Five male observers, including the author, were used, and all had a binocular acuity of 6/4. Five target faces were used, three male and two female, having no visible blemishes, facial hair or spectacles. Each target face was subjected to the same operations, in which certain features were moved by defined amounts. The maximum excursion of the chosen features on one of the targets is shown in Fig 1, the intermediate excursions having been omitted, to save space. The total number of target pictures amounted to 39 per individual target head, and each experimental session included 5 one-second presentations of each of the 39 variations, in the centre of the screen, with the rest of the screen masked electronically. Selection of the variations was random, and the observer registered his response to the question "Is this picture of the original target or is it a modified target?" by pressing one of two buttons. The screen was blanked until the observer responded, and when the computer had registered the response, the original target picture was re-presented towards one corner of the screen, for 2 or 3 seconds, while the computer selected and positioned the next presentation. All 5 observers undertook 40 such sessions, and the detailed results are tabulated in Haig (1984). However, Fig 2 shows a graphical summary of the 50% correct responses, summed across observers and summed across targets. The two sets of results are gratifyingly similar, showing that the observers apparently used similar judgemental strategies, and also indicating that the different targets aroused similar perceptual effects.

In summary, the greatest sensitivity is to Mouth Up, where observers noticed a mere 1.2 pixels movement, corresponding to nearly 1 min of arc, which is close to the visual acuity limit. I feel that this is a ratiometric effect, to do with upper lip depth or area, since downward mouth movement is less noticeable. This is testable by comparing results for Nose down and up, where the upper lip depth is varied similarly, and the same thing happens. Sensitivity to vertical shifts of eyes/eyebrows is also high and a possible criterion based on the ratio of forehead height to cheek area is supportable by comparing this with vertical movement of the entire face. Notice that

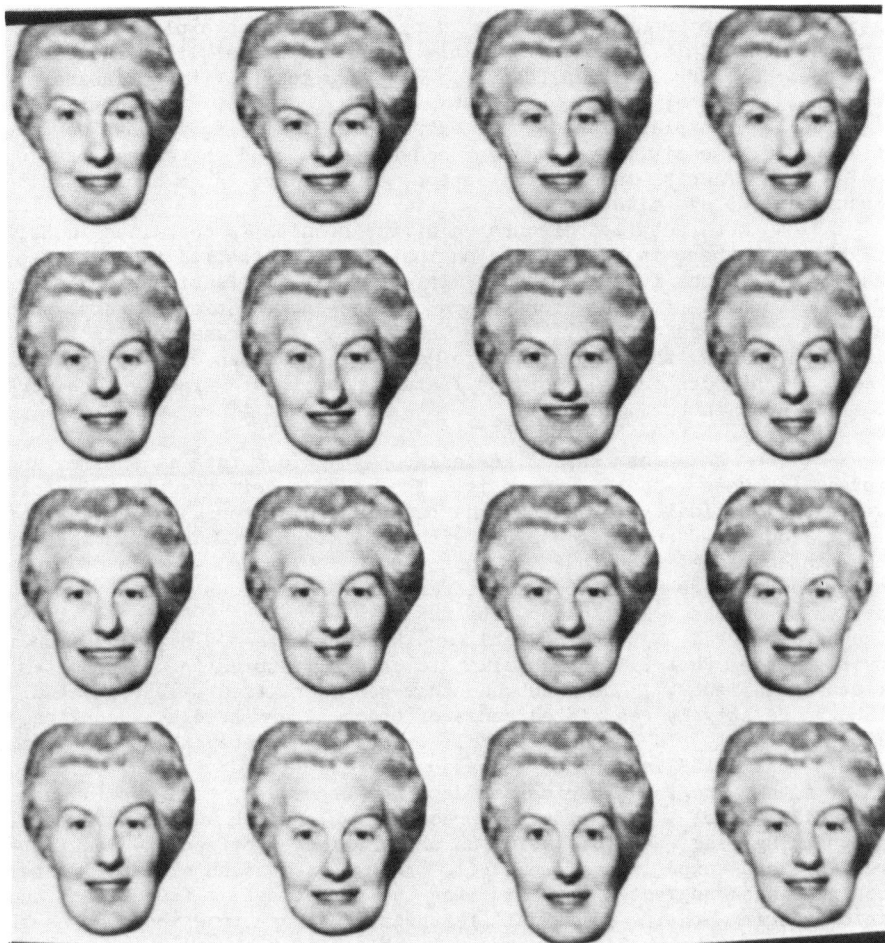

Fig 1. Photograph of the monitor screen,showing the extremes of
feature displacement applied to one target. Reading from left to
right, the distortions are;(Top row) Eyes Up, Eyes Down, Eyes Narrow,
Eyes Wide,(Second row) Nose Up, Nose Down,Mouth Up, Mouth Down,(Third
row) Mouth Wide, Mouth Narrow,Original,Reversed,(Bottom row) Face Up,
Face Down, Head Narrow, Head Wide.Each of these pictures, together
with the intermediate distortions, were only ever presented singly, at
or near the middle of the screen.

sensitivity to mouth width is very low, which is explicable on the
grounds that this is a very variable quantity in real life, and cannot
be used as a recognition feature. However, sensitivity to inward eye
movement is very high, yet outward eye movement is, relatively,
ignored! My explanation of this extraordinary finding is that we have
a powerful sensitivity to eye convergence (and therefore fixation
point) in face-to-face conversation, but there is no corresponding
mechanism for eye divergence.

A more detailed discussion of the results is contained in Haig
(1984) but there is one conclusion that I feel compelled to emphasise,
and to which I will return later; the implications of these
face-distortion results for users of face-construction systems, such
as Identikit and Photofit, are serious. A perusal of Fig 1 will
illustrate how the appearance of a single face can change, for even
very slight distortions of the feature positions. Clearly more work
must be done in this area.

4. FEATURE INTERCHANGE EXPERIMENTS

The previous set of experiments took one face at a time, and
moved features around within it. The next experiments, that I shall
describe, logically extended the technique by interchanging features
among four different faces, but without distortion. The principle of
the interchange technique is not new, but some aspects of these
experiments were significantly different from previously-reported work
of this nature. Particular note was taken of work by Davies, Ellis &
Shepherd (1977), Matthews (1978), and Walker-Smith (1978), all of whom
used either Photofit or Identikit to change features in order to test
feature saliency. One drawback, that was identified by Davies et al,
is the relatively restricted range of changes permitted by such kits.
It was partly in response to this caveat, and partly the belief that
more "realistic" imagery is necessary for modelling purposes, that led
this author to the experiments described hereunder. The considerable
versatility of the image processor, coupled with thoughtful
programming and careful stimulus preparation, promised the requisite
realism and experimental control. A further measure of experimental
control was suggested by limiting the target set to four faces, and
interchanging their principal features, rather than the more usual
practice of constructing numerous slightly different variations around
a single original face. The aim of these experiments, then, was to
construct a feature saliency list. The target set comprised four
faces, male, no spectacles, facial hair or blemishes, and the heads
were masked off by a plain surround, allowing no background
distractions. Using programs that I had previously written for the
INTELLECT, I was able to designate rectangular areas of any size, and
rewrite them into corresponding positions on any other target. The
features that I chose to interchange were eyes (as a pair), nose,
mouth (HENM) together with complete head outlines. The original
target set is shown in the top row of Fig 3, while a representative
set of single-feature interchanges is shown in the bottom row. Now,
with 4 targets, each having 4 features capable of interchange, there
is a possibility of 256 different feature combinations. Such a large
number of 128 x 128 pixel pictures would have taken up a considerable
volume of tape-store, quite apart from the very long time that would
have been absorbed in merely transferring that data from tape to
framestore. It was decided to limit the stimulus material to
single-feature-changes only, which gave 48 combinations plus 4

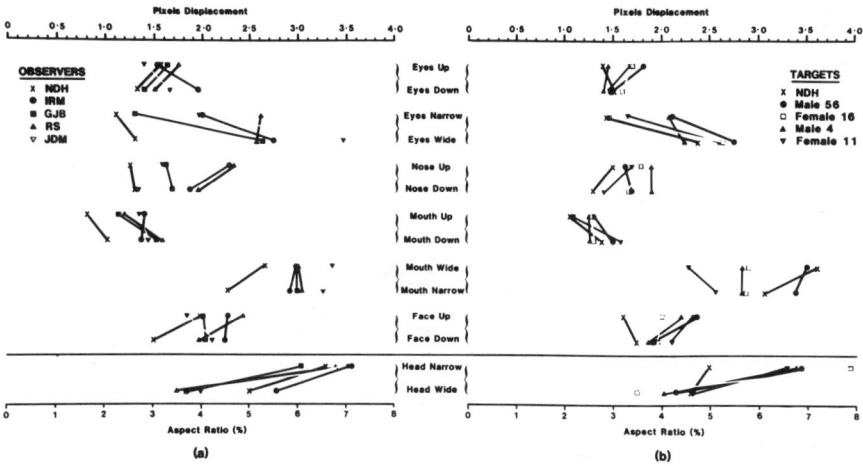

Fig 2. Plots of just-noticeable feature displacement(50% level) for each feature.(a) Results for each of the observers, summed over all the targets, and (b) results for each target, summed over all observers.

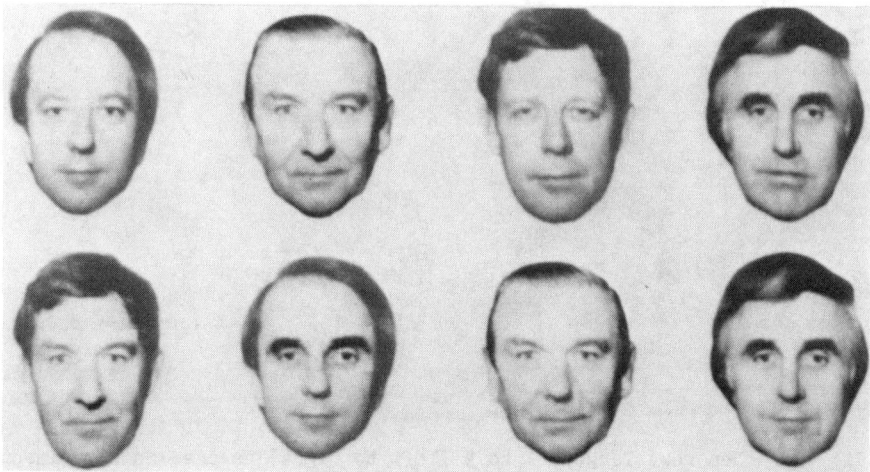

Fig 3. (Top row) Targets 1 to 4 (left to right),photographed as they appeared on the monitor screen for experiment HENM.(Bottom row) A representative selection of interchanged features;(First left) Head 3+Eyes,Nose,Mouth 2;(Second left) Eyes 4+Head,Nose,Mouth 1;(Third left) Nose 1+Head,Eyes,Mouth 2;(Right) Mouth 1+Head,Eyes,Nose 4.

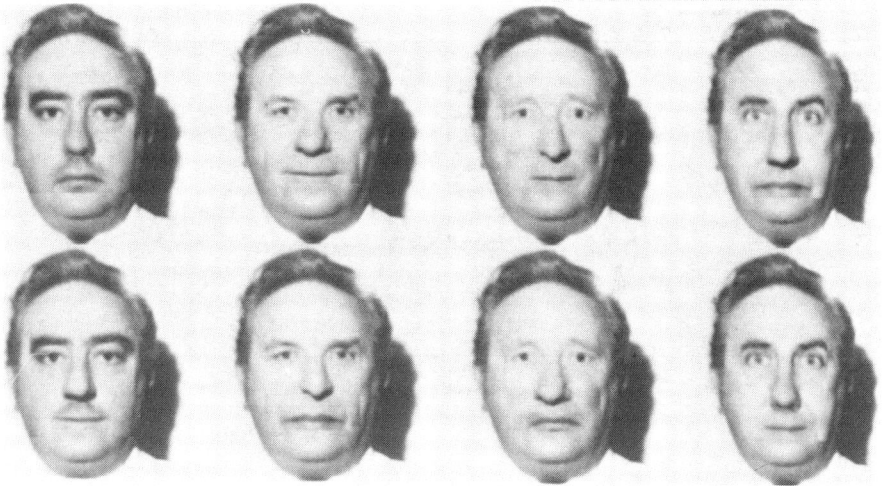

Fig 4. (Top row) Targets 1 to 4(left to right) as used in experiment ENM. Each face was superimposed on the same head.(Bottom row) A selection of interchanged features;(First left) Eyes 1, Nose 4, Mouth 2,(Second left) Eyes 2, Nose 3, Mouth 4,(Third left) Eyes 3, Nose 2, Mouth 1,(Right) Eyes 4, Nose 1, Mouth 3.

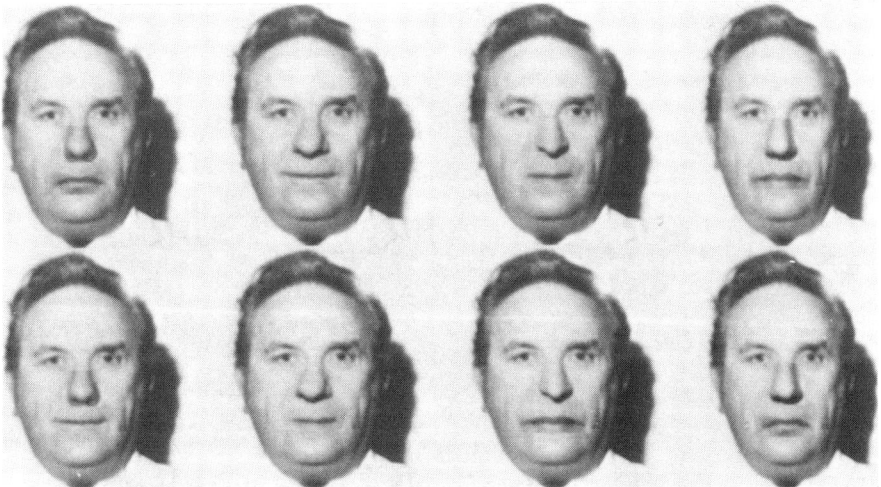

Fig 5. (Top row) Targets 1 to 4 (left to right) as used in experiment NM. The different noses and mouths were superimposed on Target 2 of Fig 4.(Bottom row) A selection of interchanged features;(First left) Nose 1, Mouth 2,(Second left) Nose 2, Mouth 3,(Third left) Nose 3, Mouth 4,(Right) Nose 4, Mouth 1.

originals, making 52 pictures overall. Each observing session consisted of four cycles of each of the 52 pictures, selected at random, and five observers were used for ten sessions each.

A similar style of presentation to the previous experiment was used; namely a one-second unmasking of a single target, followed by a blank screen until the observer responded. On this occasion, however, the observer had four buttons, corresponding to the four targets, and his memory was refreshed subsequent to each response by displaying the four targets at the bottom of the screen. The question that the observers had to answer was "Which of the four target faces does this face remind you of the most?". The computer then recorded four things; (1) the list of features displayed (for instance, Head 1, Eyes 4, Nose 1, Mouth 1), (2) the observers' response, (3) the accumulated number of times that each feature scored a "hit", and (4) the accumulated number of times that each generic feature combination scored a "hit".

The results from this experiment will be published, in detail, elsewhere. For the moment, it must suffice to indicate that, of the four interchangeable features, the Head clearly formed the major focus of attention. Summing across all five observers and all four targets, the Head scored 28.7% correct responses, with the Eyes and Mouth each scoring 24.3% and the Nose scoring 22.7%. Looking at the pattern of correct responses as a function of the "changed" single-feature, changed Heads scored 34.0%, changed Mouths 8.9%, changed Eyes 8.3%, and changed Noses 0.5%. Clearly, a change of Head, while maintaining the inner features constant, very strongly influenced observers' responses. Conversely, none of the observers seems to have paid much attention to Noses.

In view of the marked Head dominance, I decided to eliminate the Heads and test the interchangeability of the inner features alone. This was done by selecting four new faces and writing them all onto the same head. In this way, the head cannot be used as a recognition feature, thereby allowing the inner features to be permuted. Since we now had only to combine Eyes, Noses and Mouths (ENM) from four targets, the total number of permutations was 64, which was a much more manageable number from the data handling and storage aspect. The opportunity was taken to abandon single-feature changes, and Fig 4 shows a few multiple feature combinations, below the original target set. Once again, the five observers completed ten sessions of four complete feature-change cycles each. The results from this ENM experiment may be summarised briefly, across all four targets and all five observers, as favouring Eyes (58.7%) over Mouths (24.0%), followed by Noses (17.3%). In addition, the response pattern, that is the overall observer respose to generic feature combinations, demonstrated a most gratifying consistency: Response to changed Eyes only was 80.3%, to changed Mouth only was 13.8%, and to changed Nose only was 1.3%. Compare these figures with the overall pattern correct response to "all different" feature combinations, where the Eyes scored 81.0%, the Mouth was 13.8% and the Nose was 2.3%. It would appear, from these results, that the ENM experiment could have omitted all single-and double-feature changes, in favour of the "all different" feature mixtures. Nevertheless, it was necessary to use the complete combination set in order to prove the point. Note the very low correct response to Noses, which was directly comparable to the residual responses. This prompted me to continue the experiment, as before, by fixing the dominant feature and forcing a choice between the minor features.

Thus, the NM experiment was conceived and undertaken in order to confirm, unequivocally, the inferior status of the Nose as a frontal recognition feature. Fig 5 shows the target set on the top row again, with four representative Nose and Mouth combinations, below. This time, the Head and Eyes remain constant, and the observers were required to identify the most similar original target. The results clearly showed the dominance of the Mouth over the Nose, by a factor of approximately two to one.

These three feature-interchange experiments, HENM, ENM and NM established a clear hierarchy of feature saliency in which the Head outline played the major role, with the Eyes following close behind. The Mouth seems not to be very important, but the Nose seems to play almost no measurable part at all in frontal face recognition. This broad result agrees well with several published studies that employed other different techniques (for an excellent review of the field, see Table 2 in Chapter 6 of Davies Ellis & Shepherd, 1981). Furthermore, it will be shown, below, that there is stong support for this view of face recognition strategy from an entirely different type of experiment. Before moving on, however, it is appropriate to remark that all three of these experiments produced a number of "incorrect" responses that were not true errors. By way of explanation, all the experiments were 4 AFC, and yet there were some occasions when particular feature combinations aroused in the observers the impression of a "new face". Such a "new face" could not be fitted into the target set, even though it was derived directly from it. All the observers commented on this phenomenon, from time to time, since it forced them to press a button at random. This is surely further evidence of the need to treat face identification kits with a great deal of circumspection.

5. DISTRIBUTED APERTURE EXPERIMENTS

The previous exeriments, concerned with feature interchange, were well suited to an image-processing computer, although they could have been undertaken with a face identification kit. The experiments described hereunder would be very difficult to attempt, without the aid of such a system, both from the point of view of setting up the stimulus material and also from the data processing aspect. All the experiments described so far in this paper have been founded on the implicit assumption that we know what constitutes a "feature", and these designated "features" have beenmanipulated, in some systematic way, to enable conclusions to be drawn concerning their relative importance to the process of recognition. Consider, though, what a feature could be; it might be, for example, an eye, an eyebrow, a very high or very low contrast eye pupil, a bloodshot eye, a skin blemish or perhaps bags under the eyes. On the other hand, it may not be an identifiable mark at all, but merely the space between two or more marks. The face distortion experiment, in particular, raised a number of questions of this nature; we seem to be sensitive to the relative positions of certain "features" by virtue of the distances or areas between them, rather than to the "features" themseves. In such a case, surely the spaces themselves constitute features? The Distributed Aperture technique was devised in order to answer such questions directly, and it occurred to me as a result of careful consideration of the masking experiment of such workers as Goldstein &

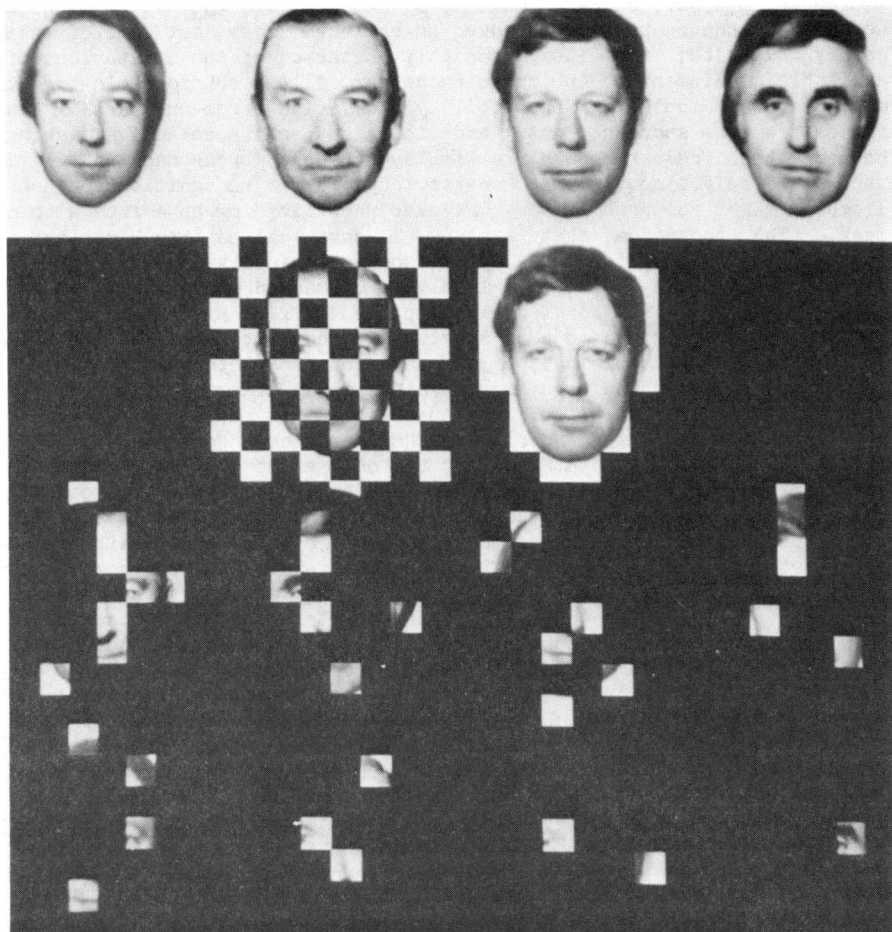

Fig 6. Photograph to illustrate the Distributed Aperture Technique.(Top row) Targets 1 to 4, as for experiment HENM.(Second row) Target 2 segmented into an 8 x 8 chequerboard array, to show the size and positions of the apertures. Target 3 illustrates the actual extent of the apertures used in the experiment(38 in all).The next two rows demonstrate the effect of exposing the different targets behind diminishing numbers of randomly positioned apertures.

Mackenberg (1966), Fisher & Cox (1975) and McKelvie (1976). All these
workers presented partially masked or occluded faces, but none of them
really exploited the idea, possibly because of the limitations of
available equipment. An image-processor allows considerable target
manipulation, including the ability to write from one part of the
framestore to another part, and it also permits selective masking
between the framestore and the display screen. I reasoned that, if I
were to truly discover what constituted a facial recognition feature,
I must make no assumptions whatever when dividing up a face with a
mask. The technique that evolved I have called the Distributed
Aperture technique, because my reasoning logically implies that all
parts of the face are equally likely to be masked or unmasked, in any
combination. I therefore divided up the 128 x128 pixel face picture
into a square grid of 8 x 8 "apertures", and programmed the computer
to replicate any combination of such apertures into another part of
the framestore, where the resultant sampled face picture could be
masked or unmasked at will. The top row of Fig 6 shows the target set
(the same target as for experiment HENM), and the chequerboard picture
in the second row demonstrates how the entire 128 x 128 squares could
be apertured. Notice, however, that many peripheral apertures contain
only white background, of no relevance to the experimental aims, and
so I programmed them out of the selection routine. This left the 38
apertures containing parts of faces, as shown in the right hand
picture in the second row of Fig 6. The next task was to program the
computer to select one of the four target faces, at random, and to
display a random selection of its 38 apertures in a chosen square with
the object of trying to identify which face is being displayed. Some
preliminary experiments quickly established that very few apertures
would be required to achieve reliable recognition. The third and
fourth rows of Fig 6 illustrate typical impressions of the target
faces viewed through varying numbers of randomly positioned apertures,
from which it may be appreciated that no more than 8 apertures would
be needed, in general, even with a presentation time of one second.
Even up to 8 apertures, however, when combined randomly over any of
the 38 available spaces for four targets gives more than 250 million
possible combinations of presentations.

Obviously, it was not possible to undertake an experiment that
presented all such possible combinations, and so a program was written
that selected (a) one of the four target faces, at random, (b) the
random number of apertures of that target to be presented, and (c) the
actual addresses of those apertures, selected at random for the 38
possible addresses. The program then recorded all of these details on
floppy discs, together with the observer's name code and his response
to each presentation. An additional program was written to retrieve
the data from the discs and process it to reveal the response patterns
for the observers, separately and together, and for the target faces,
separately and together. Even before the experiment began, it was
clear that there would be a very considerable data handling problem,
resulting in many tables of figures, that would be almost
unintelligible to all but the most diligent researcher. In other
words, an easily digestible data presentation technique was required.
It occurred to me that, since each aperture on each target was to be
exposed for a large number of times, I could normalise the correct
responses by taking the percentage correct, and then I could
re-present each aperture as a square having a brightness that was a

linear function of the percentage correct at that aperture address.

The results of this experiment, using the bright/correct display method, are shown in Fig 7 for each target separately, but summed over all four observers, and corrected for chance. The printed photographs of these results are not quantitatively correct, due to the degrading effect of the photographic and printing processes, but a clear qualitative view of the results may be obtained at a glance. It is hoped to publish these data in full, elsewhere, together with a more complete analysis of target and observer variations. For convenience, I have included Fig 8 in which I have superimposed the target results onto the respective target faces, in the top row. The picture at bottom right is the four target faces, superimposed on each other, while the bottom left pictures are the overall result, summed across all targets and observers, both raw and enhanced (for visual effect). The picture at bottom centre-right is the composite target face, overlaid with the enhanced overall result.

Fig 8 is a picture of considerable interest and a few salient points should be noted, before we move on. Firstly, looking at the overall result, notice the very high proportion of correct responses across the eyes/eyebrows and across the hairline at the forehead. Rather fewer correct responses may be seen around the side of the temples and at the mouth, while the lower chin area is clearly not a strong recognition feature. Notice, also, the two dark squares in the middle of the forehead, indicating that this area was virtually indistinguishable, from one target to the next, and providing a useful check on the validity of the data. Once again, as found in the HENM feature-exchange experiments, the noses do not influence frontal face recognition. Remembering that brightness indicates correctness of response, the most recognisable face, in the upper row, is number four. The faces were chosen for their mixture of differing features, and this target was chosen for his prominent eyebrows and distinctive hair style, both of which figure prominently in the observer's response. Number one and number three had similar eyes, giving strong and similar responses, but they had very different hairlines, giving a rather different distribution of responses that were similar in overall magnitudes. Target number two had a distinctive hairline and parting, which clearly emerged as a recognition feature. His mouth also appears prominent, being rather dissimilar to the others. Although there is insufficient space to present further data, it is pertinent at this point, to observe that the response differences between the targets were of a similar order to the response differences between the observers. Indeed, the variation was such that the whole concept of feature saliency lists seems inappropriate, to this author at least. This point, with supporting data, is developed in another paper. Finally, the median number of apertures required for a correct response, corrected for chance was 2.25. In other words, an average of only 5.9% of a target face was necessary for recognition purposes. Despite the small target set, this is still a remarkable result.

6. HIGHER RESOLUTION DISTRIBUTED APERTURES EXPERIMENT

The results from the Distributed Apertures experiments, above, were very interesting indeed, but they really only provided tantalising clues as to the precise features that influence recognition. What was required, it seemed to me, was a finer focus. As noted above, there was a possible problem in attaining a

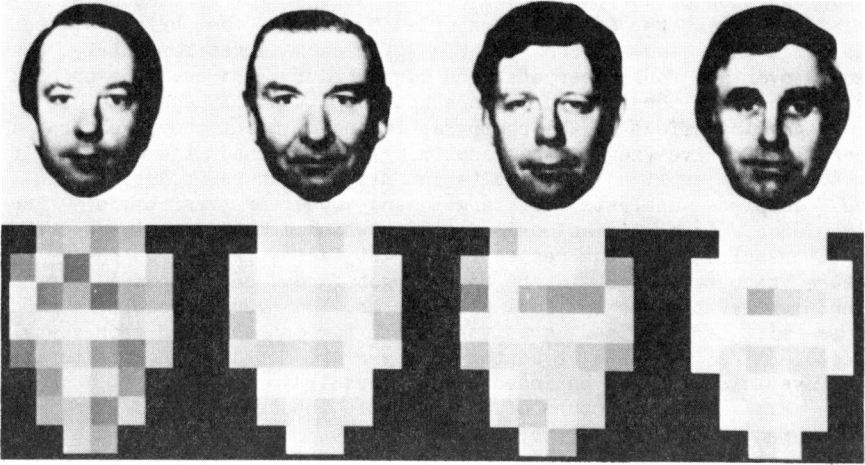

Fig 7. The bottom row consists of the aperture response maps for the target faces above. On the original display, the brightness of each aperture was made proportional to the percentage of correct responses registered for that aperture, summed over all observers and corrected for chance-correct responses. (Reprographic processes render these particular pictures only qualitative.)

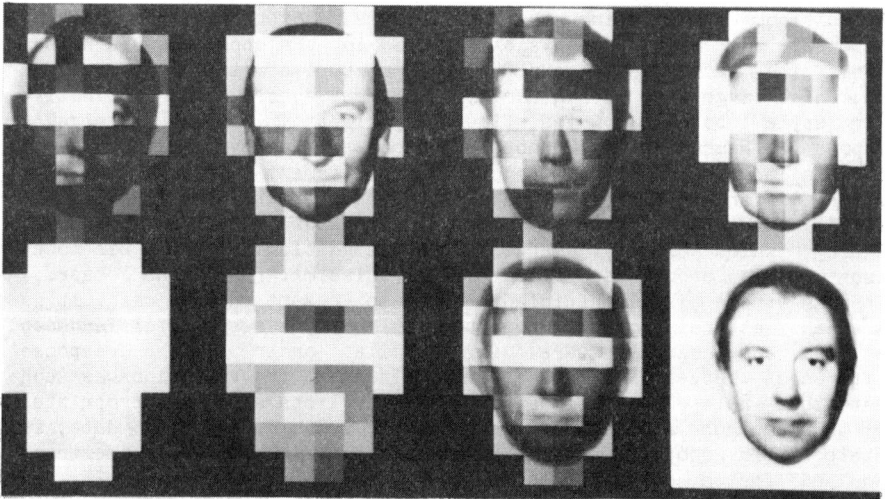

Fig 8. (Top row) The targets are shown superimposed directly on their corresponding response maps, to assist with precise feature identification. (Bottom left) This shows the original overall response map, covering all targets and all observers. Next to it is shown the same map, but contrast-enhanced, to exaggerate the relative feature response differences. (Bottom right) The face, shown on a white background, is the composite of all four target faces, added in the computer. Next to it is shown the composite face superimposed on the (enhanced) overall response map.

sufficiently significant result, if the number of apertures was increased too much, coupled with a distinct lack of storage space within the computer. It was eventually determined that the resolution could be doubled, in each (orthogonal) direction, and this would allow a total of 162 usable apertures on each target. In order that this higher resolution experiment could be directly comparable with the previous lower-resolution experiment, the identical target set was employed, albeit with four different observers. Each observer possessed 6/4 vision, corrected in two cases, and each one undertook 25 sessions of 300 presentations, making a grand total of 30,000 presentations. As before, the target was selected randomly, as were the number of apertures per presentation (up to a maximum of 24), together with the aperture addresses. All other details were as for the previous experiment. As a running check on the significance of the results, I arranged to display the current result every ten sessions or so. The final patterns established themselves surprisingly quickly, which permits the overall results to be presented with confidence, although a rigorous mathematical analysis has not yet been attempted.

It will be recalled that the median face area required for recognition in the previous experiment was 5.9%. Using the same criterion as before, the median number of apertures per presentation required for this experiment was 6.4/162 = 4.0%. I believe that the reason for an even lower threshold, for this experiment than for the previous one, lies in the greater variety of aperture positions and combinations. This conclusion, alone, justifies a rather different approach to the data-handling in future experiments of this type, and this will be elaborated upon below. With regard to the main results of this experiment, Fig 9 shows the separate target identification maps, in the middle row beneath the corresponding targets. The overall result, summed over all targets and observers, is shown in the 3rd row left, with a contrast-enhanced version next to it. As before, the composite target face (third row right) is then superimposed on the overall result, to assist in identifying the precise nature of the key features. The very bottom row is a composite of the top two rows, to assist in feature localisation.

Looking first at the individual target results in the second row, notice that Target 4 is brightest overall, denoting general ease of identifcation, followed by Target 2, then Target 3, with Target 1 being the least identifiable. Notice also how the response maps clearly mark out the differences in the individual hair outlines. Comparison with Fig 8 show a gratifying agreement, despite different observers, but the greater resolution of the later experiment reduces the contrasts between neighbouring apertures. Nevertheless, it is possible to see that the area of the eyes and eyebrows seems to attract the next greatest response. An interesting individual difference appears in this region; notice how the greater response for Targets 1, 2 and 4 is for the eyebrows, while Target 3 has a more prominent eye response. Responses in the mouth region are not so strong or so consistent, while responses in the nose region are almost at chance level.

Turning to the overall result in the third row, particularly the superimposed picture, the dominance of the hair is obvious, and most striking. Perhaps the most fascinating result of all, however, is the very clear response to the inner eyebrows. Looking at the

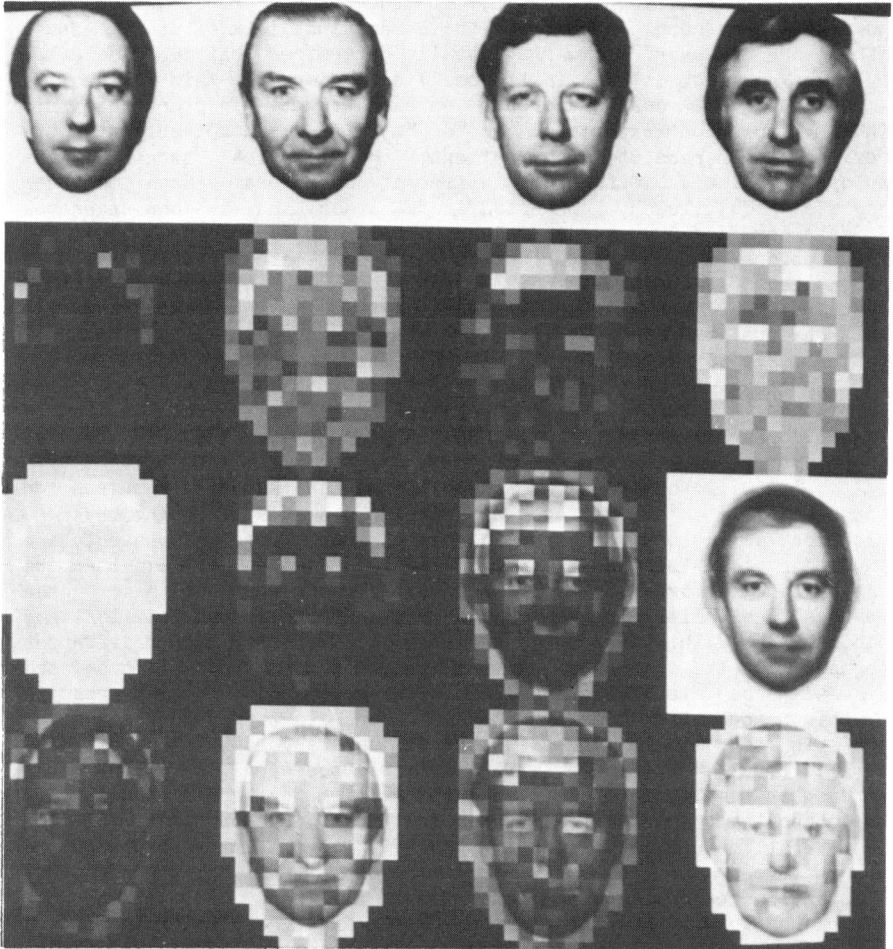

Fig 9. Photograph summarising the results of the high-resolution Distributed Apertures experiment. The top two rows correspond directly to the arrangement of Fig 7,while the bottom two rows correspond to Fig 8. Notice particularly the overall result (third row, middle two pictures); the greatest correct response was to the hairline,followed by the inner eyebrows. Note also the response at the upper lip, but not the mouth.

individual response maps, in the second row, it is not immediately obvious that those two apertures will predominate; yet they do, and in almost identical measure. This is a most remarkable result, and one that does not appear to have been discovered elsewhere. That this is true result, and not an artefact, can scarcely be questioned, since the two apertures in question were entirely independent in the experiment, yet they have so clearly emerged with similar values.

My brief review of this remarkable experiment would be incomplete without also mentioning the virtual absence of positive responses to the nose, and more surprisingly, the poor response to the mouth. Notice, however, the marked response to the upper lip area, which agrees very closely with the results of the Distortion experiments. The analysis of the data from this latest experiment is incomplete, and it is hoped to publish a more comprehensive account at a later date. It is possible to indicate that inter-observer variation between targets was considerable, as for the original Distributed Apertures experiment. This fact reinforces the objections to simple feature-listing, as a means of understanding the recognition of faces, and reminds us of the infinite variety of our targets.

7. CONCLUSIONS

This paper was intended to illustrate the usefulness of even a very simple image processing system for psycho-visual experimentation. Images may be generated, stored, manipulated and displayed in a great variety of ways that allow the research worker to break free of the shackles of non-linear photographic processes, limited and slow processing, stop watches, manual data recording, tedious experimental sessions and poor mechanical reliability. On the other hand, image processors can be expensive, although they need not be, and they demand a considerable investment of time for the writing of your own particular programs. In addition, a considerable time may be taken up in checking and validating your programs, to make sure that they are doing precisely what you think they are. Once a routine has been perfected, though, it is simple to run, and may usually be tuned very accurately to your needs, or those of your subjects. The data from all of the experiments, described above, is now permanently recorded on floppy discs, and may be recovered for retrospective investigation at any future date, particularly if some future discovery is made that may currently be obscured. In addition, the experiments could all be re-started and continued from the point where they were stopped, and next year's presentations would be essentially identical to last year's. The computer does not tire. As noted above, it is hoped to publish the results of all the experiments described here in a more complete form; the first experiment has already been published (Haig 1984).

PRACTICAL FACE RECOGNITION AND VERIFICATION WITH WISARD.

T. J. STONHAM

1. INTRODUCTION

WISARD (Wilkie, Aleksander, and Stonham's Recognition Device) is a general purpose pattern recognition machine with a special semi-parallel structure unlike that of conventional single instruction single data computers. The machine is self-adapting. It does not require programming where an explict set of rules, defining the operations to be performed on the data, have to be supplied. The behaviour of the system is established by a learning process whereby a representative set of patterns from the class of data to be recognised, is input to the machine. A wide range of pattern recognition problems can be solved with this approach, they include industrial inspection, speech recognition, medical pattern recognition and artificial vision.

In this paper, the processing of faces will be considered. Two objectives are sought - face recognition and face verification. Face recognition can be defined as the labelling of the face with an identifier. It is equivalent to asking the question 'Who am I?'. In the author's case, the label required to be associated with his face is John Stonham. Face verification on the other hand involves supplying the face together with the label, to the machine and requiring a confirmation or otherwise. The question now being asked is 'Am I John Stonham?', to which the answer is either 'Yes' or 'No'.

2. PATTERN RECOGNITION

The discipline of pattern recognition concerns the labelling of well-defined and recognisable images, sounds or measurements obtained from objects or processes in the real world environment. It is an essential operation in automation and information processing. Industry is striving towards machines capable of automatic assembly and inspection which must manipulate and make decisions on physical objects. The so called 'Fifth Generation' computer program is intended to communicate directly with the real world without having to transfer information via the keyboard. Speech and image recognition will be vital operators in the real world/machine interface.

Pattern recognition, its implementation and inherent problems have been grossly underestimated over the past twenty years. This is primarily due to the fact that humans, and even animals, are exceedingly good at interpreting images. We recognise faces, understand scenes, interpret speech and respond to smells, without knowing how we do it. So, as we do not have a detailed knowledge of human pattern recognition processes, the emulation of recognition in a machine is a somewhat intractable problem. The difficulties are exacerbated by the vast amounts of data present in an image or a sound signal. A television camera is used as a transducer to convert an image into an electronic form. The video signal from the camera represents the values of the image intensity, scanned line by line, and lasts for about forty milliseconds. It can contain frequency components exceeding 20MHz. Converting this data into numerical form results in an image comprising some quarter of a million picture cells (Pixels) each having an intensity value. If we assume each pixel can have one of two hundred and fifty six intensity values, this amounts to two million bits of information in every frame - a data rate of fifty million bits per second. If the images are in colour, the data rate will be higher. The images can be binarised so that each pixel can only be black or white (logical values 0 or 1). The data rate is then reduced but still amounts to 6.25 million bits per second. Given that conventional computers have an instruction time of the order of one microsecond, (DEC-VAX 11/780) and any processing of an image will involve tens if not hundreds of instructions per pixel, they cannot keep pace with the data rate of images at television picture resolution.

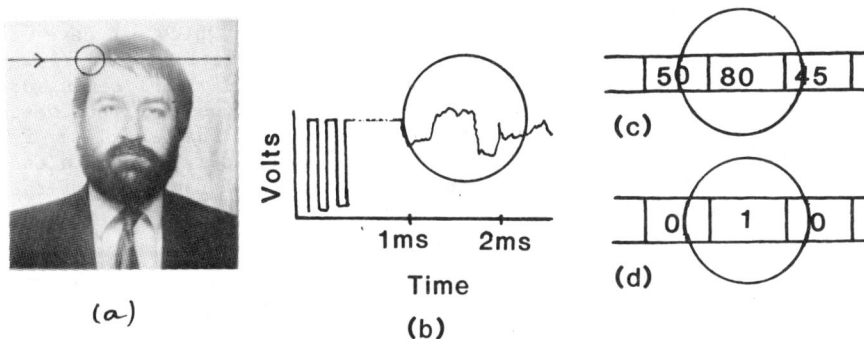

FIGURE 1. a) An input image being time scanned, b) The video signal from the line - a time dependent voltage waveform. c) the video signal averaged over fixed time intervals to produce pixels. 3 pixels shown out of the 250,000 which make up the image. d) The pixels thresholded to produce a binarised image with pixels either black (1) or white (0).

The evaluation of images which are in electronic or numerical form is far more complex than at first imagined. In conversation we may say 'this is one face, and that is another' when describing a sequence of video, implying that there are two different faces being observed. In terms of the data being collected there are countless millions of images of the two faces. Each image is unique and will result in vastly differing video signals and pixel images. These differences arise from changes in expression, position, and orientation of the faces. Other variants are introduced due to changes in lighting conditions and electronic and optical distortions in the camera and data acquisition equipment. The human is able to take in images of the two people in question and distinguish between them. It is an information processing task of extreme complexity which we take for granted and have very little understanding of how it is done.

3. HOW CAN WE ATTEMPT RECOGNITION BY A MACHINE?
The single instruction single data computer structure first laid down by John Von Neumann, in 1944, and still the dominant computer architecture, is unsuitable for pattern recognition on two counts. a) it needs to be programmed, and we do not understand the recognition process sufficiently well to be able to write a program. b) it is not fast enough to process television pictures in real time, that is, as fast as the camera supplies the data, (typically, one picture every twenty five milliseconds).
The speed problem may be overcome by new technologies. A computer

that calculates with light, rather than electrons, is being researched (1), and in these optical computers achievable instruction times of a few femtoseconds (10^{-15} second) have been suggested. However, the problem of determining what instructions have to be carried out on the data – the programming constraints – will still remain.

As humans are excellent at pattern recognition, it is not surprising that much attention has been paid over the past 30 years to natural processing systems in order to elucidate methods for pattern recognition. The complexity of the human brain, generally regarded to be composed of a vast interconnected network of some 10^{10} cells, some of which can have up to five thousand inputs, defies any analytical investigation, even if we had readily available access to the structure. The individual cells, or neurons, however, have been studied in depth, and various electronic and mathematical models have been proposed. One of the earliest is attributed to McCulloch and Pitts, 1944, (2) and has resulted in the linear discriminator method of pattern recognition which forms one of the earliest learning machine approaches (see Fig. 2)

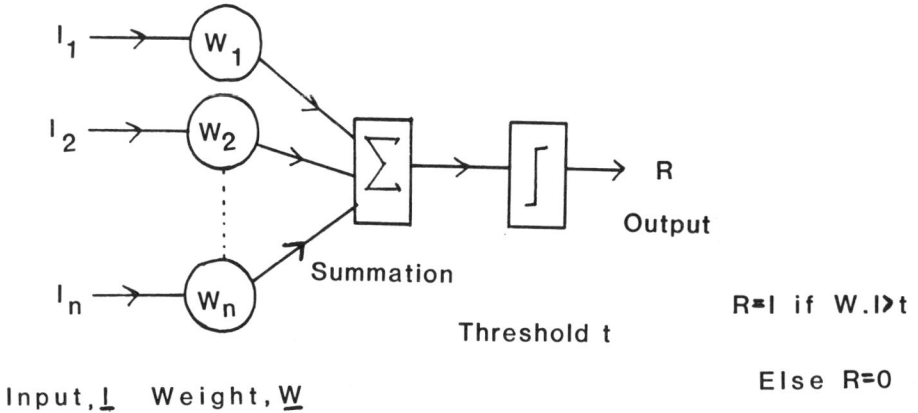

FIGURE 2. The McCulloch and Pitts Neuron Model

If we cannot resolve the structure of natural processing systems, at least some general observations can be made. The brain is clearly not a Von Neumann structure. We do not have a central processor unit and a memory which stores discrete packets of information in a type of biochemical filing cabinet. Instead, we have a distributed parallel processor where large number of neurons are processing samples of data simultaneously, reacting to input stimulii and passing on responses to subsequent neurons. The functions the neurons perform are not supplied externally in the form of a program of instructions, but evolve or adapt by being exposed to stimulii. An encouraging aside for the electrical engineer, is that the input/output information within neural systems, is in the form of firing patterns – electrical signals and potentials – which can be measured. If the inputs are assumed to be in either a firing or a non-firing state, in other words binary, and likewise the outputs, then the latter can be modelled as a combinational or a sequential logical function of the inputs. Such systems can be built using electronic components.

In developing distributed parallel processors we are not aiming to make a neural network model, although the networks still have loose similarities with natural systems. The primary objective is to develop a processing architecture which is suitable and capable of performing pattern recognition. The networks are tailored towards this goal but nevertheless they do exhibit interesting behaviours and can offer models, insights and certain explanations of the mechanisms of intelligent-like behaviour in natural systems.

4. A SELF-ADAPTING OR LEARNING NETWORK FOR PATTERN RECOGNITION.
4.1 The Organisation of the Network

A self-adapting single layer network of processors is shown in Fig.3. The input is derived from the television camera, and reduced to a binary image where the individual pixels are either black or white. In order to clarify the operation of the network, the resolution of the input has been reduced to 3 bits x 3 bits. (the resolution of a T.V. picture would normally be 512 x 512 bits). Each processor samples the input space where the image is stored. The input space has a dimensionality N, the number of pixels in the image. (nine in Fig.3). The size of the sample (the n-tuple) in this example is three or in general n, which has a lower bound of one, and an upper bound of N. Both these limits lead to trivial behaviour, and a practical range of n is between two and ten.

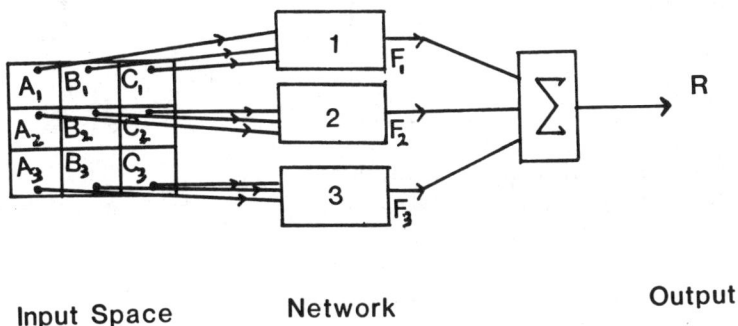

Input Space   Network   Output

FIGURE 3. A Single Layer Network.

The number of processors in a network is $\underline{N}$ if each pixel is connected n

to a processor, giving a cover of 100%. The cover can be reduced or increased. In the former case, certain pixels are ignored. Any cover beyond 100% means that some pixels will be connected to more than one processor.

The grouping together of pixels to form the n-tuples is known as the mapping of the image. In the example, a linear row-by-row mapping, with n-tuple size three has been chosen. This gives one n-tuple per row of the image and is easy to follow in the example. In practice, the mapping can be linear, but is more often random, so as to be sensitive to global features occurring across the images. Alternatively, if the precise structure of the data is known, the mapping can be tailored to detect specific features.

The system needs some data on which to form its response characteristics. This data must be representative of the class of images to which it belongs and is referred to as the teaching or training set. The class of the image is the name given to the data group as a whole. In face recognition it would be the name of the person in the image. In character recognition it may be the ASCII code of the letter being observed.

4.2 The Behaviour of the Network

Suppose the network in Fig. 3 is to be trained to recognise the letter T, (characters are being used in the explanation of the behaviour of the network because a 3 x 3 bit resolution is too low to represent a face). Three examples of the letter T, shown in Fig.4, are available to train the net.

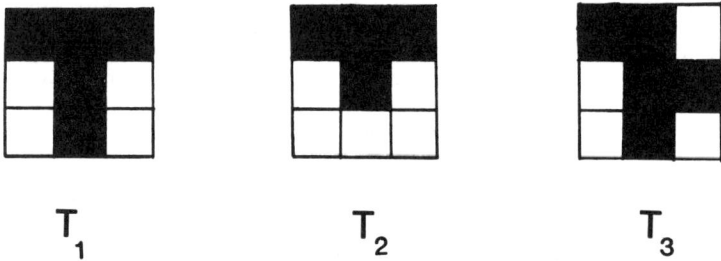

$$T_1 \qquad\qquad T_2 \qquad\qquad T_3$$

FIGURE 4. Three examples of the letter T.

If the first pattern is input to the net, as shown in Fig. 5, and we require each function to fire (respond with logical 1), the functions needed are:

$$F_1 = A_1\ B_1\ C_1$$

$$F_2 = \overline{A}_2\ B_2\ \overline{C}_2$$

$$F_3 = \overline{A}_3\ B_3\ \overline{C}_3$$

The equation for F_1 reads:F_1 is logical 1 if A_1 is 1 and B_1 is 1 and C_1 is 1.
Function F_2 reads: F_2 is 1 if A_2 is 0 and B_2 is 1 and C_2 is 0. ($\overline{A}_2$ means A_2 = 0)

Those familiar with digital hardware will recognise these functions as combinational logic operators, with the n-tuple samples being minterms of the appropriate functions. If the second training pattern T_2 is now applied to the network, and the functions changed so that it also causes all processors to respond with a logical 1, F_1 and F_2 need not change, but the third function F_3 becomes:

$$F_3 = \overline{A}_3\ B_3\ \overline{C}_3 + \overline{A}_3\ \overline{B}_3\ \overline{C}_3$$

which reads F_3 equals not A_3 and B_3 and not C_3 or not A_3 and not B_3 and not C_3.

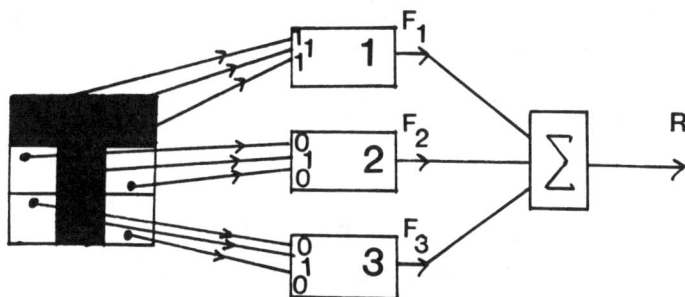

FIGURE 5. A Net receiving an Input Pattern.

The inclusion of pattern T_3 in the training sequence will result in the functions

$$F_1 = A_1 \ B_1 \ C_1 + A_1 \ B_1 \ \overline{C}_1$$

$$F_2 = \overline{A}_2 \ B_2 \ \overline{C}_2 + \overline{A}_2 \ B_2 \ C_2$$

$$F_3 = \overline{A}_3 \ B_3 \ \overline{C}_3 + \overline{A}_3 \ \overline{B}_3 \ C_3$$

The network can now be exposed to patterns and asked to react. A numerical response can be obtained by summing the outputs, which in this example gives a maximum response of three.

Fig. 6 shows some typical 3 x 3 bit patterns and the scores they produce. Those patterns which contain 'T'- like components, obtain scores of three, whereas, 'H and 0'- like patterns, which are by human inspection obviously not members of the 'T' class, give very low scores.

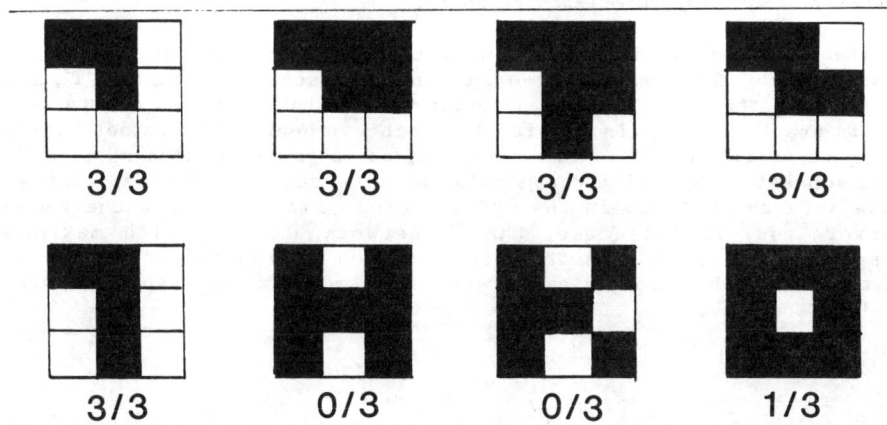

FIGURE 6. Some 3 x 3 bit test patterns and their responses.

In more general terms, the behaviour of a net can be represented by a set diagram (Fig. 7.) The universe of patterns is 512 (this is the total number of different binary patterns which can be displayed on a 3 x 3 bit grid). The training set (three patterns) applied to the network in the teach mode when the functions are built up, produces a system which generalises and will respond to a total of eight patterns. This is the generalisation set which contains G_T patterns.

$$G_T = \prod_{i=1}^{N/n} m_i$$

where M_i is the number of minterms in the function, F_i determined by the number of different input n-tuples seen by F_i during training.

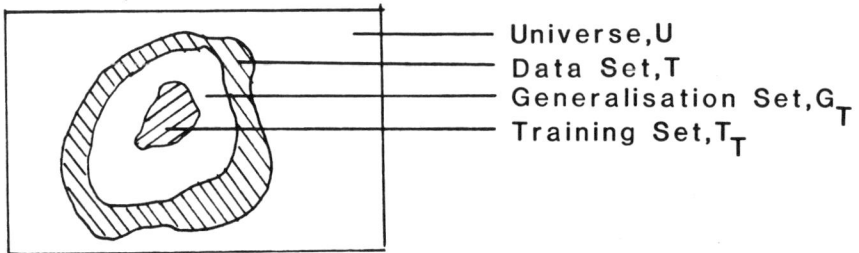

FIGURE 7. Set Diagram of Pattern Space.

The total number of patterns which can be regarded as versions of the letter 'T', by the human observer, can be represented by the set 'T', and on training the net, the generalisation set G_T should match the data set T. In practice, this is difficult to achieve because 'T' is not known. The generalisation set is therefore made as large as possible so that 'T' is a sub-set of G_T, with the proviso that G_T does not overlap another data set, as patterns in the overlay area will cause both their own network and, in this case, the 'T' network, to fire with maximum response. (see Fig. 8). If this happens, then the identification of the pattern cannot be resolved as we will have two networks responding with maximum score.

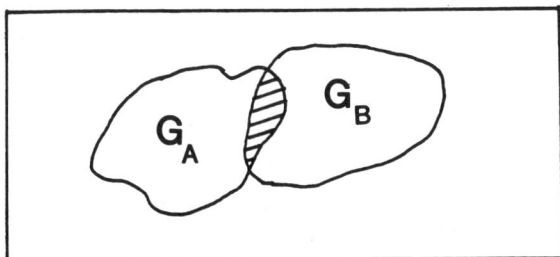

FIGURE 8. Patterns in the overlay area of generalisation sets **A** and **B** cannot be recognised. They will respond equally to class A and B networks.

A network trained as outlined above, can detect one class of patterns. If a recogniser is needed in which data is partitioned into k categories, then k networks are required. Each net is trained individually on members of its own class, and when the system is used in the classify mode, image data is applied to all the k networks in parallel. Each net provides a score, and the input can be associated with the net giving the highest score, and a confidence figure can be obtained by comparing the highest score with the second highest response.

4.3 Practical Networks

In a practical system, an input resolution would be typically 512 x 512 bits. Given an n-tuple size of four, this implies a total of $\frac{512 \times 512}{4}$ or 65,536 processors in each net. This appears to be a massively parallel system in terms of the number of processors and the connections to the input space which would number in excess of 250,000 lines. The system is however quite easily fabricated using currently available very large scale integrated electronic components. The individual processor functions can be programmed into memory circuits. Take the function F_1 from the letter 'T' detector. The function fires when input n-tuple A_1 B_1 C_1 is either 111 or 110. Now taking a random access memory (RAM) with three address lines, three being the n-tuple size, the RAM will contain 8 bits of storage. (see Fig. 9) If the memory is initially cleared and then set into the write mode and the 3-tuple (111) applied to the address lines, a logical 1 can be written into location 7. Similarly, when 3-tuple 110 is applied to the addresses, location 6 will be set to 1. At the end of teaching, memory is set to read, and the data applied to the address lines now accesses the stored information which then appears on the output lines. The memory will only output 1 when either 111 or 110 is input. All other inputs (000 to 101) will access locations 0 to 5 and output 0. The input/output behaviour of the memory is identical to that of the function F_1. The memory is acting as a Boolean logical operator.

434

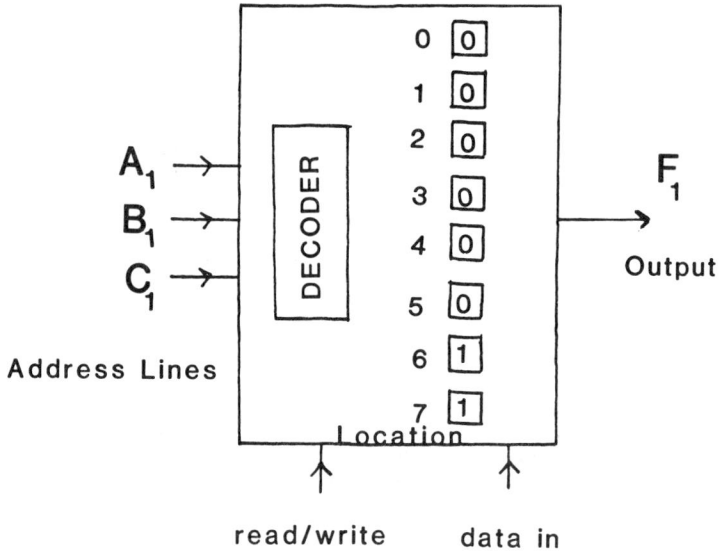

FIGURE 9. An 8-bit memory programmed as a combinational logic function.

It must be stressed to those readers not familiar with digital electronics, that the use of memory circuits as processors does not involve the storage of input images. The samples of the input patterns are never ever stored in the memory. It is the response to those samples that is stored away. The input data only stimulates the functions. The size of the memory is dependent only on the sample size n and does not vary with the number of training patterns used to set up the network. It is the contents of the memory, and hence the function of the processor which changes and ultimately stabilises with continued training.(3).

The development of hardware is facilitated by two further factors. Very large memories are now available at low cost. Two hundred and fifty six thousand bit memories currently cost around $10, and two million bit devices are under development. The second factor is the speed of these devices. The access time required to address a memory location and route its contents onto the output line, is of the order of fifty nanoseconds (5×10^{-8} seconds).

A large memory can be organised as a series of smaller memories by partitioning the address field into n-tuple and function addresses. Fig. 9 shows a 1 mega-bit memory having 20 address lines. The first four address lines receive the samples from the image, in this case a 4-tuple. Lines five to twenty are the function address lines driven from a counter. When the first n-tuple is applied, the counter is set to zero and a unique location addressed in memory (1 of 16 possible locations depending on the value of the n-tuple for that function address). The second n-tuple is sampled from the input and applied to the n-tuple address and the function address counter is increased to 00......01 giving access to one of another block of 16 possible cells. The process can be repeated for each new sample taken from the image and the total number of functions of four variables that can be accommodated in the 1 mega-bit memory is 2^{16} or 65,536.

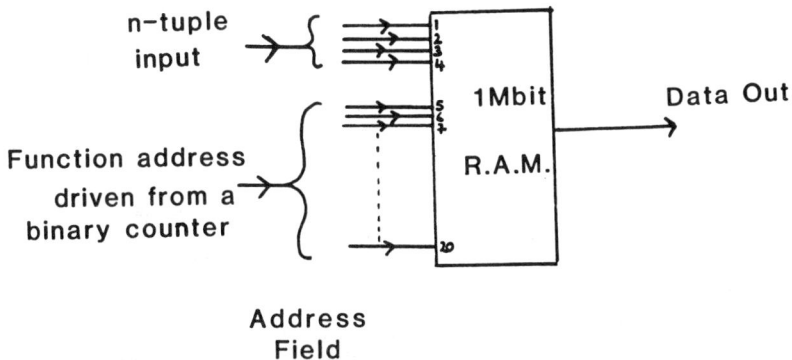

FIGURE 10. A 1 megabit memory with an address field partitioned to be programmed to perform sequentially 2^{16} different functions of 4 variables.

The cost of the electronic components for a 1 mega-bit memory is only a few tens of dollars and the access time of the memory has already been stated to be of the order 50 nanoseconds per bit. To access 65,536 functions one after another in the serial fashion will take approximately 50×10^{-8} x 65,536 or about 4 milliseconds. Given that it takes 25 milliseconds for a T.V. camera to grab an image, the serial organisation within a practical network appears to be adequate to process images at T.V. frame speed. This architecture has other practical advantages. By addressing functions within the network serially, access to the frame store only needs to be 1 bit at a time. The problem of massively parallel input connections is therefore avoided. Furthermore, this system is highly fault-tolerant as malfunctions in individual processors will not corrupt the overall network response. The architecture has been developed commericially and a general purpose adaptive pattern recognition machine - CRS WISARD - is being marketed by Computer Recognition Systems of Wokingham U.K.

5. FACE RECOGNITION
5.1. Recognition of unconstrained faces of 16 subjects.
A recognition system was set up for 16 individuals. Each person had his own network as described in sec 4. The n-tuple sample size was 4 and the input resolution 153x214, bits giving a total of 8185 functions in each network. The images were mapped onto the network using a random mapping, but constrained so that each pixel was connected to one and only one function input. The mapping was repeated for each network.
The training cycle for each discriminator involved the subject appearing before the camera, face on, and remaining within the field of view. A test/train scheme was used whereby a reponse was obtained from the network before each input image was used for training. By observing the build-up of the responses, an estimate of the progress of the training was obtained. Training continued until the network consistently

gave in excess of 95% of maximum response, ragardless of the position of the subject or his expression, provided he was face-on in the field of view. On average 200-400 images were required, but at a processing rate of 25 images per second, the training of each discriminator was completed in less that 20 seconds.

Figure 11 shows a single frame of each of the 16 subjects used in recognition tests. During testing, each person was shown to all of the 16 discriminators, each of which generated a response. Typical response profiles are shown in Fig. 12, in the form of histograms with responses normalised in the range 0.0 to 1.0. Classification of an image is achieved by determining which discriminator gives the highest response for that input image and associating it with the class of patterns used to train the highest responding discriminator. The system has been shown to function in real time without error within the bounds of the 16 class problem.

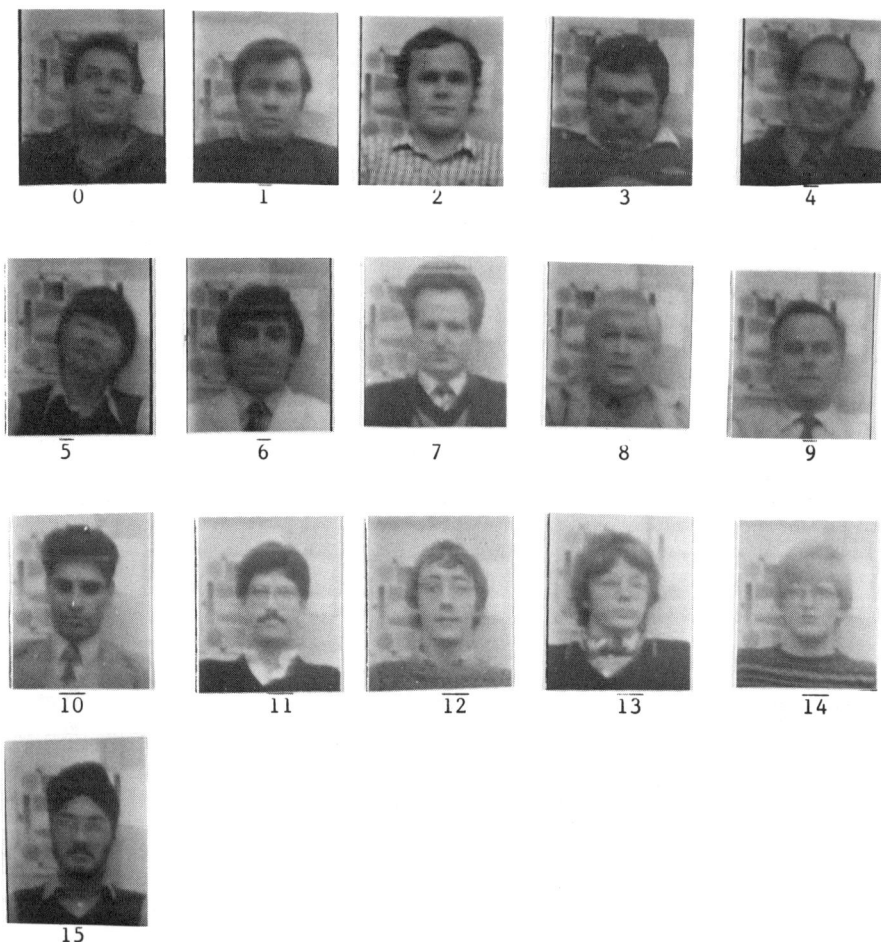

FIGURE 11. A single frame of each of the 16 subjects.

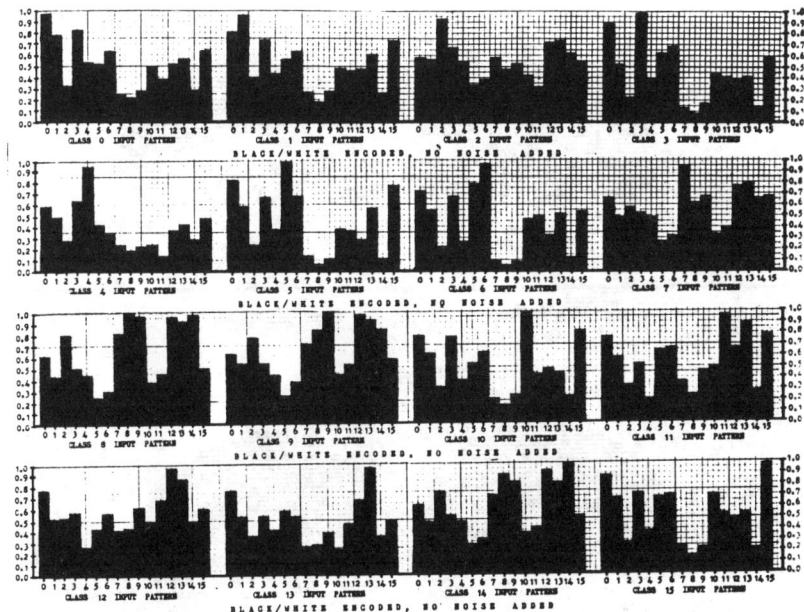

FIGURE 12. Typical response profiles for a 16 class recogniser.

5.2. Expression Recognition

In order to test the discriminant ability of the method, a two-category experiment was carried out. Only one person was involved in the experiment. The first detector was trained on the person with a smiling expression on his face, whilst for the second detector, the person was required to look serious. The n-tuple sample size in this experiment was increased to 8. This has the effect of increasing the sensitivity of the network so that it can discriminate between highly similar patterns. (4). Typical digitised frames of the smiling and serious faces are shown in Fig. 13. Real-time expression recognition was achieved and the decision could be switched between the two detectors by the subject alternatively smiling and frowning.

The system needs no prior knowledge. This is one of the significant aspects of the technique. No data analysis has to be undertaken either before or during the operation of the system. A large number $(N/_n)$ of arbitary samples of the image is used and there is consequently a high probability that some sampling n-tuples will prove to have a unique set of values for each class of data. It is the functions driven by these n-tuples which provide the discrimination properties. Other functions

438

which receive samples which are common to two or more classes will respond in the same way to images from those classes. These are redundant functions and will not contribute to the recognition process.

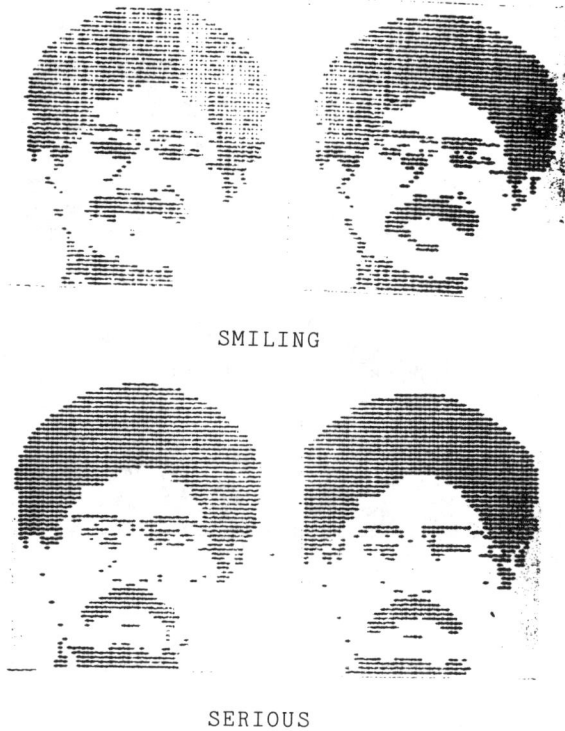

SMILING

SERIOUS

FIGURE 13. Examples of a smiling and serious face (binarised).

Various strategies have been developed in order to optimise the networks and remove the redundant processors (5) by deleting the appropriate connections. If this is done to the expression recogniser, the cover of the image can be reduced to approximately 30%, whilst the response separation between the two categories is enhanced by some 50%. The system again maintains correct recognition when tested in real time and this amounts to rates in excess of 1000 images per minute via the T.V camera.

The optimised mapping for the expression recogniser in shown in Fig. 14. An asterisk (*) indicates a useful pixel site in the input space, whereas the blank areas are to be ignored. It can be seen that the useful information is occurring around the mouth, eye region and hairline, which are the areas we, as human observers, might expect relevant expression information to occur. It should however be noted that by optimising a mapping, the hardware becomes specific to a particular problem or application. It loses its general purpose applicability.

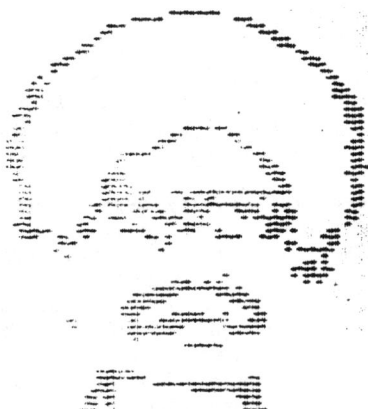

FIGURE 14. An optimsed mapping for the expression recogniser (* are useful pixel sites - the blank areas are ignored).

6. FACE VERIFICATION

The learning network approach to face recognition appears to present a novel and viable solution. The experiment using 16 subjects can be set up by using relatively modest hardware or by using software simulation if high speeds are not required. Each data category however has its own discriminator or network and if the number of categories is increased to thousands or tens of thousands as may be necessary in commercial security applications, the hardware requirements become prohibitivly large. In practice, however, the problem quite often is not one of recognition but verification - Is the person who (s)he says (s)he is?

Considering the 16 class recogniser, when tested on, say class 0 (see Fig. 12) the class 0 detector should respond with near maximal response. The other detectors which are not related to class 0 will respond, depending on the similarity between their training set images and the class 0 images. The response range in this case is between 0.3 and 0.8 of maximum. If a class of images not belonging to the 16 categories used in the experiment (ie a face from somebody other that the 16 subjects in Fig. 11) is input, each network will still respond and the system will

440

provide an overall response profile. This profile has been observed to be stable to a significant degree for a given person stimulating the system.

A profile can be obtained by any person appearing before the camera. If the profile is regarded as a transformed representation of the image verification can be achieved as follows:-

Suppose a network is trained on a relatively small set of people - say 16 as in section 5.1. The face of a person not belonging to the training categories is them input and the response profile observed. The profile is then converted into a numerical representation based on the magnitude of the detector responses and this forms the basis of a unique personal identification code. When the individual is subsequently verified at a later date, they appear before the camera and supply the system with their personal identification code. The system generates the response profile from the face and transforms it into the format of the identification code. If the supplied code correlates within prescribed limits to that generated directly from the face , the person is accepted, otherwise (s)he is rejected.

The approach has a twofold security aspect. It incorporates the use of a unique identification code and is also face driven, which is a unique image form. There are also significant hardware advantages. Whereas the recognition system can resolve K classes, where K is the number of discriminators, the verification scheme has an upper bound of K factorial categories, which, in the case of K=16, exceeds 10^{10}. Whilst it is not expected that the upper bound will be approached, as the responses of individual detectors are not independent, the method will certainly offer a verification potential for a population far in excess of the lower bound of K, when using a discriminator system.

7. FACE COMPONENT RECOGNITION.

The learning network can be adapted to assign identities to components of faces and thereby enhance computer based face retrieval systems. Suppose we wish to recognise subsets of faces such as eyes, noses, hairlines, mouths and chins. There components can be input to a learning system simply by windowing the appropriate area of the face. Suppose we assume five broad types of each component, giving a total of 5^5 or 15,625 combinations. The faces can be searched by scanning a database of 5 element vectors of the face.

$$\underline{V} = (e, n, h, m, c)$$
$$\text{where } e, n, h, m, c \in (1,2,3,4,5,)$$

Preliminary results suggest that the face components can be recognised with a learning system. The face can be transposed from a pixel image to the vector form $\underline{V}$ which is used for file searching. The automatic recognition of the face components will clearly have significant applications in the 'photo-fit' types of identification procedures which are currently based largely on human pattern recognition decisions.

8. CONCLUSIONS

The adaptive learning network offers a alternative architecture which is more suited to processing real world images and data that the conventional computer structure. The system is based very loosely on neural modelling but is principally a data processing structure. It has significant speed and programming advantages.

Initial investigations suggest that it is particularly pertinent to face processing and can be used to implement both recognition and verification strategies. Whilst there is much further research to be carried out in this area, there appears to be a strong case for considering self-adapting parallel systems for face processing and other data interpretation tasks. The problems are all fuzzy or non-deterministic and the prospects of deriving algorithms which map the data directly into its recognition category seem to be remote. The tasks can however be done -humans are excellent pattern recognisers and their information processing behaviour is generally regarded as being intelligent

The learning network described in this paper can be regarded as showing some embryonic form of artificial intelligence and represent a significant departure from the predefined algorithmic image processing hitherto available in computer based vision.

9. ACKNOWLEDGEMENTS

The author wishes to acknowledge the funding of the WISARD project provided by the U.K. Science and Engineering Research Council. Thanks are also due to Dr. B.A. Wilkie and M. Patel for carrying out and making available, experimental data.

11. OVERVIEW

PLENARY SESSION. AN OVERVIEW. COMPLEMENTARY APPROACHES TO COMMON PROBLEMS
IN FACE RECOGNITION.

M. A. JEEVES

1. INTRODUCTION

Taken together the papers presented at this Conference underlined the
major lines of research being pursued today in studies of face recognition.
On the one hand, they included a large input from cognitive psychologists
who are being increasingly successful in their attempts to fractionate the
processes involved in perceiving and recognising faces.   On the other
hand, they highlighted how much is yet to be learned about the biological
substrates of face recognition, how it develops, how it is represented in
neural structures and how such knowledge can reciprocally inform the work
of cognitive psychologists.   Thus at many points it became evident that
knowledge derived from each of these complementary approaches to common
problems could and should inform and modify the models and techniques
developed primarily within the other framework.   Whilst the papers
presented were wide ranging in their scope it is possible, nevertheless
with some slight oversimplifications, to identify several recurring issues
which may help to map out the most likely profitable lines of investigation
for future work.   In the final plenary session I identified what seemed to
me to be these recurring issues and this paper summarises that presentation
together with the reactions to it in the ensuing open discussion.   It also
looks back at the preceding papers and shows how the various contributions
indicated   actual   or   potential   links   at   the   interface   between
neuropsychology and cognitive psychology, whilst acknowledging that the
dichotomy is a useful rather than a very substantive one.

2. PROSOPAGNOSIAS

In the past lines have been fairly sharply drawn between those such as
Bodamer, 1947, Bornstein, 1963, 1969, De Renzi and Spinnler, 1966, 1969,
Benton and Van Allen, 1968, and Yin, 1970, who opt for a perceptual
hypothesis and those such as Charcot, 1883, Wilbrand, 1892, Hecaen and
Angelergues, 1962, Damasio et al, 1982, and Bruyer, 1983, who opt for a
memory hypothesis.   De Renzi underlined the dangers inherent in treating
prosopagnosia as if it were a single unitary disorder.   Instead the
meaningful thing is to speak of the prosopagnosias, thus indicating that
difficulties in face recognition do not have a unitary cause but will vary
from patient to patient.   What is now needed is a taxonomy of
prosopagnosias.   Such a taxonomy will need to distinguish between
metamorphopsic and prosopagnosic difficulties, between apperceptive and
associative forms of prosopagnosia, between difficulties involving familiar
and unfamiliar faces and will also need to identify any special
difficulties involved in the analysis of expression.   This provisional list
should be capable of further subdivision as it is guided by the theoretical
inputs of cognitive psychologists.   At the same time it is important in
every case to gain as comprehensive a description of the patients abilities
and disabilities as possible and not to try and make the observations fit a

predetermined taxonomic scheme. What seems likely is that just as the fractionation of language disorders witnessed over the past decade has immeasurably helped our understanding of the aphasias (not aphasia) so a similar fractionation of face processing will begin to enrich our understanding of disorders of face recognition. De Renzi also addressed the question of whether it is conceivable that a mechanism specialised in processing and/or storing facial data is selectively disrupted. In his view, supported by evidence from further patients, it is not likely that prosopagnosia is only a particular aspect of a more general disorder involving evoking the previously learned context of a visual stimulus. His paper underlines the need to study patients with prosopagnosia and free from perceptual impairments and in particular to pay attention to their ability to recognise personal objects. Since the patients he studied can recognise their personal objects (e.g. wallet) from other people's (wallets) then this challenges Damasio's view that prosopagnosic recognition losses extend to all classes of objects.

In discussion the cognitive psychologists present (for example Parkin and Thomson) queried whether it was any longer useful to retain what was probably an outdated dichotomy. They believe that by retaining the dichotomy there is a danger that it will be used in a way that stultifies new thinking and forces experimental data into a straitjacket. Others felt that a distinction which had been conceptually useful in the past in neurological studies of prosopagnosia should not be lightly discarded. Certainly, for the clinician the distinction remains a useful one; there are patients whose disorder presents as primarily perceptual but there are others whose perceptual capabilities from a standpoint of what they can achieve are quite normal. The perceptual/memory dichotomy used in this way is useful in providing a shorthand way of describing what a particular patient can and cannot do. Providing we keep in mind that it is merely a useful shorthand we shall not go far wrong. At the same time it was accepted that it may not be useful to cling to the idea that prosopagnosic disorders must be either perceptual or memorial, but that it would be better to follow De Renzi and others (for example, Damasio) in recognising that there may be two groups, at least, of prosopagnosics and that their aetiology may involve different neural substrates. Thus, those involving associative disorders may involve bilateral lesions whereas non-memorial ones may involve only unilateral lesions (Damasio). Since there are so few cases of prosopagnosics available, the challenge today is to ensure that those that are available are examined comprehensively. The paper by Davidoff et al in this volume provides a model of what can be achieved by such in depth studies. The data thus gathered should then enable us to rethink some of our information processing flow diagrams of face recognition. The issue of whether the cerebral damage in prosopagnosia is unilateral or bilateral was also taken up by De Renzi. As with the perception versus memory issue there are distinguished advocates of the unilateral and bilateral damage hypotheses respectively. Thus for the unilateralists we have Charcot (1983), Hecaen and Angelergues (1962) and Benton and Van Allen (1968) and for the bilateralists we have Wilbrand (1892), Bodamer (1947), Meadows (1974), Damasio (1982) and Bruyer (1983). De Renzi reminded the Conference that there are in the literature six case reports with surgical evidence showing the involvement of the right hemisphere alone. He added two further cases to these, and believed that these taken together with the Landis et al (in press) and Tiberghien (1985) patients constitute a strong support for the view that prosopagnosia may occur with unilateral damage. Damasio's earlier publications and,

reviews, on the other hand, lead to the view that there is always some
bilateral involvement. De Renzi accepts that the last word must be left to
autopsy studies. Whilst I suspect that we are arriving at a position where
the weight of evidence is in favour of bilateral lesions, it needs to be
remembered that this question does not stand apart from the analyses of the
cognitive psychologists using information processing models. This was well
illustrated at the Conference by the contribution by Umilta who argued
convincingly that the logic underlying the majority of experiments claiming
to study lateralisation of cerebral functions, including studies of face
perception, is open to question. Even if one accepts some form of
structural explanation of observed laterality affects, there still remains
the question of the detailed features of an information processing model
which best makes sense of the experimental data. Umilta believed that in
the past models have too readily ignored interhemispheric processes and he
presented a "conditional interhemispheric transmission" model which he
believed was the best fit for the available evidence from psychological
experiments, as well as doing justice to what we know about the anatomy and
physiology of the neocortical commissures. Once again, therefore, the
cognitive models cannot stand apart from the neurological data. It is at
their interface that each can, with benefit, be scrutinised afresh and
refined. This point was clearly brought out by Bauer who elegantly
demonstrated that prosopagnosics who are totally incapable of consciously
identifying any faces can nevertheless reliably discriminate facial
identity at the psychophysiological level. His data moreoever indicated a
degree of hypoarousal to visual stimuli suggesting subtly impaired
perception in prosopagnosics. Evidence of this kind is necessary and
helpful in attempting to decide whether distinctions made by cognitive
psychologists unconcerned with neural substrates find support or otherwise
from physiological and anatomical data. This underlines again how careful
studies of selected prosopagnosics can in principle do for cognitive
psychological models of image processing what HM has done for the study of
memory.

Umilta's paper makes a natural transition from the more neurologically
oriented papers to those by cognitive psychologists. Before doing so,
however, we may note that hemispheric lateralisation was taken up again by
Parkin who, like Umilta, underlined the involvement of both cerebral
hemispheres in face processing. He further argued that a consideration of
the different stages of processing of facial stimuli could be handled in
part by recognising the distinctive processing modes of the two cerebral
hemispheres.

3. MODELS OF FACE PROCESSING - COGNITIVE AND NEUROPSYCHOLOGICAL
3.1 Cognitive

Cognitive theoretical models of the processes which underlie face
recognition (e.g. Bruce, 1979, 1983; Baron, 1981; H. Ellis, 1981, 1983; Hay
and Young, 1982) were taken as the common starting point for discussions on
this topic. Bruce's identification of seven different types of information
code involved in handling facial information was generally accepted (see
papers by Young, Hay and Ellis, and Klatsky, this volume). Bruce has
distinguished the following codes: pictorial, structural, visually derived
semantic, identity specific semantic, name, expression and facial speech
codes. The components of such models are functional and are hypothesised
without any necessary regard to whether or not they are mirrored in
specific neural substrates. This is not to say that evidence from
neuropsychological investigations cannot help to refine and modify such

cognitive models. Bruce has several times emphasised how the results which are obtained from for example, experiments studying the processing of familiar faces strongly mirrors those processes found at work and described in the literature on word recognition. Her view reflected also in the paper of Hay and Young underlines the benefits gained from such approaches to the study of face recognition. They wrote "Our position is that the similarities observed reflect fundamental similarities in the way in which processes of perceptual classification and semantic classification are organised with respect to each other". They believe, moreoever, that the "recognition unit" metaphor is useful in understanding such processes even though it runs into difficulties in handling the results gained from studies of priming effects. Young and Hay in their presentation also underlined the need to make a distinction between processes involved in the recognition of familiar faces as compared with those involved with unfamiliar faces. Thus they point out that identity-specific semantic codes and name codes are only available to familiar faces and not available to unfamiliar faces. A further necessary distinction to bear in mind when formulating models of facial processing was brought out in the contribution of Davies. Reviewing the literature on the competence and completeness of facial recall and comparing this with those associated with face recognition, Davies concluded that while the existing findings generally suggest an identity mechanism mediating both recognition and recall, there appear to be a number of areas where discrepancies occur. Identifying these discrepancies and the reasons for them should provide another avenue for formulating a comprehensive theory of face memory.

One of the things which emerged clearly from consideration of the papers presented addressing the question of face recognition was, as we noted above, the way in which different approaches enable one to fractionate the process in different ways. Sergent, for example, elegantly demonstrated how the visual system provides the brain with several descriptions of facial information. The usefulness of a particular description depends upon the operations to be carried out. Low frequency information is the most resilient to degradation and the visual system can generate such information subjectively even when it has objectively been filtered out in the display. At the same time her results demonstrated that high frequencies are not redundant. Depending on the nature of the operations or the task to be performed they may benefit performance in some tasks particularly those that require accessing the identity of a face. In turn these different ways of handling low and high frequency information may be reflected in the differential sensitivity of the two hemispheres to such information. The critical role of low frequencies in any processing of faces points to the right hemisphere making the dominant contribution to perception and recognition whilst the left hemisphere may begin to add its important contribution when the process of identification becomes necessary. Such a suggestion is open to empirical investigation by applying it to the performance of prosopagnosics.

In order for recognition to take place faces must be represented in some way in human memory. Klatzky addressed this question and examined the possibility that the representation was incorporated at several different levels of abstraction. It was clear from her data (this volume) that the three levels that she identified, which she labelled as according to content, to form and to encoding process of the mapping from visual world memory, all might be used to represent human faces. She further believes that these representations differ in their contributions to episodic memory recognition. Her suggestion that the effective representation in recognition may be a visual abstraction conveying properties of the face that remain constant over variations in viewing echoed findings from a very different area reported at the Conference by Perrett. A complementary approach to the understanding of facial recall was presented by Laughery, Duvall, Wogan and Wogalter who reported work investigating some of the dynamics of facial memory. Once again their results distinguished between feature and holistic processing and the analyses revealed three technique-dependent recall strategies.

Still with the seven different types of encoding identified by Bruce in mind, it was interesting that Calis and Mens reported data which led them to the conclusion that there is a predominant way of processing expressions which is neither a normalising stage nor a part of the identification or recognition of the face. Malpass and Hughes identified three possible models whereby facial prototypes were built up which they labelled central tendency models, attribute frequency models, and interval storage models. Their evidence gave little support to the first or third of these models and pointed to the attribute frequency model as being the most plausible. Concerned about the possibility of artefacts creeping into the study of processing purely through laboratory methods, Mueller et al reported studies of spontaneous deep processing under natural conditions. It is clear from their results that the process of stereotyping may take place according to different strategies and that depending on the strategy, the encoding may differ in each case.

3.2 Neuropsychological models

The possibility of fractionating the total process involved in face recognition so clearly demonstrated by the cognitive psychologists was paralleled by the development of neuropsychological models of the same processes, for example Marzi et al made it clear that the observed hemispheric asymmetries in a face perception task depend upon the cognitive requirements of that task. Thus face recognition with advance information given might induce holistic and right hemisphere processing rather than the single feature processing which sometimes occurs in such tasks. Likewise a face naming task induces a left hemisphere superiority, providing a concomitant right hemisphere involvement is not brought about by the prior tendency for holistic processing stimulated by pre-exposure of the faces. In similar vein, Parkin presented evidence to suggest that the different stages of the face recognition process might be handled by different cerebral hemispheres. Thus the classification stage of models of face recognition would appear to be a right hemisphere process, whereas the feature extraction stage may be left-lateralised. In this way we see that stage processing models as constructed by the cognitive psychologists begin to be mapped onto neuropsychological models. Supporting evidence of a neurological kind implicating the two cerebral hemispheres but to different extents and in different ways was presented at the Conference by others including De Renzi and Umilta. And it is not only cortical processes that are involved because Crawford et al presented clinical evidence highlighting the importance of subcortical structures as well as cortical structures in face processing. This important finding links in with some of the work on monkeys not reported at the Conference but coming from Rolls' Laboratory in Oxford, where Leonard et al have recorded from cells in the amygdala and demonstrated their involvement in face processing (Leonard et al, 1985).

Bruyer's review of the literature on the kinds of experimental material used to study face perception and recognition with both unilaterally brain damaged and normal subjects once again stressed the asymmetry of cerebral functioning in processing facial material. The same point was emphasised from a complementary point of view by Small, who demonstrated that when evoked potentials were recorded in response to coloured slides of scenes and of people there was a marked asymmetry in the responses to people not evident in the response to scenes. Moreover, when a group of left-handed people was given the same task, the clear and consistently greater right hemisphere response to facial material observed in right-handers was no longer present.

That the method of responding required of subjects in face identification recognition tasks can indicate differential involvement of the two cerebral hemispheres was brought out by Thomson. He showed that the automatic-template-matching and the feature-retrieval methods that he used produced very similar results to those identified by other contributors such as Marzi and Parkin and they produce a different visual field superiority. He also demonstrated that these different ways of responding are age-related, the feature-retrieval method not emerging until 12 years of age.

Whilst the crucial heuristic role played by theories such as Marr's was underlined many times at the Conference it was equally emphasised that they need constant examination and revision. It was clear, for example, from Millward et al's work that Marr's primal sketch stage needed re-examination. They presented data using stimuli consisting of photographs of human faces but presented with low band or high band pass filters and the results provided information on which substages of Marr's primal sketch theory can best be considered to provide input into memory systems. In similar vein Perrett et al's data suggested a re-examination of stages of processing between the two and a half D representation and the three D stage in the same theory.

4. SPECIFICITY OF FACES

The question of whether there is something specific and unique about faces and the way they are processed by the brain is an issue with a distinguished pedigree (e.g. those in favour Bodamer, 1947, Hecaen and Angelergues, 1962, Yin, 1970, and those against Charcot, 1883, Wilbrand, 1892, Bornstein, 1963, 1969, De Renzi and Spinnler, 1966) and remains a live issue. It was addressed a number of times at the Conference. Thus, for example, De Schonen and Mathiert reported a developmental study of infants from four to nine months old. Their results suggested that the perception and discrimination of shapes (other than faces) are controlled in a different way from processes involved in the perception of stimuli such as faces. This could certainly be interpreted as further evidence for face specific mechanisms and would be consistent with work referred to in discussion by Ellis which had shown selective responding to faces by neonates within minutes of birth. This view would also agree with that expressed by Newcombe in discussion where she suggested that it was not unreasonable to imagine that there may be for faces a prewiring analogous to that believed to exist in the planum temporale for language (Geschwind and Levitsky, 1968). Such a view would also tie in with Salzen's comment that it makes sense to consider the possible relevance here of the evidence from imprinting studies and to at least entertain the possibility of there being a "facial" releaser present at birth. That there may be something special about faces was also drawn attention to by Tiberghien's results on the effect of context in remembering faces. These results suggested that the effects of context were greater in face memory than in verbal memory and this raised again the question of whether there is something special or even specific about faces. Certainly the neurophysiological evidence reported by Perrett is interpretable in these same terms. In addition, the evidence reported by Perrett et al produced a model of hierarchical processing which could well be the neuropsychological analogue of similar cognitive models. Having pointed to several contributions interpretable as in favour of face specific processing mechanisms it was clear from Winograd's contribution that the issue is far from settled. His results suggested that the proper dichotomy to make was between verbal and visual memory tasks and did not support a trichotomy of verbal, picture and face tasks. There was no evidence from his data for a factor dealing with faces alone and it did not support the hypothesis of a specialised system for encoding faces.

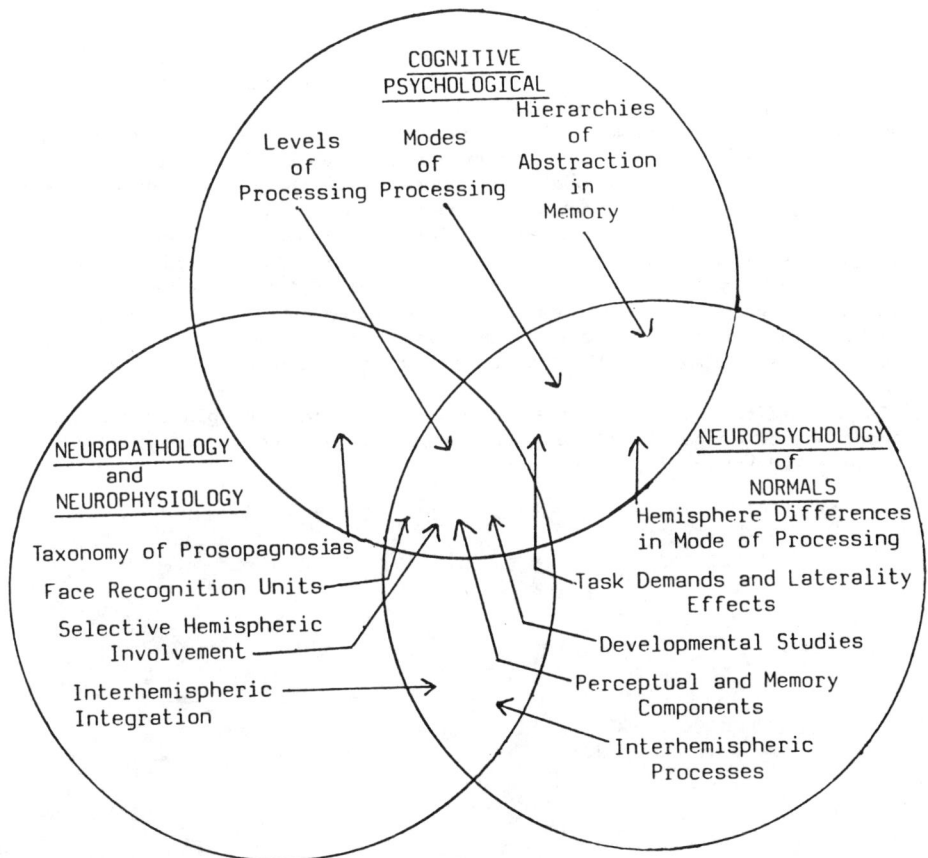

FIGURE 1. A territorial map of complementary approaches to common problems in face recognition.

5. THE WAY AHEAD

In our Preface we indicated that during the Conference plans for joint research began to emerge. The more productive of these will probably be found at the interfaces between hitherto relatively self-contained areas. We may grossly oversimplify the total research landscape by representing it in the form of a Venn diagram (see Fig. 1). The three interlocking areas are broadly described as cognitive psychological approaches, neuropsychological studies of normals and neurological studies including neurophysiological and neuropathology.

The answers sought by workers from each of the three areas to seemingly common questions will, when available, be couched in different language. Thus whether there is something special (? unique) about face perception may be answered in terms of (a) a specific neural substrate dedicated to face processing (neurological approach) (b) a particular pattern of hemispheric collaboration involved in processing faces (neuropsychological approach) or (c) a set of encoding stages special to the processing of faces and not applicable to the processing of other visual inputs (cognitive psychological approach).

Or again, cognitive and neuropsychological approaches to the question of modes of processing will be characterised in the one case (cognitive) by, for example, specifying the distinctive features of holistic vs. feature identification mechanisms and in the other case (neuropsychological) by indicating the relative involvement of each cerebral hemisphere in face processing. Both will probably be concerned with how task demands affect processing mode and hemispheric involvement.

Whether the levels of processing (Bruce) or hierarchy of abstractions (Klatsky) will have any neurological analogue in, for example, cortical to subcortical pathways and whether the search for such analogues is a fruitful task must as yet remain an open question. In the meantime each can benefit from cross comparison so that the need for parsimony of explanations prevents the unnecessary proliferation of explanatory constructs.

In all of this I suspect that a crucial role will be played as cognitive psychologists cooperate closely with neurologists and neuropsychologists in the detailed study of prosopagnosics.

12. REFERENCES

REFERENCES

Abdi, H.   Additive tree representations of verbatim memory.   In E. Terouanne (Ed.), New trends in mathematical psychology. II. New York: Elsevier, 1986.

Abdi, H., Barthelemy, J. P., Luong, X.   Tree representations of associative structures in semantic and episodic memory research.   In E. Degreef, J. Van Bugennhaut (Eds).   New trends in mathematical psychology. New York: Elsevier, 1984.

Abdi, H., Barthelemy, J. P., Luong, X.   Representations arborees et categories naturelles (to appear).

Adams, J. K.   Laboratory studies of behavior without awareness. Psychological Bulletin, 1957, 54, 383-405.

Adams, R. D., Victor, M.   Principles of neurology 2nd ed. New York: McGraw Hill, 1981.

Adams-Webber, J., & Mancusco, J. C.   Applications of personal construct theory.   New York: Academic Press, 1983.

Agnetti, V., Carreras, M., Pinna, L., & Rosati, G.   Ictal prosopagnosia and epileptogenic damage of the dominant hemisphere.   A case history.   Cortex, 1978, 14, 50-57.

Albert, M. S., Butters, N., & Levin, J.   Temporal gradients in the retrograde amnesia of patients with alcoholic Korsakoff's disease. Archives of Neurology, 1979, 36, 211-216.

Aleksander, I.   Emergent intelligent properties of progressively structured pattern recognition nets.   Pattern Recognition Letters Vol. 1. No. 3, 1985.

Aleksander, I., & Stonham, T. J.   A guide to pattern recognition using random access memories. IEE Journal, Comp. Digit. Tech. Vol. No. 1, 1979.

Alexander, M. P., Stuss, D. T., & Benson, D. F.   Capgras Syndrome : a reduplicative phenomenon.   Neurology, 1979, 29, 334-339.

Allport, D. A., Antonis, B., & Reynolds, P.   On the division of attention: A disproof of the single-channel hypothesis.   Quarterly Journal of Experimental Psychology, 1972, 24, 225-235.

Allport, G. W.   The nature of prejudice.   New York: Doubleday, 1954.

Amir, Y.   Contact hypothesis in ethnic relations.   Psychological Bulletin, 1976, 71, 319-342.

Anderson, E., & Parkin, A. J.   On the nature of the left visual field advantage in facial processing.   Cortex (in press), 1985.

Anderson, J. R.   Language, Memory and Thought.   Hillsdale: N.J., Erlbaum Associates, 1976.

Anderson, J. R.   The Architecture of Cognition.   Cambridge: M.A., Harvard University Press, 1983.

Anderson, J. R., & Bower, G. H.   Recognition and retrieval processes in face recall.   Psychological Review, 1972, 85, 249-277.

Anderson, N. H.   On the role of context effects in psychophysical judgment.   Psychological Review, 1975, 82, 462-482.

Anderson, N. H.   Algebraic rules in psychological measurement.   American Scientist, 1979, 67, 555-563.

Antes, J. R., Metzger, R. L.   Influence of picture context on object recognition.   Acta Psychologica, 1980, 44, 21-30.

Arendt, I., Bigl, V., Arendt, A., Tennstedt, A.   Loss of neurons in the nucleus basalis of Meynert in Alzheimer's, paralysis agitans and Korsakoff's disease.   Acta Neuropathologica, 1983, 61, 101-108.

Aslin, R. N., & Salapatek, P.   Saccadic localization of visual targets by the very young human infant.   Perception and Psychophysics, 1975, 17, 293-302.

Assal, G.   Regression des troubles de la reconnaissance des physionomies et de la memoire topographique chez un malade opere d'un hematome intra-cerebral parieto-temporal droit.   Revue Neurologique, 1969, 121, 184-185.

Assal, G., & Favre, C.   An observation of animal agnosia concerning cows.   Second European Workshop on Cognitive Neuropsychology.   Bressanone, Jan. 1984.

Assal, G., Favre, C., & Anderes, J. P.   Non-reconnaissance d'animaux familiers chez un paysan.   Revue Neurologique, 1984, 140, 580-584.

Atkinson, R. C., & Juola, J. F.   Search and decision processes in recognition memory.   In D. H. Krantz, R. C. Atkinson, R. D. Luce & P. Suppes (Eds.), Contemporary developments in mathematical psychology. (Vol. 1). Learning, memory and thinking.   San Francisco : Freeman, 1974.

Attneave, F., & Arnoult, M. D.   The quantitive study of shape and pattern perception.   Psychological Bulletin, 1956, 53, 452-471.

Baddeley, A. D. Applied cognitive and cognitive applied psychology : The case of face recognition, In L. G. Nilsson (Ed.), Perspectives in Memory Research : Essays in honor of Uppsala University, Hillsdale, NJ.: Erlbaum Associates, 1979.

Baddeley, A. D. Domains of recollection. Psychological Review, 1982, 89, 708-729.

Baddeley, A. D., Woodhead, M. Depth of processing context and face recognition. Canadian Journal of Psychology, 1982, 36, 148-164.

Bahrick, H. P. Memory for people. In J. Harris (Ed.), Everyday memory, actions, and absentmindedness. (pp.19-34). London: Academic Press, 1983.

Bahrick, H. P. Semantic memory content in permastore: Fifty years of memory for Spanish learned in school. Journal of Experimental Psychology: General, 1984, 113, 1-29.

Bahrick, H. P., Bahrick, P. O., & Wittlinger, R. P. Fifty years of memory for names and faces: A cross-sectional approach. Journal of Experimental Psychology: General, 1975, 104, 54-75.

Bain, A. The emotions and the will. London: Longmans, 1859.

Barkowitz, P., & Brigham, J. C. Recognition of faces: Own-race bias, incentive, and time delay. Journal of Applied Social Psychology, 1982, 12, 255-268.

Baron, R. J. Mechanisms of human facial recognition. International Journal of Man-Machine Studies, 1981, 15(2), 137-178.

Barry, R. The effect of significance upon indices of Sokolov's orienting response: A new conceptualization to replace the OR. Physiological Psychology, 1977, 5, 209-214.

Bartlett, F. C. Remembering: A study in experimental and social psychology. London: Cambridge University Press, 1932.

Bartlett, J. C., Hurry, S., & Thorley, W. Typicality and familiarity of faces. Memory & Cognition, 1984, 12, 219-228.

Bassili, J. N. Emotion recognition: The role of facial movement and the relative importance of upper and lower areas of the face. Journal of Personality and Social Psychology, 1979, 37, 2049-2058.

Bauer, R. M. Visual hypoemotionality as a symptom of visual-limbic disconnection in man. Archives of Neurology, 1982, 39, 702-708.

Bauer, R. M. Autonomic recognition of names and faces in prosopagnosia: A neuropsychological application of the Guilty Knowledge Test. Neuropsychologia, 1984, 22, 457-469.

Bauer, R. M., & Rubens, A. B. Agnosia. In K. M. Heilman and E. Valenstein (Eds.), Clinical Neuropsychology. (2nd Ed.), pp.187-241. New York: Oxford University Press, 1985.

458

Bauer, R. M., & Trobe, J. D. Visual memory and perceptual impairments in prosopagnosia. Journal of Clinical Neuro-Opthalmology, 1984, 4, 39-46.

Bauer, R. M., & Verfaellie, M. Autonomic recognition in prosopagnosia depends upon premorbidly stored facial information, (in press).

Bauer, R. M., Rediess, S., Verfaellie, M., Bowers, D., Walker, V., & Hendlin, R. Verbal and autonomic aspects of recognition memory in two forms of human amnesia, (in press).

Bay, E. Agnosie und Funktionswandel. Monographien aus dem Gesamtgebiete der Neurologie und Psychiatrie, 1950, 73, 1-94.

Bay, E. Disturbances of visual perception and their examination. Brain, 1953, 76, 515-551.

Beaumont, J. G. (Ed.) Divided Visual Field Studies of Cerebral Organisation. London: Academic Press, 1982.

Beaumont, J. G., Young, A. W., & McManus, I. C. Hemisphericity: A critical review. Cognitive Neuropsychology, 1984, 1, 191-212.

Begg, I., & Sikich, D. Imagery and contextual organization. Memory & Cognition, 1984, 12, 52-59.

Benson, D. F., Segarra, J., & Albert, M. L. Visual agnosia-prosopagnosia: A clinicopathological correlation. Archives of Neurology, 1974, 30, 307-310.

Bentin, S., & Gordon, H. W. Assessment of cognitive asymmetries in brain-damaged and normal subjects: validation of a test battery. Journal of Neurology, Neurosurgery, and Psychiatry, 1979, 42, 715-723.

Benton, A. L. The neuropsychology of facial recognition. American Psychologist, 1980, 35, 176-186.

Benton, A. L., & Van Allen, M. W. Impairment in facial recognition in patients with cerebral disease. Cortex, 1968, 4, 344-358.

Benton, A. L., & Van Allen, M. W. Prosopagnosia and facial discrimination. Journal of Neurological Sciences, 1972, 15, 167-172.

Benton, A. L., & Gordon, M. C. Correlates of facial recognition. Transactions of the American Neurological Association, 1971, 96, 91-96.

Benton, A. L., Hamsher, K., Varney, N. R., & Spreen, O. Contributions to Neuropsychological Assessment. New York: Oxford University Press, 1983.

Berlyne, D. Conflict, Arousal, and Curiosity. New York: McGraw-Hill, 1960.

Bernstein, A. S. The orienting response as novelty and significance detector: Reply to O'Gorman. Psychophysiology, 1979, 16, 263-273.

Bernstein, A. S., Taylor, K., & Weinstein, E. The phasic electrodermal response as a differentiated complex reflecting stimulus significance. Psychophysiology, 1975, 12, 158-169.

Beyn, E. S., & Knyazeva, G. R.   The problem of prosopagnosia.   Journal of
Neurology, Neurosurgery and Psychiatry, 1962, 25, 154-159.

Bhat, M. V., & Haupt, A.   An efficient clustering algorithm. IEE Transaction
on Systems, Man, and Cybernetics, 1976, 6, 61-64.

Biber, C., Butters, N., Rosen, J., Gerstman, L., & Mattis, S.   Encoding
strategies and recognition of faces by alcoholic Korsakoff and other
brain-damaged patients.   Journal of Clinical Neuropsychology, 1981, 3,
315-330.

Bidault, J. P., Luaute, A., & Tzavaras, A.   Prosopagnosia and the Delusional
Misidentification syndromes.   Biblotheca Psychiat, No. 164, Karger, Basel,
(in press).

Billig, M., & Milner, D.   A spade is a spade in the eyes of the law.
Psychology Today, (UK edition), January, 1976, 2, 13-15, 62.

Birch, E. E.   Infant interocular acuity differences and binocular vision.
Vision Research, 1985, 25, 571-576.

Birnbaum, M. H.   Using contextual effects to derive psychophysical scales.
Perception & Psychophysics, 1974, 15, 89-96.

Blanc-Garin, J.   Des faits, des concepts, des processus concernant la
perception des visages.   Seminaire de Neuropsychologie Humaine.   EHESS,
Marseille, 1980.

Blanc-Garin, J.   Perception des visages et reconnaissance de la physionomie
dans l'Agnosie des visages.   L'Annee Psychologique, 1984, 84, 573-598.

Blanc-Garin, J., Poncet, M., & Abonnel-Orlando, H.   Face and non-face
stimuli for two prosopagnosic patients.   Second European Workshop on
Cognitive Neuropsychology. Bressanone, Jan. 1984.

Blunk, R.   Recognition of emotion and physiognomy in right- and
left-hemisphere damaged patients and normals.   Communication.
International Neuropsychological Society meeting, Deauville, 1982.

Bodamer, J.   Die Prosopagnosie.   Archiv fur Psychiatrie und Nervenkrank-
heiten, 1947, 179, 6-53.

Bodis-Wollner, I.   Vulnerability of spatial-frequency channels in cerebral
lesions. Nature, 1976, 261, 309-311.

Bogousslavky, J., & Salvador, A. Le syndrome de Capgras, clinique et
problemes organiques : une reevaluation.   Annales Medico-Psychologiques
1981, 139 (9), 949-964.

Boorman, S. A., & Arabie, P.   Structural measures and the method of sorting.
In R. N. Shepard, A. K. Roney and S. Nerlove (ed.).   Multidimensional
scaling theory and applications in the behavioral science.   Vol. 1, New
York: Seminar Press, 1972.

Bornstein, B. Prosopagnosia.   In: L. Halpern (ed.).   Problems of dynamic
neurology, p.283-318. Jerusalem: Hadassah Medical Organization, 1963.

Bornstein, B., & Kidron, D. P.   Prosopagnosia.   Journal of Neurology, Neurosurgery and Psychiatry, 1959, 22, 124-131.

Bornstein, B., Sroka, H., & Munitz, H.   Prosopagnosia with animal face agnosia.   Cortex, 1969, 5, 164-1

Bothwell, R. K., Brigham, J. C., & Malpass, R. S.   A meta-analysis of eyewitness research: Cross-racial identification.   Unpublished manuscript, Florida State University, 1985.

Boudouresques, J., Poncet, M., Ali Cherif, A., & Balzamo, M.   L'agnosie des visages: un temoin de la desorganisation fonctionnelle d'un certain type de connaissance des elements du monde exterieur.   Bulletin de l'Academie Nationale de Medecine,1979, 163, 695-702.

Bousefield, W. A.   The occurrence of clustering in recall of randomly arranged associates.   Journal of General Psychology, 1953, 30, 149-165.

Bower, G. H., & Karlin, M. B.   Depth of processing of faces and recognition memory.   Journal of Experimental Psychology, 1974, 103, 751-757.

Bowey, J. A.   The interaction of strategy and context in children's oral reading performance.   Journal of Psycholinguistic Research, 1984, 13, 99-117.

Bradshaw, J. L., & Nettleton, N. C.   Human Cerebral Asymmetry.   Englewood Cliffs (NJ): Prentice-Hall, 1983.

Bradshaw, J. L., Gates, A., & Patterson, K.   Hemispheric differences in processing visual patterns.   Quarterly Journal of Experimental Psychology, 1976, 28, 667-681.

Bradshaw, J. L., Nettleton, N. C., & Patterson, K.   Identification of mirror-reversed and nonreversed facial profiles in same and opposite visual fields.   Journal of Experimental Psychology, 1973, 99, 42-48.

Bradshaw, J. L., Nettleton, N. C.   The nature of hemispheric specialization in man.   The Behavioral and Brain Sciences, 1981, 4, 52-91.

Bradshaw, J. L., & Sherlock, D.   Bugs and faces in the two visual fields: the analtyic/holistic processing dichotomy and task sequencing.   Cortex, 1982, 18, 211-226.

Bradshaw, J. L., Taylor, M. J., Patterson, K., & Nettleton, N. C.   Upright and inverted faces, and housefronts, in the two visual fields: a right and a left hemisphere contribution.   Journal of Clinical Neuropsychology, 1980, 2, 245-257.

Bradshaw, J. L., & Wallace, G.   Models for the processing and identification of faces.   Perception and Psychophysics, 1971, 9, 443-448.

Brigham, J. C.   The accuracy of eyewitness evidence: How do attorneys see it?   Florida Bar Journal, 1981, 55 (10), 714-721.

Brigham, J. C., & Barkowitz, P.   Do "they all look alike?"   The effect of race, sex, experience, and attitudes on the ability to recognize faces. Journal of Applied Social Psychology, 1978, 8, 306-318.

Brigham, J. C., Maas, A., Snyder, L. S., & Spaulding, K.   The accuracy of eyewitness identifications in a field setting.   Journal of Personality and Social Psychology, 1982, 42, 673-681.

Brigham, J. C., & Malpass, R. S.   The role of experience and contact in the recognition of faces of own- and other-race persons.   Journal of Social Issues, 1985, 41.

Brigham, J. C., Ready, D. J.   Own-race bias in lineup construction.   Law and Human Behavior, in press.

Brigham, J. C., & Williamson, N. L.   Cross-racial recognition and age: When you're over 60, do they still "all look alike?".   Personality and Social Psychology Bulletin, 1979, 5, 218-222.

Brigham, J. C., & WolfsKeil, M. P.   Opinions of attorneys and law enforcement personnel on the accuracy of eyewitness identifications.   Law and Human Behavior, 1983, 9, 337-349.

Brigham, J. C. & WolfsKeil, M. P.   Relationships between accuracy of prior descriptions and facial recognition.   Proceedings of the 91st Annual Convention of the American Psychological Association, Anaheim, CA, 1984.

Brigham, J. C., Woodmansee, J. J., & Cook, S. W.   Dimensions of verbal racial attitudes: Interracial marriage and approaches to racial equality.   Journal of Social Issues, 1976, 32 (2), 9-21.

Bruce, C. J., Desimone, R., & Gross, C. G.   Visual properties of neurones in a polysensory area in the superior temporal sulcus of the macaque. Journal of Neurophysiology, 1981, 46, 369-384.

Bruce, D.   The how and why of ecological memory.   Journal of Experiment Psychology: General, 1985, 114, 78-90.

Bruce, V.   Searching for politicians: An information-processing approach to face recognition.   Quarterly Journal of Experiment Psychology, 1979, 21, 373-395.

Bruce, V.   Visual and semantic effects in a serial word classification task. Current Psychological Research, 1981, 1, 153-162.

Bruce, V.   Changing faces: Visual and non-visual coding processes in face recognition.   British Journal of Psychology, 1982, , 105-116.

Bruce, V.   Recognizing faces.   Philosophical Transactions of the Royal Society of London, Series B, 1983, 302, 423-436.

Bruce, V., & Valentine, T.   Identity priming in the recognition of familiar faces.   British Journal of Psychology, 1985, 76, 373-383.

Bruce, V., & Valentine, T.   Semantic priming of familiar faces.   Quarterly Journal of Experiment Psychology, (in press).

Bruce, V., & Young, A. W.   A theoretical framework for understanding face recognition.   ESRC workshop on functional models of face and person recognition, Grange-over-Sands, England, March, 1985.

Bruner, J. S. On the conservation of liquids. In Bruner, J. S., Olver, R. R., Greenfield, P. M. (Eds.). Studies in Cognitive Growth. New York: Wiley, 1966.

Brunswick, E. Social perception of traits from photographs. Psychological Bulletin, 1945, 42, 5356.

Brutsche, J., Cisse, A., Deleglise, D., Finet, A., & Tiberghien, G. Effects de contexte dans la reconnaissance de visages non familiers. Cahiers de Psychologie Cognitive, 1981, 1, 85-99.   .

Bruyer, R. Le visage et l'expression faciale - approche neuropsychologique, Bruxelles : Pierra Mardaga, 1983.

Bruyer, R. Lesion cerebrale et perception de visages flous: differences hemispheriques. L'Annee Psychologique, 1980, 80, 379-390.

Bruyer, R. Lesion cerebrale et perception du visage: role des parties du visage. Psychologie Medicale, 1980, 12, 1261-1270.

Bruyer, R. Lesion cerebrale et perception du visage: etude de la symetrie faciale. Journal de Psychologie Normale et Pathologique, 1980, 85-98.

Bruyer, R., & Craps, V. Facial asymmetry: perceptual awareness and lateral differences. Canadian Journal of Psychology, 1985, 39, 54-69.

Bruyer, R., & Dussart, T. Lateral differences in the race effect in face recognition. International Journal of Neuroscience, 1985, 25, in press.

Bruyer, R., & Gadisseux, C. La reconnaissance du visage chez l'enfant normal: comparaison avec l'adulte cerebrolese. Enfance, 1980, 3, 95-106.

Bruyer, R., Laterre, C., Seron, X., Feyereisen, P., Strypstein, E., Pierrard, E., Rectem; D. A case of prosopagnosia with some preserved covert remembrance of familiar faces. Brain and Cognition, 1983, 2, 257-284.

Bruyer, R., & Stroot, C. Lateral differences in face processing: task and modality effects. Cortex, 1984, 20, 377-390.

Bruyer, R., & Velge, V. Lesions cerebrales et reconnaissance visuelle du visage humain: une etude preliminaire. Psychologica Belgica, 1980, 125-139.

Bruyer, R., & Velge, V. Lesion cerebrale unilaterale et trouble de la perception des visages: specificite du deficit? Acta Neurologica Belgica, 1981, 81, 321-332.

Buffery, A. W. H. Asymmetrical lateralization of cerebral functions and the effects of unilateral brain surgery in epileptic patients. In S. Dimont & J. Beaumont (Eds.), Hemisphere function in the human brain. London, Elek Science, 1974.

Bull, R. C. H., Green, J. The relationship between appearance and criminality. Medical Science Law, 1980, 20, 79-83.

Bullock, M. & Russell, J. A. Preschool children's interpretation of facial expressions of emotion. International Journal of Behavioral Development, 1984, 7, 193-214.

Bushnell, I. W. R. Discrimination of faces by young infants. Journal of Experiment Child Psychology, 1982, 33, 298-308.

Butters, N. Alcoholic Korsakoff's Syndrome: Some unresolved issues concerning etiology, neuropathology and cognitive deficits. Journal of Clinical and Experimental Neuropsychology, 1985, 7 (2), 181-210.

Cacioppo, J. T., & Petty, R. E. The need for cognition. Journal of Personality and Social Psychology, 1982, 42, 116-131.

Calis, G. J. J. Concerning Gibson's 'On the Face of It': Immediate Perception and Single-Glance Face Recognition. Acta Psychologica, 1984, 55, 195-214.

Calis, G. J. J., & Leeuwenberg, E. L. M. Grounding the figure. Journal of Experimental Psychology, HPP, 1981, 7, 1386-1397.

Calis, G. J. J. J., Sterenborg, J., & Maarse, F. Initial microgenetic steps in single-glance face recognition. Acta Psychologica, 1984, 55, 215-230.

Capgras, J., & Reboul Lachaux, J. L'illusion des "sosies" dans un delire systematique chronique. Bull. Soc. Clin. Med. Ment., 1923, II, 6-16.

Carey, S. The development of face perception. In G. M. Davies, H. D. Ellis & J. Shepherd (Eds.), Perceiving and remembering faces. London: Academic Press, 1981.

Carey, S., & Diamond, R. From piecemeal to configurational representation of faces. Science, 1977, 195, 312-314.

Carey, S., Diamond, R., & Woods, B. Development of face recognition - a maturational component? Developmental Psychology, 1980, 16, 257-269.

Carlson, C. R., Gantz, F. P., & Masters, J. C. Adults' emotional states and recognition of emotion in young children. Motivation and Emotion, 1983, 7, 81-101.

Carrillo, M. Contexts et Amnesia. Unpublished thesis material, University of Grenoble, 1985.

Cavanaugh, J. P. Holographic and trace strength models of rehearsal effects in the item recognition task. Memory and Cognition, 1976, 4, 186-199.

Chance, J. E., & Goldstein, A. G. Recognition of faces and verbal labels. Bulletin of the Psychonomic Society, 1976, 7, 384-386.

Chance, J. E., & Goldstein, A. G. Reliability of face recognition performance. Bulletin of the Psychonomic Society, 1979, 14, 115-117.

464

Chance, J. E., & Goldstein, A. G.   Depth of processing in response to own-
and other-race races.   Personality and Social Psychology Bulletin, 1981,
7, 475-480.

Chance, J., Goldstein, A. G., & McBride, L.   Differential experience and
recognition memory for faces.   Journal of Social Psychology, 1975, 97,
343-253.

Charcot, J. M.   Un cas de suppression brusque et isole de la vision mentale
des signes et des objects (formes et couleurs).   Progr Med, 11, 568, 1883.

Chave, F.   Contexte Prosodique et contexte semantique dans la
reconnaissance de visages non familiers.   Unpublished thesis material,
University of Grenoble, 1982.

Christen, L., Davidoff, J., Landis, T., & Regard, M.   Opposite hemifield
advantage for "face" and "nonsense face" decisions.   Communication,
International Neuropsychological Society meeting, Copenhagen, 1985.

Christen, L., & Landis, T.   Prosopagnosia.   A model for alternative
processing of the left hemisphere.   Second European Workshop on Cognitive
Neuropsychology.   Bressanone, Jan. 1984.

Christen, L., Landis, T., & Regard, M.   Left hemispheric functional
compensation in prosopagnosia - A tachistoscopic study with unilaterally
lesioned patients.   Human Neurobiology, 1985, 4, 9-14.

Christie, D. F. M., Davies, G. M., Shepherd, J. W., & Ellis, H. D.
Evaluating a new computer-based system for face recall.   Law and Human
Behavior, 1981, 5, 209-218.

Christie, D. F. M., & Ellis, H. D.   Photofit constructions versus verbal
descriptions of faces.   Journal of Applied Psychology, 1981, 66, 358-363.

Christodoulou, G. N.   The syndrome of Capgras.   British Journal of
Psychiatry, 1977, 130, 556-564.

Church, V. E.   Comparison of the Unique and Common Processing Hypotheses in
Picture and Word Memory.   Dissertation Abstracts Internation, 44, 3221B.
(University Microfilms No. ADG83-28054, 300 North Zeeb Road, Ann Arbor,
Michigan), 1984.

Clarke, R., & Morton, J.   Cross modality facilitation in tachistoscopic word
recognition.   Quarterly Journal of Experimental Psychology, 1983, 35A,
79-96.

Clark, H. H., & Carlson, T. B.   Context for comprehension.   In J. Long & A.
Baddeley (Eds), Attention and Performance IX.   Hillsdale NJ: Erlbaum
Associates, 1981.

Clark, M. S., Milberg, S., & Ross, J.   Arousal cues, arousal-related
material in memory :   implications for understanding effects of mood on
memory.   Journal of Verbal Learning and Verbal Behavior, 1983, 22,
633-649.

Clifford, B. R.   Police as eyewitnesses.   New Society,   April 22, 1976, pp.176-177.

Clifford, B. R., & Richards, V. J.   Comparison of recall by policemen and civilians under conditions of long and short duration of exposure. Perceptual and Motor Skills, 1977, 45, 503-512.

Cohen, G.   Theoretical Interpretations of Lateral Symmetries.   In Divided Visual Field Studies of Cerebral Organisation, J. G. Beaumond (Ed.), London: Academic Press, 1982.

Cohen, J.   Statistical power analysis for the behavioral sciences, (revised ed). New York: Academic Press, 1977.

Cohen, L. B., Deloache, J. S., & Pearl, R. A.   An examination of interference effects in infants' memory for faces.   Child Development, 1977, 48, 88-96.

Cohen, M. E., & Nodine, C. F.   Memory processes in facial recognition and recall.   Bulletin of the Psychonomic Society, 1978, 12, 317-319.

Cohn, R., Neumann, M. A., & Wood, D. J.   Prosopagnosia: A clinicopathological study.   Annals of Neurology, 1977, 1, 177-182.

Cole, M., Perez-Cruet, J. Prosopagnosia. Neuropsychologia, 1964, 2, 237-246.

Coles, M. G. H., Gratton, G., Bashore, T. R., Eriksen, C. W., & Donchin, E. A psychophysiological investigation of the continuous flow model of human information processing.   Journal of Experimental Psychology: Human Perception and Performance, 1985, , 529-533.

Collins, A. M., & Loftus, E. F.   A spreading-activation theory of semantic memory. Psychological Review, 1975, 82, 407-428.

Consoli, S.   Les sosies de Claire.   Topique, 1975, 16, 81-114.

Cook, S. W.   Motives in a conceptual analysis of attitude-related behavior. In W. J. Arnold, D. Levine, (eds),   Nebraska Symposium on Motivation, 1969 Lincoln, NE: University of Nebraska Press, 1970.

Corteen, R. S., & Wood, B.   Autonomic responses to shock-associated words in an unattended channel.   Journal of Experimental Psychology, 1972, 94, 308-313.

Courtois, M. R., & Mueller, J. H.   Processing multiple physical features in facial recognition. Bulletin of the Psychonomic Society, 1979, 14, 74-76.

Courtois, M. R., & Mueller, J. H.   Target and distractor typicality in face recognition. Journal of Applied Psychology, 1981, 66, 639-645.

Coyle, J. T., Price, D. L., & De Long, M. R.   Alzheimer's disease : A disorder of cortical cholinergic innervation.   Science, 1983, 2, 1184-1190.

Craik, F. I. M., & Lockhart, R. S.   Levels of processing: A framework for memory research. Journal of Verbal Learning and Verbal Behavior, 1972, 11, 671-684.

Craik, F. I. M., & Watkins, M. J. The role of rehearsal in short-term memory. Journal of Verbal Learning and Verbal Behavior, 1973, 12, 599-607.

Crick, F. H. Thinking about the Brain. Scientific American, 1979, 181.

Critchley, M. The Divine Banquet of the Brain. Raven Press, NY, 1979.

Cross, J. F., Cross, J., & Daly, J. Sex, race, age, and beauty as factors in recognition of faces. Perception and Psychophysics, 1971, 10, 393-396.

Damasio, A. R. Disorders of complex visual processing: agnosias, achromatopsia, balint syndrome and related difficulties of orientation and construction. In: M. M. Mesulam (Ed.), Principles of Behavioral Neurology, pp.259-288.

Damasio, A. R. Prosopagnosia. Trends in Neurosciences, 1985, 8, 132-135.

Damasio, A. R., Damasio, H., & Van Hoesen, G. W. Prosopagnosia: Anatomical basis and behavioral mechanisms. Neurology, 1982, 32, 331-41.

Damasio, A. R., Eslinger, P. J., Damasio, H., Van Hoesen, C. W., & Cornell, S. Multimodal Amnesic Syndrome Following Bilateral Temporal and Basal Forebrain Damage: The Case of Patient DRB. Archives of Neurology, 1985, 42, 252-259.

Damasio, A. R., Lima, P. A., & Damasio, H. Nervous function after right hemispherectomy. Neurology, 1975, 25, 89-93.

Dannenbring, G. L., & Briand, K. Semantic priming and the word repetition effect in a lexical decision task. Canadian Journal of Psychology, 1982, 36, 435-444.

Davidoff, J. B. Studies with Non-Verbal Stimuli. In: J. G. Beaumont (Ed.), Divided Visual Field Studies of Cerebral Organisation. London: Academic Press, 1982.

Davidoff, J. Specificity of face processing: the neuropsychological evidence. In: F. Denes, C. Semenza, P., Bisiacchi and E. Andreesky (Eds), Perceptives in Cognitive Neuropsychology. Hillsdale, New Jersey: Lawrence Erlbaum Associates, 1986.

Davidoff, J. B. Specificity of brain processes for face perception in normals. In: R. Bruyer (Ed.) The Neuropsychology of Face Perception and Facial Expression. Hillsdale, New Jersey: Lawrence Erlbaum Associates, 1986.

Davies, G. M. Face recognition: Issues and theories. In: M. M. Gruneberg, P. E. Morris & R. V. Sykes (Eds.), Practical Aspects of Memory. New York: Academic Press, 1978.

Davies, G. M. Face recall systems. In G. M. Davies, H. D. Ellis and J. W. Shepherd (Eds.), Perceiving and remembering faces. London: Academic Press, 1981.

Davies, G. M. Forensic face recall. In B. R. Clifford and S. Lloyd-Bostock (Eds), Evaluating witness evidence. Chichester: Wiley, 1983.

Davies, G. M. The recognition of persons from drawings and photographs. Human Learning, 1983, 2, 237-249.

Davies, G. M. Training skills in police Photofit operators. Manuscript submitted for publication, 1985.

Davies, G. M. Capturing likeness in police composites: The police artist and his rivals. Manuscript submitted for publication, 1985.

Davies, G., Ellis, H., & Shepherd, J. (Eds), Perceiving and Remembering Faces. London: Academic Press, 1981.

Davies, G. M., Ellis, H. D., & Shepherd, J. W. Cue saliency in faces assessed by the Photo-fit technique. Perception, 1977, 6, 263-269.

Davies, G. M., Ellis, H. D., & Shepherd, J. W. Face identification: The influence of delay upon accuracy of Photofit construction. Journal of Police Science and Administration, 1978, 6, 35-42.

Davies, G. M., Ellis, H. D., & Shepherd, J. W. Face recognition accuracy as a function of mode of representation. Journal of Applied Psychology, 1978, 63, 180-187.

Davies, G., & Milne, A. Recognizing faces in and out of context. Current Psychological Research, 1982, 2, 235-246.

Davies, G. M., & Milne, A. D. Eyewitness composite production: A function of mental or physical reinstatement of context. Criminal Justice and Behavior, 1985, 12, 209-220.

Davies, G. M., Shepherd, J. W., & Ellis, H. D. Similarity effects in face recognition. American Journal of Psychology, 1979, 92, 507-523.

Davies, G. M., Shepherd, J. W., & Ellis, H. D. Effects of interpolated mugshot exposure on accuracy of eyewitness identification. Journal of Applied Psychology, 1979, 64, 232-237.

Deffenbacher, K. A., Carr, T. H., & Leu, J. R. Memory for words, pictures and faces: retroactive interference, forgetting and reminiscence. Journal of Experimental Psychology : Human Learning and Memory, 1981, 7, 299-305.

Deffenbacher, K., & Horney, J. Psycho-legal aspects of face identification. In: G. Davies, H. Ellis and J. Shepherd (Eds.), Perceiving and Remembering Faces. London: Academic Press, 1981.

de Groot, A. M. B. Primed lexical decision: combined effects of the proportion of related prime-target pairs and the stimulus-onset asynchrony of prime and target. Quarterly Journal of Experimental Psychology, 1984, 36A, 253-280.

Delis, D. C., Kramer, J., Kaplan, E., & Ober, B. A. California Verbal Learning Test. Martinez, CA: Life Science Associates, 1983.

Dennett, D. C.   Content and consciousness.   London: Routledge Kegan Paul, 1969.

Dennis-Staton, R., Brumback, R. A., & Wilson, H.   Reduplicative paramnesia: a disconnection syndrome of memory.   Cortex, 1982, 18, 23-26.

De Renzi, E., Faglioni, P., & Spinnler, H.   The performance of patients with unilateral brain damage on face recognition tasks.   Cortex, 1968, 4, 17-34.

De Renzi, E., Scotti, G., & Spinnler, H.   Perceptual and associative disorders of visual recognition. Relationship to the side of the cerebral lesion.   Neurology, 1969, 19, 634-642.

De Renzi, E., & Spinnler, H.   Facial recognition in brain-damaged patients.   Neurology, 1966, 16, 145-152.

De Renzi, E., & Spinnler, H.   Visual recognition in patients with unilateral cerebral disease.   Journal of Nervous and Mental Disease, 1966, 142, 513-525.

Desimone, R., Albright, T. D., Gross, C. G., & Bruce, C.   Selective properties of inferior temporal neurons in the macaque.   Journal of Neuroscience, 1984, 4, 2051-2068.

De Valois, R. L., & De Valois, K. K.   Spatial vision.   Annual Review of Psychology, 1980, 31, 117-153.

Devine, P. G., & Malpass, R. S.   Orienting strategies in differential face recognition. Personality and Social Psychology Bulletin,, 1985, 11, 33-40.

Devlin, Rt. Hon. Lord.   Report to the Secretary of State for the Home Department of the Departmental Committee on Evidence of Identification in Criminal Cases.   Her Majesty's Station Office, London, 1976.

Diamond, R., & Carey, S.   Developmental changes in the representation of faces.   Journal of Experimental Child Psychology, 1977, 23, 1-22.

Dion, K., Berscheid, E., & Walster, E.   What is beautiful is good.   Journal of Personality & Social Psychology, 1972, 24, 285-90.

Dixon, N. F.   Preconscious processing.   London: J. Wiley, 1981.

Dolinsky, R., & Zabrucky, K.   Effects of environmental context changes on memory.   Bulletin of the Psychonomic Society, 1983, 21, 423-426.

Donaldson, W.   Context and repetition effect in recognition memory.   Memory & Cognition, 1981, 9, 308-316.

Ducci, L.   Reaction times in the recognition of facial expressions of emotion.   Italian Journal of Psychology, 1981, 8, 183-193.

Duda, P. D., & Brown, J.   Lateral asymmetry of positive and negative emotions.   Cortex, 1984, 20, 253-261.

Duda, R. O., & Hart, P. E.   Pattern Classification and Scene Analysis.   New York: Wiley, 1973.

Dukes, W. F., & Bevan, W.   Stimulus variation and repetition in the acquisition of naming responses.   Journal of Experimental Psychology, 1967, 74, 178-181.

Dunbar, K. & MacLeod, C. M.   A horse race of a different color: Stroop interference patterns with transformed words.   Journal of Experimental Psychology : Human Perception and Performance, 1984, 10, 622-639.

Ebmeier, K. P., Besson, J. A. O., Crawford, J. R., Palin, A. N., Gemmell, H. G., Sharp, P. F., Cherryman, G. R., & Smith, F. W.   Regional T1 changes in white matter on NMR and regional cerebral blood flow in dementia.   Paper presented at the 2nd Congress of the European Society of Magnetic Resonnance in Medicine, Montreaux, 1985.

Efran, L.   The effect of physical appearance on the judgement of guilt, interpersonal attraction, and severity of recommended punishment in a simulated jury task.   Journal of Research in Personality, 1974, 8, 45-54.

Eich, J. M.   Levels of Processing, Encoding Specificity, Elaboration and CHARM. Psychological Review, 1985, 92, 1-38.

Eich, M. A.   A composite holographic associative recall model. Psychological Review, 1982, 89, 627-661.

Ekman, P. (Ed.)   Emotion in the Human Face. 2nd edition. Cambridge/Paris: Cambridge University Press/Maison des Sciences de l'Homme, 1982.

Ekman, P., & Friesen, W. V.   Constants across cultures in the face and emotion. Journal of Personal and Social Psychology, 1971, 17, 124-129.

Ekman, P. & Friesen, W. V.   Unmasking the Face.   Englewood Cliffs, NJ: Prentice Hall, 1975.

Ekman, P., & Friesen, W. V.   Measuring facial movement. Environmental Psychology and Nonverbal Behaviour, 1976, 1, 56-75.

Ekman, P., Friesen, M. V., & Ellsworth, P.   Emotion in the human face.   New York: Pergamon Press, 1972.

Elliott, E. S., Wills, E. J., & Goldstein, A. G.   The effects of discrimination training on the recognition of white and Oriental faces. Bulletin of the Psychonomic Society, 1973, 2, 71-73.

Ellis, A. W., Young, A. W., & Hay, D. C.   Modelling the recognition of faces and words.   In: P. E. Morris (Ed.),   Models of cognition.   London: Wiley (in press).

Ellis, H. D.   Recognizing faces.   British Journal of Psychology, 1975, 66, 409-426.

Ellis, H.   Theoretical aspects of face recognition.   In G. Davies, H. Ellis and J. Shepherd (Eds.),   Perceiving and Remembering Faces.   London: Academic Press.

Ellis, H. D. The role of the right hemisphere in face perception. In A. Young, (Ed.), Functions of the right hemisphere. London: Academic Press, 1983.

Ellis, H. D. Practical aspects of face memory. In G. L. Wells & E. F. Loftus (Eds.), Eyewitness testimony: Psychological perspectives. (pp.12-37). New York: Cambridge University Press, 1984.

Ellis, H. D. Processes underlying face recognition. In: R. Bruyer (Ed.). The neuropsychology of face perception and facial expression. New Jersey: Lawrence Erlbaum, (in press).

Ellis, H. D. Disorders of face recognition. In: K. Poeck (Ed.). Neurology: Proceedings of the 13th world congress on neurology. Springer-Verlag (in press).

Ellis, H. D., Davies, G. M., & Shepherd, J. W. Experimental studies of face identification. National Journal of Criminal Defence, 1977, 3, 219-234.

Ellis, H. D., Davies, G. M., & Shepherd, J. W. A critical examination of the Photofit system for recalling faces. Ergonomics, 1978, 21, 297-307.

Ellis, H. D., & Deregowski, J. B. Within-race and between-race recognition of transformed and untransformed faces. American Journal of Psychology, 1981, 94, 27-35.

Ellis, H. D., & Shepherd, J. Recognition of upright and inverted faces presented in the left and right visual fields. Cortex, 1975, 11, 3-7.

Ellis, H. D., Shepherd, J. W., & Davies, G. M. An investigation of the use of the Photofit technique for recalling faces. British Journal of Psychology, 1975, 66, 29-37.

Ellis, H. D., Shepherd, J. W., & Davies, G. M. Identification of familiar and unfamiliar faces from internal and external features: some implications for theories of face recognition. Perception, 1979, 8, 431-439.

Ellis, H. D., Shepherd, J. W., & Davies, G. M. The deterioration of verbal descriptions of faces over different delay intervals. Journal of Police Science and Administration, 1980, 8, 101-106.

Endo, M. Cue saliency in upside down faces. Tohoku Psychologica Folia, 1982, 4, 116-122.

Endo, M. Cue saliency in briefly presented faces: A comparison with cue saliency in upside down faces. Tohoku psychologica Folia, 1983, 4, 85-91.

Endo, M., Takahashi, K., & Maruyama, K. The effects of observer's attitude on the familiarity of faces: using the difference in cue value between central and peripheral facial elements as an index of familiarity. Tohoku Psychologica Folia, 1984, 43, 23-34.

Enlow, D. H. Handbook of facial growth. (Second Edition). Philadelphia: W. B. Saunders, 1982.

Erdelyi, M. H.   A new look at the New Look: Perceptual defense and vigilance. Psychological Review, 1974, 81, 1-25.

Eslinger, P. J., & Benton, A. L.   Visuo-perceptual performances in aging and dementia: clinical and theoretical implications.   Journal of Clinical Neuropsychology, 1983, 5, 213-220.

Etcoff, N. L.   Selective attention to facial identity and facial emotion. Neuropsychologia, 1984, 22, 281-294.

Ettlinger, G.   Sensory deficits in visual agnosia.   Journal of Neurology, Neurosurgery, and Psychiatry, 1956, 19, 297-308.

Eysenck, M. W.   Age differences in incidental learning.   Developmental Psychology, 1974, 10, 936-941.

Fagan, J. F.   Infants' recognition for faces.   Journal of Experimental Child Psychology, 1972, 14, 453-476.

Fagan, J. F.   Recognition memory and forgetting.   Journal of Experimental Child Psychology, 1973, 16, 424-450.

Fagan, J. F.   Infants' recognition of invariant features of faces.   Child Development, 1976, 47, 627-638.

Fagan, J. F.   Infant recognition memory : Studies in forgetting.   Child Development, 1977, 48, 68-78.

Fairweather, H., Brizzolara, D., Tabossi, P., & Umilta, C.   Functional cerebral lateralisation: dichotomy or plurality?   Cortex, 1982, 18, 51-66.

Farah, M. J.   The neurological basis of mental imagery: A componential analysis.   Cognition, 1984, 18, 245-272.

Faust, C.   Die zerebralen Herdstoerungen bei Hinterhauptverletzungen und ihre Beurteilung.   Stuttgart:Thieme, 1955.

Feingold, G. A.   The influence of environment on identification of persons and things.   Journal of Criminal Law and Police Science, 1914, 5, 49-51.

Feinman, S., Entwisle, D. R.   Children's ability to recognize other children's faces.   Child Development, 1976, 47, 306-310.

Felleman, E. S., Barden, R. C., Carlson, C. R., Rosenberg, L., & Masters, J. C.   Children's and adults' recognition of spontaneous and posed emotional expressions in young children.   Developmental Psychology, 1983, 19, 405-413.

Feltz, D. L., & Landers, D. M.   The effects of mental practice on motor skill learning and performance: A meta-analysis.   Journal of Sport Psychology, 1983, 5, 25-57.

Feyereisen, P. Production and comprehension of emotional facial expressions in brain-damaged subjects. In: R. Bruyer (Ed.). The Neuropsychology of Face Perception and Facial Expression. Hillsdale, NJ: Lawrence Erlbaum Associates, in press.

Feyereisen, P., & de Lannoy, J. D. Psychologie du Geste. Bruxelles/Liege: P. Mardaga, 1985.

Findlay, J. N. Saccadic eye movements and visual cognition. L'annee Psychologique, 1985, 85, 1010-136.

Finlay, D. C., & French, J. Visual field differences in a facial recognition task using signal detection theory. Neuropsychologia, 1978, 16, 103-107.

Fiorentini, A., Maffei, L., & Sandini, G. The role of high spatial frequencies in face perception. Perception, 1983, 12, 195-201.

Fischer, M., Koch, B. Szondi-Portrats und Alltagsmensch. Eine Untersuchung der Bilder und des Bildwahlverhaltens. Szondiana, 1985, 5, 3-108.

Fisher, G. H., & Cox, R. L. Recognizing human faces. Applied Ergonomics, 1975, 6, 104-109.

Flin, R. H. Age effects in children's memory for unfamiliar faces. Developmental Psychology, 1980, 16, 373-374.

Fodor, J. A. The Modularity of Mind. Cambridge, Mass: The MIT Press, 1983.

Forsyth, F. The Fourth Protocol, 1984.

Fowler, C. A., Wolford, G., Slade, R., & Tassinary, L. Lexical access with and without awareness. Journal of Experimental Psychology: General, 1981, 110, 341-362.

Friedman, A., & Campbell Polson, M. Hemispheres as Independent Resource Systems: Limited-Capacity Processing and Hemispheric Specialization. Journal of Experimental Psychology: Human Perception and Performance, 1981, 7, 1031-1058.

French, J. W., Ekstrom, R. B., & Price, L. A. Kit of reference tests for cognitive factors. Princeton, NJ: Educational Testing Service, 1963.

Frijda, N. H. The understanding of facial expression of emotion. Acta Psychologica, 1953, 9, 294-362.

Frijda, N. H. De betekenis van gelaatsexpressie. Amsterdam: Van Oorschot, 1956.

Frijda, N. H. Recognition of emotion. In: L. Berkowitz (Ed.). Advance in Experimental Social Psychology, Vol. 4, pp.167-223. New York/London: Academic Press, 1969.

Frijda, N. H. The emotions. New York: Cambridge University Press, in press.

Frijda, N. H., & Kroon, R. M. C. Categories in face descriptions. Report Psychology Department, Amsterdam University. In preparation.

Frith, D. C. The detection of structure in visual displays. Acta Psychologica, 1976, 40, 115-125.

Frith, C. D., & Frith, U. Feature selection and classification: a developmental study. Journal of Experimental Child Psychology, 1978, 25, 413-428.

Froelich, W. D., Smith, G., Draguns, J. C., & Hentschell, U. Psychological processes in cognition and personality. Washington/London: Hemisphere McGraw-Hill, 1984.

Gaffan, D. Recognition memory in animals. In: J. Brown (Ed.), Recall and Recognition. New York, Wiley, 1976.

Galper, R. E. "Functional race membership" and recognition of faces. Perceptual and Motor Skills, 1973, 37, 455-462.

Galper, R. E., & Hochberg, J. Recognition memory for photographs of faces. American Journal of Psychology, 1971, 84, 351-359.

Gates, G. S. An experimental study of the growth of social perception. Journal of Experimental Psychology, 1923, 14, 449-461.

Gazzaniga, M. S., & Smylie, C. S. Facial recognition and brain asymmetries: clues to underlying mechanisms. Annals of Neurology, 1983, 13, 537-540.

Geffen, G., Bradshaw, J. L., & Nettleton, N. C. Attention and Hemispheric Differences in Reaction Time During Simultaneous Audiovisual Tasks. Quarterly Journal of Experimental Psychology, 1973, 25, 404-412.

Geffen, G., Bradshaw, J. L., & Wallace, G. Interhemispheric effects on reaction times to verbal and non-verbal stimuli. Journal of Experimental Psychology, 1971, 87, 415-422.

Gemmell, H. G., Sharp, P. F., Evans, N. T. S., Besson, J. A. O., Lyall, D., Smith, F. W. Single photon emission tomography in Alzheimer's disease and multi-infarct dementia. Lancet, 1984, 2, 1348.

Gertsmann, J., Problem of imperception of disease and of impaired body territories with organic lesions. Archives of Neurological Psychiatry, 1942, 8, 890-913.

Gervais, M. J., Harvey, L. O., & Roberts, J. O. Identification confusions among letters of the alphabet. Journal of Experimental Psychology: Human Perception and Performance, 1984, 10, 655-666.

Geschwind, N. Specializations of the human brain. Scientific American, 1979, 241, 180-199.

Geschwind, N., & Levitsky, W. Left-right asymmetries in the temporal speech region. Science, 1968, 161, 166.

Glaser, W. R., & Dungelhoff, F. J. The time-course of picture word interference. Journal of Experimental Psychology, 1984, 10, 640-654.

Glen, A. I. M., & Christie, J. E. Early diagnosis of Alzheimer's disease: working definitions for clinical and laboratory criteria in A. I. M. Glen and L. J. Whalley (Eds). Alzheimer's Disease, early recognition of potentially reversible deficits. Edinburgh: Churchill Livingstone, 1979.

Gibson, J. J. The ecological approach to visual perception. Boston: Houghton Mifflin, 1979.

Gilbert, C., & Bakan, P. Visual asymmetry in perception of faces. Neuropsychologia, 1973, 11, 355-362.

Gil de Diaz, M. Developpement d'une asymetrie fonctionnelle interhemispherique chez l'enfant de 4 a 12 mois: reconnaissance des visages. These de doctorat de 3eme cycle, Universite d'Aix-Marseille II, unpublished manuscript, 1983.

Gillund, G., & Shiffrin, R. M. A retrieval model for both recognition and recall. Psychological Review, 1980, 91, 1-67.

Ginsburg, A. P. Visual information processing based on spatial filters constrained by biological data. AMRL Technical Report 78-129, Ohio, 1978.

Ginsburg, A. P. Specifying relevant spatial information for image evaluation and display design: An explanation of how we see objects 1980, Proceedings of the SID, 21, 219-227.

Gloning, I., Gloning, K., Hoff, H., & Tschabitcher, H. Zur Prosopagnosie. Neuropsychologia, 1966, 4, 113-132.

Gloning, I., Gloning, K., Jellinger, K., Quatember, R. A case of "prosopagnosia" with necropsy findings. Neuropsychologia, 1970, 8, 199-204.

Godden, D., & Baddeley, A. D. When does context influence recognition memory?. British Journal of Psychology, 1980, 71, 99-104.

Goldberg, E., Costa, L. D. Hemisphere differences in the acquisition and use of descriptive systems. Brain & Language, 1981, 14, 144-173.

Goldstein, A. G. Race-related variation of facial features. Anthropometric data I. Bulletin of the Psychonomic Society, 1979, 13, 187-190.

Goldstein, A. G. Facial feature variation: Anthropometric data II. Bulletin of the Psychonomic Society, 1979, 13, 191-193.

Goldstein, A. G. Behavioral scientists' fascination with faces. Journal of Non Verbal Behavior, 1983, 7, 223-255.

Goldstein, A., & Chance, J. Measuring psychological similarity of faces. Bulletin of the Psychonomic Society, 1976, 7, 407-408.

Goldstein, A. G., & Chance, J. Memory for faces and schema theory. Paper presented at the Meetings of the Psychonomic Society, Phoenix, 1979.

Goldstein, A. G., & Chance, J.   Laboratory studies of face recognition.   In:
G. M. Davies, H. D. Ellis, and J. W. Shepherd (Eds.), Perceiving and
remembering faces. (pp.81-104). London: Academic Press, 1981.

Goldstein, A. G., & Chance, J. E.   Effects of training on Japanese face
recognition: Reduction of the other-race effect.   Bulletin of the
Psychonomic Society, 1985, 23, 211-214.

Goldstein, A. G., Chance, J. E., & Gilbert, B.   Facial stereotypes of good
guys and bad guys: A replication and extension.   Bulletin of the
Psychonomic Society, 1984, 22, 549-552.

Goldstein, A. G., Johnson, K. S., & Chance, J. E.   Does fluency of face
description imply superior face recognition?   Bulletin of the Psychonomic
Society, 1979, 13, 15-18.

Goldstein, A. G., & Mackenberg, E. J.   Recognition of human faces from
isolated facial features: A developmental study.   Psychonomic Science,
1966, , 149-150.

Goldstein, A. J., Harmon, L. D., & Lesk, A. E.   Identification of human
faces.   Proceedings of the IEEE, 1971, , 748-760.

Gombrich, E.   The mask and the face.   In E. Gombrich, J. Hochburg and M.
Black (Eds.).   Art perception and reality.   Baltimore, MD: John Hopkins
Press, 1972.

Gomori, A. J., & Hawryluk, G. A.   Visual agnosia without alexia.   Neurology,
1984, 34, 947-950.

Goodglass, H., Klein, B., Carey, P. & Jones, K.   Specific semantic word
categories in aphasia.   Cortex, 1966, 1, 74-89.

Gorea, A., Findlay, J. N., & Levy-Schoen, A.   Changing attention along the
horizontal meridian; a study of oculomotor latencies.   Paper presented at
the AVA Meeting on Eye Movements and Vision, Durham, March 1980.

Graham, F. K.   Habituation and dishabituation of responses innervated by the
autonomic nervous system.   In H. V. S. Peeke & M. J. Herz (Eds.).
Habituation: Behavioral Studies (Vol. 1).   New York: Academic Press,
1973.

Greer, K. L., Green, D. W.   Context and motor control in handwriting.   Acta
Psychologica, 1983, 54, 205-215.

Gross, C. G., Bender, D. B., & Gerstein, G. L.   Activity of inferior
temporal neurons in behaving monkeys.   Neuropsychologia, 1979, 8, 215-229.

Gross, C. G., Desimone, R., Albright, T. D., & Schwartz, E. L.   Inferior
temporal cortex as visual integration area.   In Reinoso-Suarez and
Ajmone-Marsan (Eds.).   Cortical Integration.   Raven Press, New York, 1984.

Grusser, O. J.   Face recognition within the reach of neurobiology and beyond
it.   Human Neurobiology, 1984, 3, 183-190.

Grusser, O. J., & Kirchoff, N. Face recognition and unilateral brain lesions. Communication, International Neuropsychological Society meeting, Deauville, 1982.

Haber, R. N., & Hershenson, M. The effects of repeated brief exposures on the growth of a percept. Journal of Experimental Psychology, 1965, 69, 40-46.

Hachinski, V. C., Cliff, L. D., Zilka, E., Du Boulay, G. H., McAllister, V. L., Marshall, J., Russell, R. W. R., & Symon, L. Cerebral blood flow in dementia. Archives of Neurology, 1975, 32, 632-637.

Hacker, M. J., & Ratcliff, R. A revised table of d' for M-alternative forced choice. Perception & Psychophysics, 1979, 26, 168-170.

Haig, N. D. The effect of feature displacement on face recognition. Perception, 1984, 13.

Haig, N. D. How faces differ - a new comparative technique. Perception, in press, 1985.

Hall, D. F. Obtaining eyewitness identifications in criminal investigations: Two experiments and some comments on the Zeitgeist in forensic psychology. Paper presented at the American Psychology - Law Conference, Snowmass, CO, 1977.

Hamsher, K., Levin, H. S., & Benton, A. L. Facial recognition in patients with focal brain lesions. Archives of Neurology, 1979, 36, 837-839.

Harmon, L. D. The recognition of faces. Scientific American, 1973, 227, 71-82.

Harris, G. J., & Fleer, R. E., Recognition memory for faces by retardates and normals. Perceptual and Motor Skills, 1972, 34, 755-758.

Hart, J., Berndt, R. S., & Caramazza, A. Category-specific naming deficit following cerebral infarction. Nature, 1985, 316, 439-440.

Harvey, L. O. Jr., & Sinclair, G. P. On the quality of visual imagery. Investigative Opthalmology and Visual Science, 1985, 26, 281.

Hay, D. C. Asymmetries in face processing: evidence for a right hemisphere perceptual advantage. Quarterly Journal of Experimental Psychology, 1981, 33A, 267-274.

Hay, D. C., & Young, A. W. The human face. In A. W. Ellis (Ed.), Normality and Pathology in Cognitive Functions. New York: Academic Press, 1982.

Hay, D. C., Young, A. W., & Ellis, A. W. Routes through the face recognition system. In preparation.

Hayman, M. A., & Abrams, R. Capgras Syndrome and cerebral dysfunction. British Journal of Psychiatry, 1977, 130, 68-71.

Hecaen, H., & Albert, M. Human Neuropsychology. New York: Wiley, 1978.

Hecaen, H. T., Angelergues, R. Agnosia for faces (prosopagnosia). Archives of Neurology, 1962, 7, 92-100.

Hecaen, H., Angelergues, R., Bernhardt, C., & Chiarelli, J. Essai de distinction des modalities cliniques de l'agnosie des physionomies. Revue Neurologique, 1957, 96, 125-144.

Hecaen, H., & Masure, M. C. L'agnosie des physionomies (prosopagnosie) et ses differentes varietes. In: Centenario de la Neurologia en Espana. Barcelona: Servicio de Neurologia del Hospital de la Santa Creu i Sant Paul, 517-526, 1983.

Hecaen, H., & Tzavaras, A. Etude neuropsychologique des troubles de la reconnaissance des visages humains. Bulletin de Psychologie , 1969, 22, 754-762.

Heilman, K. M., Satz, P. (Eds.). Neuropsychology of human emotion. New York: Guilford, 1983.

Heilman, K. M., Schwartz, H. D., & Watson, R. T. Hypoarousal in patients with neglect syndrome and emotional indifference. Neurology, 1978, 28, 229-232.

Hellige, J., Corwin, W., & Jonsson, J. Effects of perceptual quality on the processing of human faces presented to the left and right cerebral hemisphere. Journal of Experimental Psychology: Human Perception and Performance, 1984, 10, 90-107.

Henderson, L., & Chard, J. Semantic effects in visual word detection with visual similarity controlled. Perception and Psychophysics, 1978, 23, 290-298.

Hinton, G. E., & Anderson, J. A. Parallel Models of Associative Memory. Hillsdale, NJ: Lawrence Erlbaum Associates, 1981.

Hintzman, D. L., Stern, L. D., Contextual variability and memory for frequency. Journal of Experimental Psychology : Human Learning and Memory, 1978, 4, 539-549.

Hirschman, R. S., & Safer, M. A. Hemisphere differences in perceiving positive and negative emotions. Cortex, 1982, 18, 569-580.

Hockey, G. R. J., Davies, S., & Gray, M. M. Forgetting as a function of sleep at different times of day. Quarterly Journal of Experimental Psychology, 1972, 24, 386-393.

Hoffman, C., & Kagan, S. Field dependence and facial recognition. Perceptual and Motor Skills, 1977, 44, 119-124.

Hoffman, R. R. Context and contextualism in the psychology of learning. In: G. Tiberghien (Ed.), Context and Cognition, Cahiers de Psychologie Cognitive, in press, 1986.

Homa, G. The law enforcement composite sketch artist. West Berlin, NJ: privately printed, 1983.

Honkavaara, S. The psychology of expression. Dimensions in human perception. British Journal Psychology, Monogr. Suppl., 1961, 31, 1-96.

Horel, J. A., & Keating, E. G. Recovery from a partial Kluver-Bucy syndrome in the monkey produced by disconnection. Journal of Comparative and Physiological Psychology, 1972, 79, 105-114.

Horton, D. L., & Mills, C. B. Human learning and memory, Annual Review of Psychology, 1984, 35, 361-394.

Hosch, H. M., & Platz, S. J. Self-monitoring and eyewitness accuracy. Personality and Socialy Psychology Bulletin, 1984, 10, 289-292.'

Huaang, M., & Byrne, B. Cognitive style and lateral eye movements. British Journal of Psychology, 1978, 69, 85-90.

Hubel, D. H., & Wiesel, T. N. Receptive fields and functional architecture of monkey striate cortex. Journal of Physiology, 1968, 195, 215-243.

Hubel, D. H., & Wiesel, T. N. Brain mechanisms in vision. Scientific American, 1979, 241, 130-144.

Hulin, W. S., & Katz, D. The Frois-Wittman pictures of facial expression. Journal of Experimental Psychology, 1935, 18, 482-498.

Humphrey, N., & McManus, C. Status and the left cheek. New Scientist, 1973, 59, 437-439.

Huppert, F. A., & Piercy, M. In search of functional locus of amnesic syndromes. In L. S. Cermak (Ed.), Human Memory and Amnesia. Hillsdale, NJ: Lawrence Erlbaum Associates, 1982.

Inui, T., & Miyamoto, K. The effect of changes in visual area on facial recognition. Perception, 1984, 13, 49-56.

Izard, C. E. The face of emotion. New York: Appleton-Century-Crofts, 1971.

Jacoby, L. L., & Dallas, M. On the relationship between autobiographical memory and perceptual learning. Journal of Experimental Psychology : General, 1981, 110, 306-340.

Jacoby, L. L., & Witherspoon, D. Remembering without awareness. Canadian Journal of Psychology, 1982, 36, 300-324.

Jenkins, F. Interference to facial memory through exposure to misleading composite pictures. Unpublished doctoral dissertation, Aberdeen University, 1985.

Jenkins, F., & Davies, G. M. Contamination of facial memory through exposure to misleading composite pictures. Journal of Applied Psychology, 1985, 70, 164-176.

Jenkins, J. J. Remember that old theory of memory? Well, forget it!. American Psychologist, 1974, 29, 785-795.

Johnson, M. K. A multiple-entry, modular memory system. In G. H. Bower (Ed.), The psychology of learning and motivation: Advances in research and theory: Vol. 17, New York: Academic Press, 1983.

Johnston, W. A., Dark, V. J., & Jacoby, L. L. Perceptual fluency and recognition judgments. Journal of Experimental Psychology : Learning, Memory and Cognition, 1985, 11, 3-11.

Jones, A. C. Influence of mode of stimulus presentation on performance in racial recognition tasks. Cortex, 1969, 5, 290-301.

Jones, E. G., & Powell, T. P. S. An anatomic study of converging sensory pathways within the cerebral cortex of the monkey. Brain, 1970, 93, 793-820.

Jones, G., & Mishkin, M. Limbic lesions and the problem of stimulus-reinforcement association. Experimental Neurology, 1972, 36, 362-377.

Jones, G. V. Recognition failure and dual mechanism in recall. Psychological Review, 1978, 85, 464-469.

Jones, L. E., Hirschberg, N., Rothman, J., & Malpass, R. S. The Face Atlas: Anthropometric, Cosmetic and Physiognomic Measurements of 200 Male Faces. Technical Report No. 1, NSF GS-42801. Champaign, Illinois: Department of Psychology, University of Illinois, 1976.

Jost, A. Die Assoziationsfestigkeit in ihrer Abhangigkeit von der Verteilung der Wiederholungen. Zeitschrift fur Psychologie, 1897, 14, 436-472.

Kahneman, D. Attention and Effort. Englewood Cliffs, NJ: Prentice Hall, 1973.

Keegan, J. F. Hemispheric frequency analysis: facial recognition. Text of a communication. International Neuropsychological Society meeting, Bergen, 1981.

Keer, N. H., & Winograd, E. Effects of contextual elaboration on face recognition. Memory & Cognition, 1982, 10, 608-609.

Kellogg, R. T. Is conscious attention necessary for long-term storage? Journal of Experimental Psychology: Human Perception and Performance, 1980, 6, 379-390.

Kievit, J., & Kuypers, H. G. J. M. Basal forebrain and hypothalamic connections to frontal and parietal cortex in the rhesus monkey. Science, 1975, 187, 660-662.

Kimura, D. Right temporal lobe damage. Archives of Neurology, 1963, 8, 264-271.

Kinsbourne, M. The Mechanism of Hemispheric Control of the Lateral Gradient of Attention. In P. M. A. Rabbit, & S. Dornic (Eds.), Attention and Performance V. London: Academic Press, 1975.

Kinsbourne, M., & Warrington, E. A disorder of simultaneous form perception. Brain, 1962, 85, 461-486.

Kintsch, W. Models for free recall and recognition. In D. A. Norman (Ed), Models of human memory. New York: Academic Press, 1970.

Kiphart, M. J., Sjogren, D. D., & Cross, H. A. Some factors involved in complex-picture recognition. Bulletin of the Psychonomic Society, 1984, 22, 197-199.

Kirouac, G., & Dore, F. Y. Accuracy and latency of judgment of facial expressions of emotions. Perceptual and Motor Skills, 1983, 57, 683-686.

Kirouac, G., & Dore, F. Y. Judgement of facial expressions of emotion as a function of exposure time. Perceptual and Motor Skills, 1984, 59, 147-150.

Kitson, A., Darnbrough, M., & Shields, E. Lets face it. Police Research Bulletin, 1978, No. 30, 7-13.

Klatzky, R. L. Visual Memory: Definitions and Functions. In R. S. Wyer Jr. & T. K. Srull (Eds.). Handbook of Social Cognition, Vol. 2. Hillsdale, NJ: Erlbaum, 1984.

Klatzky, R. L., & Forrest, F. H. Recognizing familiar and unfamiliar faces. Memory & Cognition, 1984, 12, 60-70.

Klatzky, R. L., Martin, G. L., & Kane, R. A. Influence of social-category activation on processing of visual information. Social Cognition, 1982, 1, 95-109.

Klatzky, R. L., Martin, G. L., & Kane, R. A. Semantic interpretation effects on memory for faces. Memory and Cognition, 1982, 10, 195-206.

Klee, M., Leseaux, M., Malai, C., & Tibergien, G. Nouveaux effets de contexte dans la reconnaissance de visages non familiers. Revue de Psychologie Appliquee, 1982, 32, 109-119.

Kluver, H., & Bucy, P. C. Preliminary analysis of functions of the temporal lobes in monkeys. Archives of Neurology, 1939, 42, 979-1000.

Kohonen, T., Oja, E., & Lehtio, P. Storage and processing of information in distributed associative memory systems. In G. E. Hinton & J. A. Anderson (Eds.), Parallel Models of Associative Memory. Hillsdale, NJ: Lawrence Erlbaum Associates, 1981.

Kolb, B., Milner, B., & Taylor, L. Perception of faces by patients with localized cortical excisions. Canadian Journal of Psychology, 1983, 37, 8-18.

Kolers, P. A. Remembering operations. Memory & Cognition, 1973, 1, 347-355.

Konorski, J. Integrative activity of the brain. An interdisciplinary approach. University of Chicago Press, Chicago, 1968.

Kunst-Wilson, W. R., & Zajonc, R. B. *Affective discrimination of stimuli that cannot be recognized. Science, 1980, 207, 557-558.*

Kurucz, J., & Feldmar, G. *Prosopo-affective agnosia as a symptom of cerebral organic disease. Journal of the American Geriatrics Society, 1979, 27, 225-230.*

Kurucz, J., Feldmar, G., & Werner, W. *Prosopo-affective agnosia associated with chronic organic brain syndrome. Journal of the American Geriatrics Society, 1979, Vol. 27, 2, 91-95.*

Ladavas, E., Umilta, C., & Ricci-Bitti, P. E. *Evidence for sex differences in right-hemisphere dominance for emotions. Neuropsychologia, 1980, 18, 361-366.*

Landis, T., Assal, G., & Perret, E. *Opposite cerebral hemispheric superiorities for visual associative processing of emotional facial expressions and objects. Nature, 1979, 278, 739-740.*

Landis, T., Christen, L., & Cummings, J. *Prosopagnosia and associated symptoms in unilateral right posterior lesions: clinical and radiological findings in five patients. Second European Workshop on Cognitive Neuropsychology. Bressanone, Jan., 1984.*

Landis, T., Cummings, J. L., Christen, L., Bogen, J., & Imhof, H. G. *Are unilateral right posterior cerebral lesions sufficient to cause prosopagnosia? Clinical and radiological findings in six additional patients. Cortex, 1985, in press.*

Langdell, T. *Recognition of faces: An approach to the study of autism. Journal of Child Psychology and Psychiatry, 1978, 19, 255-268.*

LAPD. *Revised field interview. Training Bulletin, 1974, 6, Issue 9.*

Lasky, R. E., & Spiro, D. *The processing of tachistoscopically presented visual stimuli by 5-month-old infants. Child Development, 5, 1292-1294.*

Laughery, K. R., Alexander, J. F., & Lane, A. B. *Recognition of human faces: Effects of target exposure time, target position, pose position, and type of photograph. Journal of Applied Psychology, 1971, 55, 477-483.*

Laughery, K. R., Duval, G. C., & Folwer, R. H. *An analysis of procedures for generating facial images. Mug File Project (Report Number UHMUG-2). University of Houston, 1977.*

Laughery, K. R., & Fowler, R. H. *Sketch artist and Identikit procedures for recalling faces. Journal of Applied Psychology, 1980, 65, 307-316.*

Laughery, K. R., Rhodes, B., & Batten, G. *Computer-guided recognition and retrieval of facial images. In: G. M. Davies, H. D. Ellis & J. W. Shepherd (Eds), Perceiving and remembering faces. London, Academic Press, 1981.*

Laughery, K. R., & Smith, V. I. *Suspect identification following exposure to sketches and Identikit composites. Proceedings of the Human Factors Society 22nd Annual Meeting, Detroit, 1978.*

Lautrey, J. Diversite comportementale et developpement cognitif. psychologie Francaise, 1984, 29, 16-22.

Lavrakas, P. J., Buri, J. R., & Mayzner, M. S. A perspective on the recognition of other-race faces. Perception and Psychophysics, 1976, 20, 475-481.

Lawson, N. C. Inverted writing in right- and left-handers in relation to lateralization of face recognition. Cortex, 1978, 14, 207-211.

Lazarus, R. S. On the primacy of cognition. American Psychologist, 1984, 39, 124-129.

Lazarus, R. S., & McCleary, R. A. Autonomic discrimination without awareness: A study of subception. Psychological Review, 1951, 58, 113-122.

Lecocq, P., Tiberghien, G. Memoire et Decision, Lille, Presses Universitaires de Lille, 1981.

LeDoux, J. E., Wilson, D. H., & Gazzaniga, M. S. A divided mind: observations on the conscious properties of the separated hemispheres. Annals of Neurology, 1977, 2, 417-421.

Leehey, S. Face recognition in children: Evidence for the development of right hemisphere specialization. Ph.D Dissertation, Department of Psychology, Massachusetts Institute of Technology.

Leehey, S. C., Carey, S., Diamond, R., & Cahn, A. Upright and inverted faces: the right hemisphere knows the difference. Cortex, 1978,14, 411-419.

Leeuwenberg, E., Mens, L., & Calis, G. Knowledge within perception: Masking caused by incompatible interpretations. Acta Psychologica, 1985, 59, 91-102.

Leight, K. A., Ellis, H. C. Emotional mood states, strategies, and state-dependency in memory. Journal of Verbal Learning and Verbal Behavior, 1981, 20, 251-266.

Lenorovitz, D. R., & Laughery, K. R. A witness-computer interaction system for searching mug-files. In: G. L. Wells & E. F. Loftus, Eyewitness testimony. Cambridge, Cambridge University Press, 1979.

Leonard, C. M. Ross, E. T., Wilson, F. A. W., & Baylis, G. C. Neurones in the amygdala of the monkey with responses selective for faces. Behavioural Brain Research, 1985, in press.

Levin, H. S., Hamsher, K., & Benton, A. L. A short form of the test of facial recognition for clinical use. Journal of Psychology, 1975, 91, 223-228.

Levine, D. N. Prosopagnosia and visual object agnosia: a behavioral study. Brain and Language, 1978, 5, 341-365.

Levy, J., Trevarthen, C., & Sperry, R. W. Perception of bilateral chimeric figures following hemispheric disconnection. Brain, 1972, 95, 61-78.

Ley, R. G., & Bryden, M. P.   Hemispheric differences in processing emotions and faces. Brain and Language, 1979, 7, 127-138.

Lezak, M. D.   Neuropsychological assessment.   2nd Edition.   Oxford University Press, 1983.

Lhermitte, F., Chain, F., Escourolle, R., Ducarne, B., Pillon, B.   Etude anatomo-clinique d'un cas de prosopagnosie.   Revue Neurologique, 126, 329-346.

Lhermitte, F. Chedru, F., Chain, F.   A propos d'un cas d'agnosie visuelle, 19.   Revue Neurologique, 1973, 128, 301-322.

Lhermitte, F., & Pillon, B.   La prosopagnosie.   Role de l'hemisphere droit dans la perception visuelle.   (A propos d'un cas consecutif a une lobectomie occipitale droite).   Revue Neurologique, 1975, 131, 791-812.

Lieury, A.   La memoire episodique est-elle emboitee dans la memoire semantique? L'Annee Psychologique, 1979, 79, 123-142.

Light, L. L., Kayra-Stuart, F., & Hollander, S.   Recognition memory for typical and unusual faces.   Journal of Experimental Psychology: Human Learning and Memory, 1979, 5, 212-228.

Lindeman, R. H., Merenda, P. F., & Gold, R. B. Introduction to Bivaviate and Multivariate Analysis. Glenview, Illinois: Scott, Foresman & Co., 1980.

Lindsay, R. C. L., & Wells, G. L.   What do we really know about cross-race eyewitness identification? In S. M. A. Lloyd-Bostock, B. R. Clifford (Eds.).   Evaluating witness evidence: Recent psychological research and new perspectives (pp.219-234). New York: Wiley, 1983.

Linville, P. W.   The complexity-extremity effect and age-based stereotyping.   Journal of Personality and Social Psychology, 1982, 42, 193-211.

Lipps, T. Das Wissen von fremden Ichen. Psychol. Untersuchungen, Vol. 1, 1907.

Lissauer, H.   Ein Fall von Seelenblindheit nebst conem Beitrage zur Theorie derselben.   Archiv Psychiatrie, 1889, 21, 222-270.

Liston, E. H., & La Rue, A.   Clinical differentiation of primary degenerative and multi-infarct dementia : A critical review of the evidence.   Part 1 : clinical studies.   Biological Psychiatry, 1983, 18, 1451-1465.

Loftus, E. F.   Leading questions and the eyewitness report.   Cognitive Psychology, 1975, 7, 560-572.

Loftus, E. F.   Eyewitness testimony.   Cambridge, MA: Harvard University Press, 1979.

Loftus, G. R.   Evaluating forgetting curves.   Journal of Experimental Psychology: Learning, Memory, and Cognition, 1985, 11, 397-406.

Lorsbach, T. C., & Mueller, J. H.   Encoding tasks and free recall in children. Bulletin of the Psychonomic Society, 1979, 14, 169-172.

Luaute, J., Bidault, E., & Thionville, M. Syndrome de Capgras et organicite cerebrale. Annales Medico-Psychologiques, 1978, 5, 803-815.

Luaute J. P., Bidault, E., Zampa, P., Forray, J. P. A propos d'une variete de fausse reconnaissance avec illusion de sosie. Annales Medico-Psychologiques, 1982, 4, 461-465.

Luce, T. S. Blacks, whites, and yellows: They all look alike to me. Psychology Today, 1974, 8(11), 105-108.

Luria, A. R. Disorders of "simultaneous perception" in a case of bilateral occipitoparietal brain injury. Brain, 1959, 83, 437-449.

Luria, A. R. The Working Brain. Harmondsworth: Penguin Books, 1973.

Luria, A. R. Les fonctions corticales superieures de l'homme. Paris : P.U.F., 1978.

Lykken, D. T. The GSR in the detection of guilt. Journal of Applied Psychology, 1959, 43, 385-388.

Lykken, D. T. Psychology and the lie detector industry. American Psychologist, 1974, 29, 725-738.

Lykken, D. T. The detection of deception. Psychological Bulletin, 1979, 86, 47-53.

Lynch, J. C. The functional organization of the posterior parietal association cortex. Behavioral and Brain Sciences, 1980, 3, 485-534.

Maccoby, E. E., & Jacklin, C. N. The Psychology of Sex Differences. Standford, California: Stanford University Press, 1974.

Macrae, D., & Trolle, E. The defect of function in visual agnosia. Brain, 1956, 79, 94-110.

Mair, W. G. P., Warrington, E. K., & Weiskrantz, L. Memory disorder in Korsakoff psychosis. A neuropathological and neuropsychological investigation. Brain, 1979, 102, 749-783.

Malmi, R. A. Context effects in recognition memory. Memory & Cognition, 1977, 5, 123-130.

Malone, D. R., Morris, H. H., Kay, M. C., & Levin, H. Prosopagnosia: a double dissociation between the recognition of familiar and unfamiliar faces. Journal of Neurology, Neurosurgery and Psychiatry, 1982, 45, 820-822.

Malpass, R. S. Towards a theorical basis for understanding differential face recognition. In: J. Chance, Faces: How do we perceive and remember them? Symposium conducted at the meeting of the Midwestern Psychological Association, Chicago, 1975.

Malpass, R. S. Training in face recognition. In: G. Davies, H. Ellis, & J. Shepherd (Eds.). Perceiving and remembering faces, (pp.271-285). London: Academic Press, 1981.

Malpass, R. S. *Effective size and defendant bias in eyewitness identification lineups.* Law and Human Behavior, 1981, 5, 299-309.

Malpass, R. S., & Kravitz, J. *Recognition for faces of own- and other-race.* Journal of Personality and Social Psychology, 1969, 13, 330-334.

Malpass, R. S., Lavigueur, H., & Weldon, D. E. *Verbal and visual training in face recognition.* Perception and Psychophysics, 14, 285-292, 1973.

Maltzman, I. *Orienting in classical conditioning and generalization of the galvanic skin response to words: An overview.* Journal of Experimental Psychology: General, 1977, 106, 111-119.

Mandler, G. *Organization and Recognition.* In: E. Tulving & W. Donaldson (Eds.), New York, Academic Press, 1972.

Mandler, G. *Mind and Emotion.* New York: John Wiley, 1975.

Mandler, G. *Memory research reconsidered : a critical view of traditional methods and distinctions,* CHIP 64, San Diego, Center for Human Information Processing, 1976.

Mandler, G. *Recognizing : the judgment of previous occurrence.* Psychological Review, 190, 87, 252-271.

Mandler, J. M., & Parker, R. E. *Memory for Descriptive and Spatial Information in Complex Pictures.* Journal of Experimental Psychology: Human Learning and Memory, 1976, 2, 38-48.

Manson, V. Brathwaite, 432, US 98, 1977.

Marr, D. *Vision.* San Francisco: W. H. Freeman and Company, 1982.

Marr, D., & Nishihara, H. K. *Representation and recognition of the spatial organization of three-dimensional shapes.* Proc. R. Soc. Lon. B, 1978, 200, 269-294.

Matthews, M. L., *Discrimination of Identi Kit constructions of faces: Evidence for a dual processing strategy.* Perception & Psychophysics, 1978, 23, 153-161.

Matthews, W. B., Small, D. G., Small, M., & Pountney, E. *Pattern reversal evoked potential in the diagnosis of multiple sclerosis.* Journal of Neurology, Neurosurgery & Psychiatry, 1977, 40, 1009-1014.

Marzi, C. A., & Berlucchi, G. *Right visual field superiority for accuracy of recognition of famous faces in normals.* Neuropsychologia, 1977, 15, 751-756.

Marzi, C. A., Tassinari, G., Tressoldi, P. E., Barry, C., & Grabowska, A. *Hemispheric asymmetry in face perception tasks of different cognitive requirement.* Human Neurobiology, 1985, 4, 15-20.

Mauldin, M. A., & Laughery, K. R. *Composite production effects on subsequent facial recognition.* Journal of Applied Psychology, 1981, 66, 351-357.

Mayes, A. R., Meudell, P. R., & Pickering, A.   Is organic amnesia caused by a selective deficit in remembering contextual information.   Cortex, 1985, 21, 167-202.

McCloskey, M., & Egeth, H.   Eyewitness identification: What can a psychologist tell a jury? American Psychologist, 1983, 38, 550-563.

McCulloch, W. S., & Pitts, W. H.   A logical Calculus immanent in nervous activity. Bull. Math. Biophys., 1943, 5, p.115-133.

McDuff, T., & Sumi, S. M.   Subcortical degeneration in Alzheimer's Disease. Neurology, 1985, 35, 123-126.

McKelvie, S. J.   The role of eyes and mouth in recognition memory for faces. American Journal of Psychology, 1976, 89, 311-323.

McKelvie, S. J.   Sex differences in facial memory.   In M. M. Gruneberg, P. E. Morris & R. N. Sykes (Eds.).   Practical Aspects of Memory.   New York: Academic Press, 1978.

McKelvie, S. J.   Sex differences in memory for faces.   The Journal of Psychology, 1981, 107, 109-125.

McKelvie, S. J.   Effects of lateral reversal on recognition memory for photographs of faces. British Journal of Psychology, 1983, 74, 391-407.

Meadows, J. C.   The anatomical basis of prosopagnosia.   Journal of Neurology, Neurosurgery and Psychiatry, 1974, 37, 489-501.

Medin, D. L., & Schaffer, M.   Context theory of classification learning. Psychological Review. 1978, 85, 207-208.

Meltzoff, A. N., & Moore, M. K.   Imitation of facial and manual gestures by human neonates. Science, 1977, 198, 75-78.

Memon, A.   Recognition of unfamiliar faces : effects of pose, context and delay.   Paper presented at the Meaning of Faces conference, Cardiff, 1985.

Memon, A., & Bruce, V.   The effects of encoding strategy and context change on face recognition. Human Learning, 1983, 2, 319-326.

Memon, A., & Bruce, V.   Context effects in episodic studies of verbal and facial memory. Current Psychological Research & Reviews, 1985, in press.

Messick, S., & Damarin, F.   Cognitive styles and memory for faces.   Journal of Abnormal and Social Psychology, 1964, 69, 313-318.

Mesulam, M. M., Van Hoesen, G. W., Pandya, D. N., & Geschwind, N.   Limbic and sensory connections of the inferior parietal lobule (Area PG) in the rhesus monkey: A study with a new method for horseradish peroxidase histochemistry. Brain Research, 1977, 136, 393-414.

Meyer, D. E., Schvaneveldt, R. W., & Ruddy, M. G.   Loci of contextual effects in visual word recognition.   In P. M. A. Rabbitt & S. Dornic (Eds.). Attention and Performance V. London: Academic Press, 1975.

Michel, F., Sieroff, E., Perenin, M. T. *Prosopagnosie sans hemianopsie par lesion unilaterale droite.* Revue Neurologique, 1985, in press.

Michotte, A. E. *La perception de la causalite.* Louvain: Publ. Univ. de Louvain, 1946.

Michotte, A. E. *The emotions as functional connections.* In M. Reymert (Ed.). *Feelings and emotions.* New York: McGraw-Hill, 1950.

Milner, A. D., & Dunne, J. J. *Lateralised perception of bilateral chimaeric faces by normal subjects.* Nature, 1977, 268, 175-176.

Milner, B. *Visual recognition and recall after right temporal-lobe excision in man.* Neuropsychologia, 1968, 6, 191-209.

Mishkin, M. *Visual mechanisms beyond the striate cortex.* In R. W. Russell (Ed.), *Frontiers in Physiological Psychology.* New York: Academic Press, 1966.

Mooney, C. M. *Age in the development of closure ability in children.* Canadian Journal of Psychology, 1957, 11, 219-226.

Mooney, C. M. *Recognition of ambiguous and unambiguous visual configurations with short and longer exposures.* British Journal of Psychology, 1960, 51, 119-125.

Moreland, R. L., & Zajonc, R. B. *Exposure effects may not depend on stimulus recognition.* Journal of Personality and Social Psychology, 1979, 37, 1085-1089.

Morgan, C. L. *An Introduction to Comparative Psychology.* W. Scott: London, 1894.

Morris, P. E. *Frequency and imagery in word recognition: Further evidence for an attribute model.* British Journal of Psychology, 1978, 69, 69-75.

Morris, P. *Imaging faces.* Unpublished manuscript, 1985.

Morton, J. *Interaction of information in word recognition.* Psychological Review, 76, 165-178.

Morton, J. *Facilitation in word recognition: Experiments causing change in the logogen model.* In P. A. Kolers, M. F. Wrolstad & H. Bouma (Eds.), *Processing of Visible Language,* Vol. 1 (pp.259-268). New York: Plenum, 1979.

Morton, J. *Word recognition.* In J. Morton and J. C. Marshall (Eds.), *Psycholinguistics Series 2: Structures and Processes.* London: Elek, 1979.

Morton, J. *Will cognition survive?* Cognition, 1981, 10, 227-234.

Morton, J., Hammersley, R. H., & Bekerian, D. A. *Headed records: A framework for remembering and its failures.* Cognition, in press.

Moscovitch, M. *Information processing and the cerebral hemispheres. In: M. S. Gazzaniga (Ed.), Handbook of behavioral neurobiology, Vol. 2. Neuropsychology, New York: Plenum Press.*

Moscovitch, M. *Unpublished manuscript, 1985.*

Moscovitch, M., Scullion, D., & Christie, D. *Early vs. late stages of processing and their relation to functional hemispheric asymmetries in face recognition. Journal of Experimental Psychology: Human Perception and Performance, 1976, 2, 401-416.*

Mosher, F. A., & Hornsby, J. R. *On asking questions. In J. S. Bruner, R. R. Olver & P. M. Greefield (Eds.), Studies in cognitive growth. New York: Wiley, 1966.*

Mountcastle, V. B. *An organizing principle for cerebral function: the unit module and the distributed system. In: G. H. Edelman & V. B. Mountcastle (Eds.), The mindful brain. Cambridge, Massachusetts, MIT Press, pp.7-50.*

Mueller, J. H., & Courtois, M. R. *Test anxiety and breadth of encoding experiences in free recall. Journal of Research in Personality, 1980, 14, 458-466.*

Mueller, J. H., Heesacker, M., Ross, M. J., & Nicodemus, D. R. *Emotionality of encoding activity in face memory. Journal of Research in Personality, 1983, 17, 198-217.*

Munn, N. L. *Psychology : the fundamentals of human adjustment 4th ed. London: Harrap, 1961.*

Munsterberg, H. *On the witness stand: Essays on psychology and crime. New York: Clark, Boardman, 1908.*

Murdock, B. B. Jr. *Convolution and correlation in perception and memory. In: L. Nilsson (Ed.), Perspectives on Memory Research. Hillsdale, NJ: Lawrence Erlbaum Associates, 1979.*

Murdock, B. B. *A theory for the storage and retrieval of item and associative information. Psychological Review, 1982, 89, 609-626.*

Murdock, B. B. *A distributed memory model for serial order information. Psychological Review, 1983, 90, 316-338.*

Murri, L., Arena, R., Siciliano, G., Mazzotta, R., & Muratorio, A. *Dream recall in patients with focal cerebral lesions. ARchives of Neurology, 1984, 41, 183-185.*

Nardelli, E., Buonanno, F., Coccia, G., Fiaschi, A., Terzian, H., Rizzuto, N. *Prosopagnosia: Report of four cases. European Neurology, 1982, 21, 289-297.*

Navon, D. *Forest before Trees: The precedence of global features in visual perception. Cognitive Psychology, 1977, 9, 353-383.*

Nebes, R. D.   Direct examination of cognitive function in the right and left hemispheres.   In M. Kinsbourne (Ed.).   Asymmetrical Function in the Brain. Cambridge: Cambridge University Press, 1978.

Neely, J. H.   Semantic priming and retrieval from lexical memory: evidence for facilitatory and inhibitory processes.   Memory and Cognition, 1976, 4, 648-654.

Neil v. Biggers, 409 US 188, 93 S. Ct. 375, 34 L. Ed. 2d 401, 1972.

Neisser, U.   An experimental distinction between perceptual process and response.   Journal of Experimental Psychology, 1954, 47, 399-402.

Nettleton, N. C.   Models of Hemispheric Specialization.   Unpublished Doctoral Dissertation, Monash University, 1983.

Neuman, P. G.   An attribute frequency model for the abstraction of prototypes.   Memory & Cognition, 1974, 2, 241-248.

Neumann, P. G.   Visual prototype formation with discontinuous representation of dimensions of variability.   Memory & Cognition, 1977, 5, 187-197.

Neville, H., Snyder, E., Woods, D, & Galambos, R.   Recognition and surprise alter the human visual evoked response.   Proc. Natl. Sci. USA 79: 212-2131, 1982.

Newcombe, F.   Selective deficits after focal cerebral injury.   In S. J. Dimond & J. G. Beaumont (Eds.), Hemisphere Function in the Human Brain. London: Elek, 1974.

Newcombe, F.   The processing of visual information in prosopagnosia and acquired dyslexia: functional versus physiological interpretation.   In: D. J. Oborne, M. M. Gruneberg & R. E. Eiser (Eds.), Research in Psychology and Medicine.   London: Academic Press, 1979.

Newcombe, F., Oldfield, R. C., Ratcliff, G. G., & Wingfield, A.   Recognition and naming of object-drawings by men with focal brain wounds.   Journal of Neurology, Neurosurgery, & Psychiatry, 1971, 34, 329-340.

Newcombe, F., & Russell, W. R.   Dissociated visual perceptual and spatial deficits in focal lesions of the right hemisphere.   Journal of Neurology, Neurosurgery, and Psychiatry, 1969, 32, 73-81.

Newell, A.   You can't play 20 questions with nature and win.   In W. G. Chase (Ed.), Visual Information Processing.   New York: Academic Press, 1972.

Newell, A., & Simon, H. A.   Human Problem Solving.   Englewood Cliffs, NJ: Prentice-Hall, 1972.

Nielsen, G., & Smith, E. E.   Imaginal and verbal representations in short-term memory recognition of visual forms.   Journal of Experimental Psychology, 1973, 101, 375-378.

Norman, D. A.   Memory and Attention.   New York, Wiley, 1969.

North, P., & Cremel, N.   Observation d'un cas de prosopagnosie chez un enfant.   Societe de Neuropsychologie de langue francaise, Paris, Dec. 1981.

Ohman, A.   The orienting response, attention, and learning.   An information-processing perspective. In: H. Kimmel, E. Van Olst & J. Orlebeke (Eds.), The Orienting Reflec in Humans. Hillsdale, NJ: Lawrence Erlbaum, 1979.

O'Keefe, J., & Nadel. The Hippocampus as a Cognitive Map. London, Oxford University Press, 1978.

Olivos, G. Response delay, psychophysiologic activation, and recognition of one's own voice. Psychosomatic Medicine, 1967, 29, 433-440.

Oltman, P. K., Ehrlichman, H., & Cox, P. W.   Field independence and laterality in the perception of faces. Perceptual and Motor Skills, 1977, 45, 255-260.

O'Toole, A. J.   Recognition memory for Familiar and Unfamiliar Spatial Frequency Filtered Faces: A Physical System Approach. MS thesis, Brown University, Providence, RI, 02912, 1985.

Paivio, A. Imagery and Verbal Processes. New York: Holt, Rinehart, and Winston, Inc., 1971.

Paivio, A.   Imagery and deep structure in the recall of English nominalizations. Journal of Verbal Learning and Verbal Behaviour, 1971, 10, 1-12.

Paivio, A., Yuille, J. C., & Madigan, S.   Concreteness, imagery, and meaningfulness values for 925 nouns. Journal of Experimental Psychology Monograph Supplement, 1968, 76(1, Pt. 2).

Pallis, C. A. Impaired identification of faces and places with agnosia for colours.   Report of a case due to cerebral embolism.   Journal of Neurology, Neurosurgery and Psychiatry, 1955, 18, 218-224.

Palmer, S. E.   Fundamental Aspects of Cognitive Representation.   In: E. Rosch & B. B. Lloyd (Eds.), Cognition and Categorization. Hillsdale, NJ: Erlbaum, 1978.

Pandya, D. M., & Kuypers, H. G. J. M.   Cortico-cortical connections in the rhesus monkey. Brain Research, 1969, 13, 13-36.

Park, R., & Rothbart, M. Perception of out-group homogeneity and levels of social categorization: Memory for the subordinate attributes of in-group and out-group members.   Journal of Personality and Social Psychology, 1982, 42, 1051-1068.

Parkin, A. J., & Goodwin, E.   The influence of different processing strategies on the recognition of transformed and untransformed faces. Canadian Journal of Psychology, 1983, 37, 272-277.

Patel, M. Self-organisation and optimisation of adaptive learning net. PhD Thesis (in preparation). Faculty of Technology, Brunel University, UK.

Patterson, K. E., Baddeley, A. D. When face recognition fails. *Journal of Experimental Psychology*, 1977, *3*, 406-417.

Patterson, K., & Bradshaw, J. Differential hemispheric mediation of non-verbal visual stimuli. *Journal of Experimental Psychology: Human Perception and Performance*, 1975, *1*, 246-252.

Peris, J. L. Le role du contexte dans la reconnaissance. *Unpublished thesis material*, University of Grenoble, 1982.

Peris, J. L. A la poursuite des effets de contexte : L'utilisation de l'arriere-plan et d'un accessoire dans la reconnaissance de portraits. *Unpublished thesis material*, University of Grenoble, 1983.

Peris, J. L., & Tiberghien, G. Effet de contexte et recherche conditionnelle dans la reconnaissance de visages non familiers. *Cahiers de Psychologie Cognitive*, 1984, *4*, 323-333.

Perlmuter, L. C., & Monty, R. A. Contextual effects on learning and memory. *Bulletin of the Psychonomic Society*, 1982, *20*, 290-292.

Perrett, D. I., Rolls, E. T., & Caan, W. Visual neurones responsive to faces in the monkey temporal cortex. *Exp Brain Res*, 1982, *47*, 329-342.

Perrett, D. I., & Rolls, E. T. Neural mechanisms underlying the visual analysis of faces. In: J. P. Ewert, R. R. Capranica & D. J. Ingle (Eds.), *Advances in Vertebrate Neuroethology*. New York, Plenum Press, pp.543-566, 1983.

Perrett, D. I., Smith, P. A. J., Potter, D. D., Mistlin, A. J., Head, A. S., Milner, A. D., & Jeeves, M. A. Visual cells in the temporal cortex sensitive to face view and gaze direction. *Proc Roy Soc B*, 1985, *223*, 293-317.

Perrett, D. I., Smith, P. A. J., Potter, D. D., Mistlin, A. J., Head, A. S., Milner, A. D., & Jeeves, M. A. Neurones responsive to faces in temporal cortex: studies of functional organization sensitivity to identity and relation to perception. *Human Neurobiology*, 1984, *3*, 197-208.

Perrett, D. I., Smith, P. A. J., Mistlin, A. J., Chitty, A. J., Head, A. S., Potter, D. D., Broennimann, R., Milner, A. D., & Jeeves, M. A. Visual analyses of body movements by neurones in the temporal cortex of the macaque monkey: a preliminary report. *Behav. Brain Research*, 1985, *in press*.

Perry, E. K., Tomlinson, B. E., Blessed, G., et al. Correlation of cholinergic abnormalities with senile plaques and mental test scores in senile dementia. *British Medical Journal*, 1978, *2*, 1457-1459.

Perry, R., & Perry, E. The ageing brain and its pathology. In R. Levy & F. Post (Eds.), *The psychiatry of late life*. Oxford: Blackwell Scientific Publications, 1982.

Pettigrew, T. F. The measurement and correlates of category width as a cognitive variable. *Journal of Psychology*, 1958, *6*, 532-544.

Pettigrew, T. F. *Cognitive style and social behavior: A review of category width.* In: L. Wheeler (Ed.), *Review of Personality and Social Psychology* (Vol. 3, pp.199-223). Beverley Hills, CA: Sage, 1982.

Phillips, R. J. *Recognition, recall and imagery of faces.* In: M. M. Gruneberg, P. E. Morris, & R. N. Sykes (Eds.), *Practical aspects of memory* (pp.270-277). New York: Academic Press, 1978.

Piaget, J. *Plays, dreams and imitation in childhood.* New York: Noriten, 1951.

Piaget, J. *The construction of reality in the child.* New York: Basic Books, 1954.

Pike, R. *Comparison of convolution and matrix distributed memory systems for associative recall and recognition.* Psychological Review, 1984, 91, 281-294.

Pilowsky, I., Thornton, M., & Stokes, B. *A microcomputer based approach to the quantification of facial expressions.* Australasian Physical & Engineering Sciences in Medicine, 1985, 8, 70-75.

Pittenger, J. B., & Shaw, R. E. *Aging faces as viscal-elastic events: Implications for a theory of non-rigid shape perception.* Journal of Experimental Psychology: Human Perception and Performance, 1975, 104, 374-382.

Pizzamiglio, L., Zoccolotti, P., Mammucari, A., & Cesaroni, R. *The independence of face identity and facial expression recognition mechanisms: Relationship to sex and cognitive style.* Brain and Cognition, 1983, 2, 176-188.

Poizner, H., Kaplan, E., Bellugi, U., & Padden, C. A. *Visual-spatial processing in deaf brain-damaged signers.* Brain and Cognition, 1984, 3, 281-306.

Polans, A. R. *The effects of repression-sensitization classification and stress on eyewitness recall.* Bulletin of the Psychonomic Society, 23, 181-184.

Pollen, D. A., Nagler, M., Daugman, J., Kronauer, R., & Cavanagh, P. *Use of Gabor elementary functions to probe receptive field substructure of posterior inferotemporal neurons in the owl monkey.* Vision Research, 1984, 24, 233-241.

Poncet, M. *L'agnosie des visages.* Seminarie de Neuropsychologie Humaine. EHESS, Marseille, 1980.

Posner, M. I., Goldsmith, R., & Welton, K. E. Jr. *Perceived distance and the classification of distorted patterns.* Journal of Experimental Psychology, 1967, 73, 28-38.

Posner, M. I., & Snyder, C. R. R. *Attention and cognitive control.* In: R. L. Solso (Ed.), *Information Processing and Cognition: The Loyola Symposium.* Hillsdale: Erlbaum, 1975.

Potter, M. C., & Faulconer, B. A. Time to understand pictures and words. Nature, 1975, 253, 437-438.

Rapaczynski, W., & Ehrlichman, H. Opposite visual hemifield superiorities in face recognition as a function of cognitive style. Neuropsychologia, 1979, 20, 129-144.

Ratcliff, R. A theory of memory retrieval. Psychological Review, 1978, 85, 59-108.

Ratcliff, G., Newcombe, F. Object recognition: some deductions from the clinical evidence. In: A. Ellis (Ed.), Normality and pathology in cognitive functions. London: Academic Press, 147-171, 1982.

Read. J. D. Rehearsal and recognition of human faces. American Journal of Psychology, 1979, 92, 71-85.

Ready, D. R., Brigham, J. C. Experience, attitudes, and the own-race bias in lineup construction. Manuscript in preparation, Florida State University, 1985.

Reason, J. T., & Lucas, D. Using cognitive diaries to investigate naturally occurring memory blocks. In: J. Harris and P. E. Morris (Eds.), Everyday memory, actions and absentmindedness. London: Academic Press, 1984.

Reeve, T. G., Mainor, R. Jr. Effect of movement context on the encoding of kinesthetic spatial information. Research Quarterly for Exercise and Sport, 1983, 54, 352-363.

Reichenbach, L., & Masters, J. C. Children's use of expressive and contextual cues in judgments of emotion. Child Development, 1983, 54, 993-1004.

Reuchlin, M. Processus vicariants et differences individuelles. Journal de Psychologie Normale et Pathologique, 1978, 75, 133-145.

Reuter-Lorenz, P., & Davidson, R. J. Differential contributions of the two cerebral hemispheres to the perception of happy and sad faces. Neuropsychologia, 1981, 19, 609-613.

Reuter-Lorenz, P., Givis, R. P., & Moscovitch, M. Hemispheric specialization and the perception of emotion: Evidence from right-handers and from inverted and non-inverted left-handers. Neuropsychologia, 1983, 21, 687-692.

Rheingold, H. L. Development as the acquisition of familiarity. Annual Review of Psychology, 1985, 36, 1-17.

Rhodes, G. Lateralized processes in face recognition. British Journal of Psychology, 1985, 76, 249-271.

Rhodes, G. Perceptual asymmetries in face recognition. Brain and Cognition, 1985, 4, 197-218.

Rizzolatti, G.   Interfield Differences in Reaction Times to Lateralized Visual Stimuli in Normal Subjects. In: I. Steel Russell, M. W. van Hoff, & G. Berlucchi (Eds.), Structure and Function of Cerebral Commisures. London: Macmillan, 1979.

Rizzolatti, G., Umilta, C., & Berlucchi, G.   Opposite Superiorities of the Right and Left Cerebral Hemispheres in Discriminative Reaction Time to Alphabetical and Physiognomical Material. Brain, 1971, 94, 431-442.

Rock, I.   Orientation and Form. New York: Academic Press, 1973.

Rock, I.   The perception of disoriented figures. Scientific American, 1974, 230, 78-85.

Rock, I., Halper, F., Clayton, T.   The perception and recognition of complex figures. Cognitive Psychology, 1972, 3, 655-673.

Roediger, H. L.   Memory metaphors in cognitive psychology.   Memory & Cognition, 1980, 231-246.

Rollins, H. A., & Thibadeau, R.   The effects of auditory shadowing on recognition of information received visually. Memory and Cognition, 1973, 1, 164-168.

Rolls, E. T.   Neurons in the cortex of the temporal lobe and in the amygdala of the monkey with responses selective for faces.   Human Neurobiology, 1984, 3, 209-222.

Rolls, E. T., Perrett, D., & Thorpe, S. J.   The influence of motivation on the responses of neurons in the posterior parietal association cortex. Behavioral and Brain Sciences, 1980, 3, 514-515.

Rolls, E. T., Perrett, D., Thorpe, S. J., Puerto, A., Roper-Hall, A., & Maddison, S. Responses of neurons in area 7 of the parietal cortex to objects of different significance. Brain research, 1979, 169, 194-198.

Rondot, P., Tzavaras, A., & Garcin, R.   Sur un cas de prosopagnosie persistant depuis quinze ans. Revue Neurologique, 1967, 117, 424-428.

Rondot, P., & Tzavaras, A.   La Prosopagnosie apres vingt annees d'etudes cliniques et neuropsychologiques.   Journal de Psychologie Normale et Pathologique, 1969, 66, 133-165.

Rosch, E., Mervis, C. B., Gray, W. D., Johnson, D. M., & Poyes-Braem, P. Basic objects in natural categories.   Cognitive Psychology, 1976, 8, 382-439.

Rosen, W. G., Terry, R. D., Fuld, P. A., Katsman, R., & Peck, A. Pathological verification of ischaemic score in differentiation of dementias. Annals of Neurology, 1980, 7, 486-488.

Rosenthal, R.   Combining results of independent studies.   Psychological Bulletin, 1985, 85, 185-193.

Rosenthal, R.   The "file drawer problem" and tolerance for null results. Psychological Bulletin, 1979, 86, 638-641.

Rosinski, R. R. Picture-word interference is semantically based. *Child Development*, 1977, 48, 643-647.

Ross, E. D. Sensory-specific and fractional disorders of recent memory in man: I. Isolated loss of visual recent memory. *Archives of Neurology*, 1980, 37, 193-200.

Ross, P., & Turkewitz, G. Changes in hemispheric advantage in processing facial information with increasing stimulus familiarization. *Cortex*, 1982, 18, 489-499.

Rothbart, M. Memory processes and social beliefs. In D. Hamilton (Ed.), *Cognitive processes in stereotyping and intergroup perception* (pp.146-181). Hillsdale, NJ: Lawrence Erlbaum, 1981.

Rothbart, M., & John, O. Social categories and behavioral episodes: A cognitive analysis of the effects of intergroup contact. *Journal of Social Issues*, 1985, 41.

Rubens, A. B., Benson, D. F. Associative visual agnosia. *Archives of Neurology*, 1971, 24, 305-316.

Rubin, D. C. On the retention function for autobiographical memory. *Journal of Verbal Learning and Verbal Behavior*, 1982, 21, 21-38.

Ryback, R. S., Weinert, J., & Fozard, J. L. Disruption of short-term memory in man following consumption of ethanol. *Psychonomic Science*, 1970, 20, 353-354.

Sackett, G. P. Monkeys reared in visual isolation with pictures as visual input: Evidence for an innate releasing mechanism. *Science*, 1966, 154, 1468-1472.

Saida, S., Ikeda, M. Useful visual field size for pattern perception. *Perception & Psychophysics*, 1979, 25, 119-125.

Salasoo, A., Shiffrin, R. M., & Feustel, T. C. Building permanent memory codes: codification and repetition effects in word recognition. *Journal of Experimental Psychology*, General, 1985, 114, 50-77.

Salzen, E. A. Perception of emotion in faces. In G. M. Davies, H. D. Ellis & J. W. Shepherd (Eds.), *Perceiving and Remembering Faces*. London: Academic Press, 1981.

Scarborough, D. L., Cortese, C., & Scarborough, H. S. Frequency and repetition effects in lexical memory. *Journal of Experimental Psychology: Human Perception and Performance*, 3, 1-17.

Schiffman, H. R. Sensation and perception: An integrated approach. New York: Wiley, 1976.

Schonen, S. de, McKenzie, B., Bresson, F., & Maury, L. Central and peripheral object distances as determinants of the effective visual field in early infancy. *Perception*, 1978, 7, 499-506.

Schulman-Galambos, C., & Galambos, R. *Cortical responses from adults and infants to complex visual stimuli. Electroenceph. Clin. Neurophysiol.,* 1978, 45, 435-435.

Schwartz, M., & Smith, M. L. *Visual asymmetries with chimeric faces. Neuropsychologia,* 1980, 18, 103-106.

Seamon, J. G., Stolz, J. A., Bass, D. H., & Chatinover, A. I. *Recognition of facial features in immediate memory. Bulletin of the Psychonomic Society,* 1978, 12, 231-234.

Secord, P. F. *Facial features and inference processes in interpersonal perception. In R. Taguiri & L. Petrullo (Eds.), Person perception and interpersonal behavior. Stanford: Stanford University Press,* 1958.

Semmes, J. *Hemispheric specialization: a possible clue to mechanism. Neuropsychologia,* 1968, 6, 11-26.

Sergent, J. *About face: left-hemisphere involvement in processing physiognomies. Journal of Experimental Psychology: Human Perception and Performance,* 1982, 8, 1-14.

Sergent, J. *Theoretical and methodological consequences of variations in exposure duration in visual laterality studies. Perception and Psychophysics,* 1982, 31, 451-461.

Sergent, J. *Role of the input in visual hemispheric asymmetries. Psychological Bulletin,* 1983, 93, 481-512.

Sergent, J. *An investigation into component and configural processes underlying face perception. British Journal of Psychology,* 1984, 75, 221-242.

Sergent, J. *Configural processing of faces in the left and right cerebral hemispheres. Journal of Experimental Psychology: Human Perception and Performance,* 1984, 10, 554-572.

Sergent, J. *Inferences from unilateral brain damage about normal hemispheric functions in visual pattern recognition. Psychological Bulletin,* 1984, 96, 99-115.

Sergent, J. *Face Perception : underlying processes and hemispheric contribution, pre-print,* 1985.

Sergent, J. *Methodological constraints on neuropsychological studies of face perception in normals, pre-print,* 1985.

Sergent, J., Bindra, D. *Differential hemispheric processing of faces: Methodological considerations and reinterpretation. Psychological Bulletin,* 1981, 89, 541-554.

Sergent, J., & Switkes, E. *Differential hemispheric sensitivity to spatial-frequency components of visual patterns. Society for Neuroscience Abstracts,* 1984, 10, 317 (97.3).

Seymour, P. H. K. *Human Visual Cognition. London: Collier-McMillan,* 1979.

Shapiro, P. N., & Penrod, S.   A meta-analysis of facial identification studies.   Paper presented at the August meeting of the American Psychological Association, Toronto, Canada, 1984.

Sharp, P. F., Gemmell, H. G., Cherryman, G., Besson, J. A. O., Crawford, J. R., & Smith, F. W.   The application of 123 I iodine labelled isopropyl amphetamine imaging to the study of dementia.   Submitted to Journal of Nuclear Medicine.

Shepherd, J.   Social factors in face recognition.   In G. Davies, H. Ellis & J. Shepherd (Eds.), Perceiving and remembering faces (pp.55-79).   New York: Academic Press, 1981.

Shepherd, J. W., Davies, G. M., & Ellis, H. D.   How best shall a face be described?   In M. M. Gruneberg, P. E. Morris & R. N. Sykes (Eds.), Practical aspects of memory. London: Academic Press, 1978.

Shepherd, J. W., Davies, G. M., Ellis, H. D.   Studies of cue saliency.   In G. M. Davies, H. D. Ellis & J. W. Shepherd (Eds.), Perceiving and Remebering Faces. London: Academic Press, 1981.

Shepherd, J. W., & Deregowski, J. B.   Races and faces: A comparison of the responses of Africans and Europeans to faces of the same and different races. British Journal of Social Psychology, 1981, 20, 125-133.

Shepherd, J. W., Deregowski, & J. B., Ellis, H. D.   A cross-cultural study of recognition memory for faces.   International Journal of Psychology, 1974, 9, 205-211.

Shepherd, J. W., & Ellis, H. D.   The effect of attractiveness on recognition memory for faces. American Journal of Psychology, 1973 86, 627-633.

Shepherd, J. W., Ellis, H. D., & Davies, G. M.   Perceiving and remembering faces.   Technical report to the Home Office, contract no. POL/73/1675/24/1, 1977.

Shepherd, J. W., Ellis, H. D., & Davies, G. M.   Identification evidence: A psychological evaluation. Aberdeen, Scotland: Aberdeen University Press, 1982.

Shepherd, J. W., Ellis, H. D., McMurran, M., & Davies, G. M.   Effect of character attribution on photofit construction of a face.   European Journal of Social Psychology, 1978, 8, 263-268.

Shiffrin, R. M., & Schneider, W.   Controlled and automatic human information processing: II. Perceptual learning, automatic attending and a general theory. Psychological Review, 1977, 84, 127-190.

Shoemaker, D. J., South, D. R., Lowe, J.   Facial stereotypes of deviants and judgements of guilt or innocence. Social Forces, 1973, 427-433.

Shraberg, D., Weitzel, W. D.   Prosopagnosia and the Capgras syndrome. Journal of Clinical Psychiatry, 1979, 40, 313-316.

Shuttleworth, E. C., Syring, V., & Allen, N.   Further observations on the nature of prosopagnosia. Brain and Cognition, 1982, 1, 307-322.

Small, M.   Asymmetrical evoked potentials in response to face stimuli. Cortex, 1983, 19, 441-450.

Smith, M. C., & Magee, L. E.   Tracing the time course of picture-word processing. Journal of Experimental Psychology: General, 1980, 109, 373-392.

Smith, S. M.   Remembering in and out of context. Journal of Experimental Psychology, 5, 460-471.

Smith, S. M., Glenberg, A., & Bjork, R. A.   Environmental context and human memory. Memory & Cognition, 1978, 6, 342-353.

Sobel, N. R.   Eyewitness identification: Legal and practical problems. New York: Clark Boardman Co., 1972.

Sokolov, V. N.   Perception and the Conditioned Reflex.   Oxford: Pergamon, 1963.

Solso, R. L., & McCarthy, J. E.   Prototype formation of faces: A case of pseudo-memory. British Journal of Psychology, 1981, 72, 499-503.

Sorce, J. F., & Campos, J. J.   The role of expression in the recognition of a face. American Journal of Psychology, 1974, 87, 71-82.

Stalans, L., & Wedding, D.   Superiority of the left hemisphere in the recognition of emotional faces. International Journal of Neuroscience, 1985, 25, 219-223.

Standing, L. G., Conezio, H., & Haber, R. N.   perception and memory for pictures: single-trial learning of 2,500 visual stimuli.   Psychonomic Science, 1970, 19, 73-74.

Stern, L. D.   A review of theories of human amnesia. Memory and Cognition, 1981, 9, 247-262.

Stern, R. M., & Anschel, C.   Deep inspirations as stimuli for responses of the autonomic nervous system. Psychophysiology, 1968, 6, 132-141.

Strauss, E., & Moscovitch, M.   Perception of facial expressions.   Brain and Language, 1981, 13, 308-332.

Stroop, J. R.   Studies of interference in serial verbal reactions.   Journal of Experimental Psychology, 1935, 18, 643-662.

Synodinou, C., Christodoulou, G., Tzavaras, A.   Capgras' Syndrome and prosopagnosia. British Journal of Psychiatry, 1977, 132, 413-414.

Szentagothai, J.   The neurons network of the cerebral cortex: a functional interpretation. The Ferrier Lecture. Proc. Roy. Soc. Lond. B, 1978, 201, 219-248.

Szondi, L.   Experimenteele Triebdiagnostik. Bern: Huber, 1947.

Teuber, H. L. Alteration of perception and memory in man. In L. Weiskrantz (Ed.), Analysis of Behavior Change. New York: Harper & Row, 1968.

Thompson, W. B., & Mueller, J. H. Face memory and hemispheric dominance: Emotionality and extraversion. Brain and Cognition, 1984, 3, 239-248.

Thomson, B. G., & Laughery, K. R. Facial memory: Effects of recall efforts on subsequent recognition. Paper presented at the Annual Meeting of the Psychonomics Society, Phoenix, AZ, 1979.

Thomson, D. M. Person identification: Influencing the outcome. Australian and New Zealand Journal of Criminology, 1981, 14, 49-55.

Thomson, D. M. Context effects in recognition memory: developmental aspects. Paper presented at the Experimental Psychology Conference, Deakin University, Australia, 1984.

Thomson, D. M., Robertson, S. L., & Vogt, R. Person recognition: the effect of context. Human Learning, 1982, 1, 137-154.

Thomson, J. K. Visual field, exposure duration and sex as factors in the perception of emotional facial expressions. Cortex, 1983, 19, 293-308.

Thorndike, E. L., & Lorge, I. The Teacher's Word Book of 30,000 Words. New York: Teachers College Press, Columbia University, 1944.

Thorndike, R. M. Correlational Procedures for Research. New York: Gardner Press, 1978.

Thornton, G. R. The effect upon judgements of personality traits of varying a single factor in a photograph. Journal of Social Psychology, 1943, 18, 127-148.

Thornton, M. The mathematical modelling of facial expressions. Adelaide: University of Adelaide (unpublished dissertation), 1979.

Thornton, M., & Pilowsky, I. Facial expressions can be modelled mathematically. British Journal of Psychiatry, 1982, 140, 61-63.

Thorwald, J. The marks of Cain. London: Thames and Hudson, 1965.

Tiberghien, G. Reconnaissance a long term. Pourquoi ne pas chercher? In: S. Ehrlich & E. Tulving (Eds.), La memorie semantique. Paris: Bulletin de Psychologie, 1976.

Tiberghien, G. La memorie des visages. L'Annee Psychologique, 1983, 83, 153-198.

Tiberghien, G. Just how does ecphory work? The Behavioral and Brain Sciences, 1984, 7, 255-256.

Tiberghien, G. Mais ou sont les stimulus d'antan?. Psychologie Francaise, 1985, 30, 177-183.

Tiberghien, G., Cauzinille, E., & Mathieu, J. Pre-decision and conditional search in long-term recognition memory. Acta Psychologica, 1979, 43, 329-343.

Tiberghien, G., & Clerc, I. The cognitive locus of prosopagnosia. In R. Bruyer (Ed.), The Neuropsychology of Face Perception and Facial Expression. Hillsdale NJ: Lawrence Erlbaum Associates, in press, 1986.

Tiberghien, G., & Lecocq, P. Rappel et Reconnaissance. Lille, Presses Universitaires de Lille, 1983.

Tickner, A. H., & Poulton, E. C. Watching for people and actions. Ergonomics, 1975, 18, 35-51.

Tieger, T., & Ganz, L. Recognition of faces in the presence of two dimensional sinusoidal masks. Perception & Psychophysics, 1979, 26, 163-167.

Torii, H., & Tamai, A. The problem of prosopagnosia: report of three cases with occlusion of the right posterior cerebral artery. Abstracts of the XIII World Congress of Neurology. Journal of Neurology, 1985, Supplement to Vol. 232, p.140.

Tranel, D., & Damasio, A. R. Knowledge without awareness: An autonomic index of facial recognition by prosopagnosics. Science, 1985, 228, 1453-1454.

Tucker, D. M. Lateral brain function, emotion, and conceptualization. Psychological Bulletin, 1981, 89, 19-46.

Tulving, E. Cue-dependent forgetting. American Scientist, 1974, 62, 74-82.

Tulving, E. Ecphoric processes in recall and recognition. In: J. Brown (Ed.), Recall and Recognition. New York: Wiley, 1976.

Tulving, E. Similarity relations in recognition. Journal of Verbal Learning and Verbal Behavior, 1981, 20, 479-496.

Tulving, E. Synergistic ecphory in recall and recognition. Canadian Journal of Psychology, 1982, 36, 130-147.

Tulving, E. Elements of Episodic Memory. New York, Oxford University Press, 1983.

Tulving, E. Precis of elements of episodic memory. The Behavioral and Brain Sciences, 1984, 7, 223-268.

Tulving, E. How many memory systems are there? American Psychologist, 1985, 40, 385-398.

Tulving, E., & Thomson, D. M. Encoding specificity and retrieval processes in episodic memory. Psychological Review, 1973, 80, 352-373.

Tversky, A. Features of similarity. Psychological Review, 1977, 84, 327-352.

Tversky, B., & Hemenway, K. Categories of Environmental Scenes. Cognitive Psychology, 1983, 15, 121-149.

Tzavaras, A., Hecaen, H., & Lebras, H. Le probleme de la specificite du deficit de la reconnaissance du visage humain lors des lesions hemispheriques unilaterales. Neuropsychologia, 1970, 8, 403-416.

Ullman, S. The Interpretation of Visual Motion. Cambridge Mass.: MIT Press, 1979.

Umilta, C., Brizzolara, D., Tabossi, P., & Fairweather, H. Factors affecting face recognition in the cerebral hemispheres: familiarity and naming. In J. Requin (Ed.), Attention and Performance VII. Hillsdale, NJ: Erlbaum, 1978.

Umilta, C., Rizzolatti, G., Anzola, G. P., Luppino, G., & Porro, C. Evidence of Interhemispheric Transmission in Laterality Effects. Neuropsychologia, 1985, 23, 203-213.

Underwood, B. J. Individual differences as a crucible in theory construction. American Psychologist, 1975, 30, 128-134.

Underwood, B. J. Attributes of memory. Glenview, IL: Scott, Foresman, 1983.

Underwood, G. Contextual facilitation from attended and unattended messages. Journal of Verbal Learning and Verbal Behavior, 1977, 16, 99-106.

Ungerleider, L. G., & Mishkin, M. Two cortical visual systems. In D. J. Ingle, R. J. W. Mansfield & M. A. Goodale (Eds.), The Analysis of Visual Behavior. Cambridge, MA: MIT Press, 1982.

Valentine, T., & Bruce, V. G. The effect of race, inversion and encoding activity upon face recognition. Acta Psychologica, 1985 (in press).

Venner, B. R. Facial identification techniques. Police Research Bulletin, 1969, No. 13, 17-20.

Versace, R. Specialisation hemispherique et effets de contexte. Doctoral thesis material, University of Grenoble, 1983.

Versace, R., & Tiberghien, G. Specialisation hemispherique et frequences spatiales. L'Annee Psychologique, 1985, 85, 249-273.

Victor, M., Adams, R. D., Collins, G. H. The Wernicke-Korsakoff syndrome. Philadelphia: Davis, 1971.

Walker-Smith, G. J. The effects of delay and exposure duration in a face recognition task. Perception & Psychophysics, 1978, 24, 63-70.

Wall, P. M. Eyewitness identification in criminal cases. Springfield, IL: Charles C. Thomas, 1965.

Waltz, D. L. (Ed.) Special issue: Connectionist Models and Their Applications. Cognitive Science, 1985, 9, 1-69.

Warren, C., & Morton, J. The effects of priming on picture recognition. British Journal of Psychology, 1982, 73, 117-129.

Warrington, E. K. Neuropsychological studies of object recognition. Phil. Trans. R. Soc. Lond., 1982, B 298, 15-33.

Warrington, E. K., & Ackroyd, C. The effect of orienting tasks on recognition memory. Memory & Cognition, 1975, 3, 140-142.

Warrington, E. K., & James, M. Disorders of visual perception in patients with localised cerebral lesions. Neuropsychologia, 1967, 5, 253-266.

Warrington, E. K., & James, M. An experimental investigation of facial recognition in patients with unilateral cerebral lesions. Cortex, 1967, 317-326.

Warrington, E. K., & Taylor, A. M. Two categorical stages of object recognition. Perception, 1978, 7, 695-705.

Wasserstein, J., Zappulla, R., Rosen, J., & Thompson, A. L. Facial closure: interrelationships with facial discrimination, object closure and subjective contour illusion perception. Text of a communication, International Neuropsychological Society meeting, Mexico, 1983.

Wasserstein, J., Zappulla, R., Rosen, J., & Gerstman, L. Evidence for differentiation of right hemisphere visual-perceptual functions. Brain and Cognition, 1984, 3, 51-56.

Watkins, M. J., Ho, E., & Tulving, E. Context effects in recognition memory for faces. Journal of Verbal Learning and Verbal Behavior, 1976, 15, 505-517.

Wayland, S., & Taplin, J. E. Nonverbal categorization in fluent and non-fluent anomic aphasics. Brain and Language, 1982, 16, 87-108.

Weinstein, E. A., & Kahn, R. L. Denial of illness. C. C. Thomas, Springfield, Illinois, 1955.

Weiskrantz, L., Warrington, E. K., Sanders, M. D., & Marshall, J. Visual capacity in the hemianopic field following a restricted occipital ablation. Brain, 1974, 97, 709-728.

Weitzman, E. D. Memory and sleep: Neuroendocrinological considerations. In R. Drucker-Colin & J. L. McGaugh (Eds.), Neurobiology of sleep and memory, (pp.401-417). New York: Academic Press, 1977.

Wells, G. L. Applied eyewitness-testimony research: System variables and estimator variables. Journal of Personality and Social Psychology, 1978, 36, 1546-1557.

Wells, G. L., & Hryciw, B. Memory for faces: Encoding and retrieval operations. Memory and Cognition, 1984, 12, 338-344.

Wells, G. L., Leippe, M. R., & Ostrom, T. M. Guidelines for empirically aooeooing the fairness of a lineup. Law and Human Behavior, 1979, 3, 285-293.

503

Wells, G. L., & Murray, D. M.   What can psychology say about the Neil v Biggers criteria for judging eyewitness testimony?   Journal of Applied Psychology, 1983, 68, 347-362.

Whiteley, A. M., & Warrington, E. K.   Prosopagnosia: a clinical, psychological, and anatomical study of three patients.   Journal of Neurology, Neurosurgery and Psychiatry, 1977, 40, 395-403.

Wickelgren, W. A.   Trace resistance and the decay of long-term memory. Journal of Mathematical Psychology, 1972, 9, 418-455.

Wickelgren, W. A.   Single-trace fragility theory of memory dynamics.   Memory & Cognition, 1974, 2, 775-780.

Wickelgren, W. A.   Alcoholic intoxication and memory storage dynamics.Memory & Cognition, 1975, 3, 385-389.

Wickelgren, W. A.   Memory storage dynamics.   In W. K. Estes (Ed.), Handbook of learning and cognition processes (Vol. 4, pp.321-362).   Potomac, MD: Erlbaum, 1976.

Wickelgren, W. A.   Learning and memory.   Englewood Cliffs, NJ: Prentice-Hall, 1977.

Wickelgren, W. A.   Chunking and consolidation: A theoretical synthesis of semantic networks, configuring in conditioning, S-R versus cognitive learning, normal forgetting, the amnesic syndrome, and the hippocampal arousal system.   Psychological Review, 1979, 86, 44-60.

Wilbrand, H.   Ein Fall van Seelenblindheit und Hemianopsie mit Sectionsbefund.   Deutsche Zeitschrift fur Nervenheilkunde, 1892, 2, 361-387.

Wilkie, B. A.   A stand-alone high resolution adaptive pattern recognition system.   Ph.D. Thesis, Faculty of Technology, Brunel University, UK, 1983.

Wilson, R. S., Kaszniak, A. W., Bacon, L. D., Fox, J. H., & Kelly, M. P. Facial recognition memory in dementia, Cortex, 1982, 18, 329-336.

Winnick, W. A., & Daniel, S. A.   Two kinds of response priming in tachistoscopic recognition.   Journal of Experimental Psychology, 1970, 84, 74-81.

Winocur, G., & Kinsbourne, M.   Contextual cueing as an aid to Korsakoff amnesics.   Neuropsychologica, 1978, 16, 671-682.

Winograd, E.   Recognition memory for faces following nine different judgements.   Bulletin of the Psychonomic Society, 1976, 8(6), 419-421.

Winograd, E.   Elaboration and distinctiveness in memory for faces.   Journal of Experimental Psychology: Human Learning and Memory, 1981, 7(3), 181-190.

Winograd, E., & Rivers-Bulkeley, N. T.   Effects of changing context on remembering faces.   Journal of Experimental Psychology : Human Learning and Memory, 1977, 3, 397-405.

Wolfe, A. *Optical computing is beginning to take on the glow of reality.* Electronics Week, June 10th 1985, p.24.

Wolpert, I. *Die simultanagnosie: storung der gesamtauffasung.* Zeitschrift gesamte Neurol Psychiat, 1924, 93, 397-413.

Wolters, G. *Attribute models and the effect of frequency and imagery values on word recognition.* Acta Psychologia, 1980, 44, 269-279.

Woodhead, M. M., Baddeley, A. D., & Simmonds, D. C. V. *On training people to recognize faces.* Ergonomics, 1979, 22, 333-343.

Woodhead, M. M., & Baddeley, A. D. *Individual differences and memory for faces, picutres, and words.* Memory and Cognition, 1981, 9, 368-370.

Yakovlev, D. E. *Motility, behavior, and the brain: Stereodynamic organization and neural coordiantes of behavior.* Journal of Nervous and Mental Diseases, 1948, 107, 313-335.

Yamadori, A., & Albert, M. L. *Word category aphasia.* Cortex, 1973, 9, 112-125.

Yarmey, A. D. *The psychology of eyewitness testimony.* New York: The Free Press, 1979.

Yarmey, A. D. *The effects of attractiveness, feature saliency, and liking on memory for faces.* In M. Cook & G. Wilson (Eds.), Love and attraction (pp.51-53). Oxford, England: Pergamon Press, 1979.

Yarmey, A. D. *I recognize your face but I can't remember your name: further evidence on the tip-of-the-tongue phenomenon.* Memory and Cognition, 1973, 1, 287-290.

Yarmey, A. D. *Schemas and images in self-recognition.* In J. C. Yuille (Ed.), Imagery, memory and cognition. Hillsdale, NJ: Erlbaum, 1982.

Yarmey, A. D., Jones, H. P. *Is the psychology of eyewitness identification a matter of common sense?* In S. M. A. Lloyd-Bostock & B. R. Clifford (Eds.), Evaluating witness evidence: Recent psychological research and new perspectives. New York: Wiley, 1983.

Yin, R. K. *Looking at upside-down faces.* Journal of Experimental Psychology, 1969, 81, 141-145.

Yin, R. K. *Face recognition by brain-injured patients: a dissociable ability?* Neuropsychologia, 1970, 8, 395-402.

Young, A. W. *Methodological and theoretical bases of visual hemifield studies.* In J. G. Beaumont (Ed.), Divided Visual Field Studies of Cerebral Organization (pp.11-27). London: Academic, 1982.

Young, A. W. *Right cerebral hemisphere superiority for recognizing the internal and external features of famous faces.* British Journal of Psychology, 1984, 75, 161-169.

Young, A. W., & Bion, P. J. Absence of any developmental trend in right hemisphere superiority for face recognition. *Cortex*, 1980, 16, 213-221.

Young, A. W., & Bion, P. J. Accuracy of naming laterally presented known faces by children and adults. *Cortex*, 1981, 17, 97-106.

Young, A. W., & Bion, P. J. The nature of the sex difference in right hemisphere superiority for face recognition. *Cortex*, 1983, 19, 215-226.

Young, A. W., Ellis, A. W., Flude, B. M., McWeeny, K. H., & Hay, D. C. Interference between faces and written names. *EPS meeting*, London, England, January 1985.

Young, A. W., Flude, B. M., Ellis, A. W., & Hay, D. C. Interference with face naming. *Acta Psychologica*, (in press).

Young, A. W., Hay, D. C., & Ellis, A. W. The faces that launched a thousand slips: everyday difficulties and errors in recognizing people. *British Journal of Psychology*, 1985, 76, 495-523.

Young, A. W., Hay, D. C., & McWeeny, K. H. Right cerebral hemisphere superiority for constructing facial representations. *Neuropsychologia*, 1985, 23, 195-202.

Young, A. W., Hay, D. C., McWeeny, K. H., Ellis, A. W., & Barry, C. Familiarity decisions for faces presented to the left and right cerebral hemispheres. *Brain & Cognition*, 1985, in press.

Young, A. W., Hay, D. C., McWeeny, K. H., Flude, B. M., & Ellis, A. W. Matching familiar and unfamiliar faces on internal and external features. *Perception* (in press).

Young, A. W., McWeeny, K., Ellis, A. W., & Hay, D. C. Naming and categorizing faces and written names. *Quarterly Journal of Experimental Psychology*, (in press).

Young, A. W., McWeeny, K., Hay, D. C., & Ellis, A. W. Access to identity-specific semantic codes from familiar faces. *Quarterly Journal of Experimental Psychology*, (in press).

Zaidel, .E. Disconnection Syndrome as a Model of Laterality Effects in the Normal Brain. In: J. B. Hellige (Ed.), *Cerebral Hemisphere Asymmetry*. New York: Praeger, 1983.

Zajonc, R. B. Feeling and thinking: Preferences need no inferences. *American Psychologist*, 1980, 35, 151-175.

Zenhausern, R. Imagery, cerebral dominance, and style of thinking: A unified field model. *Bulletin of the Psychonomic Society*, 1978, 12, 381-384.

Zenhausern, R., & Repetti, J. A. A comparison of two measures of hemispheric dominance. Paper presented at the annual meeting of the Eastern Psychological Association, Philadelphia, 1979.

ADDRESSES OF PRINCIPAL AUTHORS

Abdi, H. Laboratoire de Psychologie, Ancienne Faculte, 36 Rue Chabot-Charny, 21000 Dijon, France

Bauer, R. Center for Neuropsychological Study, Department of Clinical Psychology, Box J-165, Gainsville, Florida 32610, USA

Blanc-Garin, J. Laboratoire de Psychophysiologie, Universite de Provence, Centre de Saint-Jerome, 13397 Marseille Cedex, France

Brigham, J. Department of Psychology, Florida State University, Tallahassie, Florida 32306, USA

Bruce, V. Department of Psychology, University of Nottingham, Nottingham, NG7 2RD, UK

Bruyer, R. Medical Department, Universite de Louvain, Avenue Hippocrate 54, NEXA 5480, B-1200, Bruxelles, Belgium

Calis, G. Department of Psychology, University of Nijmegen, PO Box 9104, 6500 HE Nijmegen, The Netherlands

Church, V. c/o E. Winograd, Department of Psychology, Emory University, Atlanta, Georgia, 30322 USA

Crawford, J. Department of Psychology, University of Aberdeen, Old Aberdeen, AB9 2UB, UK

Damasio, A. Department of Neurology, The University of Iowa Hospitals & Clinics, Iowa, USA

Davidoff, J. Department of Psychology, University College, Swansea, UK

Davies, G. Department of Psychology, University of Aberdeen, Old Aberdeen, AB9 2UB, UK

Deffenbacher, K. Department of Psychology, University of Nebraska at Omaha, Omaha, Nebraska 68182, USA

De Haan, E. c/o F. Newcombe, Neuropsychology Unit, Radcliffe Infirmary, Oxford, OX2 6HE, UK

De Renzi, E. Clinica Neurologica, Via del Pozzo, 71-41100 Modena, Italy

508

Ellis, H.   Department of Psychology, University of Aberdeen, Old Aberdeen, AB9 2UB, UK

Endo, M.   Department of Psychology, Tohoku University, Kawanchi, Sendai 980, Japan

Feyereisen, P.   Unite NEXA, UCL 5490, Avenue Hippocrate, B-1200, Bruxelles, Belgium

Fraser, I.   c/o D. Parker, Department of Psychology, University of Aberdeen, Old Aberdeen, AB9 2UB, UK

Frijda, N.   Psychology Department, University of Amsterdam, Amsterdam, The Netherlands

Haig, N.   MOD, RARDE, Fort Halstead, Sevenoaks, Kent, UK

Hay, D.   Department of Psychology, University of Lancaster, Bailrigg, Lancaster, LA1 4YF, UK

Jeeves, M.   Psychological Laboratory, University of St Andrews, St Andrews, Fife, UK

Klatzky, R.   Department of Psychology, University of California, Santa Barbara, CA 93106, USA

Laughery, K.   Psychology Department, Rice University, Houston, Texas 77251, USA

McKelvie, S.   Department of Psychology, Bishop's University, Lennoxville, Quebec J1M 1Z7, Canada

Malpass, R.   Behavioral Science Program, State University of New York, Plattsburgh, NY 12901, USA

Marzi, C.   Instituto di Psicologia, 3 Piazza Capitaniato, 35139, Padova, Italy

Millward, R.   Psychology Department, Brown University, Providence, RI 02912, USA

Mueller, J.   Psychology Department, University of Missouri, Columbia, Missouri 65211, USA

Parkin, A.   Department of Experimental Psychology, University of Sussex, Brighton, UK

Perrett, D.   MRC Cognitive Neuroscience Research Group, Psychological Laboratory, University of St Andrews, St Andrews, Fife, UK

Pilowsky, I.   Department of Psychiatry, University of Adelaide, Adelaide, South Australia

Regard, M.   Department of Neurology, University Hospital, CH-8091, Zurich, Switzerland

Salzen, E. Department of Psychology, University of Aberdeen, Old Aberdeen, AB9 2UB, UK

de Schonen, S. Laboratoire de Psychobiologie Experimentale, Institut de Neuropsychologie et Psychophysiologie, CNRS INP3, 13402, Marseille, France

Sergent, J. Department of Neurology & Neurosurgery, MNI, 3801 University Street, Montreal, PQ H3A 284, Canada

Shepherd, J. Department of Psychology, University of Aberdeen, Old Aberdeen, AB9 2UB, UK

Small, M. Department of Clinical Neurology, University of Oxford, The Radcliffe Infirmary, Oxford, OX2 6HE, UK

Stonham, T. Department of Electrical Engineering & Electronics, Brunel University, Uxbridge, Middlesex, UB4 3PH, UK

Thomson, D. Department of Psychology, Monash University, Clayton, Victoria 3168, Australia

Tiberghien, G. Laboratoire de Psychologie Experimentale, UER de Psychologie et des Sciences de l'Education Universite de Grenoble, 47X, 38040, Grenoble Cedex, France

Tzavaras, A. 130 Askilipiou Street, 114 71 Athens, Greece

Umilta, C. Istituto di Fisiologia Umana, Universita di Parma, Via Gramsci 14, 43100 Parma, Italy

Young, A. Department of Psychology, University of Lancaster, Bailrigg, Lancaster, LA1 4YF, UK